Spinal Afferent Processing

Spinal Afferent Processing

Edited by

TONY L. YAKSH
Mayo Clinic
Rochester, Minnesota

Plenum Press • New York and London

Library of Congress Cataloging in Publication Data

Main entry under title:

Spinal afferent processing.

Dedicated to the memory of Frederick William Lawson Kerr, M.D., 25 March 1923–28 August 1983.

Includes bibliographies and index.

1. Spinal cord—Addresses, essays, lectures. 2. Afferent pathways—Addresses, essays, lectures. 3. Senses and sensation—Addresses, essays, lectures. 4. Kerr, Frederick W. L. (Frederick William Lawson), 1923– . I. Yaksh, T. L. (Tony L.), 1944– . II. Kerr, Frederick W. L. (Frederick William Lawson), 1923– . [DNLM: 1. Afferent Pathways. 2. Spinal Cord—physiology. WL 400 S7568]

QP374.S65 1985 599′.0188 85-25753

ISBN 0-306-42046-5

A Division of Plenum Publishing Corporation

233 Spring Street, New York, N.Y. 10013

Printed in the United States of America

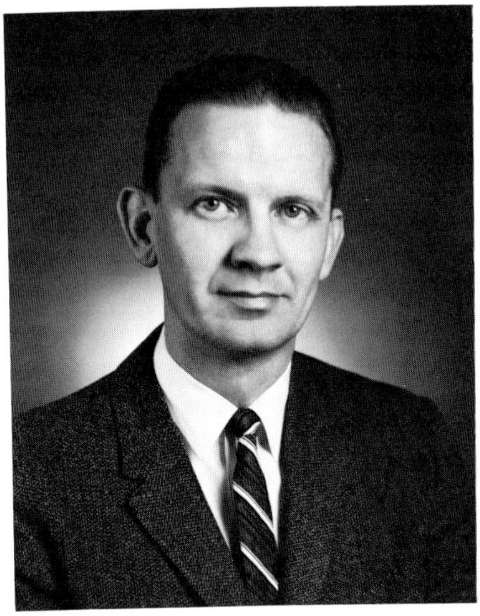

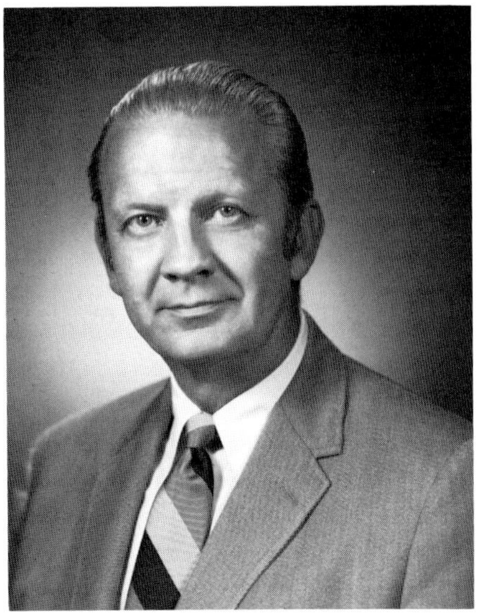

Staff photographs of Doctor Kerr taken shortly after arrival at Mayo (1960, left) and later in 1972 (right), in the prime of his research endeavors.

This is dedicated to the memory of

FREDERICK WILLIAM LAWSON KERR, M.D.

(March 25, 1923–August 28, 1983)

Let these fruits of our labor serve to remind us that in life he was a gentleman, a scholar, and a friend. At his passing he remains a light to inspire the best that is in each of us.

Contributors

JEAN MARIE BESSON, Research Unit of Pharmacological Neurophysiology of Inserm (U. 161), Paris 75014, France

M. CATHERINE BUSHNELL, Neurobiology and Anesthesiology Branch, National Institute of Dental Research, National Institutes of Health, Bethesda, Maryland 20892

JAMES N. CAMPBELL, Department of Neurosurgery and Applied Physics Laboratory, The Johns Hopkins University, Baltimore, Maryland 21205

FERNANDO CERVERO, Department of Physiology, The Medical School, University of Bristol, Bristol BS8 1TD, England

RICHARD E. COGGESHALL, Departments of Anatomy, Physiology, and Biophysics, University of Texas Medical Branch, Galveston, Texas 77550

ANTHONY H. DICKENSON, Department of Pharmacology, University College, London WC1E 6BT, England

RONALD DUBNER, Neurobiology and Anesthesiology Branch, National Institute of Dental Research, National Institutes of Health, Bethesda, Maryland 20892

GARY H. DUNCAN, Neurobiology and Anesthesiology Branch, National Institute of Dental Research, National Institutes of Health, Bethesda, Maryland 20892

PETER J. DYCK, Peripheral Nerve Laboratory, Mayo Medical School and Foundation, Rochester, Minnesota 55905

ROBERT D. FOREMAN, Department of Physiology and Biophysics, University of Oklahoma Health Sciences Center, College of Medicine, Oklahoma City, Oklahoma 73190

G. F. GEBHART, Department of Pharmacology, College of Medicine, University of Iowa, Iowa City, Iowa 52242

JOEL D. GREENSPAN, Department of Physiology, University of North Carolina School of Medicine, Chapel Hill, North Carolina 27514

DONNA L. HAMMOND, Department of Biological Research, G.D. Searle and Co., Research and Development Division, Skokie, Illinois 60077

LAWRENCE KRUGER, Departments of Anatomy and Anesthesiology and the Brain Research Center, UCLA Center for Health Sciences, Los Angeles, California 90024

CAROLE C. LAMOTTE, Sections of Neurosurgery and Anesthesiology, Yale University School of Medicine, New Haven, Connecticut 06510

DANIEL LE BARS, Research Unit of Pharmacological Neurophysiology of Inserm (U. 161), Paris 75014, France

RICHARD A. MEYER, Department of Neurosurgery and Applied Physics Laboratory, The Johns Hopkins University, Baltimore, Maryland 21205

PAUL E. MICEVYCH, Departments of Anatomy and Anesthesiology and the Brain Research Center, UCLA Center for Health Sciences, Los Angeles, California 90024

DONALD D. PRICE, Department of Anesthesiology, Medical College of Virginia, Richmond, Virginia 23298

LOUIS A. RITZ, Departments of Neurological Surgery and Neuroscience, University of Florida College of Medicine, Gainesville, Florida 32610

BARBARA E. RODIN, Departments of Anatomy and Anesthesiology and the Brain Research Center, UCLA Center for Health Sciences, Los Angeles, California 90024

M. A. RUDA, Neurobiology and Anesthesiology Branch, National Institute of Dental Research, National Institutes of Health, Bethesda, Maryland 20892

VIRGINIA S. SEYBOLD, Department of Anatomy, University of Minnesota, Minneapolis, Minnesota 55455

CHARLES J. VIERCK, JR., Department of Neuroscience and Center for Neurobiological Sciences, University of Florida College of Medicine, Gainesville, Florida 32610

LUIS VILLANUEVA, Research Unit of Pharmacological Neurophysiology of Inserm (U. 161), Paris 75014, France

WILLIAM D. WILLIS, JR., Marine Biomedical Institute and Departments of Physiology and Biophysics and Anatomy, University of Texas Medical Branch, Galveston, Texas 77550

RICHARD K. WINKELMANN, Department of Dermatology, Mayo Clinic, Rochester, Minnesota 55905

TONY L. YAKSH, Departments of Neurosurgery and Pharmacology, Mayo Clinic, Rochester, Minnesota 55905

DAVID C. YEOMANS, Department of Neuroscience and Center for Neurobiological Sciences, University of Florida College of Medicine, Gainesville, Florida 32610

Preface

Some 29 scientists from the fields of neuroanatomy, neurochemistry, neurophysiology, neuropharmacology, and behavior have contributed their efforts to this testimonial on behalf of the contributions made by Dr. F. W. L. Kerr to science and to those with whom he interacted. The intention of the contributors to this volume was to deal with the manifold advances that pertain to the substrates in spinal cord relating to the processing of sensory information, a subject that in one form or another provoked time and again Kerr's native enthusiasm for research.

The organization of the book follows a natural course from the peripheral innervation of the somatic and visceral organs (Winkelmann, Chapter 2) to the effective stimuli that activate these fibers and give rise to sensation under normal and pathological conditions (Campbell and Meyer, Chapter 3; Dubner and colleagues, Chapter 13; Dyck, Chapter 14) to the course these afferent systems take to enter the spinal cord (Coggeshall, Chapter 4) and to the organization of the systems through which this afferent information reaches the brain (Willis, Chapter 11; Vierck and colleagues, Chapter 12). Coverage is also devoted to the significant advances in immunohistochemical procedures (LaMotte, Chapter 5; Ruda, Chapter 7) and binding autoradiography (Seybold, Chapter 6) that have begun to permit us to demonstrate in a three-dimensional schema the local organization of specific neurotransmitter terminal systems and the receptors on which these neurotransmitters may act as well as the functional characteristics of the systems from which certain spinal neurotransmitters are released (Yaksh, Chapter 8). The continued efforts of those who have focused on the dorsal horn have begun to unravel the evident complexity of this region and have permitted us to add color to the otherwise black-and-white line drawings of connectivity.

Conceptually, the functional analysis of afferent processing can never be undertaken without considering the intrinsic systems that modulate its processing (Hammond, Chapter 15; Gebhart, Chapter 16). Though early behavioral experiments and the observation that such manipulations would modify Aδ/C-fiber-evoked activity led to the simplistic notion that these substrates constituted an "antipain" system, it has become increasingly apparent that these modulatory systems interact with all aspects of spinal processing. Bulbofugal and intrinsic systems not only modulate the gain of the transmission system but also serve in part to code the modality to which the cell will respond. The receptive fields of the second-order neuron are in fact the net product of those local inhibitory and excitatory inputs, which are under higher-order control. Indeed, these excitatory connections from the brainstem may provide for bilateral receptive fields in the intact spinal cord. All of these characteristics clearly indicate the complexity of the electrophysiological characteristics of dorsal horn neurons (Cervero, Chapter 9) and the complexity of the characteristics of the message that is transmitted in spinofugal axons (Foreman, Chapter 10; Willis, Chapter 11).

Such observations must clearly change the way we think of spinal coding. Thus, the early observations of a large number of wide-dynamic-range neurons and the phenomenon of polymodal convergence led many to consider simple frequency coding and labeled-line hypotheses. In fact, these multimodal systems can serve to transmit a variety of specific messages when so influenced by the modulating substrate, much as a user-defined key on a computer may mean what the user intends it to mean. The ever-changing modulation, altering gain and providing an ongoing selectivity, suggests that active processing is the theme of spinal organization. This growing appreciation of the complexity and characteristics of the underlying substrate has led naturally to major changes in the conceptualization of how these systems are organized to discretely encode the complex aspects of the stimulus environment (Price, Chapter 18; Le Bars and colleagues, Chapter 19).

Finally, one may consider whether this increasing understanding of the biochemistry and pharmacology of cord function will have tangible clinical applicability. The analgesic action of spinal opiates is one example of how basic studies on spinal pharmacology and sensory processing have led to such benefit (Yaksh, Chapter 20), but it appears certain that such insights may also apply in fields as diverse as those dealing with autonomic, bladder, and motor function. It should be recalled that in a high spinal animal, spinal reflex arcs remain intact. Changes in reflex function after transection appear to reflect changes in this spinal pharmacology, perhaps related in part to functional changes in innervation (Micevych and colleagues, Chapter 17). The possibility of modulating these spinal systems pharmacologically may provide mechanisms of ameliorating the severity of the clinical syndrome in spinal man. The very complexity of the spinal system, its discrete pharmacology, and the degree to which spinal substrates can modify peripheral function in a homeostatic fashion suggest that the future holds much promise.

This is the exciting field that we sought to address. Perhaps we attempted too much. There are many spaces, but I think an honest effort was made to cover our topics, providing both a background and an emphasis on the directions in which these areas are currently proceeding. Personally, I would like to thank the contributors to this volume. I have learned a great deal from them. I also thank Ms. Ann Rockafellow for her patience and efforts in correcting and retyping bits and pieces of every contribution.

Originally, these contributions were to form a festschrift for Kerr on his retirement from Mayo. His death prevented us from honoring him in his lifetime but cannot prevent these contributions from bearing witness to the respect and love that many had for this man.

Tony L. Yaksh

Rochester, Minnesota

Contents

Chapter 8
The Central Pharmacology of Primary Afferents with Emphasis on the Disposition and Role of Primary Afferent Substance P
TONY L. YAKSH

Chapter 9
Dorsal Horn Neurons and Their Sensory Inputs
FERNANDO CERVERO

Chapter 10
Spinal Substrates of Visceral Pain
ROBERT D. FOREMAN

Chapter 11
Ascending Somatosensory Systems
WILLIAM D. WILLIS, JR.

Chapter 12
The Spinal Pathways Contributing to the Ascending Conduction and the Descending Modulation of Pain Sensations and Reactions
CHARLES J. VIERCK, JR., JOEL D. GREENSPAN, LOUIS A. RITZ, AND DAVID C. YEOMANS

Chapter 15
Control Systems for Nociceptive Afferent Processing: The Descending Inhibitory Pathways
DONNA L. HAMMOND

Chapter 16
Modulatory Effects of Descending Systems on Spinal Dorsal Horn Neurons
G. F. GEBHART

Chapter 17

The Controversial Nature of the Evidence for Neuroplasticity of Afferent Axons in the Spinal Cord

PAUL E. MICEVYCH, BARBARA E. RODIN, AND LAWRENCE KRUGER

Chapter 18

The Question of How the Dorsal Horn Encodes Sensory Information

DONALD D. PRICE

Chapter 19

Aspects of Sensory Processing through Convergent Neurons

DANIEL LE BARS, ANTHONY H. DICKENSON, JEAN MARIE BESSON, AND LUIS VILLANUEVA

Chapter 20

The Effects of Intrathecally Administered Opioid and Adrenergic Agents on Spinal Function

TONY L. YAKSH

1
A Short Biography of F. W. L. Kerr, M.D.

Tony L. Yaksh

A. Frederick W. L. Kerr—Introduction

Frederick W. L. Kerr, after 25 years of contributing to our understanding of brain function, died on the 28th of August 1983. He was born on the 25th of March 1923 to English parents in Buenos Aires, Argentina. He received his M.D. degree from the University of Buenos Aires in 1949. He came to the United States in 1952 to begin his residency in Neurosurgery at Barnes Hospital in St. Louis under Dr. Henry Schwartz. He became an American citizen in 1961. From 1956 to 1958, after completing his residency training, he became an Assistant Professor of Neurosurgery at the State University of New York at Syracuse and was acting Chief of Neurological Surgery at the Veterans Administration Hospital there. He then came to Mayo, in his own words, to "do neurosurgery and to organize and direct a research laboratory of neurological surgery." He indeed did both. He was actually practicing neurosurgery until 1976 and was actively involved in research up to the year before his death.

B. Frederick W. L. Kerr—His Professional Career

In both his clinical and scientific career, Kerr was well recognized. As I discuss below, early in his life he developed a continuing interest in the struc-

Tony L. Yaksh • Departments of Neurosurgery and Pharmacology, Mayo Clinic, Rochester, Minnesota 55905.

ture and function of the central nervous system. It is thus perhaps not surprising that he had a reputation as a perceptive diagnostician, which I do not doubt was a direct manifestation of his continuing efforts to understand neural function. For many, however, including myself, his reputation as an investigator of CNS structure and function much preceded our appreciation of his occupational specialty. During his research career, Dr. Kerr had several principal subjects of interest. Table I shows the topical areas towards which his published research was directed. The citation list at the end of the chapter presents his published manuscripts chronologically.

In the following section, I would like briefly to review what I think are some of the salient contributions made by this individual during his 20 years of active research.

1. *The Anatomy and Functional Characteristics of the Cranial Nerves*

Doctor Kerr once indicated that to him one of the most impressive clinical syndromes was that of *tic douloureux.* He once related how early in his career several such patients had come under his care as a resident. This clinical exposure laid the groundwork for the subsequent investigations into the characteristics of the trigeminal system. As was typical of Dr. Kerr, he began to pursue this issue in the late 1950s by establishing his own rationale after what he referred to as an exhaustive consideration of the literature. Based on clinical characteristics, Dr. Kerr became convinced that certain of these paroxysmal dysfunctions had to possess peripheral ethiology (Kerr, 1962, 1963a,b, 1967a,b, 1970b). Though it was early considered by a number of investigators that the phenomenon might represent some trauma to the nerve, the prevalent thought at that time was that it was a centrally organized syndrome, perhaps comparable to a focal discharge in epilepsy.

Kerr (1963a) examined the likelihood that the effect might be related to the juxtaposition of the internal carotid artery beneath the trigeminal ganglion and the adjacent posterior rootlets. In careful and systematic autopsy studies, he demonstrated that the roof of the carotid canal was often replaced by a thin layer of connective tissue, which permitted close contact between the ventral surface of the ganglion and the underlying carotid artery. He noted that that relationship held only for the second and third divisions of the trigeminal nerve and that this correlated with the observed predominance of the involvement of the second and third divisions in the trigeminal syndrome. He demonstrated in cadavers that where the carotid canal defect was observed, pulsatile flow of saline injected into the carotid artery could be palpated through the ganglion. In subsequent microelectrode studies, he observed that those cells that lay in the ventral portion of the trigeminal ganglion had receptive fields that were distributed around the rostral areas of the face, lips, nose, and eyebrows, a distribution that corresponds with the typical distribution of trigger points (Kerr, 1963c, 1964; Kerr *et al.,* 1968). Thus, the

TABLE I
Experimental Endeavors of Frederick W. L. Kerr, MD[a]

Subject	Year: 1960 1962 1964 1966 1968 1970 1972 1974 1976 1978 1980 1982
Trigeminal systems	
Anatomy	xx ---------- x ---------- xx --------- xxxx ---------- x -------------------- x
Electrophysiology	x ---------------------------------- x ---- x
Pathology	x -------- x ---- xx
Tic	xxx ---------- xx -------------------- x -------- x -- x
Ascending sensory systems	x ---------------------------- x -------------------------- x -- x
Autonomic systems	
Pupillomotor	xx ------------- x --------------- xx
Vesico/vasomotor	x ---------- xx ------------------------ x ------------------------ xx ----- x - xx
Dorsomotor nucleus	x ------------- xx
Trauma	
Spinal cord injury (blood pressure)	x
Cerebral infarction/ischemia	xxxx
Esophageal achalasia	x
CNS sprouting	x ------------ xx
Opiate effects	
Addiction	x ---- x ---- x
Electrophysiology	x
Miscellaneous areas	
Colloidal gold	x -------------------------- x
Cerebral hypothermia	xx --- x
Head restraint	x
Brain tumors	x -------- x - xx -- x
Acupuncture	x

[a]Each "x" indicates a publication listed in the reference list.

ganglion cells whose afferents innervated regions considered typical for tic trigger points lay adjacent to the presumed source of mechanical trauma.

In a series of electron micrographic studies in normal and pathological material, he (Kerr, 1967c; Kerr and Miller, 1966) demonstrated in typical cases of tic that proliferative–degenerative changes occurred in the myelin sheath, although changes in the axon cylinder were rare. Variations on these arguments for a peripheral site of action for these neuralgias have become increasingly accepted as correct today (witness the success of the decompression procedures espoused by Janetta, 1976). It should be remembered that these experiments and their interpretations were forcefully made when many investigators and clinicians argued for a predominant central mechanism for tic.

In parallel with these studies on pathology, Kerr early began systematic investigations on the ultrastructural morphology of the sensory afferent systems, particularly as they pertained to the trigeminal nerve and the substantia gelatinosa (Kerr, 1966b, 1970a,c,d, 1971). These studies led him to speculate that selective abolition of pain might derive from lesion of the first order synapse of the primary afferent. This led him to propose the concept of spinal V nucleolysis (Kerr, 1966), a concept that was later employed successfully by Nashold (Friedman *et al.*, 1984) for certain cases of intractable pain.

An additional consideration arising from his clinical observations had to do with the phenomenon of atypical facial neuralgias, i.e., those syndromes that possess neurological signs distinct from those of known trigeminal projection systems and that have trigger points that do not correspond to the conventional dermatomes of the trigeminal system. Though many of these patients were often thought to be "hysterical," as there appeared to be no plausible anatomic basis for the reported signs, careful clinical observations by Kerr in a number of patients convinced him of the reality of the syndrome (Kerr, 1961a, 1979). By exclusion, he formed the hypothesis that suggested the likelihood of a convergence between trigeminal and cervical projections onto neurons at the C1 and C2 level. In studies with trigeminal and C1/C2 rhizotomies, he demonstrated what appeared to be a convergence between trigeminal and cervical projections on the neurons at the C1 and C2 level (Kerr, 1961b,c, 1962, 1972). Electrical recording indeed demonstrated potentials evoked at the C1 and C2 level by trigeminal stimulation.

2. *Central Autonomic Pathways*

The problems of unstable hemodynamics following acute cord compression and changes in pupil size secondary to elevated intracranial pressure were topics to which he was exposed clinically. His early experiments were among the first to examine systematically the substrate affected during elevated intracranial pressure that led to the paralytic midriasis (Kerr and Hollowell, 1964) and factors affecting the blood pressure response to acute cord compression (Alexander and Kerr, 1964). These investigations together led him to ask the more general question of what was the distribution of the descending autonomic pathways in the spinal cord. This prompted a subsequent fascinating series of papers on autonomic pathways. Using classical stimulation procedures combined with acute lesions, he was able to demonstrate the trajectory of the hypothalamic and brainstem pathways whereby brainstem stimulation would give rise to changes in pupillomotor, vasomotor, and vesicomotor function (Enoch and Kerr, 1967a,b; Lowey *et al.*, 1973). He further extended these studies to describe the spinal trajectory of these descending autonomic systems (Kerr and Alexander, 1964; Kerr and Brown, 1964).

Perhaps some of his most elegant pieces of work were his studies on the organization of the vagus (Kerr, 1967; Kerr *et al.*, 1970). Classically, the dorsomotor nucleus of the vagus was thought to be a vasomotor center. In two straightforward papers in the *Journal of Physiology* (Kerr, 1969; Kerr and Preshaw, 1969), Kerr conclusively demonstrated that chronic lesions of the dorsomotor nucleus had no effect on the vasodepressive effects produced by ipsilateral stimulation of the cervical vagi. He thus concluded "that the dorsomotor nucleus of the vagus does not supply the vagal fibers which produce contraction of the smooth muscle in bronchials, esophagus and duodenum, and that it is not the source of the cardio-inhibitory fibers." He subsequently demonstrated, however, that chronic ablation of the dorsomotor nucleus produced a "profound reduction in the gastric secretion of acid." These experiments were elegant in their simplicity and, as is typical, concisely described.

3. *Central Nervous System Regeneration and Sprouting*

Regeneration was one area that was of particular interest to Kerr. He, as were many others, was interested in the reports by Liu and Chambers (1958) that primary afferents sprouted when adjacent roots or supraspinal pathways had been chronically transected. Given his considerable experience with the projections between the trigeminal and cervical root systems, he sought to determine whether sprouting could be detected after selective lesions in those systems. In his work, Kerr was essentially unable to replicate those previous findings of Liu and Chambers. Subsequent investigations using evoked potentials also failed to show any significant evidence of either sprouting or hyperactivity following long-term trigeminal or cervical rhizotomy (Kerr, 1972b; Beckerman and Kerr, 1975). (See Micevych *et al.* for their comments on the role of sprouting in recovery of function, Chapter 17.) In all of his work, characteristically, he was careful to point out the limitations of his procedures. Moreover, in his teaching lectures to residents, he was the first to emphasize (1) that these considerations were based on normal tissue and (2) that the failure to see extensive regeneration did not exclude the fact that local sprouting could occur and that alterations in the chemical milieu might in fact alter the ability to produce the sprouting. Nevertheless, his reasoned arguments, based on analysis of embryological development, remain in my mind strong evidence that functional regeneration of long tracts is a phenomenon that, in spite of anecdotal evidence to the contrary, does not lie within our foreseeable grasp.

4. *Opiate Mechanisms of Tolerance and Dependence*

Kerr's interest in opiate tolerance and dependence arose again out of his clinical involvement in the treatment of chronic pain and his observation of the effects of chronic opiate administration on behavior in man. He was most impressed by the devastating effects that opiate abuse had and was impressed by the drive that appeared to accompany a person's will to self-administer the drug. Drawing parallels with normal vegetative function mediated by the hypothalamus, he considered the likelihood that the phenomenon of opiate drive might be found in this region. In his own words,

> The hypothesis . . . was that addiction to morphine might be due to involvement of centers concerned with appetite. It was proposed . . . that exposure of these centers to opiates over a period of time might result in substitution by these agents for the natural stimulus and that withholding of the drug would precipitate desire or craving comparable to hunger as manifested in the withdrawal syndrome (Kerr, 1971).

He demonstrated in early experiments that circumscribed lesions within the hypothalamus would significantly alter the dependence cycle in rats (Kerr and Pozuelo-Utanda, 1971). These studies were subsequently extended to investigations in primates. In the early 1970s, Dr. Kerr established a large program to produce primates that would voluntarily self-administer morphine. He carried out extensive experiments to investigate the selective effects of hypothalamic lesions on this self-administration behavior. He was able to demonstrate, as in rats, that circumscribed lesions in the hypothalamus could produce significant effects on morphine self-administration but would result in minimal effects on feeding behavior (Kerr, 1973). Indeed, his last series of experiments, incomplete at the time of his death, was directed at defining the characteristics of the effective lesion in the primate.

Further consideration of the role of opiates on hypothalamic function led Kerr to initiate studies to examine the effect of opiates on focal neuronal activity in this region. Using a locally constructed data acquisition system, which permitted triggering from several spikes of different amplitudes recorded from each of two microelectrodes, he carried out a very elegant analysis on multiple single hypothalamic units, recording concurrently in the medial and lateral hypothalamus. In this series of studies, he observed that opiates in nontolerant animals will suppress the firing of ventromedial cells and concurrently enhance the firing of lateral hypothalamic neurons. Hypothalamic tolerant animals, in contrast, showed a marked firing in the presence of opiate antagonists (Kerr *et al.*, 1974).

5. *Pain*

From the early 1960s, when he initiated his investigations on the mechanisms of *tic douloureux* and atypical facial neuralgias, the phenomenon of pain was of abiding interest to him. This interest cut across the majority of his investigations, whether the studies were directed at autonomic pathways, the use of opiates, or the pathways through which ascending information traveled. His studies on the ascending system (Kerr and Lippman, 1974; Nijensohn and Kerr, 1975; Fukushima and Kerr, 1979) led him to focus attention on the ventral portion of the spinothalamic pathway and reintroduced many who studied pain to the idea that alternate long tracts might underlie some of the recovery of function following spinal cordotomy (see Vierck *et al.*, Chapter 12).

His systematic studies on the marginal cells were inspired by the classical observations that retrograde degeneration of these marginal neurons was observed in human spinal cord following successful cordotomies. His systematic investigations at the electron microscopic level were directed by establishing the origin of the innervation of these neurons. In systematic studies, Narotzky and Kerr (1978) examinied the distribution of boutons after rhizotomy and/or lesions of the tract of Lissauer. He clearly demonstrated the predominance of afferent terminals on the distal dendrites, as those terminals lying near the cell body and the proximal dendrites all degenerated following Lissauer tractotomy. In addition, in this work, Kerr emphasized the presence of multiple vesicle profiles in the same terminal. As discussed elsewhere (see Yaksh, Chapter 8), such prescient observations preceded current thinking that multiple neurotransmitters may be found in the same terminal.

In 1975, Kerr published a review article in the journal *Pain* that emphasized the complexity of the synaptology of the dorsal horn and the multiplicity of the ascending pain pathways. Clearly, the concept of multiplicity was not uniquely attributable to Kerr, but appearing as it did, when it did, in the journal that it did, it provided a widely cited synthesis that gave a powerful impetus to the thinking regarding the coding of the ascending pain message. His thinking, based on his studies of the anatomic pathways and in consideration of the experimental literature, led him to propose what he referred to as a "postsynaptic inhibitory balance theory" (Kerr, 1975, 1979). It represented one of the first expansions of the earlier conceptualization of the dorsal horn modulatory systems made by Melzack and Wall within their "gate control theory" published in 1965. Conceptually, his formulation emphasized the importance of the marginal neuron and the likelihood that its information throughput was subject to ongoing modulation (i.e., postsynaptically) by descending and intrinsic pathways.

C. Contemplations on the Life and Career of Dr. F. W. L. Kerr

What animated Kerr into the study of brain or to become a neurosurgeon? As a medical student, he was already absorbed by the complexity of the brain as manifested in function. I believe that three things contributed to this interest. First, though there was little formal training in neuroscience in Buenos Aires at that time, and certainly none in neurophysiology, he had begun to read the monumental works of Ramon y Cajal. He once remarked that he had read the *Histologie du Système Nerveau* through at least five times and that the first time had been as a medical student. There had been assigned readings in those volumes on, interestingly, spinal tracts. So entranced, said Kerr, was he with the clarity of presentation, the order, and with the encyclopedic knowledge that he felt compelled to read it at every opportunity. Most else in the general course after that seemed, he said, pointless and superficial. Second, his medical school training placed him in the hospital. The evident differences observed in those with behavioral disorders such as tic or more subtle changes as with depression or Parkinsonlike disorders, meshing with his callow knowledge of neuroanatomy garnered from his own reading, led him to a fascination for understanding the functioning of the CNS—a fascination that he often said preceded any desire to be a surgeon.

Third, about this time, Kerr began to visit the laboratory of neuropathology at the National Hospital for Mental Diseases in Buenos Aires and eventually became a research assistant in neuroanatomy under the direction of Professor B. Moyano. As he related, at that time the predominant study of brain involved the direct study of substrate, either by fortuitous lesion (i.e., neuropathology) or by examination of its organization (i.e., neuroanatomy). He said it was at this time that he decided to devote himself to the study of the structure of the nervous system. In an early curriculum vita (1967), he noted laconically that during this period, he ". . . acquired anatomical techniques for the study of the CNS (paraffin embedding, Hortega's silver carbonate, Cajal gold chloride, etc.); prepared and drew serial sections of the brain stem including thalamus of Nissl and Weigert–Pal series."

Of even greater significance at this time than his acquisition of technical skills was the fact that his presence in an active neuropathology laboratory resulted in a repeated exposure to the inextricable relationship between form and function. He related how, after receiving a brain for processing, he would feel compelled to track down the case history and attempt to piece together the elements of the syndrome, the time at which the symptoms appeared, the degree of bleeding and the neurological sequelae, the location of the infarct, the tumor, and so on. He felt a particular pride in those instances when a former patient whom he had examined would come to autopsy and he, with his skills, was able to confirm the accuracy of his own diagnosis or suspicions. It was a learning experience that could perhaps have benefited few others as much. It was then that Kerr came to appreciate the power of systematic observations in the correlation of biological structure and function. Kerr often said that his earliest training in experimental neuroanatomy came from the examples set by Cajal in his epic series of investigations in CNS anatomy. It is hard to believe now that there was not a latent impetus for such experimentalism in Kerr's philosophy at this point. Yet, it is clear that if Fred Kerr had a hero, it was without question Ramon y Cajal. Our own generation of neurobiologists even now sense the enormous contribution of Cajal. One can only extrapolate to the earlier generations to realize how much greater would be Cajal's impact in the 1940s, particularly on a nascent neuroscientist such as Kerr.

Kerr's abiding interest in CNS function led him early to consider it as a professional subspecialty. He once said that his early goal in medical school had been to be a neurologist, but he later chose neurosurgery. He saw that specialty as a necessity to permit his ongoing management of the patient. I personally think his desire to be a surgeon was as much a manifestation of his inability to stand aside and wait while others worked at anything.

In short, I believe this early training and those experiences in Kerr's formative years as a medical student and as a resident provided an extremely fertile ground for the development of the neuroscientist. In some ways, the characteristics of his work indeed reflect the philosophy of the man. I would therefore like to take this opportunity to consider some of the common factors that appear manifested in the productive career of Kerr.

First, the starting points for virtually all of his research interests were clinical observations. In virtually every case, I can remember being told a clinical antecdote that led to this or that interest. His considerations of the trigeminal system were spurred, as I noted above, by his early exposure to patients with this syndrome, and he was aware of its devastating consequences, leading in many cases to a choice of suicide. His approach to the question of the central versus peripheral etiology of tic derived from an acute appreciation of the characteristics of the clinical symptomatology. His pursuit of the convergence at the cervical level of the trigeminal system and of other cranial nerves was brought about essentially by an appreciation of the clinical syndrome referred to indiscriminately as atypical facial neuralgia. The studies on autonomic pathways were initiated by his clinical experiences with the effects of increased intracranial pressure on pupil function and on changes in blood pressure. His persistent interest in the effects of opiates was generated by his care of patients who were dependent on morphine. Thus, in every instance that I know, Kerr's experimental endeavors were generated and directed by his close and careful observation of behavior.

Secondly, in his clinical work, the observation of a novel syndrome would lead him to the inevitable consideration of the mechanism. His first impulse was to read voluminously and critically every piece of relevant literature—to secure the facts, as he would say. A crucial point was never documented on faith or by "say so" in a review article but by perusal of the original literature—if it was in one of the six or eight languages that he read—or by complete translation if not. I remember one instance in which the question of the Law of Bell and Magendie was discussed, and it became quite apparent that all present in the room knew of the Law of Bell and Magendie, appreciated its meaning, but indeed had never read the original concepts postulated by either individual. Kerr, in his inimitable fashion, proceeded to acquire copies of the original work by Bell and by Magendie and came to the conclusion that the significant contribution as we interpret it today was indeed not controversial but belonged to Magendie.

Thirdly, in his approach to a question, he was forever seeking to correlate form and function, bringing to bear every technique that was at his disposal. His studies on the role of the dorsomotor nucleus of the vagus or the descending autonomic pathways are typical examples of his experimental methodology. He would establish the anatomic connectivity to his satisfaction and then proceed to the logical physiological experiment that would permit confirmation or rejection of the physiological relevance of that anatomic system. Although he was an anatomist, I found him at times surprisingly flippant about the significance of anatomic connectivity. He once pointed out that just about every system in the brain could be traced by one or not more than two synapses to every other system. He noted that many systems such as the spinocerebellar pathway clearly must play a role in view of their extent but that lesions had relatively little detectable effect on gross motor behavior. In contrast, the marginal neurons or locus coeruleus neurons clearly played a significant and pervasive role in pain and autonomic function, respectively, which would not otherwise be appreciated on the basis of number alone. He once noted that "structure indicates possibilities, but physiology gives us the reality."

This comment brings to mind several thoughts that I had after my initial meetings with Dr. Kerr in the early 1970s. It occurred to me at that time that he was indeed the living and breathing prototype of the neurobiologist that was fashionable in peoples' discussions in the later 1960s and early 1970s, i.e., one who pursued a problem in a methodologically eclectic fashion. In his case, his armamentarium ranged from the systematic study of behavior, whether in man or in animal, through the search for the anatomic substrate (by classical degeneration procedures or transported label and light or electron microscopy), and, finally, assessment of the role in behavior of the detected substrate by lesion, stimulation, drug intervention, or examination of single-unit activity. His goal was to solve the problem by approaching it from every side, a coordinated attack on structure and function.

Fourthly, Kerr was without question an experimentalist. Anecdotes, he would say, can provide a stimulus and a direction for one's research. They are hints and rays of light in a dark room, but such glimpses cannot replace systematic observations in well-defined systems. His own career, as noted above, was a continuing affirmation of this belief. It is therefore not surprising that Kerr was a firm believer in the use of animals in research. Once, in a local talk on the use of animals in research, he pointed to the advances made in our understanding and the management of disease. He noted that such advances did not occur as a result of a return to scholasticism or mental exercises but as a result of a combined process of thinking and doing. . . ."thinking" to direct the light of one's efforts and "doing" to test the reality of the mental exercise. In this text, he said:

> To those who would adamantly oppose research using animals, I would say that you will stand accountable for a heinous crime, not only against your own specie, but against the animals you purport to protect, for those too benefit from parallel advances in veterinary medicine.

These are clearly strong words, so, doubtless, it would surprise people of all persuasions if they were aware of the care and consideration Kerr gave to those animals in his charge and of his unswerving support for animal welfare. Kerr felt that animals, though a necessity for the advance of medical knowledge, possessed a significant intrinsic worth because of their possession of life. He maintained two dicta in the use of animals in research: (1) that every attention be made to insure that the animal did not suffer, and (2) to the degree the animals were put to some degree of discomfort, the contribution that that experiment made to medical science had to be disproportionately greater. Thus, in his eyes, the use of the unanesthetized animal was not necessarily prohibited, but that if in fact the animal were to be placed in a position where significant physical intervention would occur, the outcome had to promise disproportionate benefit to all. It was the burden of the scientist to make certain that if the animal were to be killed, its sacrifice was meaningful. There were few things, I believe, that could so enrage Kerr as to read a poorly designed experiment carried out with primates or to read of primates or dogs used in a sacrifice experiment when a rat would have served as well.

It should be noted that Kerr was forever considering the ethics of research, and it was not a foregone point to him that any given experiment should or should not be done. He once mused as to what value a man's life had versus that of a dog. "One human here," indicating one hand, and . . ."how many dogs here," gesturing with the other, emulating a scale of justice. "I don't know," he said. And then speaking of those who argued against animal research, "I don't think they know either." The recent incident of "Baby Fae" and the resistance by some of transplanting a baboon heart would, I believe, have caused him great anguish . . . the life of a human baby versus that of a baboon on his scales.

D. Frederick W. L. Kerr—The Man

Perhaps the first thing that would strike a person about Kerr was his appearance: tall, silver hair brushed starkly back, gray eyes, a stately manner, and a deep resonant voice with a slight English accent. The second factor that became apparent in subsequent conversation was his intelligence. Indeed, it would be difficult to discuss Fred Kerr's endeavors without consideration of his native intellect. I am aware that he spoke, aside from English, German, Russian, Spanish, French, Italian, and Portugese. In his acquisition of knowledge, it was my experience that Dr. Kerr was an eclectic. He read widely in literature, art, and, particularly, politics and history. At any given time, he could and would marshall his diverse resources to embellish, to support, to refute. In discussion, I felt I was watching a swordsman thrust and parry with consummate skill and finesse.

Kerr drew not only from his reading but from a lifetime of careful observation and scholarship. His memory was categorical; little seemed to escape him. This made conversations with Kerr prized episodes not to be forgotten. Not infrequently, a chance comment would lead to a morning of discussion and argument. On many a Friday afternoon, the "Happy Warrior," a local bar, was the place where the weekly weary would gather for beer and conversation. That summer of 1983, he had been listless and seemed without energy, and we actually spoke only infrequently. He attributed this lethargy to a viral infection. Several days before he died, he had not been feeling well and went home. I was concerned, but I did not appreciate the gravity of the problem. On Friday I called to ask if I could visit on Saturday or Sunday and if he needed anything from the laboratory. It turned out that Saturday morning became Saturday noon, and I thought perhaps Sunday would be more convenient. Nevertheless, I indeed did go on Saturday, and though I had intended to stay for only a short while, we chatted all afternoon. The conversation ranged from politics to gardening and sailing (two of his favorite pastimes) to science. What a marvelous conversation it was. He died early the next morning of bilateral pulmonary embolism.

As an individual, Kerr was exceedingly complex. Whatever he did or felt was always done with a passion surprising for one possessed of such a love of logic. I would note that in all he was not dogmatic. His mind could be changed with a balanced argument. If he decided he was in error, he faced no difficulty in saying so.

This intensity of emotion was made manifest in several ways. As I noted, he was born in Argentina and was a naturalized American citizen. It is no understatement, and he would concur, that he was a patriot and loved America with an intensity that caused many, I think, to smile smugly. He recounted a story once, however, that typically manifested his feelings. He had left Argentina to come to the United States for neurosurgical training.

> I took a small steamer up from Buenos Aires and arrived in Baltimore. After the medical officer in customs had processed our arrival, they left, and I was standing on deck, not really knowing what to do. I decided to venture onto the deck and to find an officer to get permission to land. I (nervously) checked to make certain that I had my documents, copies of my medical certificate, letters from Buenos Aires, letters from St. Louis, passport, visa, and so forth. I walked down the gangway looking for someone; I saw no one. I walked a bit further and still no uniform or hat appeared, no hand on my shoulder, no voice demanding my business or inten-

> tions. The air at this time seemed to be a bit too fragrant for that of a dock. I continued walking down the wharf. It seemed that the further I went the lighter my steps became. No one barred my way. There was a dawning realization that no one cared or minded what were my doings or my intentions. I will never forget that by the time that I reached the end of the dock, I was floating, literally floating, off the ground—walking on air. When I got to the end of the wharf, a taxi driver hailed, asking if I wanted a ride. I opened the door and got in. The taxi driver asked me where I wanted to go. I didn't know, I said. I was so taken aback by the sense of freedom that I didn't know. I told him to drive around so I could get my bearings. I think he thought I was on drugs—I think in a way I was.

Because of his patriotism, many thought of Fred as an extreme conservative ("somewhat to the right of Genghis Khan," quipped one colleague), but that was a glib analysis. Kerr's problem was that he was disgusted by the tyrannical extremes of either the left-wing bureaucrat or the right-wing petty dictator, as he would call them. His rearing in Argentina had given him personal experience with both. Thus, like many who cater to neither side of an argument, whether it be about communism or antivivesection or right-wing dictators, his position often appeared to be that of an extremist.

I believe that Kerr's demeanor and strongly held opinions made many people feel ill at ease in his presence and, I think, gave rise to the idea that he was a difficult man to know. He had a low tolerance for trivia, and in spite of all that is said about conversation, he was not given to accept trivial comments. A statement such as "it is well known that". . . would often elicit a request for detail. A resident or colleague who made such a generalization to cover his own lack of detailed knowledge would often find himself forced to admit that he indeed didn't know the answer. Nevertheless, to his friends and colleagues he was exceedingly loyal and ever ready to offer help where possible. Indeed, in spite of his reputation as a distant individual, there are many instances of which I am aware where Kerr went far out of his way to provide assistance to a resident or a medical student having difficulty with some aspect of neuroanatomy or neurosurgery. He was always ready to drop what he was doing to come to the laboratory to help a struggling associate get a bleeder under control or to find an aberrant vagus nerve. Whatever his opinion of the individual's native ability might be, an honest effort was generally all that was required to elicit the greatest attempts of help on his part.

Though Kerr made a significant impact by his contributions to the published literature, he influenced many peers and colleagues and contributed to their own work by his interactions. One such example of which I am personally aware is his role in the early development of the clinical use of spinal opiates at Mayo. He was a site visitor at the University of Wisconsin in 1975 when Tom Rudy and I were studying the spinal action of opiates in animal models. On seeing the data and the model, he considered it to be potentially advantageous for pain therapy. He brought the concept to the attention of Dr. Josef Wang at the Pain Clinic at Mayo. In Dr. Kerr's laboratory they then proceeded to verify the lack of toxicity associated with intrathecal opiates and obtained institutional approval for Dr. Wang to administer morphine intrathecally in man. Kerr was instrumental in obtaining the institutional approval for the first pump implant by Dr. Burton Onofrio for the chronic spinal infusion of opiates in terminal cancer patients. Other instances come to mind. In many cases, however, the true magnitude of his contributions is known only to those with whom he interacted.

Finally, when all is said and done, I must confess to what has always impressed me most about Fred Kerr. I have spoken of his intellect, his power of logic, and his experimental skills. He was a neurosurgeon of no small note. In the circles of what one calls science, he was clearly a man of considerable influence. Yet, in spite of all this, Kerr was very much what I would call a bench scientist. In spite of his power, fame, and prestige, he fully realized throughout his life that science was something that required a day-to-day involvement and that a single step forward required an inordinate investment in time and effort. It is very easy as one progresses along the ladder, as Fred Kerr did, to lose sight of this fundamental reality, that there are no shortcuts. He discovered no cure for cancer. He did not provide an ultimate therapy for *tic douloureux*. He did not produce a method for regenerating the nervous system. But, in his 25 years of science, he opened the door a bit wider to shed a bit more light on our knowledge of the sensory and autonomic nervous system and their function. About 6 months before his death, he finally had decided to retire. After several beers one Friday afternoon, I asked him if he had been satisfied with the way things had gone in his own career. There was no hesitancy in his reply. "I have done what I could do with the best of my ability," he said, "and I have enjoyed it immensely."

So long, Fred.

Chronological Citation List of Dr. Frederick W. L. Kerr

KERR, F. W. L., SCHWARTZ, H. G., AND SEAMAN, W. B. Experimental effects of radioactive colloidal gold in the subarachnoid space, clinical application in treating brain tumors. *Arch. Surg.* 69:694–706, 1954.

KERR, F. W. L., AND O'LEARY, J. L. The thalamic source of cortical recruiting in the rodent. *Electroencephalogr. Clin. Neurophysiol.* 9:461–476, 1957.

KERR, F. W. L., KING, R. B., AND MEAGHER, J. M. Brain abscess. A study of forty-seven consecutive cases. *J.A.M.A.* 168:868–872, 1958.

O'LEARY, J. L., KERR, F. W. L., AND GOLDRING, S. The relation between spinoreticular and ascending cephalic systems, in: *Reticular Formation of the Brain* (H. H. JASPER, L. D. PROCTOR, AND R. S. KNIGHTON eds.), Little, Brown, Boston, 1958, pp. 187–206.

KERR, F. W. L. Atypical facial neuralgias, their mechanism as inferred from anatomic and physiologic data. *Proc. Mayo Clin.* 36:254–260, 1961a.

KERR, F. W. L., AND OLAFSON, R. A. Trigeminal and cervical volleys, convergence on single units in the spinal gray at C-1 and C-2. *Arch. Neurol.* 5:171–178, 1961.

KERR, F. W. L. Structural relation of the trigeminal spinal tract to upper cervical roots and the solitary nucleus in the cat. *Exp. Neurol.* 4:134–148, 1961b.

KERR, F. W. L. A mechanism to account for frontal headache in cases of posterior-fossa tumors. *J. Neurosurg.* 18:605–609, 1961c.

TAUXE. W. N., SEDLACK, R. E., PITLYK, P. J., AND KERR, F. W. L. Preliminary report on the localization of brain lesions with I^{131} labeled polyvinylpyrrolidone. *Proc. Mayo Clin.* 37:109–111, 1962.

DONALD, D. E., KERR, F. W. L., FERGUSON, D. A., AND BOWRON, P. Whole-body, closed-chest perfusion in the dog. *Proc. Mayo Clin.* 37:177–179, 1962.

KERR, F. W. L. Facial, vagal and glossopharyngeal nerves in the cat, afferent connections. *Arch. Neurol.* 6:264–281, 1962a.

PITLYK, P. J., KERR, F. W. L., TAUXE, W. N., SEDLACK, R. E., AND SVIEN, H. J. Localization of brain tumors with iodine-131 polyvinylpyrrolidone. *Surg. Forum.* 13:436–437, 1962.

KERR, F. W. L., AND DONALD, D. E. Closed-chest hypothermic perfusion, cardiac arrest, and resuscitation. *Surg. Forum* 13:428–429, 1962.

KERR, F. W. L. Trigeminal neuralgia, pathogenesis and description of a possible etiology for the cryptogenic variety. *Trans. Am. Neurol. Assoc.* 87:118–123, 1962b.

KERR, F. W. L. The etiology of trigeminal neuralgia. *Arch. Neurol.* 8:15–25, 1963a.

BAKER, G. S., AND KERR, F. W. L. Structural changes in the trigeminal system following compression procedures. *J. Neurosurg.* 20:181–184, 1963.

SHORTER, R. G., TITUS, J. L., KERR, F. W. L., AND CAMPBELL, J. C. Effects of freezing and storage on survival of thyroid autografts. *Proc. Soc. Exp. Biol. Med.* 113:73–75, 1963.

KERR, F. W. L. Mechanisms, diagnosis, and management of some cranial and facial pain syndromes. *Surg. Clin. North Am.* 43:951–961, 1963b.

KERR, F. W. L. The divisional organization of afferent fibers of the trigeminal nerve. *Brain* 86:721–732, 1963c.

PITLYK, P. J., TAUXE, W. N., KERR, F. W. L., SEDLACK, R. E., AND SVIEN, H. J. Localization of brain tumors with polyvinvylpyrrolidone-I^{131}. *Arch. Neurol.* 9:437–443, 1963.

KERR, F. W. L., AND BROWN, J. A. Pupillomotor pathways in the spinal cord. *Arch. Neurol.* 10:262–270, 1964.

KERR, F. W. L., AND ALEXANDER, S. Descending autonomic pathways in the spinal cord.*Arch. Neurol.* 10:249–261, 1964.

ALEXANDER, S., AND KERR, F. W. L. Blood pressure responses in acute compression of the spinal cord. *J. Neurosurg.* 21:485–491, 1964.

DONALD, D. E., AND KERR, F. W. L. The response of dogs to perfusion and arrest of circulation at near zero cerebral temperatues. *J. Surg. Res.* 4:243–252, 1964.

KERR, F. W. L., AND HOLLOWELL, O. W. Location of pupillomotor and accommodation fibres in the oculomotor nerve, experimental observations on paralytic mydriasis.,*J. Neurol. Neurosurg. Psychiatry* 27:473–481, 1964.

KERR, F. W. L., AND LYSAK, W. R. Somatotopic organization of trigeminal ganglion neurones. *Arch. Neurol.* 11:593–602, 1964.

THOMAS, R. L., AND KERR, F. W. L. Electron microscopic studies of absorption of colloidal gold from the subarachnoid space. *Mayo Clin. Proc.* 40:603–608, 1965.

HIGGS, B., KERR, F. W. L., AND ELLIS, F. H., JR. The experimental production of esophageal achalasia by electrolytic lesions in the medulla. *J. Thorac. Cardiovasc. Surg.* 50:613–625, 1965.

KERR, F. W. L. On the question of ascending fibers in the pyramidal tract, with observations on spinotrigeminal and spinopontine fibers. *Exp. Neurol.* 14:77–85, 1966.

MAUPIN, R. A., BAKER, H. L., JR., AND KERR, F. W. L. Emulsified pantopaque, its possible application for myelography. *Radiology* 86:509–514, 1966.

KERR, F. W. L., AND MILLER, R. H. The pathology of trigeminal neuralgia, electron microscopic studies. *Arch. Neurol.* 15:308–319, 1966.

KERR, F. W. L. Spinal V nucleolysis, intractable craniofacial pain. *Surg. Forum.* 17:419–421, 1966a.

KERR, F. W. L. The ultrastructure of the spinal tract of the trigeminal nerve and the substantia gelatinosa. *Exp. Neurol.* 16:359–376, 1966b.

KERR, F. W. L. Evidence for a peripheral etiology of trigeminal neuralgia. *J. Neurosurg.* 26:168–174, 1967a.

KERR, F. W. L. Pathology of trigeminal neuralgia. Light and electron microscopic observations. *J. Neurosurg.* 26:151–156, 1967b.

KERR, F. W. L. Correlated light and electron microscopic observations on the normal trigeminal ganglion and sensory root in man.*J. Neurosurg.* 26:132–137, 1967c.

ENOCH, D. M., AND KERR, F. W. L. Hypothalamic vasopressor and vesicopressor pathways. I. Functional studies.*Arch. Neurol.* 16:290–306, 1967a.

ENOCH, D. M., AND KERR, F. W. L. Hypothalamic vasopressor and vesicopressor pathways. II. Anatomic study of their course and connection. *Arch. Neurol.* 16:307–320, 1967b.

KERR, F. W. L. Function of the dorsal motor nucleus of the vagus. *Science* 157:451–452, 1967d.

KERR, F. W. L. The pupil. Functional anatomy and clinical correlation, in: *Neuro-Ophthalmology Symposium of the University of Miami and the Bascom Palmer Eye Institute. Proceedings,* Vol. IV C. V. Mosby, St. Louis, 1968a, pp. 49–80.

KERR, F. W. L., KRUGER, L., SCHWASSMANN, H. O., AND STERN, R. Somatotopic organization of mechanoreceptor units in the trigeminal nuclear complex of the macaque. *J. Comp. Neurol.* 134:127–144, 1968.

KERR, F. W. L. Radical decompression and dural grafting in severe cerebral edema. *Mayo Clin. Proc.* 43:852–864, 1968b.

KERR, F. W. L. A brace for the management of fracture dislocation of the cervical spine: Traction, immobilization, and myelography: Technical note. *J. Neurosurg.* 30:97–101, 1969a.

KERR, F. W. L. Preserved vagal visceromotor function following destruction of the dorsal motor nucleus. *J. Physiol. (Lond.)* 202:755–769, 1969b.

KERR, F. W. L., AND PRESHAW, R. M. Secretomotor function of the dorsal motor nucleus of the vagus. *J. Physiol. (Lond.)* 205:405–415, 1969.

KERR, F. W. L., HENDLER, N., AND BOWRON, P. Viscerotopic organization of the vagus. *J. Comp. Neurol.* 138:279–289, 1970.

KERR, F. W. L. Fine structure and functional characteristics of the primary trigeminal neuron, in: *Trigeminal Neuralgia: Pathogenesis und Pathophysiology* (R. HASSLER AND A. E. WALKER, eds.), W. B. Saunders, Philadelphia, 1970a, pp. 18–21.

KERR, F. W. L. Peripheral versus central factors in trigeminal neuralgia, in: *Trigeminal Neuralgia: Pathogenesis und Pathophysiology* (R. HASSLER AND A. E. WALKER, eds.), W. B. Saunders, Philadelphia 1970b, pp. 180–190.

KERR, F. W. L. The fine structure of the subnucleus caudalis of the trigeminal nerve. *Brain Res.* 23:129–145, 1970c.

KERR, F. W. L. The organization of primary afferents in the subnucleus caudalis of the trigeminal: A light and electron microscopic study of degeneration. *Brain Res.* 23:147–165, 1970d.

KERR, F. W. L. Electron microscopic observations on primary deafferentation of the subnucleus caudalis of the trigeminal nerve, in: *Oral–Facial Sensory and Motor Mechanisms* (R. DUBNER AND Y. KAWAMURA, eds.), Appleton-Century-Crofts, New York, 1971, pp. 159–182.

KERR, F. W. L., AND POZUELO-UTANDA, J. Suppression of physical dependence and induction of hypersensitivity to morphine by stereotaxic hypothalamic lesions in addict rats: A new theory of addiction. *Mayo Clin. Proc.* 46:653–665, 1971.

LIPPMANN, H. H., AND KERR, F. W. L. Light and electron microscopic study of crossed ascending pathways in the anterolateral funiculus in monkey. *Brain Res.* 40:496–499, 1972.

KERR, F. W. L. Central relationships of trigeminal and cervical primary afferents in the spinal cord and medulla. *Brain Res.* 43:561–572, 1972a.

KERR, F. W. L. The potential of cervical primary afferents to sprout in the spinal nucleus of V following long term trigeminal denervation. *Brain Res.* 43:547–560, 1972b.

POZUELO-UTANDA, J., AND KERR, F. W. L. Suppression of craving and other signs of dependence in morphine-addicted monkeys by administration of *alpha*-methyl-*para*-tyrosine. *Mayo Clin. Proc.* 47:621–628, 1972.

LOEWY, A. D., ARAUJO, J. C., AND KERR, F. W. L. Pupillodilator pathways in the brain stem of the cat: Anatomical and electrophysiological identification of a central autonomic pathway. *Brain Res.* 60:65–91, 1973.

KERR, F. W. L. Morphine self-administration in dependent monkeys: Reduction by hypothalamic lesions. *IRCS Neuropharmacology* (73–12) 7-1-16, 1973.

KERR, F. W. L., TRIPLETT, J. N., JR., AND BEELER, G. W., JR. Reciprocal (push–pull) effects of morphine on single units in the ventromedian and lateral hypothalamus and influence on other nuclei: With a comment on methadone effects during withdrawal from morphine. *Brain Res.* 74:81–103, 1974.

LITTLE, J. R., SUNDT, T. M., JR., AND KERR, F. W. L. Neuronal alterations in developing cortical infarction. An experimental study in monkeys. *J. Neurosurg.* 40:186–198, 1974a.

KERR, F. W. L., AND LIPPMAN, H. H. The primate spinothalamic tract as demonstrated by anterolateral cordotomy and commissural myelotomy. *Adv. Neurol.* 4:147–156, 1974.

LITTLE, J. R., KERR, F. W. L., AND SUNDT, T. M., JR. The role of lysosomes in production of ischemic nerve-cell changes. *Arch. Neurol.* 30:448–455, 1975b.

LITTLE, J. R., KERR, F. W. L., AND SUNDT, T. M., JR. Synaptic alterations in developing cortical infarction: An experimental investigation in monkeys. *Stroke* 5:470–476, 1974c.

LITTLE, J. R., KERR, F. W. L., AND SUNDT, T. M., JR. Significance of neuronal alterations in developing cortical infarction. *Mayo Clin. Proc.* 827–837, 1974d.

KERR, F. W. L. The ventral spinothalamic tract and other ascending systems of the ventral funiculus of the spinal cord. *J. Comp. Neurol.* 159:335–356, 1975a.

LITTLE, J. R., KERR, F. W. L., AND SUNDT, T. M., JR. Microcirculatory obstruction in focal cerebral ischemia: Relationship to neuronal alterations. *Mayo Clin. Proc.* 50: 264–270, 1975.

NIJENSOHN, D. E., AND KERR, F. W. L. The ascending projections of the dorsolateral funiculus of the spinal cord in the primate. *J. Comp. Neurol.* 161:459–470, 1975.

GONZALEZ, G., ONOFRIO, B. M., AND KERR, F. W. L. Vasodilator system for the face. *J. Neurosurg.* 42:696–703, 1975.

BECKERMAN, S. B., AND KERR, F. W. L. Electrophysiologic evidence that neither sprouting nor neuronal hyperactivity occur following long term trigeminal or cervical primary deafferentation. *Exp. Neurol.* 50:427–438, 1975.

KERR, F. W. L. Neuroanatomical substrates of nociception in the spinal cord. *Pain* 1:325–356, 1975b.

KERR, F. W. L. Pain: A central inhibitory balance theory. *Mayo Clin. Proc.* 50:685–690, 1975c.

KERR, F. W. L. Segmental circuitry and spinal cord nociceptive mechanisms, in: *Advances in Pain Research and Therapy,* Vol. 1, (J. J. BONICA AND D. ALBE-FESSARD, eds.), Raven Press, New York, 1976, pp. 75–89.

LITTLE, J. R., KERR, F. W. L., AND SUNDT, T. M., JR. Microcirculatory obstruction in focal cerebral ischemia: an electron microscopic investigation in monkeys. *Stroke* 7:25–30, 1976.

NAROTZKY, R. A., AND KERR, F. W. L. Marginal neurons of the spinal cord: Types, afferent synaptology and functional considerations. *Brain Res.* 139:1–20, 1978.

KERR, F. W. L., WILSON, P. R., AND NIJENSOHN, D. E. Acupuncture reduces the trigeminal evoked response in decerebrate cats. *Exp. Neurol.* 61:84–95, 1978.

KERR, F. W. L. AND WILSON, P. R. Pain. *Annu. Rev. Neurosci.* 1:83–102, 1978.

KERR, F. W. L. Segmental circuitry and ascending pathways of the nociceptive system, in: *Mechanisms of Pain and Analgesic Compounds,* (R. F. BEERS, JR. AND E. G. BASSETT, eds.), Raven Press, New York, 1979, pp. 113–141.

KERR, F. W. L. Craniofacial neuralgias. *Adv. Pain Res. Ther.* 3:283–295, 1979.

FUKUSHIMA, T., AND KERR, F. W. L. Organization of trigeminothalamic tracts and other thalamic afferent systems of the brainstem in the rat: Presence of gelatinosa neurons with thalamic connections. *J. Comp. Neurol.* 183:169–184, 1979.

TYCE, G. M., SHARPLESS, N. S., KERR, F. W. L., AND MUENTER, M. D. Dopamine conjugate in cerebrospinal fluid. *J. Neurochem.* 34:210–212, 1980.

KERR, F. W. L., AND FUKUSHIMA, T. New observations on the nociceptive pathways in the central nervous system, in: *Pain,* (J. J. BONICA, ed.), Raven Press, New York, 1980, pp. 47–61.

References

FRIEDMAN, A. H., NASHOLD, B. S., JR., AND OVELMEN-LEVITT, J. Dorsal root entry zone lesions for the treatment of post-herpetic neuralgia. *J. Neurosurg.* 60:1258–1262, 1984.

JANNETTA, P. J. Microsurgical approach to the trigeminal nerve for tic douloureux, in: *Progress in Neurological Surgery,* (W. SWEET, ed.), S. Karger, Basel, 1976, pp. 180–200.

LIU, C. N., AND CHAMBERS, W. W. Intraspinal sprouting of dorsal root axons. Development of new collaterals and preterminals following partial denervation of the spinal cord in the cat. *Arch. Neurol.* 79:46–61, 1958.

MELZACK, R., AND WALL, P. D. Pain mechanisms: A new theory. *Science* 150:971–979, 1965.

2
Sensory Receptors of the Skin

RICHARD K. WINKELMANN

A. Introduction

Successive periods of investigation have produced anatomic, physiological, and psychological phases in our understanding of skin sensation. Each phase has been the result of technological improvement. The use of the electron microscope has brought about a decade of renewed anatomic study and reclassification of skin nerve endings. Correlation with single-unit recordings has produced a new awareness that anatomic simplicity may be attainable but that physiological responses remain complex and often proceed from stimulation of patterns of diverse receptor tissue. New chemical and immunochemical methods are providing a new degree of resolution of histological questions. Whole-mount preparations offer an excellent opportunity for correlation of sensation with structure and for quantitative study of receptor tissue. This review of cutaneous sensory receptors summarizes diverse approaches to the common problem of what receptors are present and on what evidence their independent existence and function rest. The chapter includes specific pertinent and current references. Exhaustive bibliographies on the subject will be found in the reviews of the last 20 years (Montagna and Brookhart, 1977; Munger, 1971; Halata, 1975; Chouchkov, 1978; Winkelmann, 1960b; Sinclair, 1981; Malinovsky and Pac, 1982).

B. Classifications of Peripheral Receptors

Early sensory receptor classifications attempted to assign specific functions to every structural variation observed. The simpler scheme proposed by

RICHARD K. WINKELMANN • Department of Dermatology, Mayo Clinic, Rochester, Minnesota 55905.

Weddell *et al.* (1954) with methylene blue methods recognized that the function of nerve was not always expressed by specialized anatomy. This was confirmed by silver studies, which emphasize such skin endings as the dermal nerve networks, hair follicle nerve networks, Meissner-type endngs, and encapsulated end organs (Winkelmann, 1960b). The studies of the Merkel cell in the last decade, largely by electron microscopy, have required expansion of these concepts to include Merkel endings of the hederiform and hair tactile (Pinkus) disk type (Winkelmann and Breathnach, 1973). The differences in sensory receptors in the skin of birds and mammals, as compared to primates, have required additional levels of classification when these subjects are discussed. The principal subject of the present discussion is the primate skin nerve endings, and where important variations occur in other animals, these are discussed in relation to the primate end organs.

The recent classification by Halata of mammalian sensory nerve endings (Table I) is based on three groups: free nerve endings, Merkel endings, and encapsulated endings (Halata, 1975). This is an appropriate basis for discussion but maintains names from anatomic antiquity. The division into epidermal and dermal nerve endings is essential, as is the division into encapsulated and nonencapsulated endings. The association of electron microscopic findings of the core of encapsulated end organs may not be of such great importance. Despite great internal variations, the chemistry of the end organs is constant from species to species. Chouchkov (1978) relied principally on electron microscopy in his discussion of encapsulated and nonencapsulated nerve endings of the skin, but he noted "denuded" nerve terminals free of lamellae and so unclassifiable by this criterion. The nonencapsulated forms include epidermal nerve and dermal nerve free endings and Merkel disks. The encapsulated forms he divided according to the internal lamellar organization. Malinovsky and Pac (1982) used much the same approach to describe 18 types of skin nerve endings. This is returning to the situation of the 1940s.

A better classification is shown in Table II; it includes epidermal and dermal forms and can be applied to all types of animal skin. This is based on

TABLE I
Classification of Skin End Organs[a]

Epidermal	Free
	Hederiform
Dermal	Free
	Hairs
	Encapsulated
	Without a lamellated core (Ruffini)
	Asymmetric, lamellated core (Meisner, Krause, Golgi–Mazzoni)
	Symmetric, lamellated core (Vater–Pacini)

[a]According to Halata (1975).

TABLE II
A Simple Classification of Types of Sensory Receptor Tissue in the Skin and Mucous Membranes

I	Nerve networks, free endings
II	Hair networks
III	Merkel cell endings
IV	Meissner corpuscle
V	Vater–Pacini corpuscle (Mammalian end organ, Herbst corpuscle, Golgi–Mazzoni body)

my perception that many of the persistent names and variations in structure are part of certain common simple patterns of nerve receptor development. My list of simple forms includes the nerve network, the Merkel cell ending, the Meissner corpuscle, and the Vater–Pacini end organ (Table III). To take an example, variations of the Vater–Pacini body such as the mammalian end organ, the Herbst corpuscle of birds, and the Golgi–Mazzoni bodies are only structural variations on a common pattern of receptor tissue development.

The advances in the neurophysiology of sensation have been remarkable and may also be used to classify sensory receptors. This approach was suggested by a classification in 1960 (Table IV) that emphasized the variability of endings associated with touch sensation and, conversely, the multiple sensations associated with the dermal nerve network (Winkelmann, 1960b). Subsequent investigations of individual receptors or receptor areas have identified neurophysiological responses of sensory nerve endings. Vibration sense has been related to the Vater–Pacini corpuscle. Iggo and Muir (1969) found the hair tactile (Pinkus) disk to be related to the type I slowly adapting sensory

TABLE III
Variations in the Basic Sensory Nerve Endings

	Variation	
Basic nerve ending	Type of skin	Nerve ending
I Nerve networks	Mammalian nasal skin	Organ of Eimer
II Hair networks	Periorificial skin	Sinus hair
III Merkel cell endings	Bird beak	Merkel corpuscle
IV Meissner corpuscle	Primate mucocutaneous or genital skin	Dermal Meissner body Mucocutaneous end organ
V Vater–Pacini corpuscle	Mammal skin	Mammalian end organ (simple Krause end bulb)
	Bird feathered skin	Herbst corpuscle
	Tendon, fascia	Golgi–Mazzoni body

TABLE IV
Classification of Dermal Nerve Endings[a]

Type of Skin	Nerve Structure for Perception of: Pain, Temperature	Touch
Hairy skin	Dermal nerve network	Hair follicle network Tactile hair disk
Glabrous skin		
General	Dermal nerve network	Papillary nerve
Distal	Dermal nerve network	Meissner corpuscle Hederiform ending
Mucocutaneous	Dermal nerve network	Mucocutaneous end organ
Mucous membrane	Dermal nerve network	Dermal nerve network

[a] From Winkelmann (1960).

receptor. It seems reasonable from current information that Meissner corpuscles are rapidly adapting receptors. Iggo (1974) has classified cutaneous physiological sensory receptors as slowly and rapidly adapting mechanoreceptors and cold and warm receptors. Horch *et al.* (1977) found 11 types of mechanoreceptive units in cat skin, and it is evident that preferential stimulus response, rapid or slow adaptive response, size of sensory field, high or low threshold, rapid or slow conductance, and type of discharge may all produce unique combinations of physiological response but are not necessarily correlated with individual anatomic structures.

A simple current classification of structure and function is that contained in Table V. This correlates the adapting response to the sensation perceived and indicates an end organ capable of this response. It must be remembered that these sensations are not uniquely or solely a function of these end organs. The mammalian end organ as a rapidly adapting lamellated corpuscle (a Vater–Pacini corpuscle) is ideally suited by its rapid adaptation and vibration responsiveness (Janig, 1971; Loewenstein, 1971) to serve in the cat skin as does the Meissner corpuscle in the skin of primates. It is important to recognize these simple forms of the endings, but it is perhaps more important to recognize that they are frequently associated together in complex sensory units such as the organ of Eimer, the hair follicle nerve end organ, or the Pinkus

TABLE V
Type of Cutaneous Mechanoreceptor Response per Sensory Unit

	Slowly adapting	Rapidly adapting
Superficial	Pinkus tactile disk Hederiform endings	Meissner corpuscle Mammalian end organ
Deep	?Hair nerve ending	Vater–Pacini corpuscle

disk and that the sensory response may be associated with multiple sensory receptor types in a specifc area.

C. Components and Patterns of Myelinated and Unmyelinated Nerve Endings

The sensory nerve fibers associated with the skin are characterized by a continual interchange or bifurcation and combination of nerves within units. This same pattern is maintained in the dermal and subcutaneous nerve networks. This peripheral geographic association of separate axons is added to the overlapping of nerve fibers in the skin to form irregular dermal nerve networks. The networks are present at the dermal–subcutaneous junction and, in association with the vascular plexuses, rise into the superficial nerve networks, particularly the subpapillary network beneath the epidermis.

The distribution of diameters is over a narrow range, and fewer large myelinated nerves are observed than in muscle nerve. Most nerve fiber diameters are 2 to 6 μm, and there is only a small component of larger fibers. Myelinization decreases as one moves from peripheral nerve to cutaneous nerve. This is the result of multiple divisions of nonmyelinated nerve and progressive loss of the myelinated layer. Cauna (1966) states that the many nonmyelinated nerves in the dermal plexus are continuations or branches of nerves that are myelinated more proximally. The density of the nerve networks varies greatly and also changes with the growth of the body part. Aging gradually reduces sensory perception and receptor density.

The specialized end organs in the skin are almost always supplied by myelinated nerve fibers that do not commonly run in the usual dermal nerve plexuses. These myelinated fibers frequently rise rectilinearly from deep plexuses through the dermis to innervate the hair follicles and the Meissner and Merkel nerve endings. This is most graphically observed in the hairy skin, where myelinated nerve will rise long distances vertically between the hair follicles to the tactile (Pinkus) disk in the epidermis or to the hair follicle end organs. Despite these differences in plexus formation, a basic principle of an anatomic overlap is maintained: the outflows of multiple sensory nerves from multiple dorsal root ganglia cells are associated together in the nerve itself, the nerve plexus, and finally at the end organs (Figure 1). This conception from 1960 has been repeated by Munger (1971) and by Montagna and Brookhart (1977) (see Ruda, Chapter 7).

The nonmyelinated nerves embedded in the cytoplasm of Schwann cells divide and disperse into superficial layers of the dermis, reaching the subpapillary zone and occasionally into the dermal papillae. The nonmyelinated nerve rarely if ever becomes a "free" ending. The Schwann cell invests the nerve axon for its entire length and along its multiple rami. Neighboring Schwann cell processes occasionally overlap. Much more rarely, a gap may occur, and the axon will be observed only with basement membrane. The last

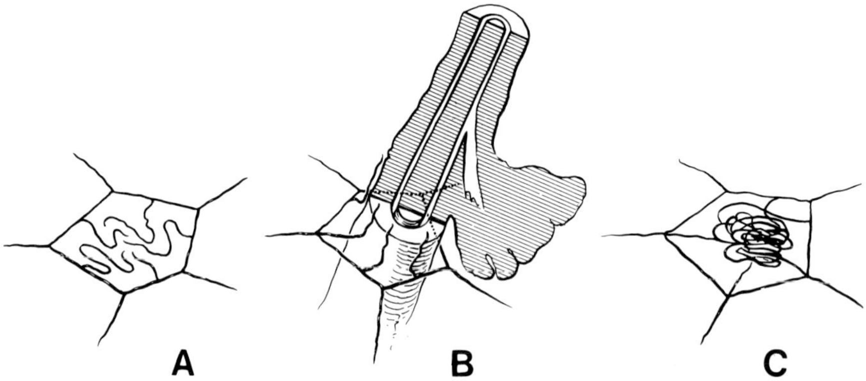

FIGURE 1. Patterns of nerve endings showing the association in common nerve trunks of the skin of the sensory nerve supply from multiple dorsal root ganglion cells. The final terminus may be free endings, organized nerve endings, or hair follicle endings. (From Winkelmann, 1960b.)

Schwann cell, usually subpapillary in location, invests all the rami of the dividing nonmyelinated nerve. Cauna (1973) termed this cell and its associated nerve fibers and terminations a penicillus, and the endings "penicillate" endings. These fine branches overlap considerably and may exchange axons with neighboring Schwann cells. These nerves are poor in organelles and usually negative for cholinesterase. Occasional subepidermal nerves are positive for cholinesterase and ATPase in my experience. It is difficult to know if these are "penicillate" nerve endings in the sense Cauna used the term. This term, "penicillate" nerve endings, seems a supernumerary name for the subepidermal nonmyelinated nerve network and its associated Schwann cells, and most authors use quotation marks with the term. Much more extensive discussion is necessasry if the term is used in general parlance.

The term *free terminal* means the end of the sensory nerve tissue. The term should not be used for the point at which perineural cells are not present. It usually describes a slight expansion of the axon that is filled with multiple cell organelles and is covered by a basement membrane and on occasion may not be completely covered by Schwann cell cytoplasm. The Schwann cell basement membrane may reduplicate and join with the basement membrane of the epidermis. Free nerve terminals are found throughout the dermis, associated with the hair follicle, and in the dermal papillary body. They may be demonstrated by silver, whole-mount cholinesterase, or electron microscopic methods (Figure 2).

Epidermal dendritic cells (Langerhans cell, indeterminate cell), which stain with silver, gold, and methylene blue, are often mistaken for intraepidermal nerve. The human embryo contains epidermal nerve, but in adult human skin it has proved difficult to show any consistent or frequent epidermal nerve structure. Electron microscopy has not changed this. Obser-

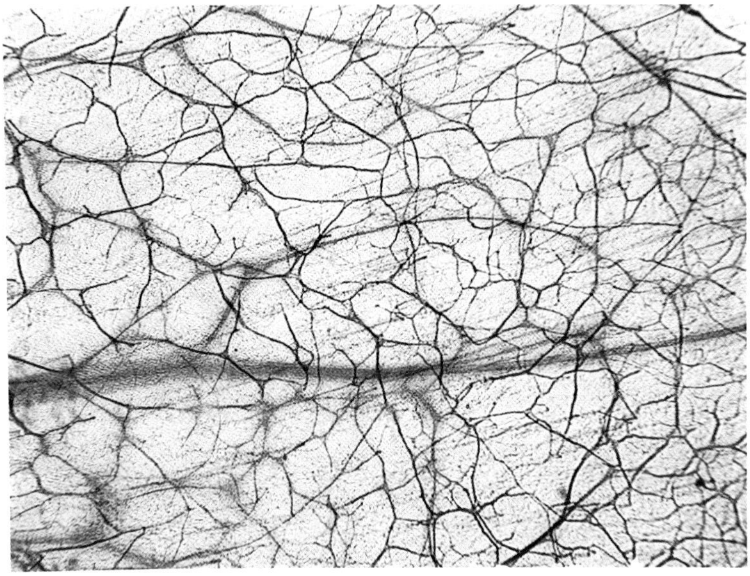

FIGURE 2. Patterns of nerve networks in the stroma of human cornea showing the size of the network and free endings. Cholinesterase whole-mount method, ×35.

vations have been made that certain hyperplastic or malignant states are associated with increased invasion of the epidermis by nerve (Fitzgerald, 1968). One needs serial sections in order to separate satisfactorily the long dendrites of epidermal dendritic cells from nerve tissue. The generally accepted principle is that only in thickened and specialized epidermis may intraepithelial nerve be anticipated. Intraepidermal nerve is part of certain complex sensory endings of the nasal skin and muzzle of many mammals (Figure 3).

D. Specialized Nerve Endings

1. Hair Follicle Nerve Endings

Myelinated nerve fibers rise from deep plexuses to innervate the hair follicle. Human hairs have from five to nine nerve trunks supplying the nerve endings. Giacometti (1965) and Giacometti and Montagna (1969) present data that there are six to eight nerves per follicle. Small hairs in small mammals may have as few as two nerve fibers, and Weddell and Pallie (1955) found as many as 20 nerves arriving at single large hairs in the rabbit. The cutaneous nerve may branch to supply as many as 120 rabbit hair follicles; no similar data are available for man.

The myelinated nerves branch and approach the follicle from all directions, forming an irregular network around the hair follicle. From this net-

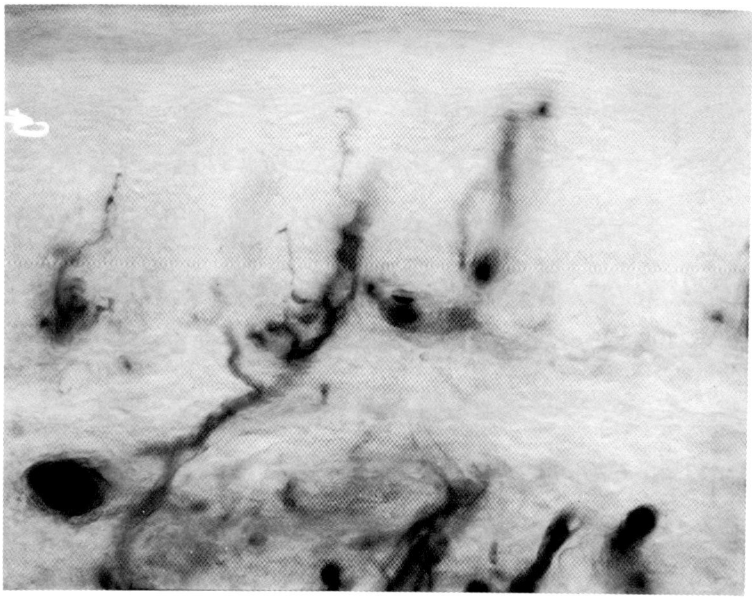

FIGURE 3. Merkel cell nerve-associated disks and intraepithelial nerve fibers. Rabbit palate. Specific cholinesterase, ×400.

work (Figure 4), the terminal nonmyelinated fibers are derived. The hair network lies in the connective tissue around the follicle, with the axons lying in Schwann cell cytoplasm. The nerve fibers encircle the follicle in a characteristic circular "collar" arrangement closely applied to the external root sheath below the sebaceous gland. Bulbous nerve terminals in the external sheath may be found in human hair, and Mahrle and Orfanos (1974) describe Merkel endings within and next to the hair follicles. The fine fibers turn and run either parallel to the external root sheath as loops or to fine terminations. The multiple parallel endings observed in large hairs were termed lanceolate endings by Andres (1966). This term has been used particularly to describe longitudinal enlarged parallel nerve fiber terminals or spindles observed to be covered externally by thick basement membrane and by bilateral flaps of Schwann cell membranes. These endings contain mitochondria and vesicles and may be demonstrated by multiple histochemical methods in individual species. The circular hair nerve network has been called a pilo-Ruffini ending, adding more confusion to the receptor terminology. Much more acceptable is the term hair nerve end organ proposed by me (Winkelmann, 1960b) and Montagna and Brookhart (1977).

The mammalian skin contains groups of multiple hair types. The sensory or sinus hair is the largest and richest in innervation. Munger and Halata (1983) have described a smaller sensory hair that they term a hemisinus hair

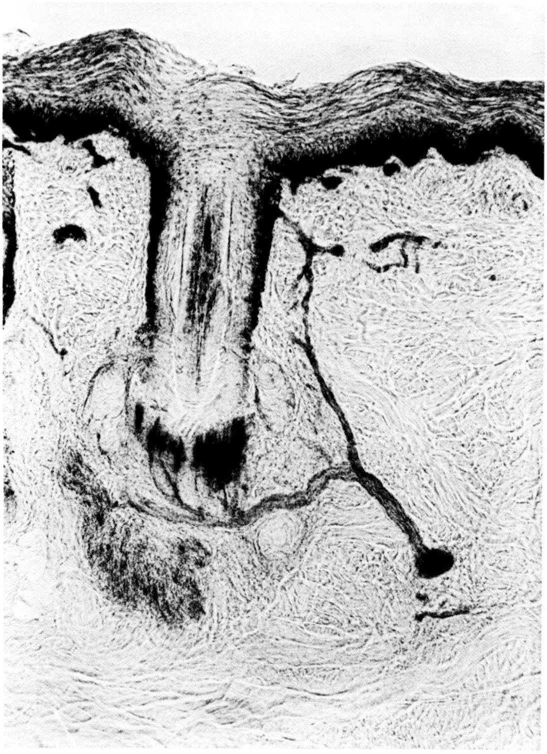

FIGURE 4. Hair follicle innervation demonstrated by cholinesterase method, demonstrating a large nerve innervating cholinesterase-positive lanceolate endings vertically along the hair follicle and a branch of the nerve rising to the neck of the follicle. Specific cholinesterase, ×100.

with a smaller, less extensive blood sinus. Mahrle and Orfanos (1974), Andres and von Duhring (1975), and Munger and Halata (1983) have noted Merkel cells in primate hair follicles. More rudimentary vellus hairs have only free nerve endings and hair nerve end organs composed of more recently named lanceolate terminals and the circular collar of nerve axons. Lanceolate terminals are readily visible in larger hairs and are often missing in small vellus or involutional hairs. The circular collar of nerve is best developed in largest hairs.

During the hair cycle, the nerve remains in place about the hair follicle below the sebaceous gland. Nerves about the lower end of the follicle involute. Giacometti and Montagna (1969) suggest that nerves about human hair follicles are very stable, with only minor changes during the hair cycle. When the follicles are absent, as in the bald scalp, the nerves may still be observed as collapsed masses, which Weddell (cited in Sinclair, 1981) and Giacometti (1965) have suggested are similar to Meissner-type corpuscles. Free nerve endings may be associated with any type of hair structure. Merkel cells are observed in the external root sheath of large hairs in the perifollicular connective tissue and in the perifollicular epithelium, specifically in the tactile Pinkus disk (Mahrle and Orfanos, 1974).

2. *The Meissner Corpuscle*

The Meissner corpuscles are lobular or multilobular nerve endings, frequently with expanded nerve terminals (Sinclair, 1981) that are found in the skin of primates and marsupials. Sinclair declares that they are to be found in "all mammals, particuarly in the dermal papillae of the friction surfaces." It is my experience that the mammalian end organ or simple end bulb is present in or adjacent to the dermal papillae of most nonprimate mammals, serving the same function as the primate Meissner corpuscle. Malinovsky and Pac (1982) also recognize that the mammalian end organ or simple end bulb is equivalent to the primate Meissner corpuscle. Wherever the Meissner corpuscle is described in nonprimate mammals, the descriptions and photomicrographs are uniformly poor and questionable. The Meissner corpuscle occurs in man and other primates on the palms, soles, and digits and on the sides of the fingers and toes. The gorilla has these endings in the dorsal knuckle pads of the hands, on which it leans (Winkelmann, 1961). The South American monkeys have Meissner corpuscles in the ventral surface of the prehensile tails (Winkelmann, 1963b).

The Meissner corpuscles measure 20×100 μm and are usually found in the dermal papillae, long axis perpendicular to the surface. One corpuscle to a dermal papilla (Figure 5) is usual (Cauna, 1956). When the epidermis is removed, the Meissner corpuscles are found to be lined up in the dermal papillary rows, which reproduce fingerprint ridges. The numbers of Meissner corpuscles drop rapidly with postfetal growth and then slowly decline with age. More complex endings may be observed in old age (Cauna, 1964).

Myelinated nerve rises to the base of one or multiple Meissner corpuscles and also separately to the smaller apical lobule of the Meissner corpuscle. On occasion, it is possible to see an individual myelinated fiber innervate and pass through one lobule to terminate in a second. The nerve loses its myelin sheath within the end organ. The nerves branch and run transversely in the ending, forming layers of nerve tissue separated by laminar cells. Hematoxylin and eosin staining demonstrates the transverse laminar cells and negative image of the interposed terminal nerve fibers and nerve endings. Nerve stains show the variable pathway of the nerve fibers wrapping around and interweaving within the corpuscle and between the terminations.

Laminar cells may be, and probably are, modified Schwann cells and are often round in simple Meissner bodies and flattened in multilobular, complex bodies. Malinovsky and Pac (1982) use the term Schwann cell in referring to laminar cells. The laminar cells are often observed as a narrow cytoplasmic strip with pinocytotic vesicles separating the axons and containing neurofilaments, neurotubules, glycogen, mitochondria, vesicles, and occasionally myelin figures. I found an isolated instance of typical granular cell degeneration in a Meissner corpuscle on one occasion. The capsule of the Meissner corpuscle is composed of perineurial cells, but the capsule is incomplete, and the con-

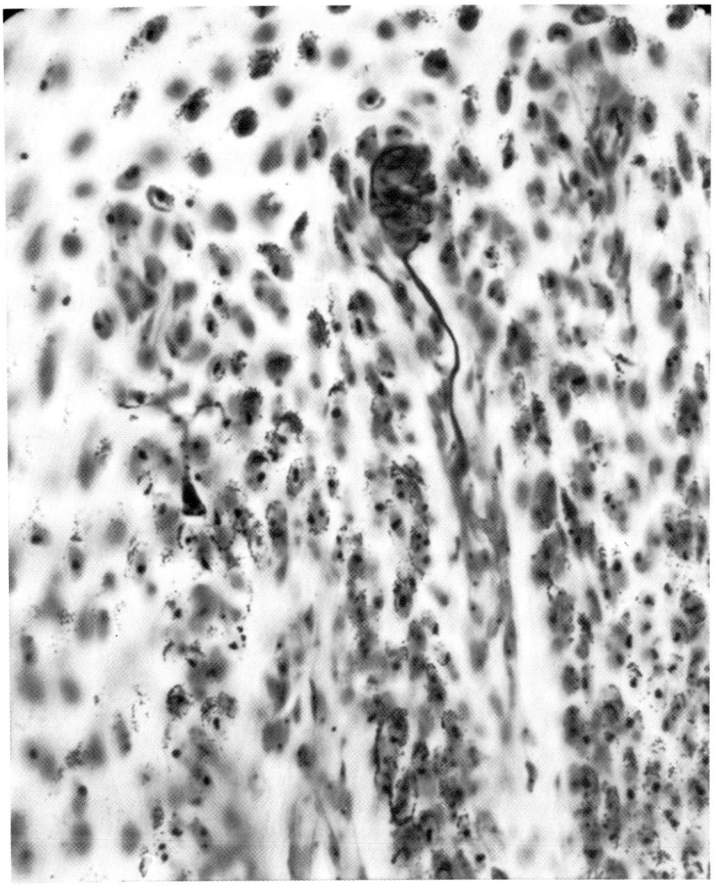

FIGURE 5. Meissner corpuscle in the apex of a papillary body. Quokka. Bielschowsky, ×500.

nective tissue found within the Meissner corpuscle connects with the connective tissue of the dermal papilla.

The Meissner corpuscles of primates and marsupials are structurally equivalent but not histochemically similar (Winkelmann, 1965). Cholinesterase is present in most Meissner corpuscles and outlines the transverse structure. The North American opossum does not have cholinesterase in its Meissner corpuscles; only alkaline phosphatase is present in the opossum ending (Winkelmann, 1964). The only primate with alkaline phosphatase in a Meissner corpuscle is the gibbon (Winkelmann, 1962b). Other hydrolytic and respiratory enzymes may be found in the Meissner corpuscle, particularly those of lesser primates (Winkelmann, 1971).

Whereas multiple Meissner corpuscles are supplied by branches from more than one myelinated nerve, the extent of cross or multiple innervation in man is not known. Quantitative studies of Meissner corpuscles show a correlation of peripheral neuropathy and Meissner receptor populations (*vide infra*).

Classifications by Halata (1975), Chouchkov (1978), and Malinovsky and Pac (1982) place the Meissner corpuscle among the encapsulated end organs. There is a connective tissue element to the central portion of the Meissner corpuscle, and the ending is clearly demarcated by a staining quality from the surrounding papillary dermal connective tissue. However, no structurally constant and distinct capsule exits, and no subcapsular space can be identified. I believe it is a mistake to include this end organ in the category with the Pacini end organ and its variants, which clearly have an inner bulb, laminated capsule, definite perineurial capsule, and subcapsular space. Yet the neurophysiology of the ending shows that it is probably a rapidly adapting mechanoreceptor, and this is also true for the Pacini end organ.

3. *The Mucocutaneous End Organ*

Krause (1860) describd an end bulb in human skin composed of a massive coil of unmyelinated nerve. Later, these endings were called mucocutaneous nerve endings, for they are found in human genital skin, lip, perianal skin, and conjunctivae (Weddell, cited by Sinclair, 1981). Because it was first described and confirmed in genital skin, it was also called the genital corpuscle.

These organs are frequently innervated in groups by two or more myelinated nerves. A myelinated nerve may enter one corpuscle, leave, and innervate a second. Such rosarylike endings are often found. The myelinated nerve wraps around the end organ, loses its myelin sheath, and ramifies into a massive coil of unmyelinated nerve (Figure 6). The myelinated nerves do not penetrate significantly as such into the body.

The mucocutaneous end organs are 40 to 140 μm in diameter (Malinovsky and Sommerova, 1973). They are usually found in glabrous transitional skin between hairy skin and true mucous membrane and are frequently found in the subpapillary dermis. The rete ridges are not as significantly developed in this skin as they are in the hands and feet. However, I have demonstrated the end organ in papillary bodies in monkey mucocutaneous skin.

Perineural cells are found in the capsule, but no complete capsule with a well-defined subcapsular space is observed. Thus, it is comparable to the Meissner corpuscle in this respect. Ultrastructural studies show a nonstructured cross-sectional mass of axons, nerve terminals, and Schwann cell lamellae. Chouchkov (1978) mentions seeing preterminals with mesaxons and nerve endings with stacks of lamellae. Within the end organ, collagen, fibroblasts, and macrophages are to be found. Malinovsky and Sommerova (1977)

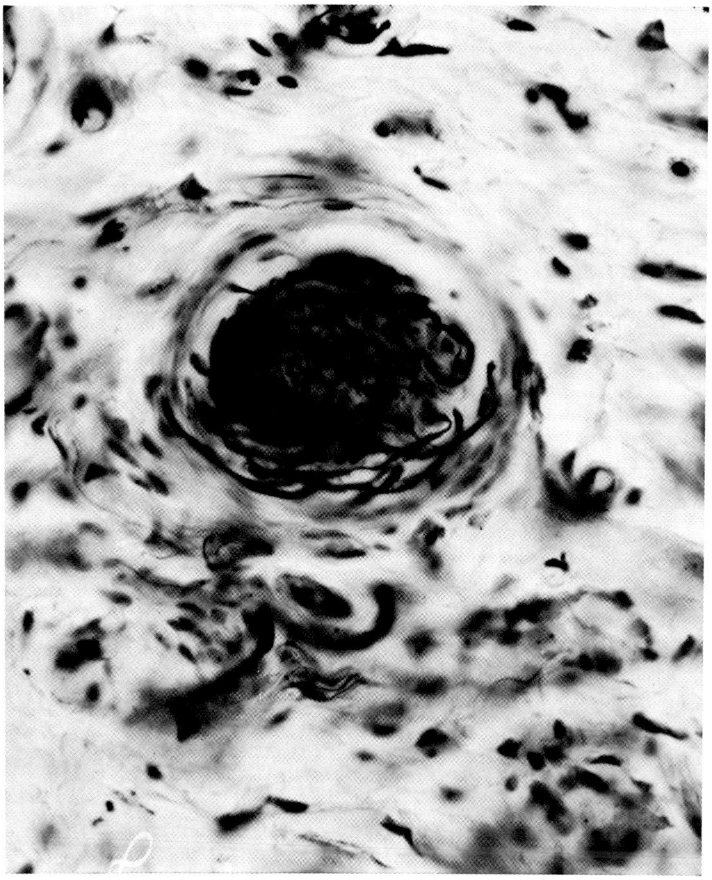

FIGURE 6. Mucocutaneous end organ of human clitoris demonstrating the rolled myelinated and unmyelinated nerves of the end organ. Winkelmann method, ×400.

showed a laminated stack of terminals in the mucocutaneous end organ of the green monkey quite similar to the Meissner corpuscle.

There is no agreement as to whether this is a distinctive nerve end organ or simply a variant of the Meissner corpuscle. The lowest lobule of the Meissner corpuscle is similar in shape, size, and components. The deeper location and the well-defined capsular spaces are only minor changes in the basic nerve ending organization. The study of receptors in primate skin has convinced me that the Meissner corpuscle and the mucocutaneous end organ are variations of the same basic receptor. This is particularly apparent in the smaller, simpler primates such as the lemuridae and lorisidae but may be also observed in New- or Old-World monkeys, as I demonstrated by silver techniques in an exhaustive comparative study (Winkelmann, 1963b). This has been confirmed by Malinovsky's studies (Malinovsky and Pac, 1982). When more physiological studies are done, I believe they will show that these end organs and the Meissner corpuscles are comparable rapidly adapting mechanoreceptors.

4. *Merkel Cell Endings*

The Merkel cell is a clear cell with an oval or reniform nucleus, cytoplasmic surface hornlike projection, and cytoplasmic membrane-bound granules 80–100 nm in diameter (Fortman and Winkelmann, 1973). Nuclear rodlets (Figure 7) have been described by Fortman and Winkelmann in this cell (Winkelmann and Breathnach, 1973). The cell may be associated with nerve in the dermis or epidermis, may occur in clusters or in characteristic nerve endings or alone, and has been associated with many types of nerve receptor structure (Table VI). The cell has been thought to be derived from the neural crest, the APUD system, or the epidermal cells (Winkelmann, 1977). The capacity to form desmosomal bridges with the epidermal cells (Figure 8) has given rise to speculation on its derivation from keratinocytes (English, 1974). Paget cells also form desmosomes with keratinocytes and are clearly derived from malignant tumor cells. At present, the derivation from neural origin appears reasonable.

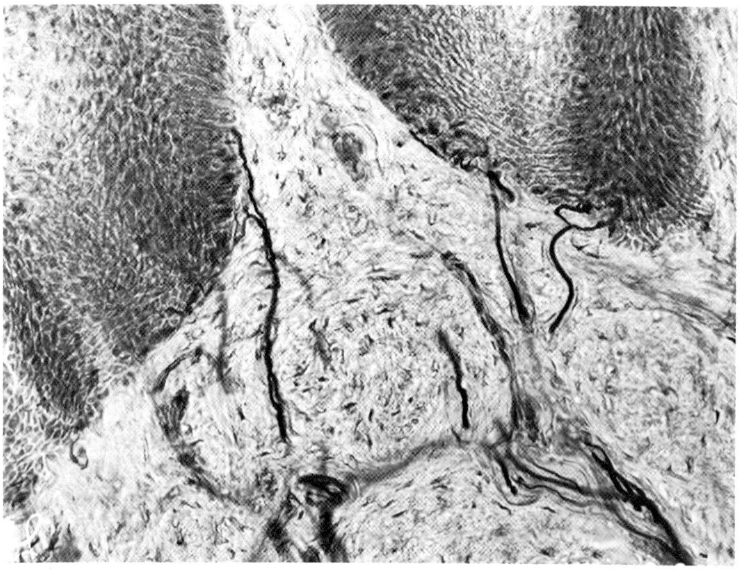

FIGURE 7. Multiple nerves rise to the epidermis and innervate the expanded nerve disks within the epidermis associated with the Merkel cells. Kangaroo palate. Winkelmann method, ×300.

TABLE VI
Merkel Cell Endings

Epidermis
Hederiform ending of Merkel–Ranvier
Organ of Eimer
Hair disk of Pinkus
Without nerve
Hair
Common and sensory hair
Dermis
With nerve
Without nerve
Merkel corpuscle

Pinkus (1902) described the hair disk containing Merkel cells in 1902, and subsequently the term Pinkus disk or Pinkus nerve end organ has been used to describe this receptor. The disks are circumscribed elevations or thickenings of the epidermis, usually in the anticline position in relation to the associated hair follicle. These epithelial thicknesses contain a cluster of Merkel

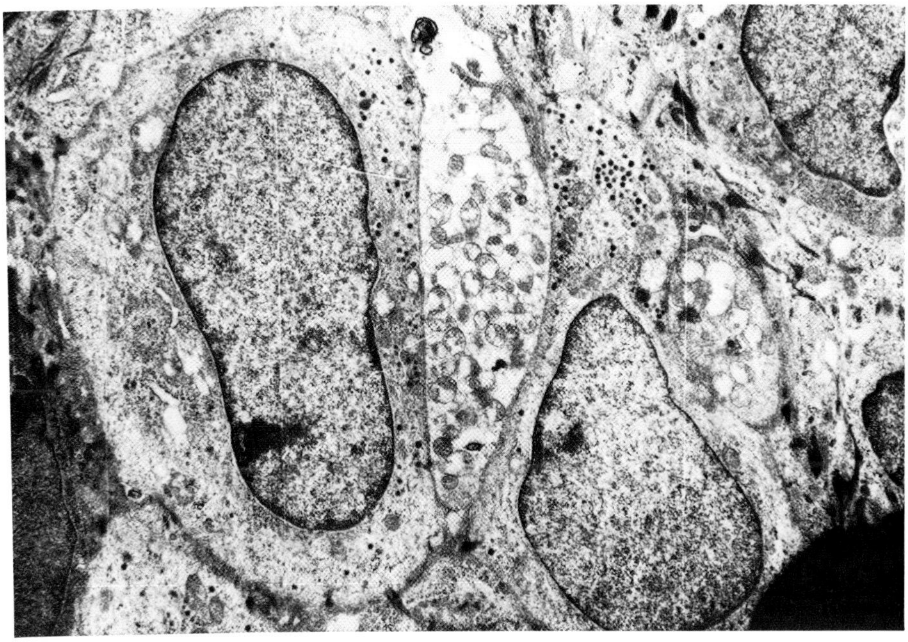

FIGURE 8. Merkel cells with an expanded nerve ending between them. The characteristic membrane-bound Merkel granules are seen in the cytoplasm facing the nerve. The nerve ending contains massive numbers of mitochondria and clear vesicles. Human palatal epidermis. ×8240.

cells associated with nerve endings. The numbers of Merkel cells vary from 20 to 50 depending on the species and disk size. The nerve ending is supplied by myelinated nerve, which loses its myelination before reaching the Merkel cells (Iggo and Muir, 1969). Nerve axons covered with Schwann membranes reach the epidermis, where the basement membranes fuse as the axons penetrate the epidermis to end in a platelike nerve expansion (Figure 9). It is this nerve expansion that stains with silver or methylene blue. Although periodic acid–Schiff may stain the receptor in rare species, there are few direct stains for the cell. Recently, antibody to the Merkel cell has been described by Saurat *et al.* (1983), which will provide for direct demonstration of it. Most of the histochemistry of the Merkel cell is associated with the nerve ending. These nerve endings have been demonstrated by cholinesterase, alkaline phosphatase, peptidase, nucleoside triphosphatase, and neuron-specific enolase in various species (Winkelmann, 1982). The cell granules resemble sympathetic granules, but no catecholamines or serotonin have been demonstrated. Hart-

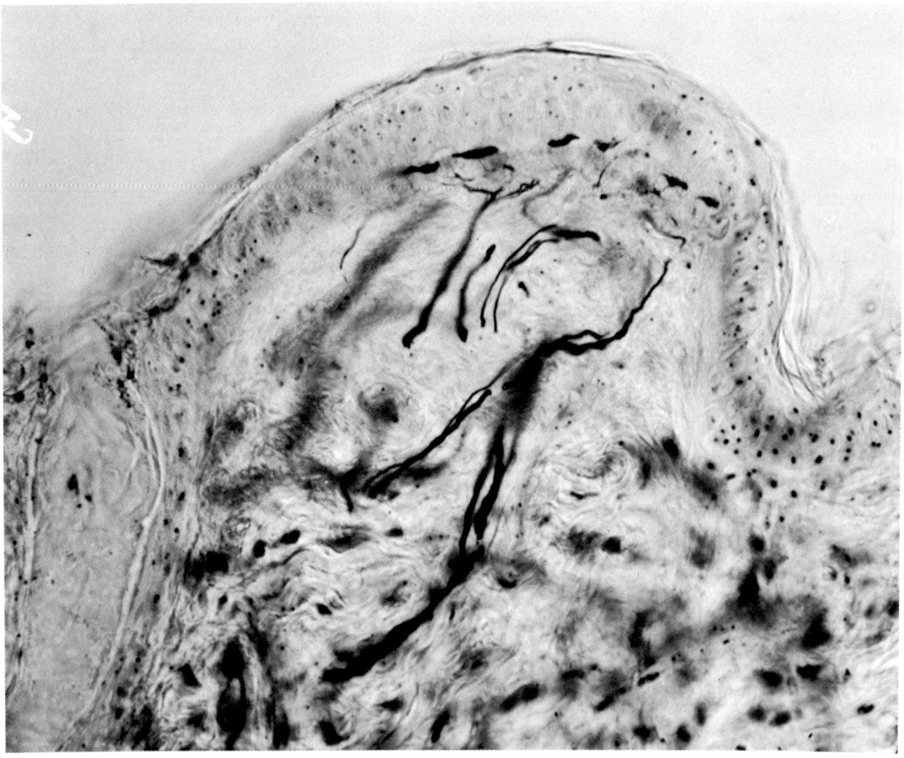

FIGURE 9. A tactile or touch dome (Pinkus disk) demonstrating the myelinated innervation that supplies the expanded nerve disks in the epidermis associated with the Merkel cells. Perivaginal skin of quokka. Winkelmann method, ×400.

schuh *et al.* (1983a,b) have demonstrated Met-enkephalin and VIP in Merkel cells from various species, confirming the peptide capacity of these cells and suggesting a close relationship to nerve tissue.

The hederiform ending was described by Merkel (1875) and named by Ranvier (1880). These endings consist of nerve rami associated with ivy-leaf clusters of Merkel cells in the bases of the rete ridges of glabrous and transitional mucous membrane epidermis. These nerve endings are frequently found in human fingers and may be found in palatal rugae. They represent the tactile equivalent of the hair disk in nonhairy skin. Iggo (1974) has associated the Merkel cell clusters in the hair disk and, by analogy, the hederiform endings with type I slowly adapting mechanoreceptors.

In all areas, the epithelial–Merkel cell complexes consist of thickened epidermis, epidermis devoid of melanocytes, whose place the Merkel cell seems to occupy, and an enlarged vascular supply. Munger (1971) called these endings Merkel–rete endings. Occasionally, intraepithelial nerve is associated with these structures.

Merkel cells have been observed by Breathnach (1980) in dermal nerves and isolated in the dermis. Mahrle and Orfanos (1974) described similar findings with relation to hair structures. I have described Merkel cells without nerve association high in the epidermis of gingiva.

Merkel corpuscles are observed only in the dermis of nonaquatic birds and are confined to the region of the beak and palate (Saxod, 1978b). These nerve endings consist of one or multiple flattened Merkel cells, usually arranged in a group or stack parallel to the surface of the epidermis, within a dermal papilla. Flattened nerve terminals and lamellar cells are the other components. Merkel cells contain dense-core granules and bundles of microfilaments. The cytoplasm of the cell has projections or horns that extend into the capsule. The nerve terminal contains mitochondria, neurofilaments and neurotubules, and clear and dense-core vesicles. Dense junctions occur on the interfaces between the nerve terminal and the Merkel cell. At low power, these end organs resemble Meissner corpuscles in location and structure.

Grandry corpuscles are receptors usually found in aquatic birds in the beak, palate, and tongue (Berkhoudt, 1980). These corpuscles are formed of two or more large specialized cells. The cells of the Grandry corpuscle are sensory cells that enclose a disk nerve ending. Capsular satellite cells that contain cholinesterase surround this ending together with collagen fibers and fibroblasts (Saxod, 1973). A single nerve fiber may branch to supply multiple Grandry corpuscles. This appears superficially to be a Merkel-type ending, but the dense-core granules are much larger than Merkel cell granules, ranging from 1000 to 3000 μm. No information about the nature of the Grandry sensory cells is available. The histochemistry of the end organ is found in the surrounding satellite cells. Unique perinuclear sensory organelles are large ovoid and fusiform structures composed of layers of granules of ribonucleic acid.

E. The Encapsulated Nerve End Organs

The Pacini corpuscle and the mammalian or simple end organ (end bulb) are the basic large and small encapsulated end organs of the skin. They are composed of the same tissue elements, which are disposed in a similar manner and have the same physiological responses, restricted, of course, by differences in size and depth of the end organs.

1. The Pacini Corpuscle

The largest nerve end organ and one phylogenetically common to most vertebrates was described by Pacini and characterized by Pease and Quilliam (1957), who demonstrated its bilateral, symmetrical inner lamellar capsule by electron microscopy. The end organ may be as small as 100 μm or as large as 1 to 4 mm in diameter. It averages 1 mm in length and 0.7 mm in width. Such a large end organ may be dissected out and visualized with the naked eye. This end organ may be found in serous membranes, lymph nodes, or pancreas, but it is most often located along nerve, fascial, or deep tendon structures. The small, coiled form with multiple axons found in the tendons has been termed the Golgi–Mazzoni body (Figure 10). I demonstrated pseudo-Golgi–Mazzoni bodies matching figures in the literature presented with this name that were clearly sections of a small Pacini corpuscle or of its stalk (Winkelmann, 1960b).

The Pacini body is found in the subcutaneous tissue of mammalian and primate skin. It may be closely associated with blood vessels, and Cauna (1976) suggests that this relationship to glomus bodies may be important in blood pressure regulation. It is noteworthy that most of the acral glomus bodies in man are in the dermis and most of the Pacini corpuscles are in the subcutaneous tissue, so without direct physiological demonstration, the role of these end organs in vascular responses is only conjecture. The gross appearance of this end organ may be smooth and even, yet this smooth outer capsule may contain an inner bulb that can be curved, U-shaped, or even coiled. The simple Pacini bodies have a straight inner bulb. Many bodies are found with the inner bulb as well as the stalk coiled. Wax reconstructions of these endings emphasize that in man the external form of the ending may also be curved (Winkelmann and Osment, 1956). Retroperitoneal end organs may be more complex.

The components of the Pacini corpuscle are the straight or coiled stalk containing the myelinated nerve supply, the inner bulb containing the axon and nerve terminal, the bilaterally symmetrical lamellar capsule, and the external capsule. The myelinated nerve runs proximally to the sensory ganglion cells directly and may serve more than one body. Although branching of the myelinated nerve is the usual nerve supply of multiple corpuscles, the myelinated nerve may run axially from one corpuscle to another (rosarylike end-

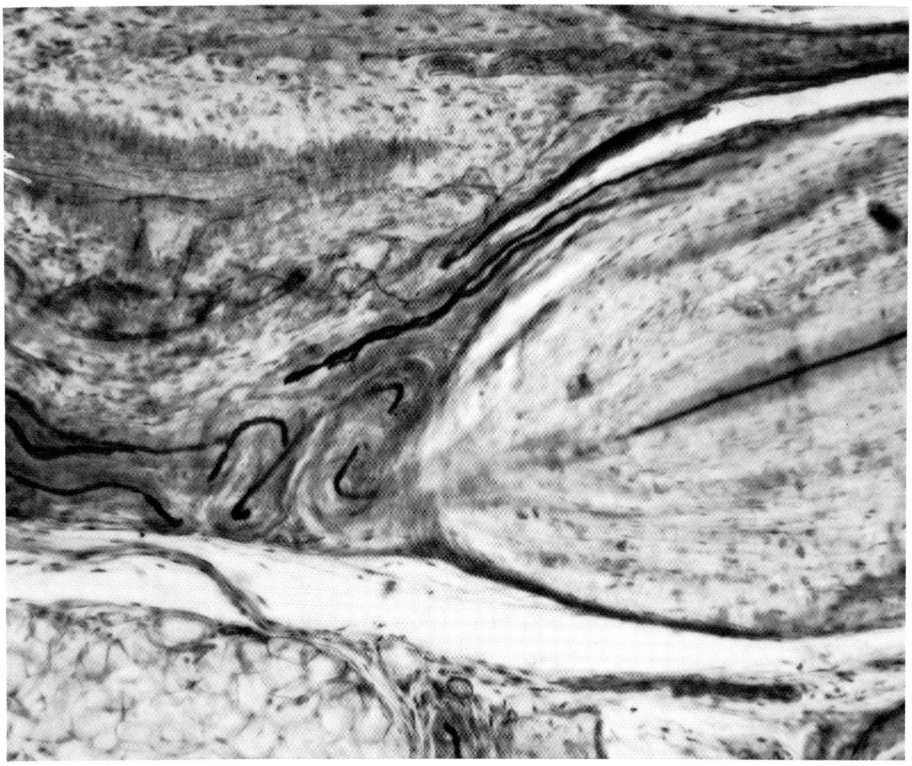

FIGURE 10. Vater–Pacini corpuscle demonstrating the axial fiber, the inner bulb, and the capsule. The convoluted stalk, which has often been mistaken for other end organs such as a Golgi–Mazzoni body, is observed to the left and resembles the simple sensory corpuscle or mammalian end organ. Human finger. Winkelmann method, ×100.

ings). The myelinated nerve contains at least one and often two nodes of Ranvier in the stalk, but the myelin sheath is lost shortly after penetration of the inner bulb. The inner bulb is an enlarged space composed of Schwann cell membranes covered by basement membranes. These membranes are pinocytotic and may show desmosomes. The axial nerve may be duplicated or complex, particularly in early development. The axial nerve is ovoid in diameter. The axon contains neurofilaments, microtubules, mitochondria, smooth endoplasmic reticulum, and rare lysosomes and myelin dense bodies.

The nerve proceeds to its termination at the distal end of the body. Along the way it protrudes cytoplasmic extensions between the bilateral clefts of the lamellar cells. These cytoplasmic extensions contain clear vesicles, as does the termination. The terminal portion is usually bifid but may be bulbous. Oval or round mitochrondria occupy the central zone of the receptor plasm and are very numerous. Glycogen granules, many lysosomes, and myelin bodies are present. The receptor plasm may have bare areas covered only by basement membrane. Projections or horns of nerve terminal axoplasm may project into the surrounding intercellular spaces. These projections are found in all other types of receptors as well as in Pacini bodies. Surrounding this axon and terminal is the inner bulb or core composed of Schwann cells, containing cholinesterase, alkaline phosphatase, or other hydrolytic or respiratory enzymes. Collagen fibers are found in the inner bulb.

The inner core lamellae vary in number from 20 to 60, and they are more widely separated towards the surface of the end organ. A basement membrane covers the inner core cells and lamellae. Desmosomal connections occur between closely opposed inner lamellae. The lamellae are also arranged in bilaterally symmetric layers. The outer lamellae are formed by circularly oriented cells widely separated in the capsule. These lamellae vary from 20 to 100 in number. The lamellae of the capsule are fluid-filled spaces that also contain collagen fibers. Blood vessels form a widely spaced network in the outer capsule. The external capsule of the Pacini body is composed of multiple layers of overlapping and closely adherent perineurial cells. The cells demonstrate active pinocytosis and are surrounded on their external and internal faces by a basement membrane. Below the external capsule is a distinct subcapsular space containing fibroblasts, macrophages, and collagen.

The Pacini end organ corresponds in location and by response to an ending for deep pressure. It is a rapidly adapting receptor and as such responds to vibration. Similar physiological responses are given by the Herbst end organ, the Pacini body variant found in glabrous and feathered skin and mucous membranes of birds. The Herbst corpuscle is smaller and has acid mucopolysaccharide in its capsule and a bilateral row of Schwann cells within the inner bulb directly opposed to the axon (Saxod, 1978b; Winkelmann and Myers, 1961). Cholinesterase is located in the inner bulb of the Herbst corpuscle.

2. *Simple or Mammalian End Organs*

Krause described cylindrical "*endkolben*" in the skin of mammals, and subsequently these have been called by a number of names: small Vater–Pacini corpuscles by Boeke; mammalian end organ by Winkelmann; paciniform corpuscles by Malinovsky; simple sensory corpuscles by Malinovsky; and simple bulboid nerve endings by Halata. All of these terms are an attempt to describe the simple corpuscular ending of the skin of mammals. Sinclair does not discuss the ending, and confusion about the ending and its significance must be resolved. It is of great importance, for most neurophysiological research is done in mammals that have the simple sensory corpuscle (or mammalian end organ) in the glabrous and acral skin, where the primates have Meissner corpuscles or their variant, the mucocutaneous end organ.

This simple corpuscular ending appears comparable to the isolated inner bulb or core of the Pacini corpuscle. The embryological studies of Pacini corpuscles show how much these bodies in the early stages of development resemble the adult simple sensory corpuscles (mammalian end organ) (Malinovsky and Pac, 1982). This nerve ending is also supplied in clusters by branching myelinated nerve fibers. Rosary-type axial innervation of a series of these endings has been described. The nerve ending is commonly found in the subpapillary or papillary dermis of the glabrous or acral skin of mammals (Figure 11; Winkelmann, 1960a). It has been described in tongue, palate, and submucosal locations as well (Winkelmann, 1962a). The hairy skin adjoining the mucocutaneous regions shows a concentration of these endings, decreasing in number rapidly as one moves away from the glabrous area (Malinovsky and Pac, 1982). The ending is observed in the tail skin in lion and kangaroo and in the dorsal and ventral hairy skin of dog, cat, mouse, and marsupials, but only in rare observation. The extensive literature is summarized by Malinovsky and Pac (1982).

The nerve ending is composed of an axial nerve, a core, and the capsule. Variations observed in the external form or in the number of axons or disposition of the central core have been used to classify these endings. Halata (1975) described three forms based on the presence of clefts in the core: two opposing clefts, one cleft, and no cleft. Malinovsky and Pac (1982) described five groups: (1) a single axial nerve with or without loops, (2) branching axons, (3) divided or partly divided bodies, (4) polyaxonal, and (5) rosary-arranged corpuscles. As has been emphasized, rosary arrangement is a variant observed in all sensory corpuscular nerve endings and is not a basis for individual variation. The mammalian end organs with multiple axons or branching axons are larger in diameter. These variations lose much of their importance when quantitative data are reviewed. Malinovsky and Pac (1982) demonstrated multiple variations of the corpuscle in foot pad, tongue, nose, and lip of the cat, but the first three minor variations actually account for 64 to 97% of the endings in the separate regions. There appears to be a basic common plan for this end organ, which is expressed predominantly and quantitatively. The fact that the foot pad has more complicated endings than other regions does not destroy the basic unity of structure visible in these studies. Similarly, Peterson *et al.* (1972) found in the cat hip joint capsule mammalian end organs that could be simple, elongated, or complex in form. But here also, the simple sensory corpuscle was the predominant form, and complex endings were only 17% of 1200 endings studied.

The more superficial the end organ, the smaller in diameter or cross section it will be. The spherical end bulbs range from 30 to 100 μm in diameter. The elongated forms are 30 to 50 μm in width and 100 to 300 μm in length. Although an elongated form may be linear, it is common for one or more curves to appear along its length. Often, the curve may be vertical to the surface of the skin. The more complex endings are found in the pads of the paws and in the nasal skin, where multiple arrays of coils may lie on or adjacent to one another.

The major portion of the nerve ending is composed of Schwann cell

A

B

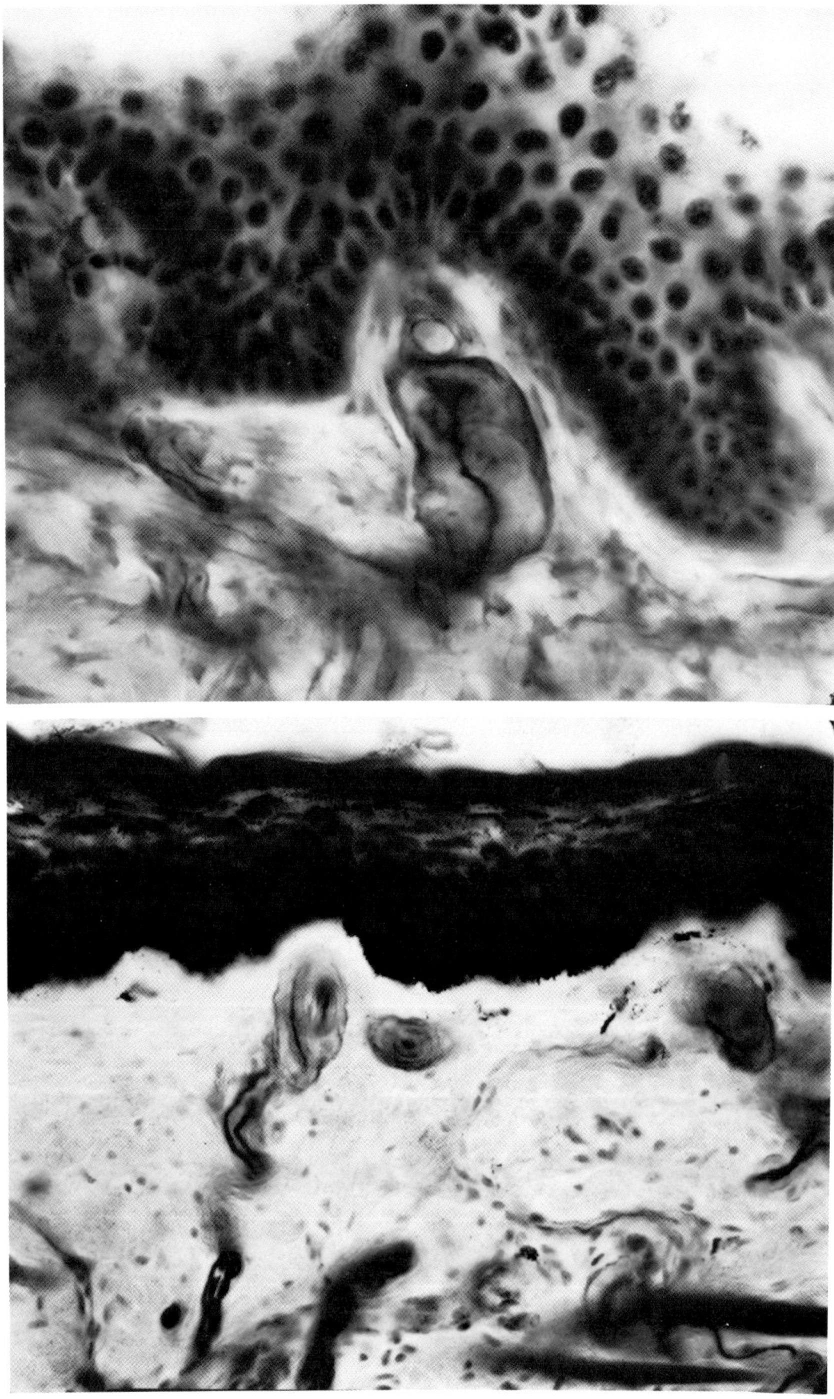

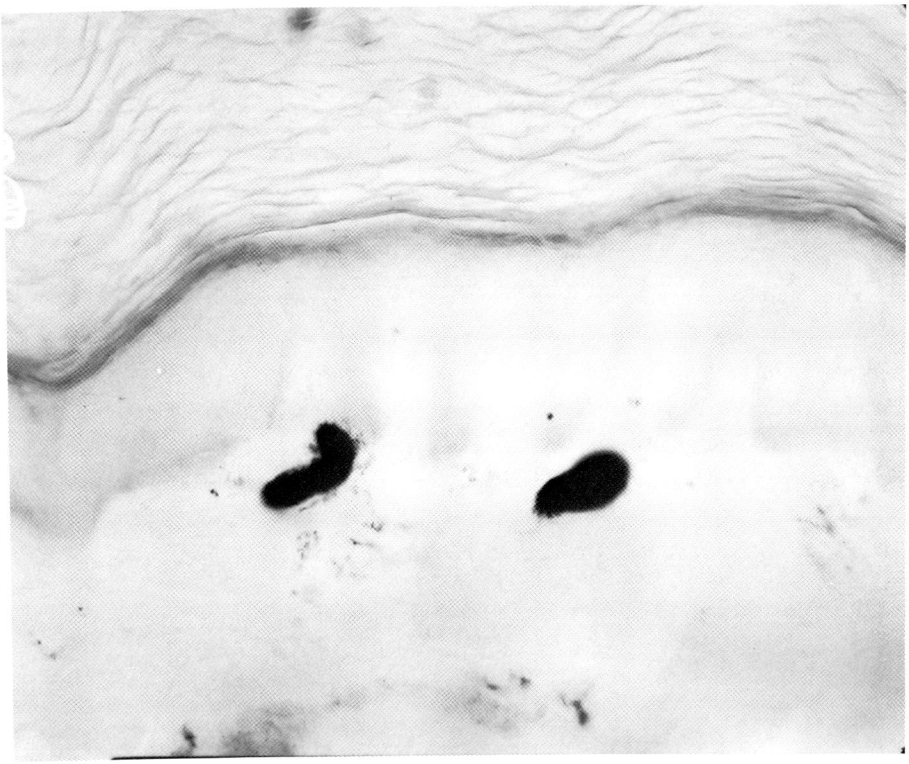

FIGURE 12. Mammalian end organs below the epidermis of cat paw. Nonspecific cholinesterase, ×250.

lamellae, which make up the inner core and most of the end organ. The largest corpuscles rarely have 30 lamellae, the average corpuscle has ten lamellae, and the smallest and most rudimentary may have only three to six lamellae. The inner core often consists of only three to five cells, whose lamellae surround the axon and terminal. Some endings show concentric or spiral lamellar structures, and larger endings show clefts and bilaterally symmetrical arrangements, as in the Pacini corpuscle. The lamellae have many pinocytotic vesicles and are covered with basement membrane that on occasion is reduplicated. The innermost lamellae have desmosome contacts with the axon and terminal. The interlamellar space contains fluid and collagen fibers and enzymes (Figures 12 and 13).

The nerve may follow a direct course to the end of the corpuscle, where

FIGURE 11. (A) Mammalian end organ. Simple sensory corpuscle in the cat paw demonstrating its superficial position, axial nerve, and capsule. Winkelmann method, ×400. (B) Coiled and elongated mammalian end organ in cat lip. Winkelmann method, ×400.

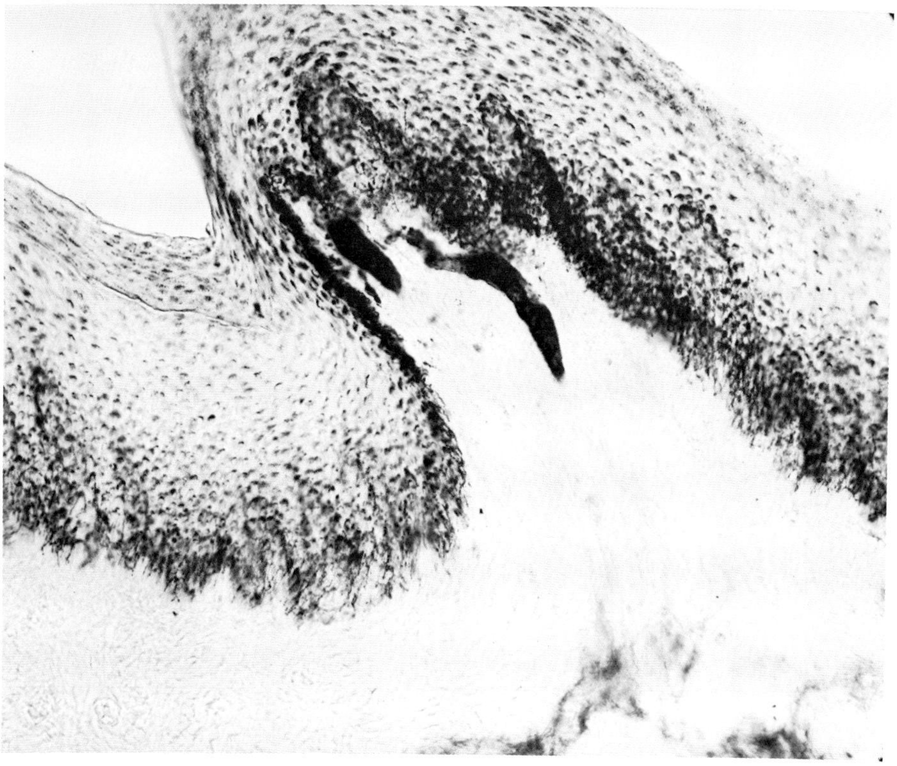

FIGURE 13. Mammalian end organs in the dermis of the palatal rugae of the cat. Nonspecific cholinesterase, ×160.

an expanded tip may be present. Bifurcation of the ending has been described. Frequently, the nerve will twist within the core. Often it is difficult not to cut multiple cross sections of an axon as it coils within the body. This does not appear to be sufficient reason to consider these anatomic variations as new types of end organ.

It is easy to agree with Malinovsky and Pac (1982) that the simple sensory corpuscles in the skin of mammals are not uniform. Complex variations of axon, terminations, and lamellar structures occur. Perhaps the most difficult to recognize are the failure of capsule formation, as in the hedgehog. Such corpuscles are found beneath the epidermis.

Janig (1971) described the simple sensory corpuscle (mammalian end organ) as a rapidly adapting receptor. This would be natural since the other encapsulated Pacini and Herbst corpuscles are rapidly adapting end organs. Since the simple corpuscle takes the position in the glabrous mammalian skin in which the Meissner corpuscle is found in the primate, one can appreciate the utility of the equivalent nerve ending also being a rapidly adapting mechanoreceptor.

Iggo and Ogawa (1977) studied the rapidly adapting receptors of glabrous skin of the cat. They associated simple encapsulated corpuscles with rapidly adapting mechanoreceptor units. Their discussion indicates that they believed that these end organs were the equivalent of Krause's cylindrical end bulb and so equal to the simple sensory corpuscle (Malinovsky) and the mammalian end organ (Winkelmann).

3. *The Ruffini Corpuscle Controversy*

Ruffini described a fusiform structure with a definite capsule in the deep cutaneous tissue of the finger. Miller *et al.* (1960) produced a methylene blue photomicrograph that they labeled a Ruffini body and noted that the nerve appeared to ramify within the capsule to expanded tips. No satisfactory silver preparation photomicrographs of this ending exist (Winkelmann, 1960b). Sinclair (1981) states "the importance of the Ruffini body remains to be established."

Chambers *et al.* (1972) described Ruffini bodies in the hairy skin of the cat by electron microscopy. These bodies were large, 0.5 to 2 mm in length and slightly broader at the center than at the poles. Because of its size, such an end organ should have been reported many times and confirmed by histochemical and other conventional methods. These Chambers end organs appear closer to the simple sensory end organ or mammalian end organ in one of the variations described by Malinovsky and Pac (1982). Electron microscopic study showed a capsule of four to five layers of perineural cells surrounding a polyaxonal core. There is a broad subcapsular space with connective tissue fibroblasts and macrophages that merges with the dermal connective tissue. Nonmyelinated axonal branches have a variable course that terminates in nerve endings, and each is invested with Schwann cell lamellae. The axon is also described as covered in part only by basement membrane. The existence of this ending is accepted by Halata, by Chouchkov, and by Malinovsky and Pac (1982) despite the lack of any serious confirmation by other techniques. Halata and Munger (1981) described a single end organ in an alopecia areata scalp and generalized to state that this is a universal end organ of the skin of man. Halata and Munger (1981) compared and described the Ruffini ending as a type of joint capsule end organ.

In 1978, further confusion was added when the term "pilo-Ruffini ending" was applied by Biemesdorfer *et al.* (1978) to the circular nerve ending about the hair follicle in the facial skin of the rhesus monkey. This use of the term has been continued by Munger and Halata (1983) speaking of hair follicle nerve endings. It is hard to justify this use of an old classic term for a new receptor area because of electron microscopic similarities in nerve terminations. Nomenclature must be justified by tradition and structure as well as by physiological response. It seems unusual that such an elusive receptor has been associated with a specific type II slowly adapting mechanoreceptor on no better evidence than that no other obvious receptor presented itself. Iggo and Gottschaldt (1974) list the Ruffini ending as existing in the subcutaneous tissue or deep dermis despite the absence of any demonstration of an ending in this location in human skin.

F. Complex Nerve Endings

The mucocutaneous skin contains multiple areas of not one nerve receptor but multiple combined forms in a small volume of tissue. These endings usually exist as a combination of Merkel cell nerve masses in the rete ridges associated with intraepidermal nerve fibers. Frequently, immediately adjacent to the epidermis is a coiled or complex mammalian end organ. This produces the typical end organ of Eimer in the nose of the hedgehog, mole, and similar animals (Figure 14; Malinovsky, 1981). In some locations, as in the horse lip,

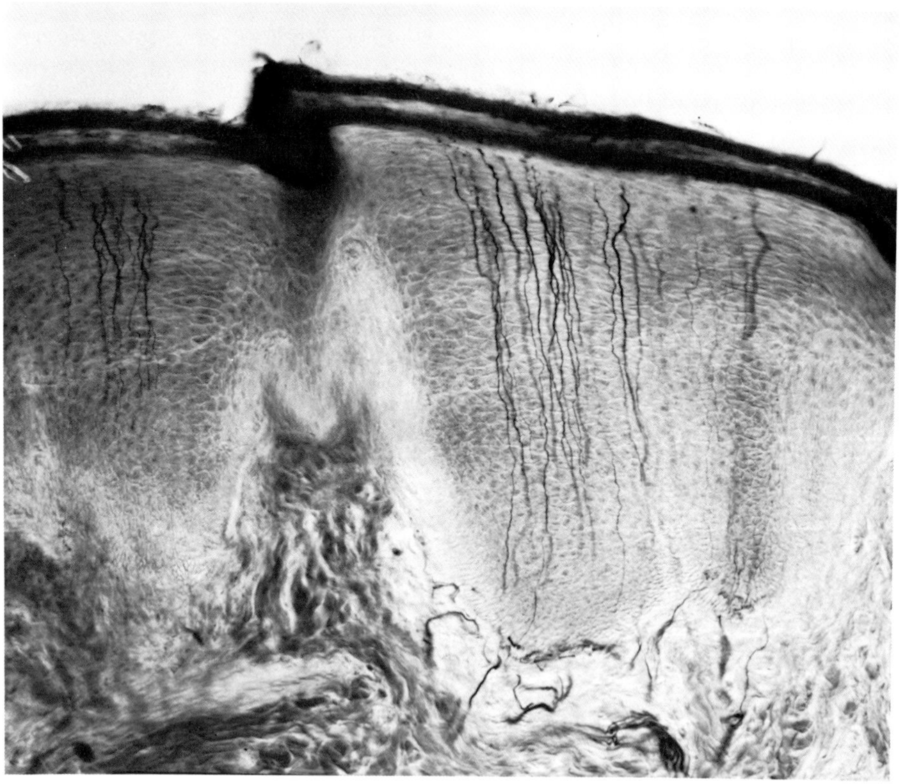

FIGURE 14. Complex nerve ending from the nose of North American opossum (*Didelphis virginiana*) showing multiple intraepithelial nerves, nerve disks associated with Merkel cells in the basal layer of the epidermis, and a simple sensory corpuscle (mammalian end organ) in the dermis. The whole ensemble is an organ of Eimer.

the intraepidermal nerve is emphasized; in areas such as the frictional skin, the Merkel cell complexes may be more prominent, as may be recognized in the palatal rugae.

The Merkel cell masses in the tactile disk (Pinkus) offer another example of an ending that appears at first to be uniform. Free nerve endings are invaribly related to it. Many species have the simple sensory corpuscle (mammalian end organ) below the tactile (Pinkus) disk. The kangaroo hairy skin has such large masses of axon approaching the disk between the hair follicles that it appears to form a giant axonal mass of distinctive nature. Yet, it is only another variation in emphasis of the basic components of the complex nerve ending related to the tactile disk.

The large hair nerve networks qualify as complex nerve endings (Munger, 1982). Halata (1975) described small bulbous endings associated with the hairs, and particularly with sensory hairs. One may find free terminals as well as the Merkel cell endings in the perifollicular and follicular tissue. The lanceolate endings along the external root sheath in a palisade and the circular nerve fibers with connective tissue relationships make the hair follicle endings more complex than other groups, yet all of these very complex masses of sensory receptor tissue are composed of essentially the same individual receptor elements: free nerve endings, Merkel cell epithelial endings, and simple corpuscular endings. Histological, histochemical, immunochemical, and electron microscopic methods now exist to identify the individual components of all of these complex organized receptors.

G. *Quantitative Studies of Cutaneous Sensory Receptors*

The existence of good histological, histochemical, and electron microscopic methods for sensory tissue in the dermis has made possible quantitative approaches to sensory receptor anatomy. Using horizontal sections and cholinesterase, Zollman and Winkelmann (1962) were able to state that the anterior paw of the raccoon had a significant increase in simple sensory corpuscles (mammalian end organs) as compared to the posterior paw.

Malinovsky and Pac (1982) studied the same sensory end organs in the cat and divided them into simple and various types of complex endings. They gave numbers of end organs per area studied in lip, paw, tongue, and nose. Similar studies gave numbers of end organs in goat, pig, sheep, and cow. They noted in all species and all areas that the simple end organ was the most frequent form observed. They studied simple corpuscles of joints and combined these data with those from Hromada and Polacek (1958) showing that simple end organs were most prominent. The highest percentage of complicated end organs (8.75%) was observed in the cat paw. Peterson *et al.* (1972) used the whole-mount technique with alkaline phosphatase and cholinesterase to study the total number and nature of end organs in the joint capsule of the hip. Three types of sensory corpuscles were found: simple, elongated, and complex. Twenty cat hip joint capsules were studied completely for nerve end organs, and a total of 1473 end organs were identified. The proportion of endings was 64% simple, 19% elongated, and 17% complex.

The number, distribution, and density of end organs could be studied (Table VII). There were from 21.9 end organs/cm^2 to 57.4 end organs/cm^2. The number of end organs for the entire capsule, 43.1/cm^2, gives a false impression because the superior capsule had half as many end organs as the posterior and inferior surface. These data may indicate that weight-bearing surfaces may have more encapsulated end organs, as was already suggested by Malinovsky and Pac (1982). Although the number of end organs varied widely from cat to cat, the right and left hip capsules were remarkably similar in most instances. Individual variation in quantity of nerve endings is a factor that must always be considered. Although an average of 73.7 end organs per hip capsule sounds reasonable, the variation is so great that some hips are over- and some underinnervated compared to this standard.

The cholinesterase whole-mount method gives a good means of gauging nerve density and end-organ density in fascia and tendon. Jackson *et al.* (1966) used this technique to show a marked diminution of sensory nerve tissue with age in the spinal ligaments. Nerve networks and no special end organs were seen at all ages in the annulus fibrosis. Becton *et al.* (1966) used the same method to study the whole innervation of the extensor hood mechanism of the human index finger. Dense nerve networks were observed in the flexor tendon vincula, and sparse nerve was observed in the other areas. The nerve tissue in the extensor fascial hood is concentrated over the joints.

Robertson and Winkelmann (1970) studied the nerve networks in the stroma of the human cornea. It is possible to view the size and number of nerve nets and also, in the whole mount, to visualize both free stroma and intraepidermal nerve endings. The mucocutaneous end organ at the limbus can be seen. This study indicated that oral mucosa could be studied. Desjardins *et al.* (1971) studied human oral gingiva from maxillary, mandibular, incisor, and molar areas at successive ages. Quantitative assessment of the nerves and

TABLE VII
Number of Encapsulated Sensory End Organs in Hip Capsule of the Cat[a]

Region[b]	Endings/cm^2
Superior	21.9
Anterior	36.5
Inferior	57.4
Posterior	56.6
Mean	43.1

[a] From Peterson *et al.* (1972).
[b] Five of ten cats had comparable values in right and left hip capsules.

nerve endings was made. The 109 specimens were treated by the sodium bromide–whole-mount–cholinesterase method so that the epithelium was removed and the papillary bodies and nerve endings could be counted. The number of mucocutaneous end organs in the gingiva increased with age in all areas. Males always had fewer nerve endings per unit area than females. The number of nerve endings decreases as one examines more posterior maxillary gingiva, but this is not true in mandibular gingiva. The presence or absence of teeth or dentures did not appear to influence the amount of nerve tissue or number of nerve endings.

Muller and Winkelmann (1969) applied the same cholinesterase whole-mount technique to the study of human chest skin in patients with herpes zoster neuralgia. Contralateral normal skin served as a control. The decrease in nerve networks and distortion of nerve networks was readily apparent and was confirmed by thick vertical sections. The areas of diminished nerve network correlated with absent histamine flare.

A study of the neuropathies by use of a frozen-section cholinesterase method by Dyck *et al.* (1966) showed a definite decrease in the end organs in patients with chronic sensory loss. The greatest decrease was found in patients with the most severe sensory loss on neurological examination. The possibility of a unique cutaneous sensory neuropathy was proposed as the result of study of a patient with good sensory conduction time and decreased to absent Meissner corpuscles (Dickens *et al.*, 1963). Cauna (1980) made a careful electron microscopic study of digital skin with graphic reconstructions. He found 80 dermal papillae per square millimeter and noted free nerve endings in 60% of them. As many as five free endings could be in one papilla.

The techniques are now available for careful controlled quantitative assessment of nerve endings in skin and correlation with physiological function. Certain restrictions must apply. The tissue must come from constant areas and be prepared by constant techniques. The tissue must be rigorously monitored for age and sex. Because it is usually not possible to compare individuals of the same species quantitatively, each study subject must serve as its own control. Large numbers of subjects must be studied, as shown by the variation in the cat hip study. Each age group must be compared with itself. Males and females cannot be grouped together. The technology is now present to provide an excellent anatomic basis for all studies. The addition of immunochemical whole-mount procedures should ensure an even greater capacity to provide answers to all the anatomic questions in sensation.

H. *Histochemistry of Nerve End Organs*

Demonstration of nerve end organs of all types is possible by histochemical methods. The reaction of the end organs is usually not confined to the axon but related to the surrounding lamellar structures. The chemical reaction defines the nerve-associated tissue, and the axon is seen as a negative line coursing through the end organ. The Meissner corpuscle may be demonstrated by respiratory enzymes. Mitchell (1965) reported the dehydrogenases in the Meissner corpuscle of the rhesus monkey, and I found that the New- and Old-World monkeys and lesser primates had Meissner and mucocutaneous end organs that were easily demonstrated by succinic dehydrogenase and cytochrome oxidase (Winkelmann, 1963b). The Meissner corpuscle mucocutaneous end organ may be demonstrated by nonspecific cholinesterase reaction in all of the primates. Alkaline phosphatase is present in this end organ in the gibbon (Winkelmann, 1962b). Steigleder and Schultis (1968) demonstrated nonspecific esterase in the Meissner corpuscle in man, and Montagna and Yun (1962) and Winkelmann (1971) have shown nonspecific esterase in the Meissner corpuscles of the galago. The Meissner corpuscles of the opossum contain alkaline phosphatase and not cholinesterase (Winkelmann, 1964). Other marsupials had cholinesterase and varying amounts of alkaline phosphatase in motor end plates and hair follicle nerve end organs (Winkelmann, 1966).

The mammalian or simple end organ common to the skin of all mammals

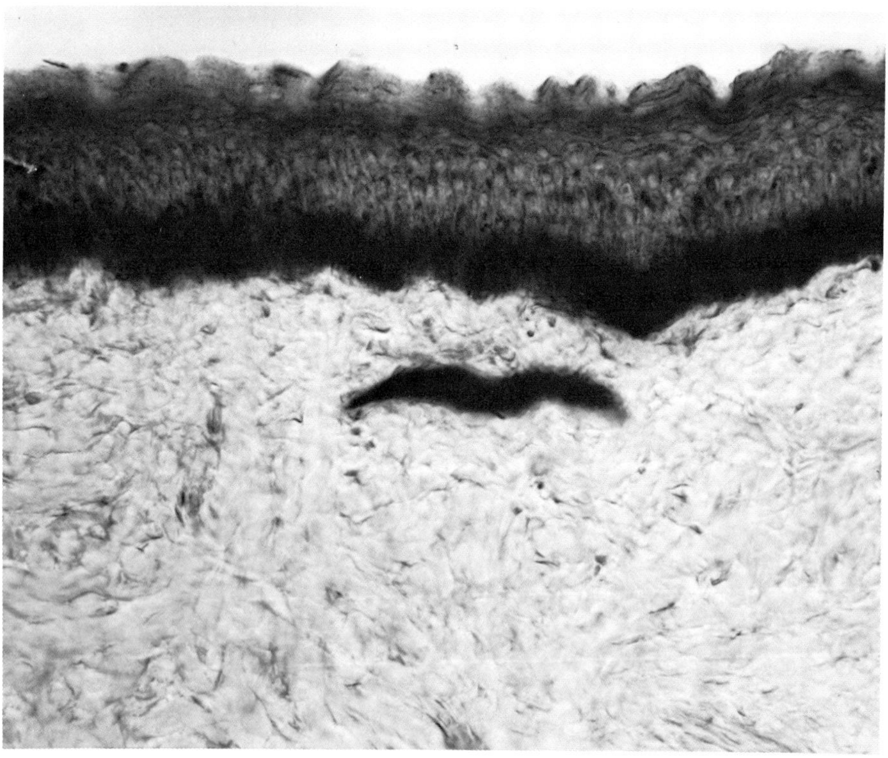

FIGURE 15. Elongated mammalian end organ in the dermis of the lion lip. Alkaline phosphatase, ×250.

was demonstrated by nonspecific cholinesterase in the skin of the cat (see Figures 12 and 13). That this end organ is comparable to the inner bulb of the Pacini corpuscle is emphasized by the histochemical demonstration of the elongated and rounded structure filled with enzyme activity through which the axon passes, entirely comparable to the inner bulb of the Pacini corpuscle. The end organ of the cat contains alkaline phosphatase as well as nonspecific cholinesterase. All other felines studied have alkaline-phosphatase-positive end organs also (Figure 15; Winkelmann, 1960a). The nerve end organs of the badger and coatimundi have indoxyl esterase (Bourlond and Winkelmann, 1966). The rabbit end organs have naphthol chloroacetic esterase (Figure 16) and leucine aminopeptidase. These histochemical techniques have stable end products, and, therefore, it is possible to use Bielschowski or Winkelmann frozen-section silver methods to demonstrate axons coursing through the mass of the end organ demonstrated by the chemical procedure.

The Pacini corpuscle found in all vertebrates has an expanded capsule containing polysaccharides in birds. The inner bulb, analogous to the mammalian end organ, contains nonspecific cholinesterase, alkaline phosphatase, or dehydrogenases according to the species studied (Malinovsky and Pac, 1982; Winkelmann, 1971).

The Merkel cell complexes of the skin demonstrate hydrolytic enzyme activity associated with the epidermal plate. Cholinesterase and ATPase may be demonstrated in many species. The tactile hair disk is cholinesterase pos-

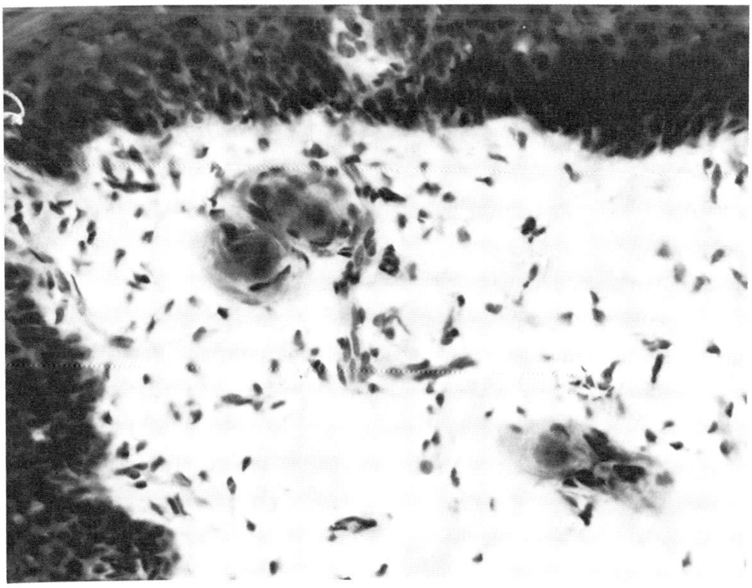

FIGURE 16. Coiled mammalian end organ within the dermis of the rabbit palatal ruga. Naphthyl chloracetate esterase, ×400.

itive in the rabbit (Winkelmann *et al.*, 1967). Alkaline phosphatase demonstrates the tactile hair disk in some marsupials and the guinea pig (Winkelmann, 1982). Merkel-rich epithelial areas occur in the palatal rugae of the rabbit, and these are positive for leucine aminopeptidase (Figure 17). The Merkel cell is not demonstrated by the enzyme techniques but may be demonstrated by periodic acid–Schiff in some species. The studies for catecholamines and serotonin in our laboratory and other laboratories have not yielded a chemical demonstration of specific material in the Merkel cell.

The hair follicle nerve network is complex, with both vertical and circular arrangements of nerve fibers. The vertical palisade of lanceolate endings and the circular collar of nerve may be demonstrated by cholinesterase in most mammals. Montagna and Brookhart (1977) has demonstrated that cholinesterase activity is not related to the hair cycle. The relative amounts of specific and nonspecific cholinesterase vary greatly from one animal family to another. Alkaline phosphatase may be observed in the lanceolate endings of the red kangaroo, and the circular mass of the hair nerve may also contain alkaline phosphatase (Winkelmann, 1966). The smaller primates have simple perifollicular nerve endings, and frequently only the circular hair network is present. Leucine aminopeptidase has been demonstrated in the galago (Winkelmann, 1971).

The nerve trunks of the skin contain mast cells and acid mucopolysaccharide, and this has been the basis for staining nerve trunks with metachro-

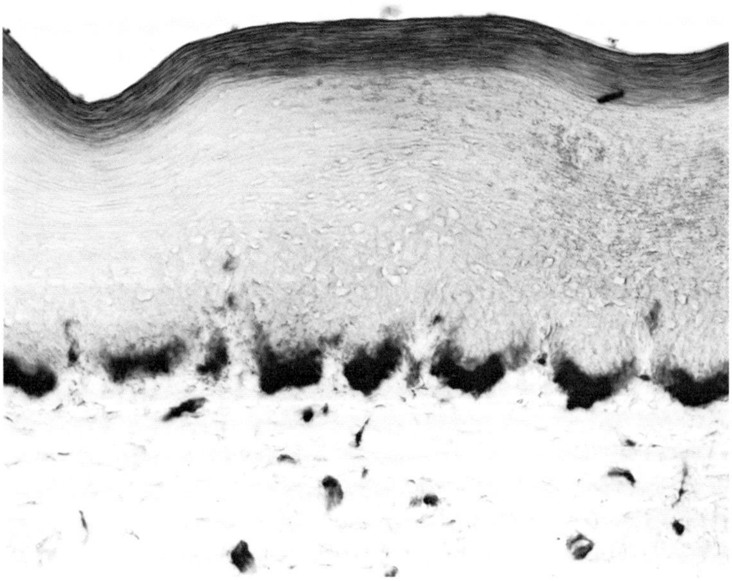

FIGURE 17. Leucine aminopeptidase activity associated with Merkel epithelial innervation of rabbit palate. 4-Methoxyleucine aminopeptidase method, ×250.

matic stains. Lipid stains, of course, may stain the myelin sheath as long as its dimensions are large enough. The sensory nerve networks may be demonstrated by cholinesterase technique. The intraepithelial nerve endings may be demonstrated only by specific cholinesterase. The use of the cholinesterase whole-mount technique after sodium bromide treatment permits the removal of the epidermis and the study of the whole dermis for the density of cholinesterase nerve networks (Winkelmann *et al.*, 1967). Free endings may be demonstrated this way, and the relationship of the specialized end organs to the nerve networks may be seen. The dermal and intraepidermal nerve networks in the cornea have been studied by whole-mount technique (Robertson and Winkelmann, 1970). The innervation of entire tendons or fascial structures has been studied by the method of the whole-mount preparation in both animals and man (Lipscomb and Winkelmann, 1961). Variable ATPase reaction occurs in human skin, particularly in subepidermal unmyelinated nerve fibers. The cholinesterase technique in the whole-mount preparations and in sections to demonstrate hair follicle nerve end organs may be followed by the whole-mount silver preparations (Winkelmann, 1971). Montagna and his colleagues (Montagna and Brookhart, 1977) have used this extensively to describe innervation of haired skin in man and primates. Saxod (1978a) has described the use of a similar whole-mount preparation for the study of density of end organs in skin innervation.

The histochemical preparations are able to define nerve end organs whatever the technique. The distinctive appearance of the mammalian end organ, lanceolate nerve endings, Meissner corpuscle, and Merkel endings when studied by these methods makes it easy to accept these as individual endings. The ability to add silver methods to the histochemistry has made it possible to define the axon and terminus in relation to the chemistry of the membranes. An end organ should have this definitive integrity before it is accepted.

I. Immunohistochemistry of Nerve Endings

The isolation of specific antigens from nerve tissue has provided an opportunity to study normal nerve tissue by using antibodies raised to these antigens and demonstrating them in fixed tissue by fluorescent or peroxidase coupling methods. The isolation of S-100 protein from cytoplasm of central nervous system cells is accomplished by solution of this acid protein in 100% saturated ammonium sulfate. This protein is found in the cytoplasm of nerve cells, melanocytes, and Langerhans cells. The antibody to it has been ued to identify pigmented nevus and melanoma cells and the cells of histiocytosis X (Rowden *et al.*, 1983). Its first use was to define neurocellular tumors of the central nervous system. It has also helped to define the granular cell Schwannoma as a nerve tumor. Clear-cell sarcoma is positive for S-100 protein, consistent with its pigment cell origin. The Meissner corpuscle is S-100 protein positive (Figure 18).

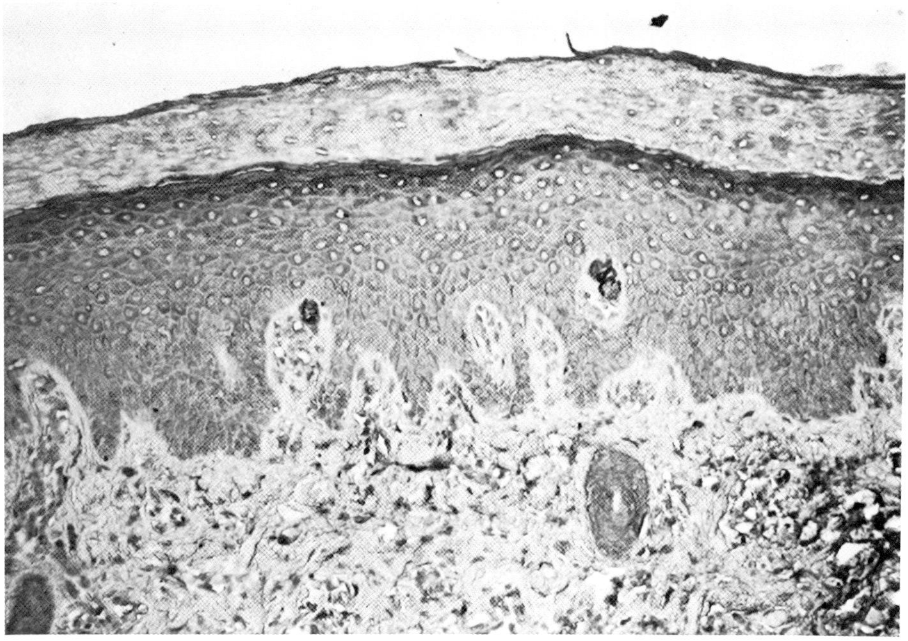

FIGURE 18. Meissner corpuscles in papillary bodies. Human foot. S-100 antibody–peroxidase method, ×40.

The separation of myelin basic protein, glial fibrillary protein, and neurofilament protein has added additional antibodies for the study of nerve tumors. The peripheral neurofibromas are positive for myelin basic protein. These antibodies are just beginning to be used in the study of anatomic problems. Studies with these antibodies should help to decide some of the problems of neural versus mesenchymal origin of the capsule material of nerve end organs. Some nonspecific tissue antigens are found on nerve tissue and may have some use. The HLA-DR antibody may demonstrate the surface of nerve fibers within nerve trunks (Figure 19). The combination of neuroimmunochemistry and electron microscopy will enhance the value of the antibody demonstrations.

The Merkel cell has been demonstrated by antibody to neuron-specific enolase (Gu *et al.*, 1981). This antibody demonstrates the content of this enzyme in neural tissue. My interpretation of the preparations published is that the nerve terminus associated with the Merkel cell may be positive. Electron microscopy will be needed to settle this problem.

Hartschuh and colleagues (1983a) have used antibodies to various peptides such as neurotensin, somatostatin, and calcitonin applied to preparations of Merkel cell epidermis. Positive results were obtained with Met-enkephalin in rodents (rat, mouse, and guinea pig). No other species was found to have

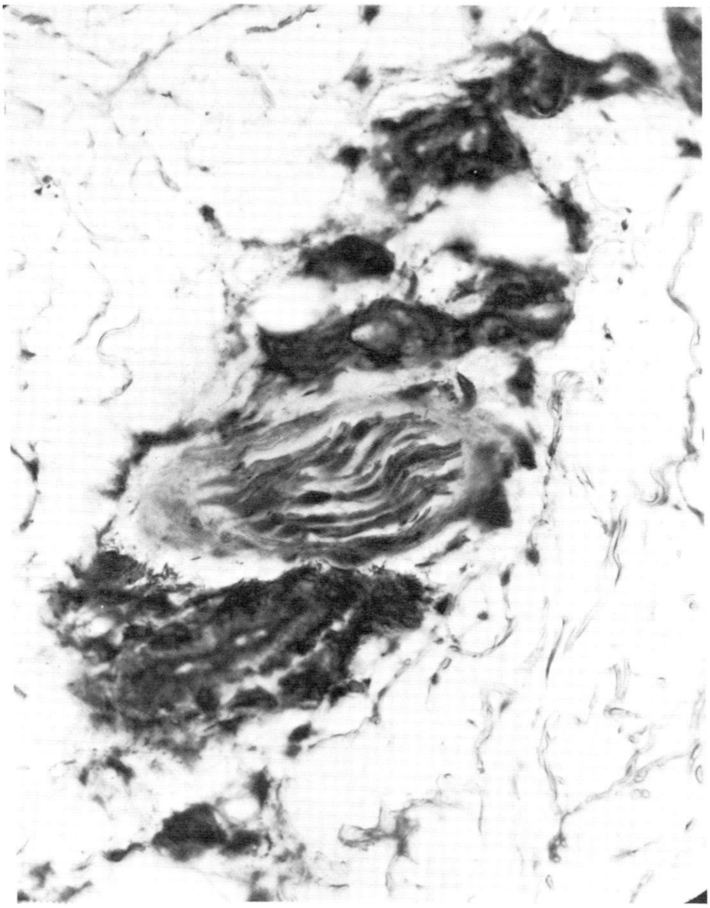

FIGURE 19. Nerve trunk in dermis of human arm skin. HLA-DR antibody–peroxidase method, ×250.

this enkephalin content. Continued study demonstrated vasoactive intestinal polypeptide (VIP) in the Merkel cells in a variety of locations in all other species studies (man, cat, dog, and pig) (Hartschuh *et al.*, 1983b). Human gingival Merkel cells contain a rodlike nuclear inclusion also observed in a VIP-containing tumor of the pancreas (Fortman and Winkelmann, 1973).

Saurat *et al.* (1983) recently described antibodies to glycoconjugates found on red blood cell membranes, which are usually traced by cold agglutinin antibodies. One of these antibodies reacted to the Merkel cell in rabbit epidermis. Its location in the Merkel cell was confirmed by electron histochemistry. Nerve fibers were not stained. The cytoplasm of the Merkel cell was intensely stained. It remains to be seen if this human cold agglutinin monoclonal antibody (μ, κ, Prh) with its affinity for glycoconjugates in the rabbit lip Merkel cell cytoplasm is expressed in other species and in other locations.

References

ANDRES, K. H. Ueber die feinstruktur der rezeptoren an sinushaaren. *Z. Zellforsch.* 75:339–365, 1966.

ANDRES, K. H. AND VON DUHRING, L. Morphology of cutaneous mechanoreceptors, in: *Handbook of Sensory Physiology,* Vol. II (A. IGGO, ed.), Springer, Berlin, 1975, pp. 3–28.

BECTON, J. L., WINKELMANN, R. K., AND LIPSCOMB, P. R. Innervation of human finger tendons, as determined by histochemical techniques. *J. Bone Joint Surg.* 48A:1519–1541, 1966.

BERKHOUDT, H. The morphology and distribution of cutaneous mechanoreceptors (Herbst and Grandry corpuscle) in bill and tongue of mallard (*Anas platyrhynchos* L.). *Neth. J. Zool.* 30:1–34, 1980.

BIEMESDORFER, D., MUNGER, B. L., BINCK, J., AND DUBNER, R. The pilo-Ruffini complex. *Brain Res.* 142:197–222, 1978.

BOURLOND, A., AND WINKELMANN, R. K. Nervenendorgane der Haut beim Dachs. *Acta Neuroveg.* 29:149–155, 1966.

BREATHNACH, A. The mammalian and avian Merkel cell in the skin of vertebrates. *Linnean Soc. Symp. Ser.* 9:283–291, 1980.

CAUNA, N. Nerve supply and nerve endings in Meissner's corpuscles. *Am. J. Anat.* 99:315–350, 1956.

CAUNA, N. The effect of ageing on the receptor organs of human dermis, in: *Aging,* Vol. 6, *Advances in Biology of Skin* (W. MONTAGNA, ed.), Permagon Press, New York, 1964, pp. 63–96.

CAUNA, N. Fine structure of the receptor organs and its probable functional significance, in: *Touch, Heat and Pain* (A. V. S. ROUCK AND J. KNIGHT eds.), J and A Churchill, London, 1966, pp. 117–127.

CAUNA, N. The free penicillate nerve endings of the human hairy skin. *J. Anat.* 115:277–288, 1973.

CAUNA, N. Morphological basis of sensation in hairy skin. *Prog. Brain Res.* 43:35–45, 1976.

CAUNA, N. Fine morphological characteristics and microtopography of the free nerve endings of human digital skin. *Anat. Res.* 198:643–656, 1980.

CHAMBERS, M. R., ANDRES, K. H., VON DURING, M., AND IGGO, A. Structure and function of the slowly adapting type III mechanoreceptor in hairy skin. *Q. J. Exp. Physiol.* 57:417–445, 1972.

CHOUCHKOV, C. N. Cutaneous receptors. *Adv. Anat. Embryol. Cell Biol.* 54:1–62, 1978.

DESJARDINS, R. P., WINKELMANN, R. K., AND GONSALEZ, D. W. Comparison of nerve endings in normal gingiva with those in mucosa covering edentulous ridges. *J. Dent. Res.* 50:867–879, 1971.

DICKENS, W. M., WINKELMANN, R. K., AND MULDER, D. W. Cholinesterase demonstration of dermal nerve endings in patients with impaired sensation. *Neurology, (Minneap.)* 13:91–100, 1963.

DYCK, P. J., WINKELMANN, R. K., AND BOLTON, C. F. Quantitation of Meissner corpuscles in hereditary sensory disorders. *Neurology (Minneap.)* 16:10–17, 1966.

ENGLISH, K. B. Cell types in cutaneous type I mechanoreceptors (Haarscheiben) and their alterations with injury. *Am. J. Anat.* 141:105–126, 1974.

FITZGERALD, M. J. T. The innervation of the epidermis, in: *Skin Senses* (D. R. KENSHALO, ed.), Charles C. Thomas, Springfield, IL, 1968, pp. 61–80.

FORTMAN, G. J., AND WINKELMANN, R. K. A Merkel cell nuclear inclusion. *J. Invest. Dermatol.* 61:334–338, 1973.

FORTMAN, G. J., AND WINKELMANN, R. K. The Merkel cell in human oral mucosa. *J. Dent. Res.* 11:1303–1312, 1977.

GIACOMETTI, L. The anatomy of the human scalp, in: *Aging,* Vol. 6, *Advances in Biology of the Skin* (W. MONTAGNA, ed.), Pergamon Press, New York, 1965, pp. 97–118.

GIACOMETTI, L., AND MONTAGNA, W. Innervation of the hair follicle, in: *Advances in Biology of the Skin,* Vol. IX, *Hair Growth* (W. MONTAGNA AND R. L. DOBSON, eds.), Pergamon Press, New York, 1969, pp. 392–398.

GU, J., POLCK, J. M., TAFIA, F. J., MARANGOS, P. J., AND PEARSE, A. G. E. Neuron specific enolase in the Merkel cells of mammalian skin. *Am. J. Pathol.* 104:63–68, 1981.

HALATA, Z. The mechanoreceptors of mammalian skin. *Adv. Anat. Embryol. Cell Biol.* 50:3–77, 1975.

HALATA, Z. AND MUNGER, B. L. Identification of the Ruffini corpuscle in human hairy skin. *Cell Tissue Res.* 219:437–440, 1981.

HARTSCHUH, W., WEIHE, E., BUCHLER, M., HELMSTAEDTER, V., FEURLE, G. E., AND FORRSSMANN, W. G. Metenkephalin-like immunoreactivity in Merkel cells, *Cell Tissue Res.* 201:343–348, 1983a.

HARTSCHUH, W., WEIHE, E., YANAIHARA, N., AND REINECKE, M. Immunohistochemical localization of vasoactive intestinal polypeptide (VIP) in Merkel cells of various mammals. *J. Invest. Dermatol.* 81:361–364, 1983b.

HORCH, K. V., TUCKETT, R. P., AND BURGESS, P. R. A key to the classification of cutaneous mechanoreceptors. *J. Invest. Dermatol.* 69:75–82, 1977.

HROMADA, J., AND POLACEK, P. A. Contribution to the morphology of encapsulated nerve endings in the joint capsule and in the periarticular tissue. *Acta Anat.* 33:187–202, 1958.

IGGO, A. Cutaneous receptors, in: *The Peripheral Nervous System* (J. I. HUBBARD, ed.), Plenum Press, New York, 1974, pp. 347–404.

IGGO, A., AND GOTTSCHALDT, K. M. Cutaneous mechanoreceptors in simple and in complex sensory structures, in: *Mechanoreception* (J. SCHWARZKOPF, ed.), Westdeutsch Verlag, Opladen, 1974, pp. 153–176.

IGGO, A., AND MUIR, A. R. The structure and function of a slowly adapting touch corpuscle in hairy skin. *J. Physiol. (Lond.)* 200:763–796, 1969.

IGGO, A., AND OGAWA, H. Correlative physiological and morphological studies of rapidly adapting mechanoreceptors in cat's glabrous skin. *J. Physiol. (Lond.)* 266:275–296, 1977.

JACKSON, H. C., WINKELMANN, R. K. AND BICKEL, W. H. Nerve endings in the human spinal column. *J. Bone Joint Surg.* 48A:1272–1281, 1966.

JANIG, W. Morphology of rapidly and slowly adapting mechanoreceptors in the hairless skin of the cat. *Brain Res.* 28:217–231, 1971.

KRAUSE, W. *Die terminalen Korperchen der Einfach sensiblen Nerven, Hahn, Hanover, 1860.*

LIPSCOMB, P R., AND WINKELMANN, R. K. A whole-mount cholinesterase technic for study of innervation of the deep structures of the limbs. *J. Invest. Dermatol.* 37:481–483, 1961.

LOEWENSTEIN, W. R. Mechano-electric transduction in the Pacinian corpuscle, in: *Principles of Receptor Physiology* (W. R. LOEWENSTEIN, ed.), Springer, Berlin, 1971, pp. 362–374.

MAHRLE, G. AND ORFANOS, C. E. Merkel cells as human cutaneous neuroreceptors. *Arch. Dermatol. Forsch.* 251:19–26, 1974.

MALINOVSKY, L. Sensory innervation in the hedgehog snout epidermis, *Erinaceus europaeus. Scripta Med.* 54:113–126, 1981.

MALINOVSKY, L., AND PAC, L. *Morphology of Sensory Corpuscles in Mammals.* Opuscular Morphologia 74, University of Brno, 1982.

MALINOVSKY, L., AND SOMMEROVA, J. Sensory nerve endings in the human labia minora pudendi and their variability. *Folia Morphol. (Praha)* 21:351–354, 1973.

MALINOVSKY, L., AND SOMMEROVA, J. Sensory nerve endings in the penis of the green monkey (*Cercopithecus aethiops*). *Z. Mikrosk. Anat. Forsch.* 91:94–104, 1977.

MERKEL, F. Tastzellen und Tastkorperchen bei den Hauttieren und beim Menschen. *Arch. Mikrosk. Anat. Entwickl.* 11:636–652, 1875.

MILLER, M. R., RALSTON, H. J., AND KASAHARA, M. The pattern of cutaneous innervation of the human hand, foot and breast, in: *Advances in Biology of Skin,* Vol. 1, *Cutaneous Innervation* (W. MONTAGNA, ed.), Pergamon Press, New York, 1960, pp. 1–16.

MITCHELL, J. C. Distribution of dehydrogenases in the skin of the rhesus monkey. *J. Histochem. Cytochem.* 13:668–676, 1965.

MONTAGNA, W., AND BROOKHART, J. M. Cutaneous innervation and modalities of cutaneous sensibility. *J. Invest. Dermatol.* 69:1–189, 1977.

MONTAGNA, W., AND YUN, J. S. The skin of primates VII. The skin of the great bush baby (*Galago grassicaudaticus*). *Am J. Phys. Anthropol.* 20:149–165, 1962.

MULLER, S. A., AND WINKELMANN, R. K. Cutaneous nerve changes in zoster. *J. Invest. Dermatol.* 52:71–77, 1969.

MUNGER, B. L. Patterns of organization of peripheral sensory receptors, in: *Handbook of Sensory Physiology*, Vol. I, *Principles of Receptor Physiology* (W. R. LOEWENSTEIN, ed.), Springer, Berlin, 1971, pp. 523–569.

MUNGER, B. L. Multiple afferent innervation of primate facial hairs: Henry Head and Max von Frey revisited. *Brain Res. Rev.* 4:1–43, 1982.

MUNGER, B. L., AND HALATA, Z. The sensory innervation of primate facial skin. I. Hairy Skin. *Brain Res. Rev.* 5(1):45–80, 1983.

PEASE, D. C., AND QUILLIAM, T. A. Electron microscopy of the Pacinian corpuscle. *J. Biophys. Biochem. Cytol.* 3:331–342, 1957.

PETERSON, H. A., WINKELMANN, R. K., AND COVENTRY, M. B. Nerve endings in the hip joint of the cat: Their morphology distribution and density. *J. Bone Joint Surg.* 54:333–343, 1972.

PINKUS, F. Ueber einen Eisher unbekannten Nebenapparat am Haarsystem des Menschen. Haarscheiben. *Dermatol Z.* 9:465–469, 1902.

RANVIER, L. Nouvelles recherches sur les organes du tact *C. R. Acad. Sci. [D] (Paris)* 91:1087–1089, 1880.

ROBERTSON, D. M., AND WINKELMANN, R. K. A whole-mount cholinesterase technique for demonstrating corneal nerves: Observations in the albino rabbit. *Invest. Ophthalmol.* 9:710–715, 1970.

ROWDEN, G., CONNELLY, E. M., AND WINKELMANN, R. K. Cutaneous histiocytosis X: The presence of S-100 protein and its use in diagnosis. *Arch Dermatol.* 119:553–559, 1983.

SAURAT, S. H., CHAVEZ, P., CARRAUX, P., AND DIDIER, J., L. A human monoclonal antibody reacting with Merkel cells: Immunofluorescence, immunoperoxidase and immunoelectron microscopy. *J. Invest Dermatol.* 81:249–252, 1983.

SAXOD, R. Activite cholinesterasique des corpuscles sensorials cutanes de Herbst et de Grandry. *Histochemie* 34:43–63, 1973.

SAXOD, R. Combination of cholinesterase staining of nerves and stereoscopic viewing for three dimensional study of skin innervation in whole mounts. *J. Invest. Dermatol.* 70:95–97, 1978a.

SAXOD, R. Development of cutaneous sensory receptors in birds, in: *Handbook of Sensory Physiology*, Vol. IX, *Development of Sensory Systems* (W. R. LOEWENSTEIN, ed.), Springer, Berlin, 1978b, pp. 338–410.

SINCLAIR, D. C. *Mechanisms of Cutaneous Sensation.* Oxford University Press, New York, 1981.

STEIGLEDER, G. K., AND SCHULTIS, K. Zur Histochemie der Meissnerchen Tastkorperchen. *Acta Neuroveg.* 18:335–343, 1968.

WEDDELL, G., AND PALLIE, W. Studies on the innervation of skin II. The number, size and distribution of hairs, hair follicles, and orifices of the rabbit ear. *J. Anat.* 89:175–188, 1955.

WEDDELL, G., PALMER, E., AND PALLIE, W. The morphology of peripheral nerve terminations in the skin. *Q. J. Micra. Sci.* 95:483–501, 1954.

WINKELMANN, R. K. The mucocutaneous endorgan. *A.M.A. Arch. Dermatol.* 76:225–235, 1957.

WINKELMANN, R. K. The endorgan of feline skin. A morphological and histochemical study. *Am. J. Anat.* 107:281–290, 1960a.

WINKELMANN, R. K. *Nerve Endings in Normal and Pathologic Skin.* Charles C Thomas, Springfield, IL, 1960b.

WINKELMANN, R. K. Nerve endings in the skin of the gorilla. *J. Comp. Neurol.* 116:145–155, 1961.

WINKELMANN, R. K. The mammalian endorgan in oral tissue of the cat. *J. Dent. Res.* 41:207–212, 1962a.

WINKELMANN, R. K. Cutaneous sensory endorgans of some anthropoid apes. *Science* 136:384–386, 1962b.

WINKELMANN, R. K. Cholinesterases. *Ann. N.Y. Acad. Sci.* 100:224–434, 1963a.

WINKELMANN, R. K. Nerve endings in the skin of primates, in: *Evolutionary and Genetic Biology of Primates*, Vol. 1 (J. BUETTNER-JANUSH, ed.), Academic Press, New York, 1963b, pp. 229–259.

WINKELMANN, R. K. Nerve endings of the North American oppossum (*Didelphis virginiana*). A comparison with nerve endings of primates. *Am. J. Phys. Anthropol.* 22:253–258, 1964.

WINKELMANN, R. K. Innervation of the skin: Notes on a comparison of primate and marsupial nerve endings, in: *Biology of the Skin and Hair Growth* (A. G. LYNE AND B. F. SHORT, eds.), Elsevier, New York, 1965, pp. 171–182.

WINKELMANN, R. K. Some unusual histochemical properties of kangaroo. *J. Invest. Dermatol.* 46:446–452, 1966.

WINKELMANN, R. K. New methods for the study of nerve endings, in: *The Skin* (E. HELWIG, ed.), Williams & Wilkins, Baltimore, 1971, pp. 112–126.

WINKELMANN, R. K. The Merkel cell system and comparison with the neurosecretory or APUD system. *J. Invest. Dermatol.* 69:44–46, 1977.

WINKELMANN, R. K. The histochemistry of the Merkel cell neuroepithelial endings of cat and rabbit skin and oral mucosa. *Acta Dermatol. Ven.* 62:383–387, 1982.

WINKELMANN, R. K. AND BREATHNACH, A. The Merkel cell. *J. Invest. Dermatol.* 60:2–15, 1973.

WINKELMANN, R. K., AND MYERS, T. T. The histochemistry and morphology of the cutaneous sensory endorgans of the chicken. *J. Comp. Neurol.* 117:27–35, 1961.

WINKELMANN, R. K. AND OSMENT, L. O. The Vater–Pacini corpuscle in the skin of the human fingertip. *Arch. Dermatol.* 73:116–122, 1956.

WINKELMANN, R. K, WOLFF, K., AND PIERCE, J. Removal of epidermis with sodium bromide for cholinesterase staining of dermal nerve. *Stain Technol.* 42:214–215, 1967.

ZOLLMAN, P. E., AND WINKELMANN, R. K. The sensory innervation of the common North American raccoon (*Procyon lotor*). *J Comp. Neurol.* 119:149–157, 1962.

3
Primary Afferents and Hyperalgesia

JAMES N. CAMPBELL AND RICHARD A. MEYER

A. *Introduction*

Pain has two aspects. The first is its function as a warning system to ward off immediate threats. It is, in a sense, a necessary evil that serves to warn the organism of injury. But pain has another face, which we term hyperalgesia—the perceptual companion of inflammation, be it from infection, the mundane abrasion, a burn of the skin, or from the causalgia that mysteriously complicates only certain nerve injuries and cripples its victim. Save for the latter condition, where the pain seems to serve no apparent purpose, hyperalgesia seems not to be part of a warning system but instead is a reminder that something is wrong. A remarkable resetting of the threshold for pain occurs: the inflamed skin may become the source of increased pain merely by being lightly touched or gently warmed. The victim arduously protects the hyperalgesic part, which we infer may ultimately promote healing.

For reasons that will become apparent, we discuss separately primary and secondary hyperalgesia. Primary hyperalgesia refers to changes that occur within the site of injury, whereas secondary hyperalgesia refers to changes that occur outside the site of injury. Both are manifest by the lowering of threshold for pain, augmented pain with suprathreshold stimuli, and spontaneous pain.

JAMES N. CAMPBELL AND RICHARD A. MEYER • Department of Neurosurgery and Applied Physics Laboratory, The Johns Hopkins University, Baltimore, Maryland 21205.

B. Peripheral Neural Substrates That Subserve Pain Sensation

Before considering mechanisms of hyperalgesia, it is useful to review peripheral neural mechanisms of pain sensation in the normal state. Studies in monkeys, humans, and other species have shown that there exists a specialized class of C and A fibers in the peripheral nerve, termed nociceptors, that encode the occurrence, intensity, duration, and location of noxious and near-noxious stimuli (Adriaensen *et al.*, 1983; Beck *et al.*, 1974; Beitel and Dubner, 1976; Bessou and Perl, 1969; Burgess and Perl, 1967; Campbell *et al.*, 1979; Croze *et al.*, 1976; Georgopoulos, 1976; Gybels *et al.*, 1979; Kumazawa and Perl, 1977; LaMotte and Campbell, 1978; Meyer and Campbell, 1981a; Torebjork and Hallin, 1974).

This section summarizes the neurophysiological studies done in anesthetized monkeys and psychophysical studies done in humans to determine the role of nociceptors in pain sensation. This correlative analysis is particularly useful for the following reasons: (1) studies of other somatosensory modalities have suggested a close correspondence between peripheral coding mechanisms in man and monkey (LaMotte and Mountcastle, 1975; Mountcastle *et al.*, 1972; Talbot *et al.*, 1968); (2) neurophysiological studies in anesthetized monkeys allow for high-quality recordings of a large number of fibers (compared, for example, to the difficulty of obtaining stable recordings for several hours in awake humans); and (3) psychophysical studies done in humans provide a richer, more reliable source of information than those possible in other species.

Pain can be produced by a variety of experimental stimuli; however, heat has been the modality chosen by most investigators. The intensity of heat stimuli can be controlled precisely (Meyer *et al.*, 1976), and the amount of pain and the response of primary afferents to heat can be reliably reproduced.

Three categories of receptors responsive to heat stimuli applied to the skin have been identified: warm fibers, C fibers responsive to heat and mechanical stimuli (CMHs), and A fibers sensitive to heat and mechanical stimuli (AMHs). The properties of warm fibers, summarized in Table I, are such that they are well suited for coding for the sensation of warmth but not pain. They show exquisite sensitivity to gentle warming of the skin (Darian-Smith *et al.*, 1979; Konietzny and Hensel, 1975). In fact, at usual ambient skin temperature, they have ongoing activity that is readily suppressed by cooling of the receptive field. Warm fibers have punctate single receptive fields and have a monotonically increasing response (Figure 1) to stimuli of increasing but nonnoxious intensity (LaMotte and Campbell, 1978). However, as shown in Figure 2, for stimuli greater than about 45°C, the response changes notably. The fiber response ends before the stimulus ends, and the total evoked response decreases. This nonmonotonic response provides evidence that warm fibers do not code for the painfulness of heat stimuli.

The CMHs and AMHs constitute the nociceptors. Intense stimuli, whether mechanical or heat, are needed to activate these receptors. Additionally, they

TABLE I
Properties of Heat-Sensitive Primary Afferents in the Monkey[a]

Property	Warm fibers	CMHs[b]	AMHs Type I[c]	AMHs Type II[d]
Receptive field area (mm^2)	<1 (302)[e]	18 ±3 (34)	37 ± 4 (44)	—
Spontaneous activity (impulses/s)	1.6 ± 0.1 at 34°C (47)[e]	None	None	None
Heat threshold (°C)	<1°C above background[b]	43.6 ±0.6 (34)	>49	43 (15)
Response to ice	Suppression of Spontaneous activity[b,e]	0–2 impulses/s	None	—
Mechanical threshold (bars)	>27 (16)[b,e]	6.0 ± 0.6 (34)	3.5 ± 0.3 (44)	0.4 g (9)
Conduction velocity (m/s)	1.2 ± 0.1 (50)[e]	0.8 ±0.1 (22)	31.1 ± 1.5 (43)	15.2 ± 9.9 (15)

[a] Values are means ± S.E.M. Numbers in parentheses are *n*.
[b] From LaMotte and Campbell (1978).
[c] From Campbell *et al.* (1979).
[d] For afferents innervating the face; from Dubner *et al.* (1977).
[e] From Darian-Smith *et al.* (1979).

have a monotonically increasing response to stimuli of increasing noxious intensity. A traditional view of the function of these two types of fibers is that AMHs encode so-called first pain, otherwise known as pricking pain, and CMHs encode burning pain, otherwise known as second pain (Campbell and Lamotte, 1983; Lewis and Pochin, 1937).

This formulation, however, has proved too simple. Instead, it appears that there are certain regional differences in the behavior of CMHs (Campbell and Meyer, 1983), and also there are at least two types of AMHs. That there are two types of AMHs was noted by Dubner and colleagues (1977) in studies of nociceptive afferents that innervate the monkey face. The properties of each type are shown in Table I. The more common type, which comprised 78% of the sample of AMHs that Dubner *et al.* (1977) studied, have a high threshold to heat. Following injury to their receptive field, however, they become remarkably sensitive to heat. We propose that these fibers be called *type I AMHs. Type II AMHs* have a much lower heat threshold. The Dubner group showed that these type II AMHs supplied the primary afferent input leading to escape responses from heat stimuli applied to the face (Dubner *et al.*, 1977). Type II AMHs probably provide the afferent input to signal first pain. This is discussed in more detail later.

In studying afferents responsive to heat stimuli that innervate the gla-

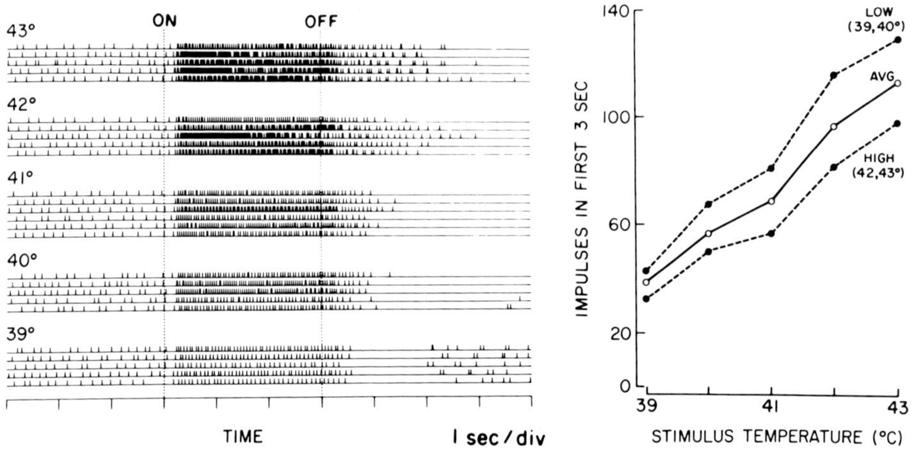

FIGURE 1. Responses of a warm fiber innervating the hand to stimuli of 39 to 43°C presented at 25-s interstimulus intervals. Each stimulus occurred with equal frequency and was preceded by every other stimulus an equal number of times. Within these constraints, the order of presentation was randomized. Left panel: Impulse train replicas (vertical tics) of responses on each trial (each horizontal line) and grouped by the temperature of the stimulus delivered. Right panel: Stimulus–response functions constructed from data shown in left panel. The solid line represents the mean cumulative impulse count during each stimulus averaged for all presentations of the same intensity. The dotted lines represent the stimulus–response functions obtained when the preceding stimulus was of low intensity (39 and 40°C) versus when the preceding stimulus was of high intensity (42 and 43°C). Base temperature was 38°C. (From LaMotte and Campbell, 1978.)

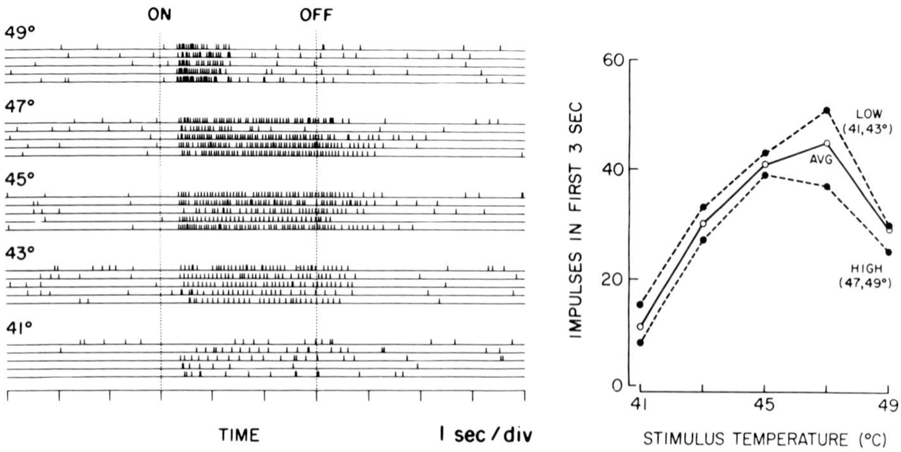

FIGURE 2. Responses of a warm fiber to stimuli of 41 to 49°C. Same paradigm and format as in Figure 1. (From LaMotte and Campbell, 1978.)

brous skin of the hand, we have found no type II AMHs. The type I AMHs, in contrast, are found readily, and, as will become clear, the characteristics of these fibers are important to consider in the discussion of hyperalgesia (Campbell *et al.*, 1979; Fitzgerald and Lynn, 1977). The conduction velocity of type I AMHs had a mean of 31 m/s and ranged as high as 55 m/s. Thus, many of these fibers might be more correctly considered to be A-β fibers rather than A-δ fibers. These fibers, though initially relatively insensitive to heat, develop a markedly enhanced sensitivity following a thermal injury to their receptive field. Figure 3 shows the development of such an enhanced response of a typical type I fiber to repeated 3-s 53°C stimuli. The heat threshold before and after injury to the receptive field of the type I AMHs is shown in Figure 4. Prior to injury, 88% had thresholds greater than 49°C, whereas after injury, 67% had thresholds less than 45°C. Thus, type I AMHs become dramatically sensitized following a heat injury.

As previously noted, innervation of the glabrous skin of the hand by type II AMHs has not been reported. The response to a 45°C stimulus of two type II AMHs that innervated the hairy skin of the arm are shown in Figure 5. In contrast to the type I AMHs, the type II AMHs have a short receptor utilization time (time between stimulus onset and initiation of the first action potential) and also show more activity at the onset of the stimulus. These type II AMHs are thus ideal candidates for coding for first pain sensation on the hairy skin. The first pain–second pain sequence in humans has not been observed for stimuli presented to the glabrous skin of the hand with stimulus intensities up to 51°C (Campbell and LaMotte, 1983). This is in keeping with the failure to find type II AMHs in the glabrous skin of monkeys.

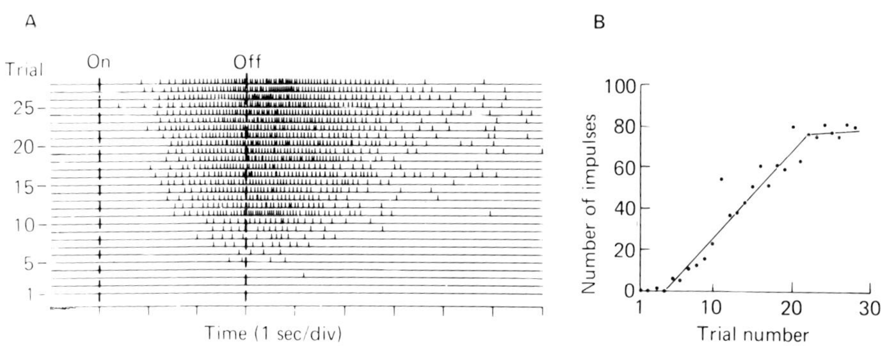

FIGURE 3. Response of a type I AMH to a stimulus of 53°C, 3 s duration, repeated every 28 s. The response increased with repeated exposures to the stimulus. The base temperature was 38°C. A: Neural impulse-train replica. Each horizontal line corresponds to one trial, and the trials are arranged in sequence from the bottom to the top. Each vertical tick corresponds to a neural impulse, and the vertical dashed lines indicate the times at which the stimulus was turned on or off. B: Sensitization curve. The total evoked response is plotted as a function of the trial number. The total evoked response is the cumulative number of impulses evoked during the 28 s following the beginning of the stimulus. (From Campbell *et al.*, 1979.)

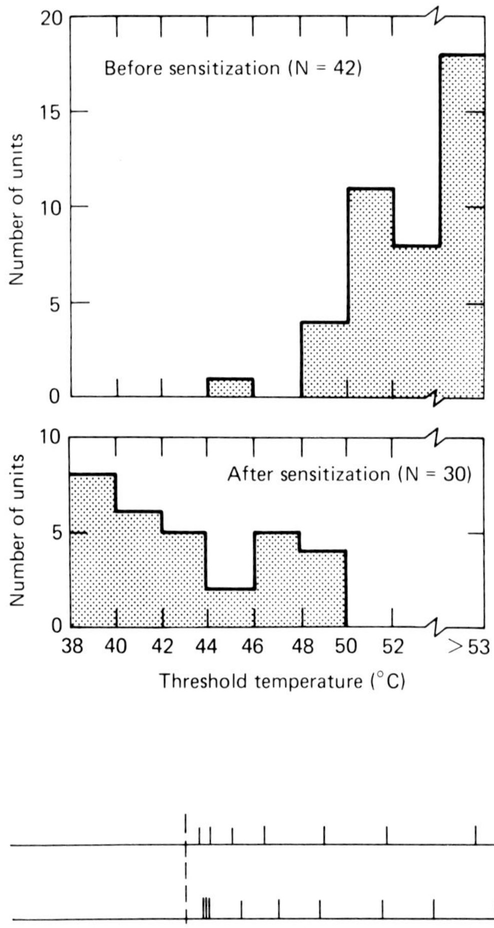

FIGURE 4. Histograms of thermal thresholds for the type I AMHs before and after sensitization. The heat thresholds of all the AMHs decreased following sensitization. The column ">53°C" corresponds to those fibers that did not respond to the maximum stimulus in the threshold series. (From Campbell *et al.*, 1979.)

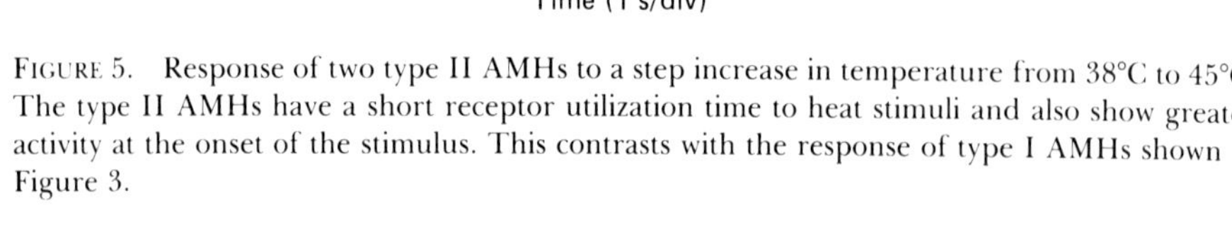

FIGURE 5. Response of two type II AMHs to a step increase in temperature from 38°C to 45°C. The type II AMHs have a short receptor utilization time to heat stimuli and also show greater activity at the onset of the stimulus. This contrasts with the response of type I AMHs shown in Figure 3.

The long receptor utilization time to heat noted in type I AMHs does not apply to mechanical stimuli. Figure 6 shows the typical response to graded constant-force mechanical stimuli of increasing intensity. Comparable studies of type II AMHs have not as yet been done.

The properties of CMHs are listed in Table I. The heat threshold (near 43°C) is less than that of type I AMHs and about the same as type II AMHs. Unlike warm fibers, CMHs display a monotonically increasing response to heat stimuli above 45°C (Figure 7). In addition, stimulus interaction is a prominent property of CMHs (LaMotte and Campbell, 1978). As shown in Figure 7, the response varies inversely with the intensity of previous stimulation.

It is likely that CMHs, not AMHs, code for the intensity of pain evoked by stimuli up to 49°C applied to the glabrous skin of the hand. This may be inferred, in part, by default, since the AMHs found on the glabrous skin of the hand are type I and typically have no responses below 50°C in the absence of injury. Another line of evidence comes from comparing the normalized stimulus–response functions of CMHs to the ratings of magnitude of pain in

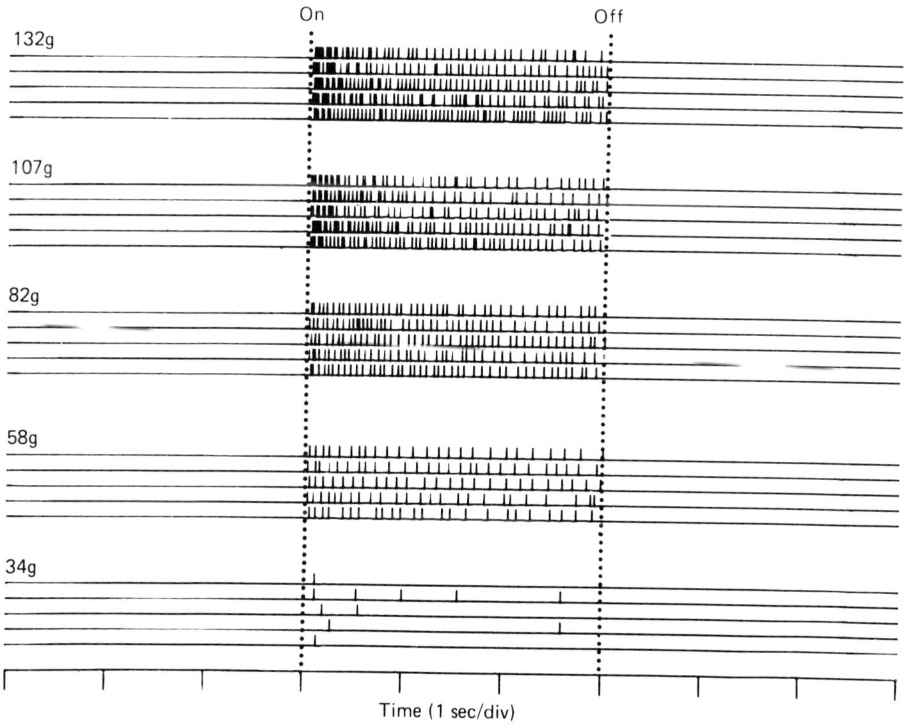

FIGURE 6. Response of a type I AMH to mechanical stimuli of constant force. Each stimulus was a step indentation of the skin of constant force lasting 3 s and presenting every 28 s. The force of indentation was varied randomly from 34 to 132 g. Base force was 10 g, and probe size was 0.8 mm diameter. Format similar to Figure 1. (From Campbell *et al.*, 1979.)

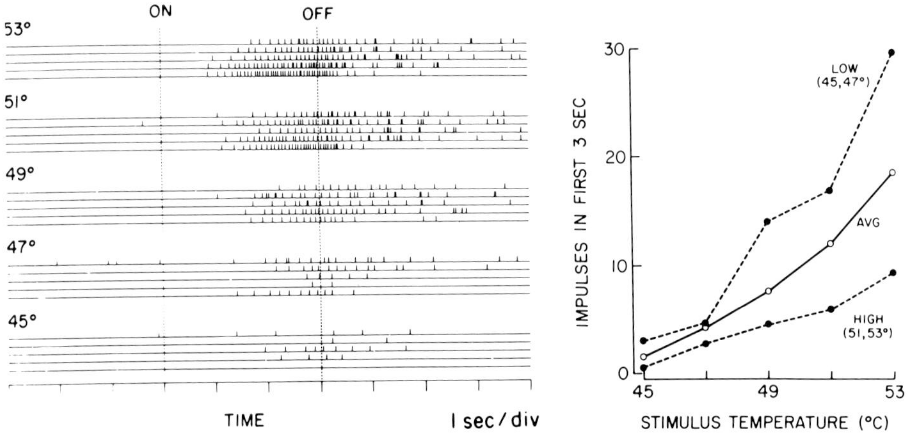

FIGURE 7. Responses of an unmyelinated nociceptive fiber (CMH) innervating the hairy skin of the forearm to stimuli of 45 to 53°C. Format same as that described for Figure 1. (From LaMotte and Campbell, 1978.)

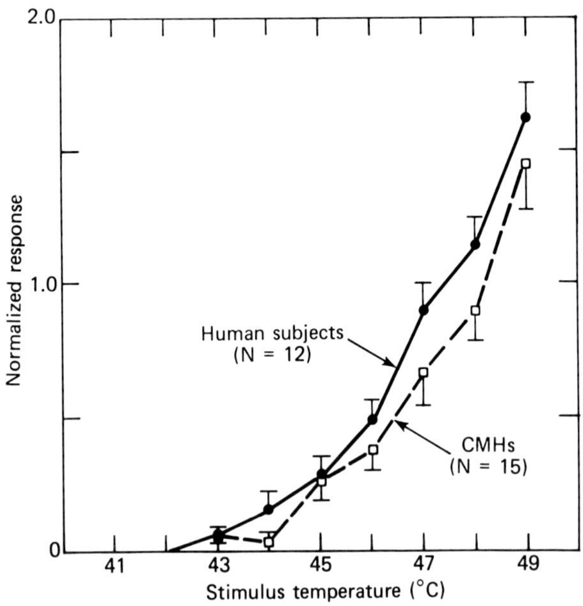

FIGURE 8. Normalized response of human subjects and CMHs exposed to identical stimuli. The first stimulus of the heat sequence was always 45°C. The remaining nine stimuli ranged from 41 to 49°C in 1°C increments and were presented in random order. The stimuli were 3 s in duration and were presented every 30 s. The response to a given stimulus was normalized by dividing by the response to the first 45°C stimulus for each subject or fiber. The close match between the curves supports a role of CMHs in pain sensation. (From Meyer and Campbell, 1981b.)

human subjects when each is given the same stimuli (Meyer and Campbell, 1981b). As shown in Figure 8, the normalized stimulus–response functions are quite similar. Additional evidence to support this concept includes the following observations:

1. Selective A-fiber (pressure cuff) or C-fiber (local anesthetic) blocks indicate that C-fiber function is necessary for thermal pain perception near pain threshold on the glabrous skin (Sinclair, 1981; Torebjork and Hallin, 1973).
2. Stimulus interaction effects observed in psychophysical experiments (LaMotte and Campbell, 1978) are also observed in recordings from CMHs (for example, see Figure 7).
3. The latency to pain sensation on glabrous skin following step temperature changes is long enough that C fibers could be responsible (Campbell and LaMotte, 1983).
4. Intraneural electrical stimulation of single identified CMHs in humans elicits pain (Torebjork and Ochoa, 1980).

C. *Afferents Encoding Primary Hyperalgesia*

This preliminary discussion of peripheral neural mechanisms of pain when stimuli are presented to the uninjured skin brings us to a discussion of the neural mechanism of hyperalgesia. An obvious issue at the outset is: Can hyperalgesia be explained by a commensurate change in the sensitivity of the nociceptors? Hints that such might be the case arose from studies of Bessou and Perl (1969), Beck *et al.* (1974), Beitel and Dubner (1976), and others who described sensitization of C-fiber nocicepetors to heat stimuli. The findings of a decrease in heat threshold, an augmented response to suprathreshold stimuli, and, on occasion, spontaneous activity correlated qualitatively with the properties of hyperalgesia (see Table II).

To resolve the issue of which if any nociceptors code for primary hyperalgesia, we performed a correlational analysis of psychophysical studies of hyperalgesia in humans with responses of nociceptors (CHMs and type I AMHs) in monkeys when each was given identical heat stimuli to the glabrous skin of the hand before and after a 53°C, 30-s burn (Meyer and Campbell,

TABLE II
Comparison of Characteristics of Hyperalgesia and Sensitization

Hyperalgesia (subject response)	Sensitization (fiber response)
Decreased pain threshold	Decreased threshold for response
Increased pain to suprathreshold stimuli	Increased response to suprathreshold stimuli
Spontaneous pain	Spontaneous activity

1981c). The burn led to prominent hyperalgesia in the human subjects (Figure 9A). The 41°C stimulus after injury was as painful as the 49°C stimulus prior to injury. The CMHs showed a decrement of response following the burn (Figure 9C), whereas type I AMHs were markedly sensitized (Figure 9B). As shown in Figure 10, the magnitude of pain during the burn was sustained at a high level. The CMHs responded vigorously during the first 3 s of the 30-s burn stimulus but then rapidly adapted. The AMHs showed the reverse pattern, being initially unresponsive but then showing a more vigorous response. In this same study, an A-fiber block after the burn resulted in a substantial decrease in the pain to heat stimulli applied to the burn site.

These data suggest two conclusions: (1) type I AMHs, not CMHs, code for the thermal hyperalgesia that follows a burn to the glabrous skin of the hand, and (2) type I AMHs probably code for the enduring pain associated with a sustained high-intensity heat stimulus such as 53°C for 30 s. These results caused confusion concerning the role of CMHs in view of previous

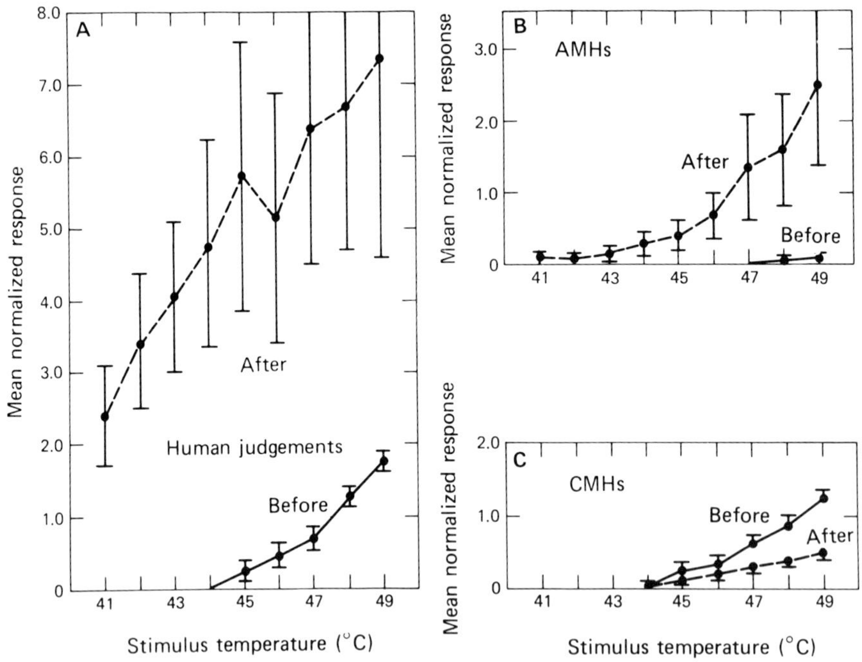

FIGURE 9. Normalized response to heat sequence (described in Figure 8) before and after a 53°C, 30-s burn to the glabrous skin of the hand. A: Human judgments ($n = 8$). B: A-fiber nociceptive afferents (type I AMHs) in monkey ($n = 14$). C: C-fiber nociceptive afferents (CMHs) in monkey ($n = 15$). Standard error bars are shown. The burn resulted in an increase in the magnitude of pain (hyperalgesia) in human subjects that was matched by an enhanced response (sensitization) in the type I AMHs. In contrast, the burn resulted in a decreased sensitivity in the CMHs. (From Meyer and Campbell, 1981c.)

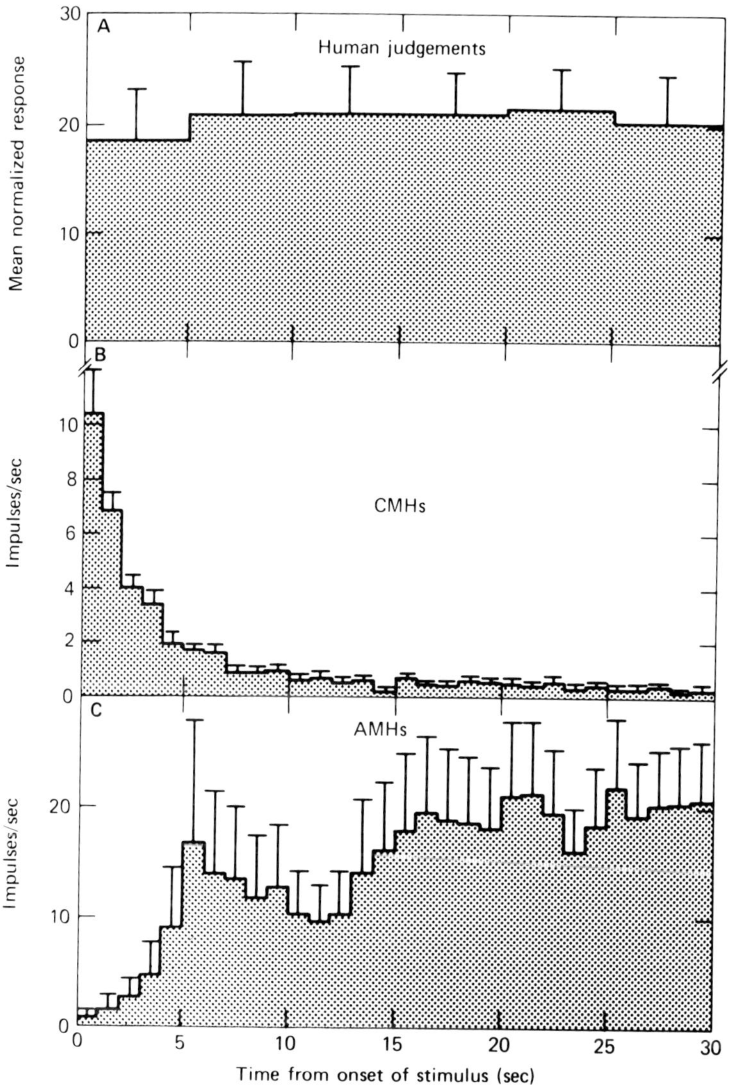

FIGURE 10. Histogram of mean responses during the 53°C, 30-s burn. A: Human judgments ($n = 8$). B: C-fiber nociceptive afferents ($n = 15$). C: A-fiber nociceptive afferents ($n = 14$). Standard error bars are shown. The pain was intense throughout the stimulus. The brisk response of the CMHs at the beginning of the stimulus adapted to a low rate after 5 s. The response of the type I AMHs increased during the first 5 s and remained at a high level throughout the stimulus. (From Meyer and Campbell, 1981c.)

observations that CMHs may, in certain instances, sensitize. This confusion seems to have been resolved by the finding that sensitization of unmyelinated nociceptive afferents in monkey varies with skin type (Campbell and Meyer, 1983). The CMHs that innervate hairy skin sensitize readily, whereas those that innervate the glabrous skin of the hand will not sensitize regardless of the stimuli used. For example, repeated application of a sequence of 41°C to 49°C 3-s stimuli resulted in sensitization of hairy skin CMHs but did not alter the response of glabrous skin CMHs (Figure 11). The difference could not be explained by a difference in the initial sensitivity of the two types of fibers. Both the heat threshold and the response to the first heat stimulus (45°C) were similar. The fact that CMHs that innervate hairy skin sensitize leads to the possibility that CMHs might play a role in primary hyperalgesia in hairy skin. In a series of papers, LaMotte and colleagues (LaMotte *et al.,* 1982, 1983) have demonstrated that the decrease in heat pain threshold following a mild heat injury (50°C, 100-s burn) to the hairy skin of human subjects correlated with the decrease in threshold of CMHs in monkey. However, the painfulness of suprathreshold stimuli (e.g., 49°C) was not greatly different before and after the injury, whereas the response of the CMHs to the 49°C was greatly

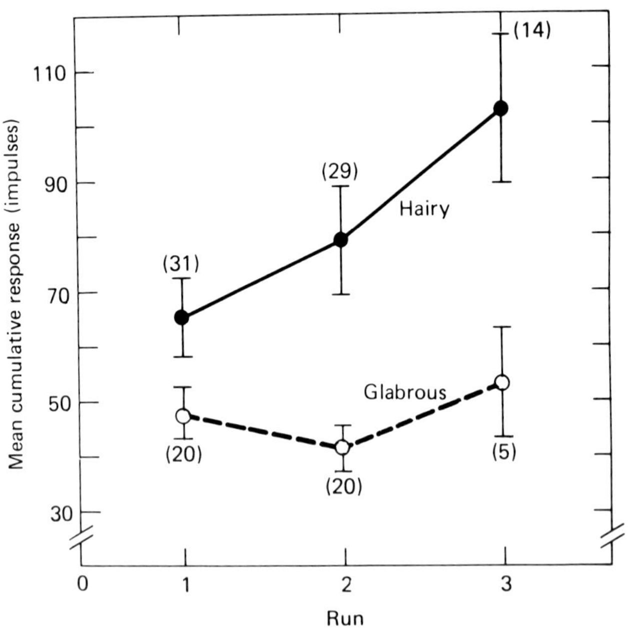

FIGURE 11. Mean cumulative response of hairy skin and glabrous skin C-fiber nociceptive afferents to the heat sequence described in Figure 8 as a function of run number. Each run was separated by a 10-min stimulus-free interval. For fibers innervating hairy skin (solid line), the cumulative response increased significantly (sensitized) with repeated runs, whereas for glabrous skin (dashed line), the response did not change significantly. (From Campbell and Meyer, 1983.)

augmented. It might be noted that type I AMHs on hairy skin, as with glabrous skin, also become sensitized by intense heat stimuli. Thus, it appears that both CMHs and AMHs play a role in signaling primary hyperalgesia in hairy skin. The relative role of CMHs and AMHs may be dictated by the intensity of the injury.

The biochemical basis for sensitization and primary hyperalgesia is not well understood. Chapman *et al.* (1961) found that kininlike substances were involved. Since hyperalgesia develops within minutes after a 53°C, 30-s burn (Meyer and Campbell, 1981c), it is probable that early events in the inflammatory process are involved. The so-called nonsteroidal antiinflammatory drugs may, at least in part, control pain by reducing inflammation (Capetola *et al.*, 1983). Presumably, prostaglandin synthesis is inhibited through inhibition of cyclooxygenase (Kuehl and Egan, 1980; Lands and Hanel, 1983). Beck and Handwerker (1974; Handwerker, 1976) reported that close arterial injection of bradykinin or prostaglandin E_2 results in sensitization of CMHs to heat stimuli. However, no similar study has been done with AMHs.

We recently determined a means to sensitize reversibly nociceptors to heat stimuli. The response properties of nociceptors were found to vary depending on the choice of general anesthetic agent (Campbell *et al.*, 1984): CMHs and AMHs studied in monkeys under anesthesia with inhaled halothane and N_2O had greater responses than those studied in monkeys under anesthesia with intravenous pentobarbital, as shown in Figure 12. Through subsequent experiments, it was determined that this difference derived from sensitizing effects of halothane. Figure 13 shows an example of varying doses of halothane on the response of a CMH to repeated 47°C, 3-s stimuli. The effect of halothane was dose related and reversible. Halothane directly affects the nociceptive receptor, as its effects could not be explained by alteration of sympathetic tone, cutaneous perfusion, or blood pressure. To date, we do not know if the effects of halothane extend to other types of primary afferent or whether other anesthetic agents exert a similar effect. An understanding of the molecular mechanism by which halothane sensitizes nociceptors could aid in understanding how skin injury causes sensitization.

D. Characteristics of Secondary Hyperalgesia

Although there is general agreement on the nature of primary hyperalgesia as described above, descriptions of secondary hyperalgesia reported by Lewis (1933, 1935, 1942) and Hardy (Hardy *et al.*, 1950, 1952) differ. Lewis found hyperalgesia to mechanical stimuli but reported that a "lowering of pain threshold to heat is suspected to occur from time to time; but the effect, when present, is slight" (Lewis, 1942, p. 70). He proposed that secondary hyperalgesia resulted from sensitization of adjoining "pain receptors" by way of the "nocifensor system." The nocifensor system was viewed to be independent of sensory afferents and autonomic nerve fibers. Activation of nocicep-

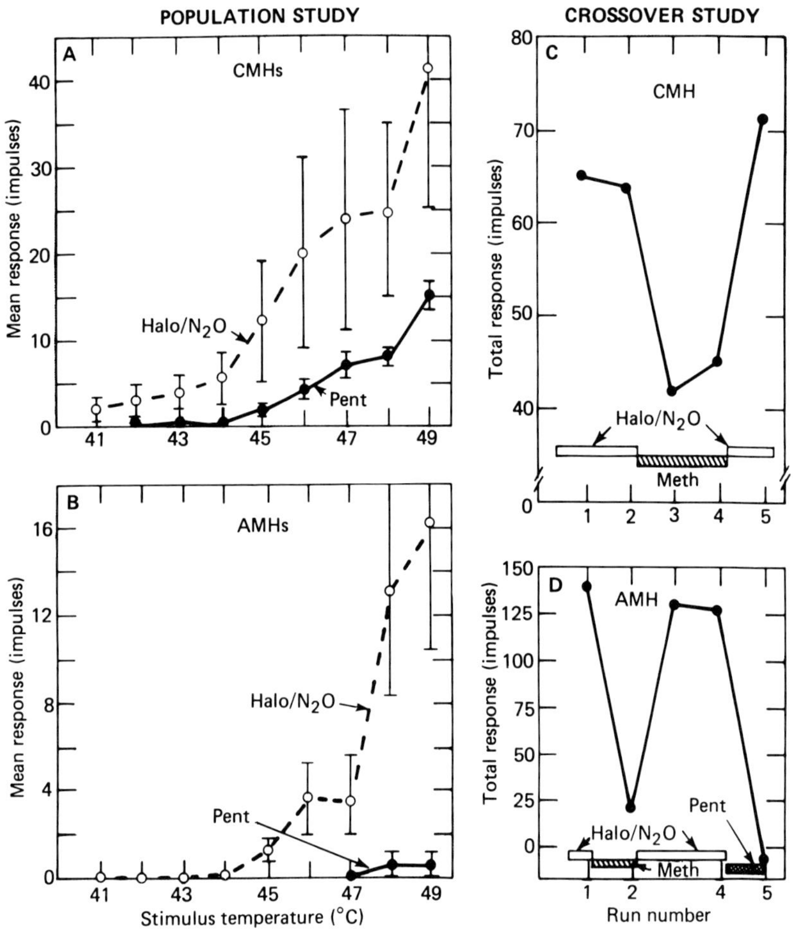

FIGURE 12. Comparison of the responses of C-fiber (CMH) and type I A-fiber (AMH) nociceptive primary afferents to heat stimuli under two different anesthetic conditions. A: The response of 32 CMHs in monkeys anesthetized with pentobarbital (3–6 mg/kg per h) was compared with that of 12 CMHs in monkeys anesthetized with a combination of halothane (0.8%) and N_2O (67%). The responses under halothane/N_2O were substantially greater. B: The response of 26 AMHs in pentobarbital-anesthetized monkeys was compared with that of 23 AMHs in halothane/N_2O-anesthetized monkeys. Again the response under halothane/N_2O was greater. C: Results of a typical anesthetic crossover study of a CMH. The cumulative response to the ten 41–49°C stimuli is shown. The sequence was repeated with 10-min stimulus-free intervals. The anesthetic conditions are indicated by the horizontal bars. After run 2, the halothane/N_2O was stopped, and anesthesia was maintained with repeated infusions of methohexital (2 mg/kg delivered approximately every 2–3 min). Immediately after run 4, the methohexital infusion was stopped, and the halothane/N_2O was restarted. The response of this CMH was about 70% greater under halothane/N_2O anesthesia. D: Results of a typical anesthetic crossover study of a type I AMH. The paradigm was similar to that described in C except after the fourth run halothane/N_2O anesthesia was replaced by intravenous infusion of pentobarbital (2 mg/kg bolus) rather than methohexital. The response of this AMH under halothane/N_2O was more than five times that under the barbiturates. (From Campbell *et al.*, 1984.)

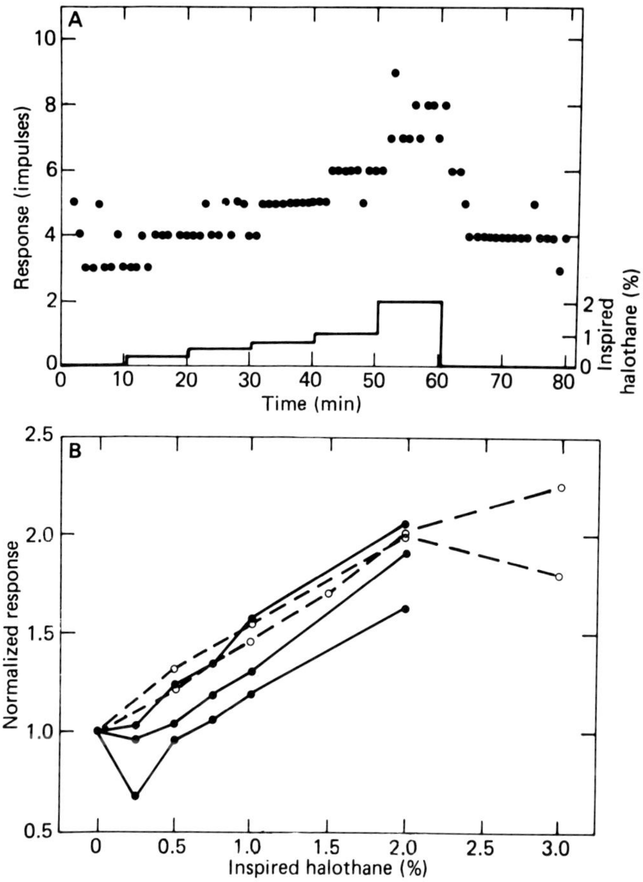

FIGURE 13. Response of CMHs to heat stimuli in monkeys anesthetized with pentobarbital as a function of different concentrations of inspired halothane. A: Response of a typical CMH to a 3-s 47°C stimulus repeated every 60 s, showing the time course of effects of halothane. As halothane was increased in steps from 0 to 2%, the response of the CMH increased with a lag period of about 3 min. When the halothane was stopped, the response of the CMHs promptly returned to base line. B: Dose–response curves showing the response of 5 CMHs to heat stimuli as a function of different halothane concentrations. Responses were normalized by dividing by the response at 0% halothane concentration. In three CMHs (solid lines), 45°C or 47°C 3-s stimuli were repeated every 60 s while the halothane concentration was changed. For two other CMHs (dashed lines), the cumulative response to the sequence of 41–49°C stimuli (see Figure 12) was obtained for each dose of halothane. For these two CMHs, the changes in halothane concentration were made at the beginning of the 10-min stimulus-free interval that separated each run. The response of the CMHs increased as a function of halothane dose regardless of the stimulus paradigm used. (From Campbell *et al.*, 1984.)

tors triggered a response reflexively (the axon reflex) in the nocifensor system, which branched into adjoining tissue. Activation of these nocifensor branches led to release from their terminals of substances that in turn sensitized and activated the nociceptors that innervated the adjoining area, thus leading to secondary hyperalgesia. By Lewis's formulation, therefore, secondary hyperalgesia was similar to primary hyperalgesia in that both resulted from sensitization of nociceptors.

In support of Lewis's contention, it is clear that there are changes associated with injury that depend on the integrity of innervation of the tissues. Notably, the flare response is neurogenic. The flare disappears several days after innervation to the skin is interrupted (Chapman *et al.*, 1961). Presumably, substances are released from nerve terminals in association with nociceptor activation that lead to surrounding vascular dilatation (thus, the flare).

Like Lewis, Hardy believed that primary hyperalgesia was caused by sensitization of what we now term nociceptors. However, Hardy believed that the threshold for pain to both mechanical heat stimuli in the secondary region was not decreased, but rather that at and above threshold pain was more evident. He discounted the so-called nocifensor system. Instead, he postulated that changes accounting for secondary hyperalgesia occurred in the dorsal horn of the spinal cord. Input of the sensitized nociceptors from the area of injury leads to activation of internuncial neurons, which in turn sensitize dorsal horn "pain" neurons that innervate the skin surrounding the region of injury. Hardy reasoned that much of the input from primary nociceptive afferents was subliminal, i.e., not sufficient to activate the second-order (or higher) neurons. This input, however, results in pain when these second-order neurons are sensitized by the input of the internuncial neurons, which in turn are activated by the sensitized neurons in the region of primary hyperalgesia.

In our psychophysical studies, light brushing of the skin caused burning pain when applied to an area next to a burn, indicating an obvious decrease in the pain threshold. However, pain in response to heat stimuli to the same area was not enhanced. Postulating that our injury was perhaps insufficient to bring our hyperalgesia to heat in the secondary area, we adopted the paradigm illustrated in Figure 14 (Raja *et al.*, 1984a). Burns consisting of 53°C for 30 s were applied to two locations (spots A and D), leaving enough room between the stimuli to do psychophysical testing on uninjured skin (spot B). The burns resulted in blisters after several hours about 50% of the time. Within minutes, the skin became tender to touch (mechanical hyperalgesia). When a nylon monofilament probe was dragged across the skin, there was a clear point of demarcation between normal and hyperalgesic skin. Light brushing of the skin never evoked pain prior to injury but consistently did so after injury both in the primary and secondary hyperalgesia area. The zone of mechanical hyperalgesia and the maximum area of flare evident to visual inspection are shown in Figure 14 for a typical subject. In all subjects tested to date, the area of mechanical hyperalgesia was larger than the area of flare. Pain thresholds were measured at sites A, B, and C using Von Frey hairs.

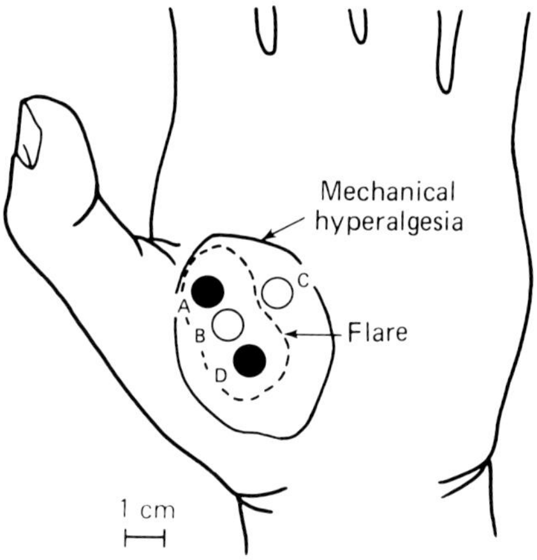

FIGURE 14. To determine the characteristics of secondary hyperalgesia, mechanical thresholds for pain and ratings of pain to heat stimuli were recorded at sites A, B, and C before and after burns at sites A and D. The burns consisted of a 53°C, 30-s stimulus at both sites. The area of flare and area of mechanical hyperalgesia following the burns in one subject is shown. In all subjects, the area of mechanical hyperalgesia was larger than the area of flare. Mechanical hyperalgesia was present even after the flare disappeared. (From Raja *et al.*, 1984a.)

The threshold was decreased in each location (from 12.0 ± 1.1 bars to 5.2 ± 0.5 bars).

Could the mechanical hyperalgesia in the secondary area be the result of stretching of the skin in the area of injury? There are three points against this. (1) Light brushing of the skin in the secondary region did not result in motion of the skin in the primary region. (2) The pain evoked in the secondary region was not mislocalized to the primary region. (3) Stretching would be expected to be less as the distance between the burn and the area mechanically stimulated increased, yet the degree of mechanical hyperalgesia did not systemically differ between the spots.

The responses to heat stimuli at sites A, B, and C were also tested. Marked hyperalgesia to heat (thermal hyperalgesia) was observed at site A, the injury site, and pain ratings increased more than fourfold. Between the two burns, the painfulness of the heat stimuli actually decreased by 50%. At site C, the ratings of pain to heat were comparable to those before injury. Thus, at both sites B and C, thermal hyperalgesia did not occur despite the observation that there was concurrent mechanical hyperalgesia. Particularly noteworthy is the finding that site B was hypalgesic to heat while being mechanically hyperalgesic.

The conclusion seems inescapable that separate mechanisms for secondary and primary hyperalgesia exist. Contrary to the postulates of Lewis, these data suggest that nociceptor sensitization does not account for secondary hyperalgesia. If it did, sensitization of nociceptors to mechanical but not heat stimuli would be expected to occur. This has not been observed in neurophysiological experiments. Hardy's claims that in the region of secondary hyperalgesia (1) the threshold to mechanical and heat stimuli is unaltered and (2) that pain to suprathreshold mechanical and heat stimuli is augmented are not consistent with our results. Instead, the changes must be considered separately for mechanical and heat stimuli. The pain threshold for mechanical stimuli is decreased, and pain to suprathreshold mechanical stimuli is increased. For heat stimuli, either no changes occur or there may be a transient period of decreased pain sensitivity (i.e., hypalgesia).

E. Primary Afferents and Secondary Hyperalgesia

A key observation in the formulation of Lewis was that electrical stimulation of a nerve trunk would lead to hyperalgesia in the distribution of that nerve even if the proximal end of the nerve was blocked with a local anesthetic during the stimulation period (Lewis, 1942). Whether he believed that hyperalgesia to heat as well as mechanical stimuli occurred is not clear.

In preliminary studies, we tested the effects of nerve trunk stimulation on the subsequent sensitivity of CMHs and AMHs. The electrical stimulus was of low frequency (2–5 Hz) and of sufficient intensity to excite C fibers. We did not observe sensitization of CMHs or AMHs to heat. A transient decrease in response to heat stimuli was noted in CMHs several minutes after the electrical stimulus, but the response generally returned to base line in time. These results are in disagreement with those of Fitzgerald (1979), who performed a similar study in cats and rabbits and found a lower heat threshold for the population of CMHs that had been antidromically stimulated. Other than the difference in species and skin type (hairy versus glabrous), we cannot account for the discrepancy in results.

Little has been mentioned thus far about the sensitization of primary afferent nociceptors with regard to mechanical stimuli. It might be expected that sensitization of nociceptors to heat stimuli following injury of their receptive field must be accompanied by sensitization to mechanical stimuli. To date, however, we have observed a decrease in threshold to mechanical stimuli as tested by Von Frey hairs infrequently (Campbell *et al.*, 1979). Responses to suprathreshold mechanical stimuli have not been tested quantitatively. To determine if an injury to half of the receptive field of a nociceptor might lead to sensitization of the other half, Thalhammer and LaMotte (1982, 1983) applied a 56°C, 7-s burn to half the receptive field of seven AMHs and nine CMHs located on hairy skin (Figure 15). Sensitization to heat was observed only in the receptive-field half that was burned and not in the other half. No significant changes in mechanical threshold were observed in either half. It may be that mechanical hyperalgesia even within the zone of injury cannot be explained by sensitization of nociceptors to mechanical stimuli. If this is the case, then mechanical hyperalgesia within and outside the zone of injury may have the same mechanism. This is supported by the observation that the decrease in Von Frey threshold to pain both within and outside the zone of injury was similar. Therefore, it may be misleading to refer to primary and secondary hyperalgesia. The more accurate designation is perhaps to distinguish mechanical from thermal hyperalgesia. The latter occurs only within the area of injury and is caused by sensitization of nociceptors, whereas the

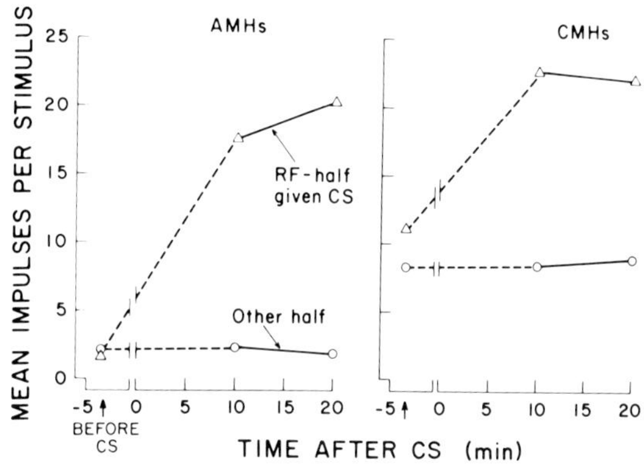

FIGURE 15. The mean responses of seven AMHs and four CMHs to a 51°C, 5-s stimulus before and after a conditioning stimulus (CS), which was a 56°C, 7-s stimulus applied to half of the receptive field. Sensitization was observed only for the receptive-field half directly exposed to the conditioning stimulus (triangles) and not for the other half (circles). (From Thalhammer and LaMotte (1983), with permission.)

former occurs both within and outside the area of injury and results from another mechanism.

What then is the mechanism of secondary hyperalgesia or, preferably, mechanical hyperalgesia? Although the mechanism is not clear at the present time, the following hypotheses deserve consideration. We have already discussed the possibility that sensitization may play a role as postulated by Lewis. Though our preliminary data do not support this mechanism, more detailed studies with more sophisticated techniques for mechanically stimulating the skin are needed.

There are a number of possible central mechanisms (Woolf, 1983) that would not require sensitization of nociceptors in the uninjured area to occur. Injury may somehow facilitate input of nociceptors from the adjoining uninjured area (Hardy *et al.*, 1950). This is plausible because the threshold for pain (5 bars) in the hyperalgesic zone (primary and secondary regions are similar in this regard) is still above the threshold of many nociceptors (see Table I). Tonic input of the sensitized nociceptors from the injured area could, via collateral sprouts, facilitate the response of central nociceptive neurons innervating the secondary hyperalgesia region. This facilitation could enhance the input of nociceptors innervating the secondary hyperalgesic zone. One problem with this hypothesis is that enhanced pain with suprathreshold heat stimulation would be expected but has not been observed. A variation of this hypothesis circumvents this problem. There is evidence that input of low-threshold mechanoreceptors masks the input of nociceptors (Bini *et al.*, 1984). Thus, a given amount of input from nociceptors would lead to less pain if there was concurrent input of low-threshold mechanoreceptors. The tonic input of sensitized nociceptors could suppress the masking effect of low-threshold mechanoreceptors, thus augmenting the input of nociceptors in response to mechanical stimulation of their receptive field. This mechanism would explain why mechanical but not thermal hyperalgesia occurs in the region of secondary hyperalgesia.

In a related hypothesis, injury would damage the low-threshold receptors such that they have decreased sensitivity. A decline of input from low-threshold fibers with mechanical stimulation would lead to decreased central masking and thus facilitate the activation of central nociceptive neurons by peripheral nociceptors. A major finding against this hypothesis is that the detection threshold in the region of mechanical hyperalgesia is less than the threshold for pain and appears not to be altered significantly by injury sufficient to evoke hyperalgesia.

It has also been postulated that low-threshold mechanoreceptors themselves may signal hyperalgesia. The sensitized peripheral nociceptors may facilitate input of low-threshold mechanoreceptors such that they can activate central nociceptive neurons. Once again, this would explain how mechanical hyperalgesia could occur in the absence of thermal hyperalgesia.

F. Hyperalgesia Following Peripheral Nerve Injury

Peripheral nerve injury can lead to chronic pain and hyperalgesia (Sunderland, 1978). In general, mechanical hyperalgesia is easy to demonstrate. In some patients, movement even of hair follicles elicits pain. Responses to heat stimuli in these patients are variable (Lindblom and Verrillo, 1979). In some cases, there seems to be exaggerated pain to suprathreshold heat stimuli, but there is no clear-cut decrease in the pain threshold. Perhaps the hyperalgesia in these patients is more like that of secondary hyperalgesia.

To determine further what fibers signal hyperalgesia in patients with nerve injuries in the upper extremities, we have applied a tourniquet inflated above systolic pressure to the affected arm (Raja *et al.*, 1984b). It is known that ischemic blocks induce an orderly loss of sensory function beginning with those functions subserved by the largest fibers. In 11 of the 13 patients (two did not tolerate application of the cuff), hyperalgesia began to disappear 7–15 min after application of the cuff. Hyperalgesia completely disappeared after 15–22 min. At this time, sensitivity to touch was altered, indicating loss of A-β-fiber function, although sensitivity to warmth and cold was unaffected.

These results suggest a prominent role of large fibers in signaling hyperalgesia in cases of nerve injury. This is opposite to the formulation that pathological pain results from loss of tonic input of large-diameter afferents. Whether the hyperalgesia results from activity in low-threshold mechanoreceptive afferents or the more rapidly conducting type I AMHs (mean conduction velocity, 31 m/s) remains to be determined.

G. Conclusions and Perspectives for the Future

Dating to early in this century, it has been suspected that the smallest of peripheral nerve fibers, the C fibers, code for the hyperalgesia arising from tissue and nerve injury. The results of a correlational analysis of psychophysical studies in humans and neurophysiological studies in monkeys suggest that A-fiber nociceptors, not C fibers, code for the hyperalgesia to heat stimuli following a burn to the hand. In other areas of the body, it is likely that both C- and A-fiber nociceptors play a role in hyperalgesia.

An argument was once waged as to whether central or peripheral mechanisms accounted for hyperalgesia. As many such arguments are resolved, it appears likely that both mechanisms are of importance. As we now are in an era in which nearly all accept that nociceptors code for the occurence, duration, location and intensity of pain, we now must consider whether that is always the case. There is reason to question the thesis that nociceptors code for the hyperalgesia manifest to mechanical stimuli within but particularly outside an area of injury.

The hyperalgesia that cripples certain victims of nerve injury seems to resemble that which accompanies inflammation of the skin following trauma. The question for the future is whether the mechanisms are similar. Large fibers, not the small fibers, signal the hyperalgesia that follows nerve injury. We need now to know which class of sensory myelinated fibers is reasonable. A-fiber nociceptors, low-threshold mechanoreceptors, or both may be involved.

Finally, the time is ripe to determine the biochemical mechanism of hyperalgesia. Curiously, the general anesthetic halothane sensitizes nociceptors. Could this finding be a clue to the biochemical mechanism of sensitization? Presumably by-products of inflammation such as the prostaglandins and leukotrienes play an integral role in the sensitization process. But which of these agents is responsible and how sensitization occurs remain challenging questions for future research.

ACKNOWLEDGMENTS. Efforts of numerous individuals contributed to this work. We in particular wish to thank Dr. Srinivasa N. Raja for his contributions to this research as well as the technical assistance of Adil Khan, Trudy Lund, and Ronald Burke. This work was supported by PHS grants NS-00519, NS-14447, and GM-32259.

References

ADRIAENSEN, H., GYBELS, J., HANDWERKER, H. O., AND HEES, J. V. Response properties of thin myelinated (A-δ) fibers in human skin nerves. *J. Neurophysiol.* 49:111–122, 1983.

BECK, P. W., AND HANDWERKER, H. O. Bradykinin and serotonin effects on various types of cutaneous nerve fibers. *Pflugers Arch.* 347:209–222, 1974.

BECK, P. W., HANDWERKER, H. O., AND ZIMMERMAN, M. Nervous outflow from the cat's foot during noxious radiant heat stimulation. *Brain Res.* 67:373–386, 1974.

BEITEL, R. E., AND DUBNER, R. Response of unmyelinated (C) polymodal nociceptors to thermal stimuli applied to monkey's face. *J. Neurophysiol.* 39:1160–1175, 1976.

BESSOU, R. E., AND PERL, E. R. Response of cutaneous sensory units with unmyelinated fibers to noxious stimuli. *J. Neurophysiol.* 32:1025–1042, 1969.

BINI, G., CRUCCU, G., HAGBARTH, K., SCHADY, W., AND TOREBJORK, E. Analgesia effect of vibration and cooling on pain induced by intraneural electrical stimulation. *Pain* 18:239–248, 1984.

BURGESS, P. R., AND PERL, E. R., Myelinated afferent fibers responding specifically to noxious stimulation of the skin. *J. Physiol.* 190:541–562, 1967.

CAMPBELL, J. N., AND LAMOTTE, R. H. Latency to detection of first pain. *Brain Res.* 226:203–208, 1983.

CAMPBELL, J. N., AND MEYER, R. A. Sensitization of unmyelinated nociceptive afferents in monkeys varies with skin type. *J. Neurophysiol.* 49:98–110, 1983.

CAMPBELL, J. N., MEYER, R. A., AND LAMOTTE, R. H. Sensitization of myelinated nociceptive afferents that innervate monkey hand. *J. Neurophysiol.* 42:1669–1679, 1979.

CAMPBELL, J. N., RAJA, S. N., AND MEYER, R. A. Halothane sensitizes cutaneous nociceptors in monkey. *J. Neurophysiol.* 52:762–770, 1984.

CAPETOLA, R. J., ROSENTHALE, M. E., and DUBINSKY, B., AND MCGUIRE, J. L. Peripheral antialgesics: A review. *J. Clin. Pharmacol.* 23:545–556, 1983.

CHAPMAN, L. F., RAMOS, A. D., GOODELL, H., AND WOLF, H. G. Neurohumural features of afferent fibers in man. *Arch. Neurol.* 4:49–82, 1961.

CROZE, S., DUCLAUX, R., AND KENSHALO, D. The thermal sensitivity of the polymodal nociceptors in the monkey. *J. Physiol.* 263:539–562, 1976.

DARIAN-SMITH, I., JOHNSON, K. O., LAMOTTE, C., SHIGENAGA, Y., KENINS, P., AND CHAMPNESS, P. Warm fibers innervating plamar and distal skin of the monkey: Responses to thermal stimuli. *J. Neurophysiol.* 42:1297–1310, 1979.

DUBNER, R., PRICE, D. D., BEITEL, R. E., AND HU, J. W. Peripheral neural correlates of behavior in monkey and human related to sensory-discriminative aspects of pain, in: *Pain in the Trigeminal Region* (D. J. ANDERSON AND B. MATHEWS, ed.), Elsevier, Amsterdam, 1977, pp. 57–66.

FITZGERALD, M. The spread of sensitization of polymodal nociceptors in the rabbit from nearby injuries and by antidromic nerve stimulation. *J. Physiol. (Lond.)* 297:207–216, 1979.

FITZGERALD, M., AND LYNN, B. The sensitization of high threshold mechanoreceptors with myelinated axons by repeated heating. *J. Physiol. (Lond.)* 365:549–563, 1977.

GEORGOPOULOS, A. P. Functional properties of primary afferent units probably related to pain mechanisms in primate glabrous skin. *J. Neurophysiol.* 39:71–83, 1976.

GYBELS, J., HANDWERKER, H. O., AND VAN HEES, J. A comparison between the discharges of human nociceptive nerve fibers and the subject's ratings of his sensations. *J. Physiol. (Lond.)* 292:193–206, 1979.

HANDWERKER, H. O. Pharmacological modulation of the discharge of nociceptive C-fibers, in: *Sensory Functions of the Skin in Primates* (T. ZOTTERMAN, ed.), Pergamon Press, Oxford, 1976, pp. 427–439.

HARDY J. D., WOLFF, H. G., AND GOODELL, H. Experimental evidence on the nature of cutaneous hyperalgesia. *J. Clin. Invest.* 29:115–140, 1950.

HARDY, J. D., WOLFF, H. G., AND GOODELL, H. *Pain Sensation and Reactions,* Williams & Wilkins, Baltimore, 1952.

KONIETZNY, F., AND HENSEL, H. Warm fiber activity in human skin nerves. *Pflugers Arch.* 359:265–267, 1975.

KUEHL, F. A., JR., AND EGAN, R. W. Prostaglandins, arachidonic acid, and inflammation. *Science* 210:978–984, 1980.

KUMAZAWA, T., AND PERL, E. R. Primate cutaneous sensory units with unmyelinated (C) afferent fibers. *J. Neurophysiol.* 40:1325–1338, 1977.

LAMOTTE, R. H., AND CAMPBELL, J. N. Comparison of responses of warm and nociceptive C-fiber afferents in monkey with human judgments of thermal pain. *J. Neurophysiol.* 41:509–528, 1978.

LAMOTTE, R. H., AND MOUNTCASTLE, V. B. Capacities of humans and monkeys to discriminate between vibratory stimuli of different frequency and amplitude: A correlation between neural events and psychophysical measurements. *J. Neurophysiol.* 38:539–559, 1975.

LAMOTTE, R. H., THALHAMMER, J. G., TOREBJORK, H. E., AND ROBINSON, C. J. Peripheral neural mechanisms of cutaneous hyperalgesia following mild injury by heat. *J. Neurosci.* 2:765–781, 1982.

LAMOTTE, R. H., THALHAMMER, J. G., AND ROBINSON, C. J. Peripheral neural correlates of magnitude of cutaneous pain and hyperalgesia: A comparison of neural events in monkey with sensory judgements in human. *J. Neurophysiol.* 50:1–26, 1983.

LANDS, W. E. M., AND HANEL, A. M. Inhibitors and activators of prostaglandin biosynthesis, in: *Prostaglandins and Related Substances* (C. PACE-ASCIAK AND E. GRANSTROM, eds.), Elsevier, New York, 1983, pp. 203–223.

LEWIS, T. Clinical observations and experiments relating to burning pain in extremities and to so-called "erythromelalgeia" in particular. *Clin. Sci.* 1:175–211, 1933.

LEWIS, T. Experiments relating to cutaneous hyperalgesia and its spread through somatic nerves. *Clin. Sci.* 2:373–423, 1935.

LEWIS, T. *Pain,* Macmillan, New York, 1942.

LEWIS, T., AND POCHIN, E. E. The double pain response of the human skin to a single stimulus. *Clin. Sci.* 13:67–76, 1937.

LINDBLOM, V., AND VERRILLO, R. T. Sensory functions in chronic neuralgia. *J. Neurol. Neurosurg. Psychiatry* 42:422–435, 1979.

MEYER, R. A., AND CAMPBELL, J. N. Evidence for two distinct classes of unmyelinated nociceptive afferents in monkey. *Brain Res.* 224:149–152, 1981a.

MEYER, R. A., AND CAMPBELL, J. N. Peripheral neural coding of pain sensation. *Johns Hopkins APL Tech. Dig.* 2:167–171, 1981b.

MEYER, R. A., AND CAMPBELL, J. N. Myelinated nociceptive afferents account for the hyperalgesia that follows a burn applied to the hand. *Science* 213:1527–1529, 1981c.

MEYER, R. A., WALKER, R. E., AND MOUNTCASTLE, V. B. A laser stimulator for the study of cutaneous thermal pain sensation. *I.E.E.E. Trans. Biomed. Eng.* 23:54–60, 1976.

MOUNTCASTLE, V. B., LAMOTTE, R. H., AND CARLI, G. Detection thresholds for vibratory stimuli in humans and monkeys: Comparison with threshold events in mechanoreceptive afferent nerve fibers inneverating the monkey hand. *J. Neurophysiol.* 35:122–136, 1972.

RAJA, S. N. CAMPBELL, J. N., AND MEYER, R. A. Evidence for different mechanisms of primary and secondary hyperalgesia following heat injury to the glabrous skin. *Brain* 107:1179–1188, 1984a.

RAJA, S. N., CAMPBELL, J. N., MEYER, R. A., AND MACKINNON, S. N. Hyperalgesia following nerve injury is signalled by myelinated fibers. *Pain* (Suppl. 2):s8, 1984b.

SINCLAIR, D. *Mechanisms of Cutaneous Sensation.* Oxford University Press, New York, 1981.

SUNDERLAND, S. *Nerves and Nerve Injuries,* Churchill Livingstone, New York, 1978.

TALBOT, W. H., DARIAN-SMITH, I., KORNHUBER, H. H., AND MOUNTCASTLE, V. B. The sense of flutter-vibration: Comparison of the human capacity with response patterns of mechanoreceptive afferents from the monkey hand. *J. Neurophysiol.* 31:301–334, 1968.

THALHAMMER, J. G., AND LAMOTTE, R. H. Spatial properties of nociceptor: Sensitization following heat injury of the skin. *Brain Res.* 231:257–265, 1982.

THALHAMMER, J. G., AND LAMOTTE, R. H. Heat sensitization of one-half of a cutaneous nociceptor's receptive field does not alter the sensitivity of the other half, in: *Advances in Pain Research and Therapy,* Vol. 5 (J. J. BONICA, U. LINDBLOM AND A. IGGO, eds.), Raven Press, New York, 1983, pp. 71–75.

TOREBJORK, H. E., AND HALLIN, R. G. Perceptual changes accompanying controlled preferential blocking of A and C fiber responses in intact human skin. *Exp. Brain Res.* 16:321–332, 1973.

TOREBJORK, H. E., AND HALLIN, R. G. Responses in human A and C fibers to repeated electrical intradermal stimulation. *J. Neurol. Neurosurg. Psychiatry* 37:653–664, 1974.

TOREBJORK, H. E., AND OCHOA, J. Specific sensations evoked by activity in single identified sensory units in man. *Acta Physiol. Scand.* 110:445–447, 1980.

WOOLF, C. J Evidence for a central-component of post-injury pain hypersensitivity. *Nature* 306:686–688, 1983.

4
Nonclassical Features of Dorsal Root Ganglion Cell Organization

RICHARD E. COGGESHALL

A. Introduction

Dorsal root ganglion cells and their cranial nerve equivalents are the primary sensory cells for general somatic sensation. The cell bodies of these neurons are located in dorsal root and certain cranial nerve ganglia. Each cell body is reported to give rise to a single stem process that branches into a proximal and a distal process, the proximal process entering the spinal cord through a dorsal root and the distal process passing to the periphery via a peripheral nerve. This organization is schematized in Figure 1, and similar pictures are seen in almost all texts dealing with the organization of the nervous system. This is an important scheme, for it imposes restraints on the way we reason about the transfer of somatic information centrally. In recent years, however, evidence has accumulated to indicate that two aspects of the above scheme are oversimplified. These are (1) that each dorsal root ganglion cell has a single process in the dorsal root and a single process in the peripheral nerve and (2) that the central processes of dorsal root ganglion cells travel only in the dorsal root. This report indicates how we arrived at the classic scheme and then presents the evidence indicating that the classic scheme needs modification. Some speculations as to the functional significance of these modifications are offered.

RICHARD E. COGGESHALL • Departments of Anatomy, Physiology, and Biophysics, University of Texas Medical Branch, Galveston, Texas 77550.

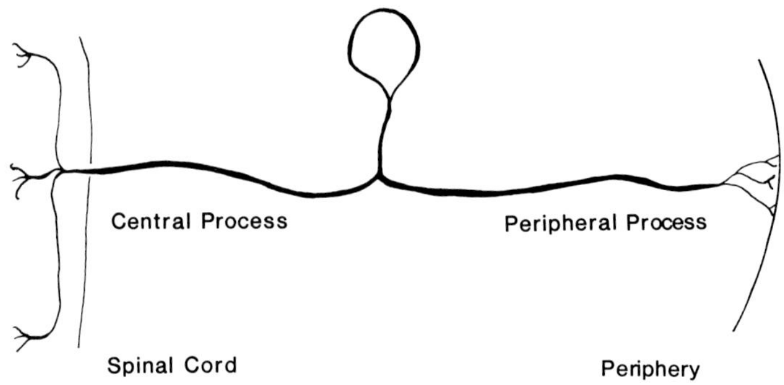

FIGURE 1. A primary sensory cell as it is classically pictured. Note that the cell body, which is located in a dorsal root or equivalent cranial nerve ganglion, is unipolar. The stem process from the cell body then divides into a peripheral process, which travels via a peripheral nerve to a receptive area at the periphery, and a central process, which travels to the central nervous system, in this case the spinal cord.

B. Branching of Dorsal Root Ganglion Cell Processes

Dorsal root ganglion cells are depicted as pseudounipolar neurons with a stem process that divides into a central process that enters the spinal cord through the dorsal root and a peripheral process that extends to the periphery in a peripheral nerve (Figure 1). One functional implication of this structural scheme is that any particular dorsal root ganglion cell brings information from the periphery via a single process and sends it towards the spinal cord via another single process. Admittedly, there is considerable branching peripherally as the peripheral process divides and redivides to innervate the receptive field and also centrally, where the central process divides into ascending and descending collaterals and these collaterals redivide into various processes passing to different parts of spinal cord and brainstem. Nevertheless, the central process of the primary cell is depicted as a single channel throughout the length of the dorsal root, and the peripheral process of the same cell is depicted as a single channel throughout much of the length of the peripheral nerve. The evidence that led to the formation of this construct is worth considering.

1. Classical Perspective

The first data, from a chronological point of view, that mammalian dorsal root ganglion cells are pseudounipolar neurons with single central and peripheral processes came from studies on ganglion architecture by investigators who used basic histological techniques, particularly the whole-cell-staining techniques such as methylene blue or variants of the Golgi reaction (e.g., Dogiel, 1908; Ramon y Cajal, 1909). Following the lead of Ranvier (1875), these investigators found the T- or V-shaped first division of the stem process and then depicted dorsal root ganglion cells as shown in Figure 1. There seems to be little doubt that the original division of the stem process is as they showed it. Nevertheless, their evidence is not definitive for the concept that the resulting processes are unbranched until they reach the periphery or spinal cord. First, there is the difficulty that these preparations are studied in histological sections and the processes bend and turn to a certain extent. Thus, for any particular cell, one cannot follow the fibers from the stem process division for any distance, and, consequently, one cannot be certain that there is no branching distal to the primary division. Second, although it is not often remembered today, Dogiel (1896, 1908) actually described and illustrated branching of the primary processes of some dorsal root ganglion cells in the dorsal root ganglion.

2. *Ratio of Ganglion Cells to Processes*

Because of the above difficulties, it was thought desirable to confirm by other methods the statement that each dorsal root ganglion cell gives rise to only a single central and a single peripheral process. Since such an arrangement, if there were no other fibers in the dorsal root, would lead to equal numbers of dorsal root axons and ganglion cells for any particular segment, many studies were undertaken to determine the numbers of dorsal root axons and dorsal root ganglion cells for the same spinal segments in various vertebrates. It might be mentioned that as numbers of dorsal root ganglion cells and dorsal root axons should be equal by this reasoning, so numbers of dorsal root ganglion cells and peripheral sensory axons should also be equal. The difficulty is that there are nonsensory fibers in the peripheral nerve, whereas it was felt that the dorsal root contains only sensory axons (see below). Presumably, this explains why studies on the dorsal root axon/ganglion cell ratios are common and studies on the peripheral sensory axon/ganglion cell ratios are rare.

Early studies reported that there was a surplus of ganglion cells over axons (e.g., Hatai, 1902), but these can be disregarded because the existence of unmyelinated fibers in the dorsal root was not appreciated. In 1911, however, Ranson developed a silver stain for unmyelinated axons in the peripheral nerves and roots and reported that there were large numbers of unmyelinated axons in dorsal roots. He speculated that these were sensory axons and that they were the processes of the small dorsal root ganglion cells. This was a major advance and is generally accepted today. Ranson's findings, since they showed the presence of nonmyelinated sensory processes, also indicated that the previously published ratios of dorsal root axons to ganglion cells were probably incorrect. Several studies then followed, and the main points of discussion concerned the adequacy of the silver stains and whether there was an accurate count of the unmyelinated axons. The issue was generally regarded as being settled by the studies of Duncan and Keyser (1938) and Holmes and Davenport (1940). These investigators agreed that there was essentially a 1 : 1 relationship of dorsal root axons to ganglion cells, and thus the suggestion that each doral root ganglion cell gives rise to only a single central process was confirmed.

With the advent of the electron microscope, however, it quickly became apparent that unmyelinated axons cannot be individually visualized in the light microscope even when they are darkened by high-quality silver stains (Gasser, 1955). Thus, the previous dorsal root axon counts are open to question. For this reason, it was necesary to repeat the axon counts with the electron microscope, where both myelinated and unmyelinated axons are clearly visible. When this was done for lumbosacral segments of the rat, approximately twice as many axons as ganglion cells were found (Langford and Coggeshall, 1979, 1981).

One possible way to explain the above results without violating the 1 : 1 ratio of sensory axons to dorsal root ganglion cells woulld be that there are efferent axons in the dorsal root. This would obviously lead to more dorsal root axons than ganglion cells even if there was one and only one dorsal root axon for each ganglion cell. The reason for focusing on this particular question is that there is a considerable literature suggesting that such fibers exist (Hinsey, 1934). The primary evidence is that axons are seen in the proximal stump of a cut dorsal root. Since axons attached to their cell bodies usually survive, it was thought that this indicated that there were axons in the spinal cord that sent their processes distally through the dorsal root. There are two problems with these studies, however. First, insufficient precautions were taken against ingrowth of axons from nearby nerves into the proximal stump, and second, the light microscope is not an adequate instrument with which to examine fine axons. When the work was repeated carefully (Hinsey, 1934), and when the electron microscope was used to examine the proximal stump (Langford and Coggeshall, 1979), it became apparent that no axons survived in the proximal stump of a cut dorsal root. Thus, it is usually accepted that there are no efferent dorsal root axons and that only sensory axons are found in the dorsal root.

If there is a surplus of dorsal root axons as compared to ganglion cells, and if there are no efferent fibers in the dorsal roots, the obvious interpretation is that some dorsal root ganglion cells must give rise to more than one central process. Since the published electron microscopic studies have been primarily concerned with lumbosacral areas in the rat, however, one might ask whether the phenomenon is general or whether the rat might be just a deviant species. To deal with this problem, we have recently completed counts of dorsal root axons and ganglion cells for sacral areas of the cat. In this material, as in the rat, there is a considerable surplus of axons to ganglion cells (Risling *et al.*,1983; Chung and Coggeshall, 1983). Thus, it seems clear that there are more dorsal root axons than ganglion cells in mammals and that earlier students of dorsal root ganglion cell structure, because of the lack of resolution of the light microscope, were misled in their axonal counts because they could not recognize all individual unmyelinated axons in dorsal roots.

Since it now seems clear that there are more dorsal root axons than dorsal root ganglion cells in mammals, it is reasonable to ask whether there are also more sensory axons than dorsal root ganglion cells in the proximal peripheral nerve. Unlike the dorsal root, however, there are other types of axons in the peripheral nerve, namely, axons to striated muscle and postganglionic sympathetic axons. These must be removed before the counts can be done. Ventral rhizotomy will remove the motor axons, and sympathectomy will remove the postganglionic sysmpathetic axons. After this surgery is performed, the counts indicate more than a two-to-one preponderance of axons to ganglion cells for sacral segments in the rat (Langford and Coggeshall, 1981). Thus, as for the dorsal root, there are more sensory axons for the same segment of the body than there are dorsal root ganglion cells in the proximal peripheral nerve.

The above data indicate that there are more sensory axons in the dorsal root and proximal peripheral nerve than there are dorsal root ganglion cells for each segment of the body. Our interpretation of these data is that a significant number of dorsal root ganglion cell processes branch distal to the primary division but still in the general vicinity of the ganglion. The obvious next question is whether there is any other evidence to support this interpretation. Probably the major suggestion that branching might occur prior to very recent work is the evidence summarized in two studies by Sinclair and colleagues (Sinclair *et al.*, 1948; Sinclair, 1949). These investigators point out that much clinical data gathered from patients who suffer from referred pain are consistent with the idea of proximal peripheral sensory axon branching. Treatment of instructive cases with local anesthetics abolished pain in such a way as to reinforce this view. These studies never seemed to make a major impact, however, probably for two reasons. First, the evidence was indirect and thus did not unambiguously prove the point, and second, everyone assumed on the basis of the classical work that sensory axons did not branch near the ganglion.

In recent years, there has been a resurgence of the ideas put forth by Sinclair and his colleagues because of a sudden spate of articles providing more direct evidence to indicate that sensory axons branch in or near the ganglion. First, there are the modern anatomic studies showing a surplus of dorsal root and peripheral sensory axons. These have been discussed above. Next, there are physiological studies showing impulses carried by processes of the same sensory cell in different peripheral nerves (Bahr *et al.*, 1981; Pierau *et al.*, 1982). It has also been shown that the same dorsal root ganglion cell is labeled with different retrogradely transported markers when each marker is applied to a different peripheral nerve (Taylor and Pierau, 1982). Furthermore, there is the work of Said (1983), which to date is published only in abstract form. This investigator teased individual dorsal root ganglion cells and their proximal processes from osmicated dorsal root ganglia and noted several instances in which dorsal root ganglion cell processes branched distal to the primary division. If all these data are accepted, and these studies seem to be well done and well controlled, there would seem to be no other explanation but that both central and peripheral processes of dorsal root ganglion cells branch.

If it is accepted that the central and peripheral processes of a significant number of dorsal root axons branch, it might be asked where this branching occurs. One would presume that it does not happen next to the primary bifurcation of the stem process or it would have been seen by the master cytologists of the 19th and early 20th centuries. In our work, however, we noted the same number of axons in the dorsal root near the ganglion as in the dorsal root near the spinal cord. Furthermore, the work of Said (1983) shows that the branching takes place within or close to the ganglion but usually not in close proximity to the primary division. Thus, it is our hypothesis that the branching takes place relatively far from the primary division but still within or close to the dorsal root ganglion. This hypothesis now needs to be confirmed and made more precise by the visualization of single dorsal root ganglion cells and their processes with morphologically visible markers that can be placed directly into individual cell bodies.

The purpose of this section of the present chapter is to indicate that there is strong and rapidly increasing evidence that a significant number of dorsal root ganglion cells have both central and peripheral processes that branch in the dorsal root ganglion. A probable arrangement of these cells is shown in Figure 2. A final question concerns the possible importance of this branching. For the peripheral branching, the obvious inference is that this arrangement might provide an explanation for referred pain. This suggestion presumes that different branches of the same dorsal root ganglion cell would innervate two different body regions, for example, the heart and the inside of the left arm. If further implies that when one of the branches is activated, the central nervous system interprets the information as coming from the other branch. It must be admitted that there is minimal evidence for these suggestions at present, but until the likelihood that dorsal root ganglion cell processes branch is appreciated, these possibilities will not even be considered.

On the central side, an interesting possibility is that different branches of the same sensory cell might pass to different parts of the central nervous system. This is, of course, what happens with ascending and descending collaterals of primary afferent fibers, but the possibility that major axonal branches of a primary afferent cell might travel to completely separate central locations should be noted. There is some evidence of information transfer failure at branch points in axons. Since the presence of branching implies the presence of branch points, this raises the possibility that the dorsal root ganglion cell

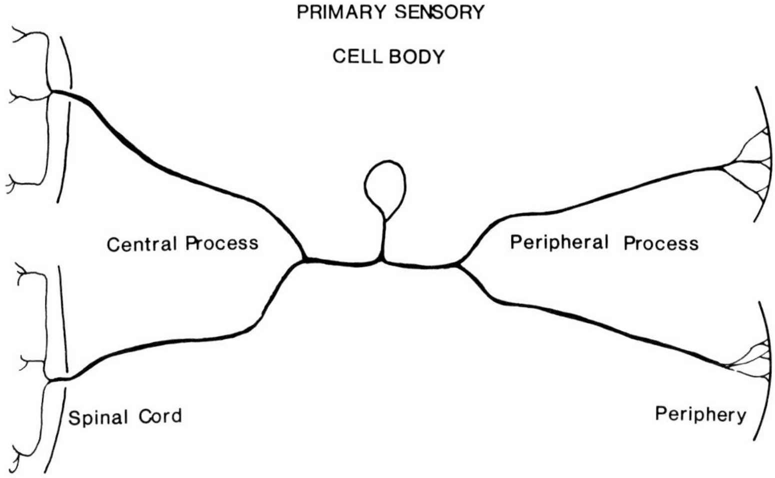

FIGURE 2. Recent evidence makes it probable that the depiction of the processes of primary sensory cells as in Figure 1 is too simple. Rather, it seems to be the case that some, perhaps many, of the primary sensory cells have central and peripheral processes that are branched, as depicted in this diagram. This arrangement may have important functional consequences such as, for example, a peripheral explanation for referred pain.

itself might modify the transfer of information from periphery to center by blockage at branch points, an idea that would probably not be considered if all dorsal root ganglion cells were thought to give rise to only a single central and a single peripheral process.

3. *Summary of the Classical View of Afferent Branching*

1. Classical work led to the description of a dorsal root ganglion cell as a pseudonunipolar neuron whose stem process divided into a single peripheral axon and a single central axon.
2. The data on which this concept is based are the depictions of dorsal root ganglion cells as they are outlined in classic histological stains and the 1 : 1 ratio of dorsal root ganglion cells to dorsal root axons as determined by light microscopy.
3. Recent electron microscope evidence indicates that the earlier axonal counts are incorrect, however, and that there are more sensory axons than dorsal root ganglion cells.
4. This surplus of axons to ganglion cells is seen both centrally in the dorsal root and peripherally in the peripheral nerve.
5. Recent physiological evidence indicates that the same sensory axon can be recorded in different peripheral nerves.
6. Recent studies using retrograde markers show that the same dorsal

root ganglion cell can be labeled by two different markers applied to different peripheral nerves.

7. Some individual neurons and their proximal processes teased free from an osmicated dorsal root ganglion show branching of both the proximal and distal processes distal to the primary branch.
8. Items 3–7 above strongly indicate that at least some dorsal root ganglion cells have central and/or peripheral processes that branch within the dorsal root ganglion.
9. One inference is that this arrangement might provide an anatomic basis for referred pain.
10. Another inference is that some dorsal root ganglion cells might transmit sensory information to different parts of the spinal cord or brainstem by separate processes.
11. A final inference is that the branching of primary sensory processes might result in a modification of information transfer from periphery to spinal cord.
12. Futher research to determine the numbers and functional types of those dorsal root ganglion cells with branched processes is obviously desirable.

C. Ventral Root Afferent Fibers

Classic work led to the idea of the separation of funtion of the spinal roots. This concept, in my opinion, was first made clear by the experiments of Magendie, and his crucial papers as well as those of Bell are reproduced in the book by Cranefield (1974). This is regarded as an extremely important generalization concerning the organization of the nervous system. The anatomic basis of the law of separation of function of the spinal roots is that only sensory axons are found in the dorsal root and only motor axons are found in the ventral root. In recent years, however, the discovery of large numbers of afferent fibers in the ventral root may necessitate a revision of this generalization.

1. Classical Perspective: Recurrent Sensibility

It would be foolish to attempt a comprehensive review of the various experiments that led to the establishment of the idea of the separation of sensory and motor functions in the spinal roots. The fundamental experiments are that section of the dorsal roots results in loss of sensation in a dermatomal pattern and section of ventral roots leads to segmental loss of muscle innervation. These experiments have been repeated with variations in a large number of different studies. Perhaps, therefore, it would be more useful to ask whether there are any studies in the older literature that are at variance with this concept. Probably the first indication that the law of separation of function of the spinal roots, as it is usually stated, might be oversimplified came from the work of Magendie himself and that of his pupil Claude Bernard (Cranefield, 1974). These investigators showed that strong stimulation of the distal stump of a cut ventral root caused animals to react as if they were suffering pain, and they further noted that if the dorsal root was then cut, the stimulation no longer had an effect. The name given to this phenomenon was recurrent sensibility. This work was extended in a dramatic way in humans by showing that stimulation of a ventral root caused intense pain and inactivation of the dorsal root application of a local anesthetic rendered the stimulus ineffective (Frykholm, 1951; Frykholm *et al.,* 1953). The interpretation of these experiments was basically that some dorsal root axons curve into and then out of the ventral root on the way from periphery to spinal cord. This arrangement was thought not to violate the law of separation of function of the spinal roots, although it did imply that some sensory axons traveled for a significant distance into the distal part of the ventral root.

The morphological basis of recurrent sensibility was discussed by Sherrington (1894), who discovered that a few myelinated fibers degenerated in the proximal stump and survived in the distal stump of a cut ventral root. This finding was confirmed by Windle (1931). Sherrington suggested that these fibers might be the anatomic basis of recurrent sensibility. This was never accepted, however, because the fibers were few and also because large myelinated axons are thought to have little to do with the transmission of pain.

2. *Current Evidence for Unmyelinated Afferent Fibers Entering the Ventral Root*

The issue of afferent fibers in the ventral root was then infrequently discussed until the discovery that there were large numbers of unmyelinated axons in cat ventral roots (Coggeshall, 1979, 1980). These axons came from dorsal root ganglion cells, so they were presumed to be sensory (Coggeshall *et al.,* 1974). They make up 15–30% of the fibers in various ventral roots (Coggeshall *et al.,* 1974; Applebaum *et al.,* 1976; Emery *et al.,* 1977). Evidence that the cells of origin of these fibers are sensory came from the demonstration that individual unmyelinated fibers in the ventral root carried information from single peripheral receptive fields (Clifton *et al.,* 1976; Coggeshall and Ito, 1977). Furthermore, unmyelinated sensory fibers in the ventral root are found not only in cats but also in rats and probably in humans (Coggeshall *et al.,* 1975, 1977). Thus, it would seem that mammalian ventral roots contain a sizable number of unmyelinated and a few myelinated sensory fibers.

3. Looping Afferents in the Ventral Root

If all the ventral root afferent fibers entered the spinal cord directly through the ventral root, it would be difficult to explain the phenomenon of recurrent sensibility. It should be remembered that the pain of recurrent sensibility occurs when the distal stump of a cut ventral root is stimulated and interruption of the dorsal root fibers eliminates the pain. Neither of these results would be expected if all ventral root afferent fibers enter the spinal cord via the ventral root. Thus, this raises the question as to whether there might be other categories of afferent fibers in the ventral root, the first being those that carry information directly into the spinal cord by the ventral root, and the others being those that are responsible for recurrent sensibility.

If there is a separate group of fibers in the ventral root that are responsible for recurrent sensibility, their most probable course is to loop into the ventral root and then back into the dorsal root as suggested, for example, by Magendie (cited in Cranefield, 1974) or Frykholm (1951). Outside of the presence of recurrent sensibility itself, what is the evidence that such looping fibers exist? First, there is physiological evidence that some myelinated fibers form loops in rat ventral roots (Bostock, 1981). There are also the observations by Risling and Hildebrand (1982) that show a steady decrease in unmyelinated axon numbers in the ventral root as one counts axons in cross sections of ventral root ever closer to the spinal cord.

Our own laboratory has obtained recent physiological evidence from single-cell recordings that also bear on this issue. We record from neurons in the dorsal horn, cut the ventral root, and place the distal stump of the ventral root on stimulating electrodes (Chung *et al.*, 1983). A certain number of neurons in the dorsal horn can then be excited by strong stimuli to the distal stump of the ventral root. The stimulus is no longer effective if the dorsal root of the same segment is crushed or cut. This stimulus is also no longer effective if the distal stump is crushed distal to the stimulus site, indicating that the results are not caused by current spread. Latencies indicate that the axons that excite the dorsal horn neurons are almost certainly unmyelinated. This evidence is clearly preliminary, but it supports the idea that there are axons that loop in the ventral root and then pass to the spinal cord via the dorsal root.

A final category of unmyelinated sensory axons in the ventral root are those that seem to innervate pia or ventral surface of spinal cord and then use the ventral root as a convenient route to reach the dorsal root ganglion (Dalsgard *et al.*, 1982). Such axons have been seen by the use of immunocytochemical stains for the possible neurotransmitter, substance P, which presumably implies that these axons are from the substance-P-containing cells in the dorsal root ganglion (see Yaksh, Chapter 8).

Thus, it would seem that there are at least three categories of primary afferent unmyelinated sensory axons in mammalian ventral root. First, there are those that enter the spinal cord through the ventral root. These are the fibers that violate the law of separation of function of the spinal roots. Second, there are those fibers that pass into the ventral root and then loop back, probably without entering the spinal cord. These are the fibers that are presumed to be the basis for recurrent sensibility. There are two possible subcategories of these latter fibers, those with central processes that loop into the ventral root and those with peripheral processes that loop into ventral root. Finally, there are those fibers that arise from receptive fields on the ventral surface of the spinal cord or surrounding meninges and then use the ventral root as a convenient pathway to reach the dorsal root ganglion. Experiments designed to determine the various proportions of these fibers are now desirable.

A final possibility that would combine the two sections of this chapter is that the ventral root afferent fibers that enter the spinal cord through the ventral root might be the result of branching of the central processes of some dorsal root ganglion cells. This inference supposes that some or all of the neurons that give rise to a ventral root afferent also give rise to a dorsal root afferent. Loeb (1976) actually recorded from such a cell, but it was large because the recorded axons had a fast conduction velocity. It will be important to record from the small dorsal root ganglion cells that give rise to unmyelinated axons to see if similar data can be obtained from these neurons.

4. Destination and Role of Ventral Root Afferents

The next obvious question concerns the central destination of these fibers. That some of these unmyelinated fibers entering through the ventral root pass into the gray matter of the spinal cord is attested to by several experimental observations. First, there is the finding that some dorsal root ganglion cells are labeled when the marker horseradish peroxidase is placed in the spinal cord after the dorsal roots are cut (Maynard *et al.*, 1977; Yamamoto *et al.*, 1977). It is difficult to interpret this in any way except that the marker is transported to the ganglion cell via an axon in the ventral root. These observations are consistent with the preliminary reports of a reduction in substance P in the dorsal horn of the spinal cord following ventral rhizotomy (Stroink *et al.*, 1983). As discussed by Yaksh in Chapter 8, substance P is thought to be a marker for small unmyelinated afferents and may be related to systems that respond to high-threshold stimuli (see comments by Campbell in Chapter 3 and Dubner *et al.*, Chapter 13). Light and Metz (1978) observed fine fibers in the dorsal laminae of the spinal gray that originated from systems in the ventral root. Second, activation of these ventral root systems has physiological effects that suggest that ventral root fibers have an excitatory influence on spinal afferent processing. Cardiovascular changes occur when strong stimulation is delivered to the sciatic nerve following dorsal root section (Longhurst *et al.*, 1980). An increased discharge of motor neurons following section of dorsal roots and intraarterial injection of bradykinin has also been reported (Voorhoeve and Nauta, 1983). There are also reports of relief of post-dorsal-rhizotomy chronic segmental pain by removal of appropriate spinal ganglia (Hosobuchi, 1980). These effects are all interpreted as being mediated by ventral root afferent fibers.

All of these findings seem to indicate that a number of ventral root afferents enter the spinal cord directly through the ventral root. I feel it is a reasonable suggestion that these fibers are at least partially responsible for the failure of dorsal rhizotomy to relieve pain and also that the existence of such fibers implies that it is impossible to denervate by dorsal rhizotomy alone. These data also suggest that in patients suffering chronic pain that is segmentally localized and unaffected by treatments such as dorsal rhizotomy, dorsal root ganglionectomy might be an operation that would be beneficial because it would remove both the dorsal and ventral root afferents (Coggeshall *et al.*, 1975).

5. *Summary of Organization of Afferent Input in the Ventral Roots*

1. The classic view is that dorsal roots contain only sensory axons and ventral roots contain only motor axons.
2. This is referred to as the "law" of the separation of function of the spinal roots.
3. As regards to the ventral root, the phenomenon of recurrent sensibility is probably the major indication from early work that the law of separation of function of the spinal roots might be oversimplified.
4. Sherrington discovered a few "wrong-way" afferent myelinated fibers in mammalian ventral roots and speculated that they might explain recurrent sensibility. Since such fibers do not carry noxious information, this speculation is unlikely.
5. Large numbers of unmyelinated sensory fibers have recently been discovered in mammalian ventral roots.
6. Some of the unmyelinated sensory fibers in the ventral root seem to enter the spinal cord directly through the ventral root.
7. The fibers mentioned in item 6 above violate the law of separation of function of the spinal roots, and they preclude complete denervation by dorsal rhizotomy alone. Presumably, they are a cause for the failure of dorsal rhizotomy to relieve pain.
8. Recent evidence indicates that other ventral root afferents loop into the ventral root and then pass to the spinal cord via the dorsal root. These are presumably the explanation for recurrent sensiblity.
9. Another population of unmyelinated ventral root afferent fibers seems to be those that innervate the ventral surface of spinal cord or surrounding meninges. At least some of these axons contain visualizable concentrations of substance P.

10. Experiments to work out the proportions and type of information by each category of ventral root afferents would be desirable.

ACKNOWLEDGMENTS. The research described in this paper is partially supported by NIH grants 10161, 17039, 11255, and 07377 and grant #82-231 from The Moody Foundation of Texas.

References

APPLEBAUM, M. L., CLIFTRON, G. L., COGGESHALL, R. E., COULTER, J. D., VANCE, W. H., AND WILLIS, W. D. Unmyelinated fibres in the sacral 3 and caudal 1 ventral root of the cat. *J. Physiol (Lond.)* 256:557–572, 1976.

BAHR, R., BLUMBERG, H., AND JANIG, W. Do dichtomizing afferent fibers exist which supply visceral organs as well as somatic structures? A contribution to the problem of referred pain. *Neurosci Lett.* 24:25–28, 1981.

BOSTOCK, H. U-turns in rat ventral roots. *J. Physiol (Lond.)* 312:49–50P, 1981.

CHUNG, J. M., LEE, K. H., ENDO, K., AND COGGESHALL, R. E. Activation of central neurons by ventral root afferents. *Science* 222:934–935, 1983.

CHUNG, K., AND COGGESHALL, R. E. The ratio of dorsal root ganglion cells to dorsal root axons in sacral segments of the cat. *J. Comp. Neurol.* 225:24–30, 1984.

CLIFTON, C. L., COGGESHALL, R. E., VANCE, W. H., AND WILLIS, W. D. Receptive fields of unmyelinated ventral root afferent fibers in the cat. *J. Physiol (Lond.)* 256:573–600, 1976.

COGGESHALL, R. E. Afferent fibers in the ventral root. *Neurosurgery* 4:443–448, 1979.

COGGESHALL, R. E. The law of separation of function of the spinal roots. *Physiol. Rev.* 60:716–755, 1980.

COGGESHALL, R. E., AND ITO, H. Sensory fibres in ventral roots L7 and S1 in the cat. *J. Physiol (Lond.)* 267:215–235, 1977.

COGGESHALL, R. E., COULTER, J. D., AND WILLIS, W. D. Unmyelinated axons in the ventral roots of the cat lumbosacral enlargement. *J. Comp. Neurol.* 153:39–58, 1974.

COGGESHALL, R. E., APPLEBAUM, M. L., FAZEN, M., STUBBS, T. G. III, AND SYKES, M. T. Unmyelinated fibers in ventral roots of humans, a possible explanation for the failure of the dorsal rhizotomy to relieve pain. *Brain* 98:157–166, 1975.

COGGESHALL, R. E., EMERY, D. G., ITO, H., AND MAYNARD, C. W. Unmyelinated and small myelinated axons in the rat ventral roots. *J. Comp. Neurol.* 173:175–184, 1977.

CRANEFIELD, P. F. *The Way In and the Way Out.* Futura, Mount Kisco, New York, 1974.

DALSGARD, C.- J., RISLING, M., AND CUELLO, C. Immunohistochemical localization of substance P in the lumbosacral spinal pia mater and ventral roots of the cat. *Brain Res.* 246:168–171, 1982.

DOGIEL, A. S. Der Bau der spinal Ganglien bei den Saugetieren. *Anat. Anz.* 12:140–152, 1896.

DOGIEL, A. S. *Der Bau der Spinalganglion des Menchen und den Saugetieren,* Fischer, Jena, 1908.

DUNCAN, D., AND KEYSER, L. L. Further determinations of the numbers of fibers and cells in the dorsal roots and ganglia of the cat. *J. Comp. Neurol.* 68:479–490, 1938.

EMERY, D. G., ITO, H., AND COGGESHALL, R. E. Unmyelinated axons in thoracic ventral roots of the cat. *J. Comp. Neurol.* 172:37–47, 1977.

FRYKHOLM, R. Cervical root compression resulting from disc degeneration and root-sleeve fibrosis. A clinical investigation. *Acta Chir. Scand. [Suppl]* 100:148–159, 1951.

FRYKHOLM, R., HYDE, J., NORLEN, G., AND SKOGLUND, C. R. On pain sensations produced by stimulation of ventral roots in man. *Acta Physiol. Scand. [Suppl]* 106:455–459, 1953.

GASSER, H. S. Porperties of dorsal root unmedullated fibers on 2 sides of the ganglion. *J. Gen. Physiol.* 38:709–728, 1955.

HATAI, S. Numbers and size of the spinal ganglion cells and dorsal root fibers in the white rat at different ages. *J. Comp. Neurol.* 12:107–124, 1902.

HINSEY, J. C. Are there efferent fibers in the dorsal roots? *J. Comp. Neurol.* 59:117–133, 1934.

HOLMES, F. W., AND DAVENPORT, H. A. Cells and fibers in spinal nerves. IV. The number of neurites in dorsal and ventral roots of the cat. *J. Comp. Neurol.* 73:1–5, 1940.

HOSOBUCHI, Y., The majority of unmyelinated afferent axons in human ventral roots probably conduct pain. *Pain* 8:167–180, 1980.

LANGFORD, L. A., AND COGGESHALL, R. E. Branching of sensory axons in the dorsal root and evidence for the absence of dorsal root efferent fibers. *J. Comp. Neurol.* 184:193–204, 1979.

LANGFORD, L. A., AND COGGESHALL, R. E. Branching of sensory axons in the peripheral nerve of the rat. *J. Comp. Neurol.* 203:745–750, 1981.

LIGHT, A. R., AND METZ, C. B. The morphology of spinal cord efferent and afferent neurons contributing to the ventral roots of the cat. *J. Comp. Neurol.* 179:501–516, 1978.

LOEB, G. E. Ventral projections of myelinated doral root ganglion cells in the cat. *Brain Res.* 106:159–165, 1976.

LONGHURST, J. C., MITCHGELL, J. H., AND MOORE, M. B. The spinal cord ventral root—an afferent pathway of the hindlimb pressor reflex. *J. Physiol (Lond.)* 301:467–476, 1980.

MAYNARD, C. W., LEONARD, R. B., COULTER, J. D., AND COGGESHALL, R. E. Central connections of ventral root afferents as demonstrated by the HRP method. *J. Comp. Neurol.* 172:601–608, 1977.

PIERAU, F.-K., TAYLOR, D. C. M., ABEL, W., AND FREDRICH, B. Dichotomizing peripheral fibres revealed by intracellular recording from rat sensory neurones. *Neurosci. Lett.* 31:123–218, 1982.

RAMON Y CAJAL, S. *Histologie du Systeme Nerveux de l'homme et des vertebres,* Institute Cajal, Madrid, 1909; reprinted 1952.

RANSON, S. W. Non-medullated fibers in the spinal nerves. *Am. J. Anat.* 12:62–87, 1911.

RANVIER, L. Des tubes nerveux en T et de leurs relations avec les cellules ganglion-naires. *C. R. Acad. Sci [D] (Paris)* 81:1274–1276, 1875.

RISLING, M., AND HILDEBRAND, C. Occurrence of unmyelinated axon profiles at distal, middle and proximal levels in the ventral root L7 of cats and kittens. *J. Neurol. Sci.* 56:219–231, 1982.

RISLING, M., ALDSKOGIUS, H., HILDEBRAND, C., AND RIMAHL, S. Effects of sciatic nerve resection on L7 spinal roots and dorsal root ganglia in adult cats. *Exp. Neurol.* 82:568–580, 1983.

SAID, G. Division of myelinated fibres issuing from dorsal root ganglion cells of the rat, in: *Proceedings of the Peripheral Nerve Study Group,* Sous l'egide de l'I.N.S.E.R.M. et du C.N.R.S., Paris, France, 1983.

SHERRINGTON, C. S. On the anatomical constitution of nerves. *J. Physiol (Lond.)* 17:211–258, 1894.

SINCLAIR, D. C. The remote reference of pain aroused in the skin. *Brain* 72:364–371, 1949.

SINCLAIR, D. C., WEDDELL, G., AND FEINDEL, W. H. Referred pain and associated phenomena. *Brain* 71:184–211, 1948.

STROINK, A., MICEVYCH, P., GO, V. L. W., AND YAKSH, T. L. Immunochemical studies of substance P in the dorsal horn following ventral root rhizotomy. *Anat. Rec.* 205:192A, 1983.

TAYLOR, D. C. M., AND PIERAUM F.-K. Double fluorescence labelling supports electrophysiological evidence for dichotomizing peripheral sensory nerve fibres in rats. *Neurosci. Lett.* 33:1–6, 1982.

WINDLE, W. F. Neurons of the sensory type in the ventral roots of man and of other mammals. *Arch. Neurol. Psychiatry* 26:791–800, 1931.

VOORHOEVE, P. E., AND NAUTA, J. Do nociceptive ventral root afferents exert central somatic effects? *Adv. Pain Res. Ther.* 5:105–110, 1983.

YAMAMOTO, T., TAKAHASHI, K., SATOMI, H., AND ISE, H. Origins of primary afferent fibers in the spinal ventral roots in the cat as demonstrated by the horseradish peroxidase method. *Brain Res.* 126:350–354, 1977.

5
Organization of Dorsal Horn Neurotransmitter Systems

CAROLE C. LAMOTTE

A. Introduction

The spinal cord dorsal horn is endowed with neural structures rich in a variety of neurotransmitters and neuromodulators, including amino acids, peptides, catecholamines, and serotonin. Many are concentrated in the superficial dorsal horn (laminae I, II, and III), with precise subregional accumulations specific for each substance.

Amino acids in dorsal horn structures include glutamate, glycine, and GABA. Glutamate may be associated with the larger-diameter, myelinated dorsal root afferents and, correspondingly, is in high concentration in the deeper regions of the dorsal horn and in the ventral horn. Glycine and GABA are present in interneurons of the substantia gelatinosa (lamina II) and in lamina III.

The peptides substance P (SP), cholecystokinin (CCK), vasoactive intestinal polypeptide (VIP), and somatostatin (SS) are found in axons and synaptic terminals of small-diameter myelinated or nonmyelinated primary afferents of the dorsal roots. Many local spinal interneurons also are peptidergic, containing SP, SS, CCK, enkephalin (ENK), or neurotensin (NT). Descending axons from the brainstem provide another source of terminals in the dorsal horn containing SP, SS, CCK, and ENK. Descending axons arising from neurohormonal peptidergic neurons in the ventral diencephalon also terminate in the dorsal horn and contain ACTH, TRH, and neurophysin.

CAROLE C. LAMOTTE • Sections of Neurosurgery and Anesthesiology, Yale University School of Medicine, New Haven, Connecticut 06510.

In addition to the descending peptidergic systems to the dorsal horn, there are significant serotoninergic, adrenergic, and dopaminergic projections arising from specific nuclei in the brainstem.

As the list of neurochemicals found in the dorsal horn grows larger each year, insight into their structural and functional organization is also growing. It is now clear that there is a precise laminar distribution of the neurochemicals, and their distribution is dependent on the segmental level assayed. Ultrastructural immunocytochemical studies have begun to identify the structures containing the neurochemicals as well as some of the target structures of the nerve terminals. Golgi-like immunostaining of dorsal horn neurons containing a particular transmitter now allows comparison of their morphology with past descriptions of cell types. Tracing techniques combined with immunostaining also aid analysis of the cell groups in the brainstem that give rise to neurochemically specific descending systems. This chapter reviews only some of the many current findings of the dorsal horn neurochemical organization. Recent reviews by Davidoff (1983) and by Salt and Hill (1983) have admirably accomplished a more comprehensive cataloguing of the neurochemical array found in the spinal cord.

B. *The Dorsal Horn Laminae: A Neurochemical Torte at the Light Microscopic Level*

When consecutive sections of the dorsal horn are immunostained for a variety of different neurochemicals, comparison of the specific patterns of labeled terminal distribution reveals that each substance produces its own unique "fingerprint" in the dorsal horn. The laminae of Rexed serve as the boundaries of the distributions, although subdivisions of the laminae are now recognized. Figure 1 presents camera lucida drawings of consecutive sections of the C6 segment of the monkey spinal cord from material immunostained with the PAP method for five different peptides and for 5-HT (de Lanerolle and LaMotte, 1983b). The peptide substance P is in high concentration in laminae I and II_O, with moderate amounts in lamina III and less in laminae IV and V. This pattern is quite similar in most species, including rat (Barber *et al.*, 1979; Hunt *et al.*, 1981), opossum (DiTirro *et al.*, 1981), cat (Hökfelt *et al.*, 1975b), monkey (de Lanerolle and LaMotte, 1983a) and man (de Lanerolle and LaMotte, 1982). Cholecystokinin has a pattern of distribution that is similar to but less dense than that of SP (Gibson *et al.*, 1981); in fact, there is considerable evidence of coexistence of SP and CCK in some neurons, including dorsal root ganglion cells (Dalsgaard *et al.*, 1982; Maciewicz *et al.*, 1984). Somatostatin, in contrast, is found in dorsal root ganglion cells (Hökfelt *et al.*, 1975a) and in fine axons and terminals in lamina I but in some species forms two distinct bands of heavy terminals in lamina II_O and in lamina III (Burnweit and Forssmann, 1979; Gibson *et al.*, 1981; Schrøder, 1984). Vasoactive intestinal polypeptide is found in laminae I, II_O, and II_i in approxi-

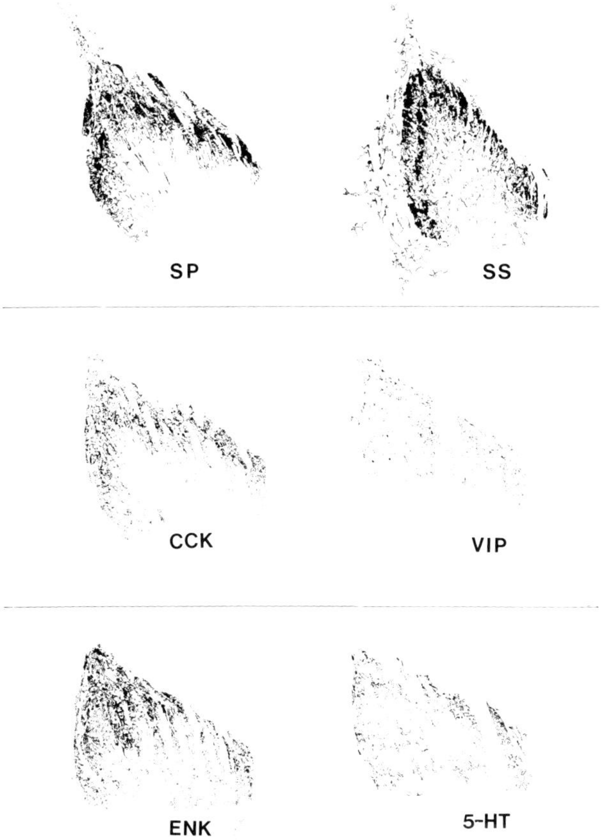

FIGURE 1. Camera lucida tracing of immunoreactive terminal fields of five peptides and 5-HT in the dorsal horn of the cervical (C6) monkey spinal cord. Each drawing represents one of a series of serial vibratome sections from the segment, each immunostained using the PAP method.

mately equal concentration. The presence of VIP in the cervical dorsal horn has previously been considered negligible, although its occurrence in the sacral cord has been commonly observed (Basbaum and Glazer, 1983; Honda *et al.*, 1983; Anaud *et al.*, 1983). The VIP immunostaining recently observed (LaMotte and de Lanerolle, 1983c) here in the cervical cord is exquisitely vulnerable to most fixatives, whereas that in the sacral cord is of such high concentration that immunostaining is reliable there despite loss from fixation.

1. *Primary Afferents*

Overall, the laminar concentrations of SP, SS, CCK, and VIP in the superficial laminae reflect their predominant localization in small-diameter primary afferents, which have been well demonstrated to terminate in these same laminae (LaMotte, 1977; Light and Perl, 1979; Ralston and Ralston, 1979; Gobel *et al.*, 1981). Substance P (Hökfelt *et al.*, 1975b), SS (Hökfelt *et al.*, 1975a), CCK (Dalsgaard *et al.*, 1982), and VIP (Lundberg *et al.*, 1978) have been localized in dorsal root ganglion cells, and acute dorsal rhizotomy results in a significant reduction in these peptides in the superficial dorsal horn (Hökfelt *et al.*, 1975b; Yaksh *et al.*, 1982a; Schrøder, 1984). Capsaicin, when given neonatally, destroys primary afferent C (nonmyelinated) fibers and, at higher doses, A-δ myelinated fibers; it produces a corresponding depletion of SP, CCK, SS, and VIP in the dorsal horn, dorsal root ganglia, and in peripheral nerves (Janséo *et al.*, 1981; Nagy *et al.*, 1981; see Yaksh, Chapter 11).

So far, peptides have not been associated with large-diameter, heavily myelinated primary afferents. Both classical and recent data support the view that certain amino acids, particularly L-glutamate and L-aspartate, may be neurotransmitters of these larger dorsal root axons. In a recent review, Salt and Hill (1983) deal with the multiple problems of interpreting experiments designed to test this hypothesis. However, some of the evidence in favor can be summarized from that review: (1) L-glutamate is in high concentration in the dorsal roots; (2) stimulation of the dorsal columns results in release of L-glutamate in the dorsal column nuclei; (3) D-aspartate injected into the dorsal horn or the dorsal column nuclei is retrogradely transported to only large dorsal root ganglion cells; (4) the excitation of dorsal horn neurons by stimulation of large myelinated dorsal root axons is antagonized by iontophoresis into the dorsal horn of antagonists to the receptors of L-glutamate and aspartate.

2. *Interneurons*

In addition to the major contribution by small-diameter primary afferents to the distribution of SP, CCK, and SS, there are also contributions from the intrinsic neurons of the dorsal horn that contain these peptides as well as contributions from descending supraspinal axons. Substance-P-positive neurons (Gibson *et al.*, 1981; Hunt *et al.*, 1981) and CCK-positive neurons have been found in laminae II, III, IV, and V (Schrøder, 1983). Somatostatin neurons also are present in I, II, IV, and V (Dalsgaard *et al.*, 1981; Hunt *et al.*, 1981; in fact, the density of SS terminals in the dorsal horn may be primarily from local neurons, as dorsal rhizotomy produces a less dramatic reduction in SS than in SP and CCK (Schrøder, 1984).

Other intrinsic neurons of the dorsal horn have been identified as containing substances not also associated with primary afferents. These neurochemicals include glycine, GABA, enkephalin, and neurotensin. Many glycine neurons appear to be located in lamina III (Aprison *et al.*, 1969), whereas GABA neurons are located more superficially. GABA interneurons and their terminals have been localized using antibodies to the GABA-synthesizing enzyme glutamate decarboxylase (GAD). In the rat dorsal horn, the heaviest distribution of GAD is in the superficial dorsal horn, with a dense band in lamina I and another in laminae II and III. Lamina I GAD-positive neurons resemble the stalked cells described in the Golgi studies of Gobel, and those in laminae II and III resemble islet cells (McLaughlin *et al.*, 1975; Barber *et al.*, 1982.)

Enkephalin-positive interneurons are present in laminae I through V (Gibson *et al.*, 1981; Glazer and Basbaum, 1981; Sumal *et al.*, 1982). Lamina I ENK neurons are large, with rostrocaudally extended dendrites (Glazer and Basbaum, 1981). Lamina II ENK cells in the outer region mainly resemble stalked cells and in deeper lamina II resemble islet cells (Bennett *et al.*, 1982) Enkephalin terminals are likewise heavily distributed in laminae I and II (Figure 1) (Aronin *et al.*, 1981; DeTirro *et al.*, 1981; LaMotte and de Lanerolle, 1983a; Charnay *et al.*, 1984).

Neurotensin cells and terminals have been found in laminae I, II, and III of the monkey, cat, and rat, with some species variation in the density of distribution within these laminae (Seybold and Elde, 1982; DiFiglia *et al.*, 1984). The NT neurons have some characteristics in common with islet, stalked, and border neurons. Neurotensin terminals are thought to arise almost entirely from these spinal neurons, as neither dorsal rhizotomy nor spinal lesions reduce the terminal fields of NT in the dorsal horn.

3. *Descending Systems*

Many of the peptides associated with either primary afferents or dorsal horn spinal neurons have also been identified in terminals and axons arising from descending fibers. Their relative contribution of terminals to the dorsal horn is small, but their functional significance is yet to be determined.

Substance P neurons in the medullary raphe have been found to project to the spinal cord in the rat, although the ventral horn appears to receive a heavier projection than the dorsal horn. These terminals may also contain serotonin, since SP and 5-HT coexist in some cells of the raphe nuclei (Bowker *et al.*, 1981).

Cholecystokinin may coexist with SP in some terminals, including both primary afferents (Dalsgaard *et al.*, 1982) and descending fibers. For example, CCK and SP neurons in the Edinger–Westphal nucleus have similar distributions, and at least some of these cells project to the spinal cord and probably contain both peptides (Maciewicz *et al.*, 1984).

Somatostatin-containing neurons of the periventricular nuclei of the hypothalamus project to the spinal cord, but their contribution is assumed to be quite minor in comparison to that from the SS primary afferents and SS dorsal horn cells (Schroder, 1984).

Although the majority of ENK terminals in the dorsal horn probably arise from local neurons, enkephalin-containing neurons that project to the spinal cord have also been identified in the brainstem, including cells in the pars gigantocellularis reticularis nucleus and the raphe nuclear complex (Hökfelt *et al.*, 1979; Bowker *et al.*, 1981).

In contrast to the above, other descending systems are the only, or at least the major, source of certain neurochemicals in the dorsal horn. Serotonin (5-HT) is found in high concentation in laminae I, II_O, IV, and V of the dorsal horn (Figure 1) (Fuxe, 1965; Ruda *et al.*, 1982; LaMotte and de Lanerolle, 1983b). Most serotoninergic terminals originate from descending axons of neurons in the raphe nuclei of the brainstem, including the medullary nuclei raphe magnus, raphe obscurus, raphe pallidus, and the ventral parts of the nucleus gigantocellularis; neurons in these nuclei project to all levels of the spinal cord. The raphe magnus projects via the spinal dorsolateral funiculus to the dorsal horn, whereas the nuclei raphe obscurus and pallidus project via the ventral funiculus to the ventral horn (Basbaum *et al.*, 1978; Basbaum and Fields, 1979).

The cervical cord also receives serotoninergic projections from the mesencephalic nucleus raphe dorsalis and the underlying tegmentum (Bowker *et al.*, 1981; Messing and Lytle, 1977 for review). Recently, serotoninergic neurons also have been found throughout the length of the spinal cord in several species, including the monkey (LaMotte *et al.*, 1982; DiTirro *et al.*, 1983; Ritchie *et al.*, 1984). Most of these spinal cells lie ventral to the central canal, although a few are found in the superficial dorsal horn; their contribution to the dorsal horn neuropil is unknown at present.

Noradrenergic terminals (NE) are found in heaviest concentration in lamina II; they arise from the locus coeruleus, and their descending axons are found in the lateral funiculus (Fuxe, 1965; Nygren and Olson, 1977; Satoh *et al.*, 1982). A dopaminergic projection from the A11 cell group of the periventricular region of the diencephalon also has been shown to project to the spinal cord (Bjorklund and Skagerberg, 1979; Anden *et al.*, 1966).

The neurosecretory cell groups of the periventricular region of the hypothalamus project to the medulla and the spinal cord (Hancock, 1976; Pittman *et al.*, 1984). In rat and monkey, axons immunopositive for oxytocin and for neurophysin are found in the dorsal part of the lateral funiculus, and terminals are found in laminae I and X and in the intermediolateral (IML) nucleus (Swanson and McKellar, 1979). Further comments on the neurotransmitter characteristics of these descending systems can be found in Chapter 15 by Hammond.

C. *Ultrastructural Localization and Functional Correlations*

1. *Primary Afferents*

Several types of SP terminals observed in laminae I and II resemble those described for primary afferents (Ralston and Ralston, 1979; Knyihar-Csillik *et al.*, 1982), i.e, C glomerular terminals with large granular vesicles (C-LGV terminals), simple terminals with large granular vesicles (LGV terminals), and a smaller number of simple terminals containing small round clear vesicles (R terminals) (de Lanerolle and LaMotte, 1983a; DiFiglia *et al.*, 1982; Barber *et al.*, 1979) (Figure 3A). Most of the SP terminals are directly presynaptic to dendrites and form asymmetric synapses; thus, they may be excitatory to dorsal horn neurons. There is considerable evidence that some SP terminals are likely to be associated with nociceptors (Olgart *et al.*, 1977). Horseradish peroxidase filling of primary afferents identified as nociceptors reveals that they often end as C terminals within laminae I and II_O; some nociceptive afferent terminals can end as non-C terminals in lamina I as well (Gobel *et al.*, 1981; Rethelyi *et al.*, 1982). Dorsal horn neurons that increase their spontaneous activity in response to iontophoresis of SP are also responsive to noxious mechanical and/or thermal peripheral stimuli and to electrical stimulation of A and C fibers (Henry, 1976); SP also facilitates the responses of neurons to noxious stimuli (Randic and Miletic, 1977; Davies and Dray, 1980). Further, stimulation of peripheral A and C fibers has been shown to release SP from the cord (Yaksh *et al.*, 1980). In contrast, units activated by low-threshold mechanical stimulation are usually less affected by SP, although excitation of nonnociceptive neurons has also been observed. Depletion or damage to SP primary afferents by systemic or intrathecal administration of capsaicin affects chemical, mechanical, and thermal nociceptive thresholds, again implying a role for these afferents in nociception (Hayes and Tyers, 1980; Yaksh *et al.*, 1979). For a further discussion of the possible role of substance P in the primary afferents, see comments by Yaksh (Chapter 8).

Target neurons of the SP primary afferents are likely to include both projection neurons (spinothalamic and spinoreticular) and spinal interneurons. Terminations onto interneurons are suspected, for some of the many spines and small dendrites within the SP C-glomerular complexes may arise from stalked and islet interneurons (Gobel, 1978a,b), and these interneurons may contain peptides such as enkephalin (Bennett *et al.*, 1982) or amino acids such as GABA (Barber *et al.*, 1982). These circuits might be a basis for modulation of dorsal horn activity through excitation of inhibitory interneurons, which in turn may either inhibit projection neurons directly or presynaptically modulate primary afferent terminals via axoaxonic contacts.

Interestingly, our preliminary EM analysis (Figure 2) also reveals that the other primary afferent peptides, CCK, SS, and VIP, are likewise localized mainly in simple LGV, LGV-C, and R terminals in laminae I and II. The morphological similarities of the terminals of these four peptides are striking. Although some coexistence is likely, such as for SP and CCK, SS and VIP are considered to represent distinct populations of dorsal root ganglion cells.

Much less is known of the actions of these peptides of primary afferents. Cholecystokinin excites both nociceptive and nonnociceptive dorsal horn neurons (Jeftinija *et al.*, Salt and Hill, 1983). Iontophoresis of SS usually suppresses the activity of dorsal horn neurons and their responsiveness to peripheral stimuli (Randic and Miletic, 1978), although excitation has also been observed

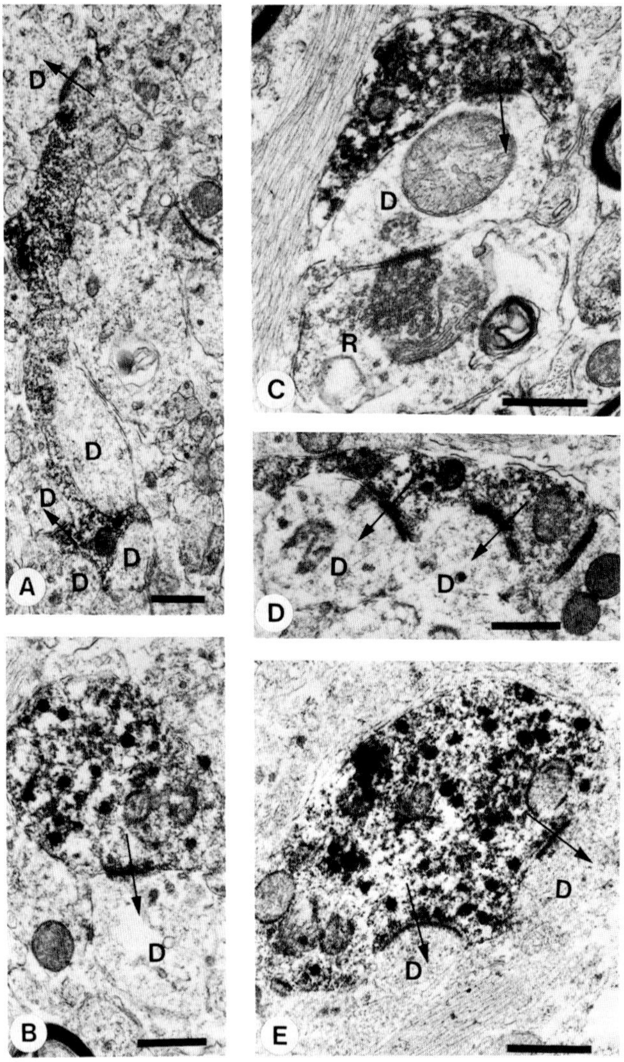

FIGURE 2. Immunostained synaptic terminals in laminae I and II_O of monkey spinal cord (C6). Bars = 0.5 μm. A: Longitudinal section through a CCK-LI process. At top, a varicosity forms a synaptic contact onto a dendrite; at bottom, a C terminal forms contacts onto four dendrites. B: A simple LGV terminal with VIP-LI that forms an asymmetric contact on a dendrite. C: A simple R terminal that is immunoreactive for CCK and an unlabeled R terminal form synaptic contacts onto the same small dendrite. D: A C terminal immunoreactive for VIP forms synaptic contacts onto two small dendrites. E: A large LGV-C terminal that is immunoreactive for SS contacts two dendrites.

(MacDonald and Nowak, 1981). Iontophoresis of VIP in the dorsal horn produces excitation of both nociceptive and nonnociceptive neurons (Jeftinija *et al.*, 1982; Salt and Hill, 1983); VIP has been mainly described in primary afferents in the lumbosacral cord and has been strongly suggested to be associated with visceral afferents, possibly nociceptive. However, its presence in all major levels of the spinal cord indicates additional functional roles for VIP.

2. *Interneurons*

The majority of GAD terminals contain pleomorphic or flattened vesicles and make symmetric synaptic contacts; they are usually presynaptic to dendrites and sometimes to cell somata, some of which also receive primary afferent terminals. In sagittal sections of laminae II and III, axoaxonal synaptic complexes are found in which the GAD terminals are presynaptic to terminals containing round vesicles and making asymmetric synaptic contacts with other profiles. It has also been demonstrated that in some cases the postsynaptic terminal is either a C-glomerular type of primary afferent or an R-type primary afferent terminal (McLaughlin *et al.*, 1975; Barber *et al.*, 1978).

Iontophoresis of GABA hyperpolarizes interneurons of the dorsal horn and also depolarizes primary afferent axons (see Barber *et al.*, 1978; Davidoff, 1983 for reviews); therefore, both postsynaptic and presynaptic effects are observed, in agreement with the axodendritic and axoaxonic contacts described for GABA.

Enkephalin terminals contain clear round vesicles and often a few large granular vesicles; they usually form asymmetric contacts with dendrites or dendritic spines (Figure 3B) (Aronin *et al.*, 1981; Glazer and Basbaum, 1983; LaMotte and de Lanerolle, 1983a). In some cases, the same dendrite has been found to receive primary afferent contacts as well (Sumal *et al.*, 1982). Enkephalin terminals have been shown to directly contact dorsal horn projection neurons (Ruda, 1982). Two types of axoaxonic complexes have been observed in lamina I in which an ENK terminal was presynaptic to another terminal (LaMotte and de Lanerolle, 1983a). One complex consists of an ENK terminal apposing an LGV terminal (Figure 3C). In the other complex, the ENK terminal is presynaptic to an R terminal (Figure 3D). In both complexes, the pre- and postsynaptic terminals often both form synapses on to the same dendrite. Both types of postsynaptic terminals resemble categories of primary afferents. A third type of axoaxonic complex has been described in which an ENK terminal is postsynaptic to a terminal containing flattened vesicles (Glazer and Basbaum, 1983).

Iontophoresis of enkephalinin the dorsal horn depresses the spontaneous activity of neurons and their responses to both nociceptive and nonnociceptive stimuli, but often preferentially to the noxious stimuli (Zieglgansberger and Tulloch, 1979; Duggan *et al.*, 1977). These are considered to be postsynaptic

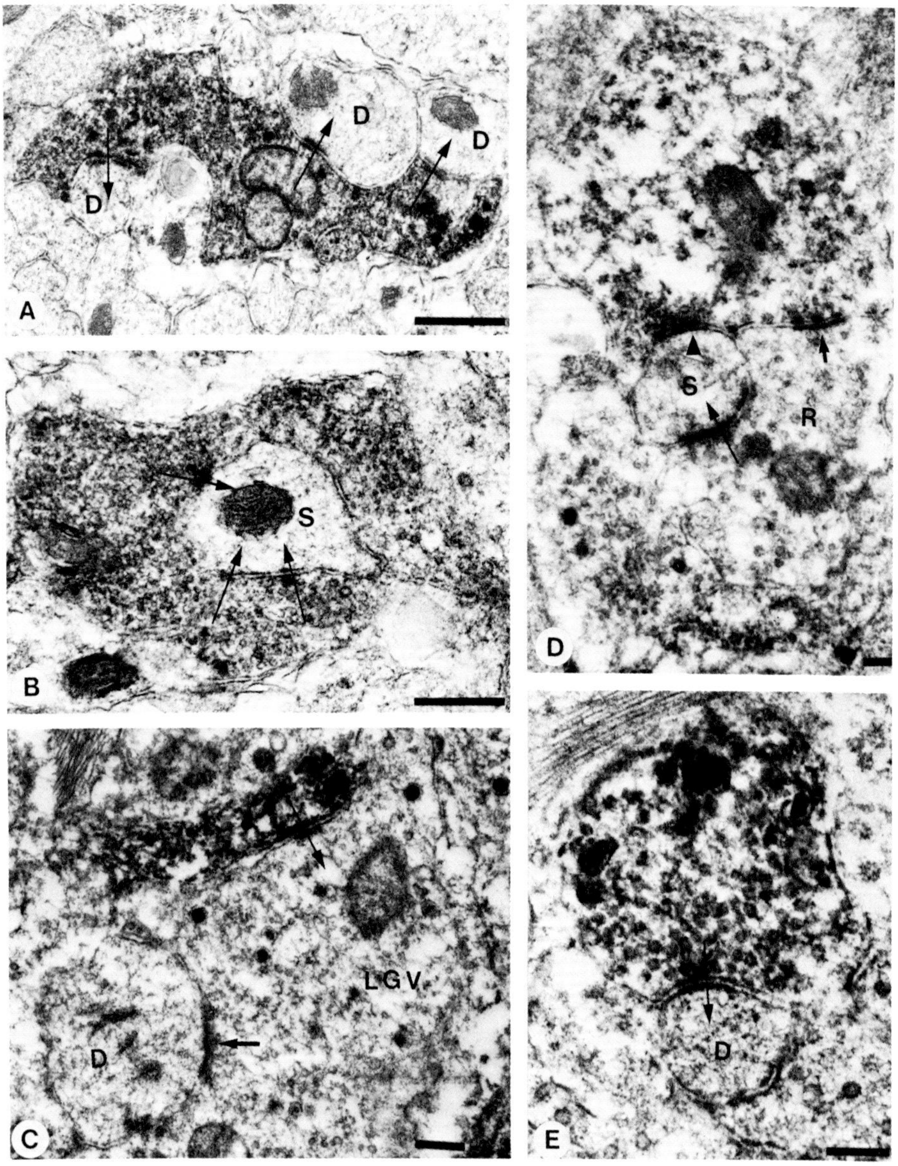

FIGURE 3. Immunostained synaptic terminals in laminae I and II_O of monkey spinal cord (C6). A: Terminal with substance-P-like immunoreactivity (SPLI). Terminal is classified as LGV-C type, forming the center of a glomerulus with synaptic contacts (arrows) onto three surrounding dendrites (D). Bar = 0.5 μm. B: A dendritic spine head (S) is surrounded by a met-enkephalin-like immmunoreactive (MELI) profile. Three synaptic contacts are indicated. Bar = 0.5 μm. C: One type of axoaxonic triplet complex involving a MELI terminal. Here a MELI profile apposes an unlabeled LGV terminal, forming a specialized contact. The LGV terminal forms an asymmetric synapse onto a small dendrite. Bar = 0.1 μm. D: Second type of MELI axoaxonic triplet. Here a MELI profile apposes an unlabeled R terminal (short arrow), forming a specialized contact. A dendritic spine (S) receives synapses from the MELI profile (arrowhead) and from the R terminal (long arrow). Bar = 0.1 μm. E: A serotonin-immunoreactive terminal (SLI) forming a synapse onto a small dentrite or spine. Terminal contains round vesicles and a few large granular vesicles and forms a symmetric junction. Bar = 0.25 μm.

effects and may be accounted for by the numerous enkephalin terminals found on dendrites, spines, and somata of dorsal horn neurons. Enkephalin presynaptic mechanisms are also suspected. Substance P release by primary afferents is suppressed by opiates (Jessel and Iverson, 1977), and degeneration of primary afferents results in a fall in opiate receptor sites in the superficial dorsal horn (LaMotte *et al.*, 1976; Ninkovic *et al.*, 1981). Primary afferent C-fiber depolarization by opiates has also been observed (Woolf and Fitzgerald, 1982). The axoaxonic contacts of ENK onto terminals resembling those arising from primary afferents, particularly the peptidergic small-diameter afferents, may provide a morphological basis for these presynaptic phenomena.

Neurotensin in laminae I and II is found in terminals containing both clear round vesicles and large granular vesicles; synaptic contacts are asymmetric onto dendrites and occasionally onto somata or somatic spines (DiFiglia *et al.*, 1984). In some cases, a terminal contacts up to three dendrites. Dorsal horn dendrites may receive several NT terminals. Some behavioral studies have reported analgesic effects of NT and possible naloxone dependence, but others have not found these results (Clineschmidt *et al.*, 1979). A similar conflict in reported physiological effects of NT exists, as both excitation and depression of dorsal horn neurons by NT have been observed in dorsal horn neuron spontaneous activity and in responses to stimuli (Henry, 1982; Miletic and Randic, 1979; Yaksh *et al.*, 1982b).

3. Descending Pathways

Serotonin terminals have been identified at the light microscope level in contact with marginal neurons, stalked cells, and islet cells; dendritic shafts were most often innervated (Hoffert *et al.*, 1983). Ultrastructural analysis reveals that 5-HT terminals contain small round clear vesicles and usually a few granular vesicles; synaptic junctions are usually symmetric (Figure 3E). Most contacts are indeed axodendritic; a few axospinous and axosomatic contacts are also present (Ruda *et al.*, 1982; LaMotte and de Lanerolle, 1983b; Light *et al.*, 1983). Additionally, axoaxonic contacts in which the 5-HT terminal is presynaptic to an LGV terminal also are found in the apical and lateral region of lamina I (LaMotte and de Lanerolle, 1983b). The small-diameter peptidergic primary afferents are one suspected source of the postsynaptic LGV terminals. Both postsynaptic and presynaptic actions of 5-HT have been observed in pharmacological studies of serotonin in the dorsal horn. Iontophoresis of 5-HT in the dorsal horn, or stimulation of the raphe, specifically suppresses the responses of high-threshold and wide-dynamic-range spinothalamic cells in laminae I, II, and V to noxious mechanical or thermal stimuli (Enberg and Ryall, 1966; Randic and Yu, 1976; Fields *et al.*, 1977; Belcher *et al.*, 1978; Jordan *et al.*, 1979; Yaksh, 1979; Gerhart *et al.*, 1981; Davies and Roberts, 1981). In addition, a presynaptic action of 5-HT on dorsal root fibers is indicated by the depolarization of both cutaneous mechanoreceptive and nociceptive primary afferents observed following stimulation of the NRM

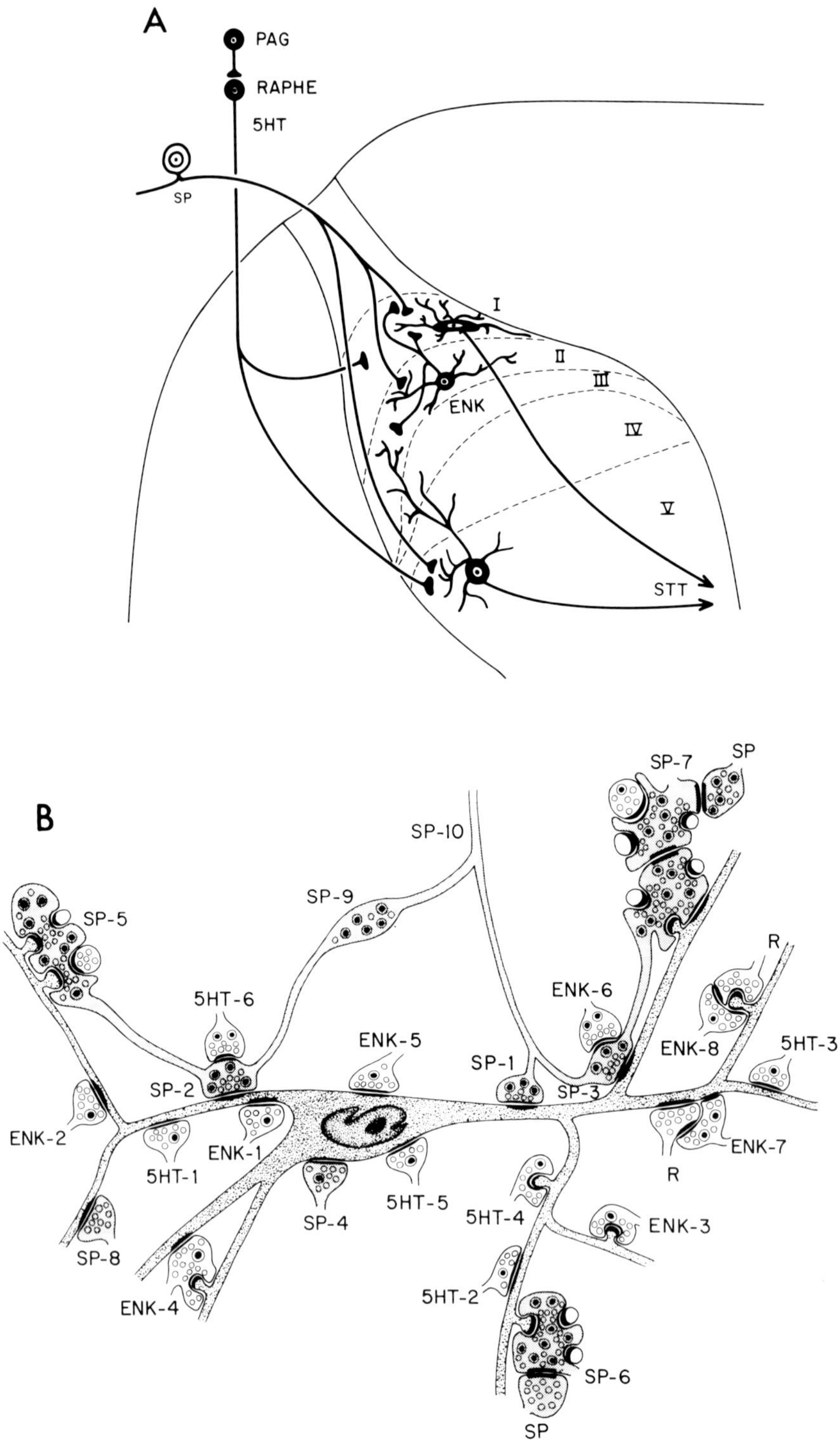
A
PAG
RAPHE
5HT
SP
I
II
III
IV
V
ENK
STT
B
SP-10
SP-7
SP
SP-5
SP-9
5HT-6
ENK-6
R
ENK-5
SP-1
ENK-8
5HT-3
SP-2
SP-3
ENK-2
5HT-1
ENK-1
ENK-7
R
SP-4
5HT-5
5HT-4
ENK-3
SP-8
ENK-4
5HT-2
SP-6
SP

(Carstens *et al.*, 1981; Martin *et al.*, 1979). Further comments by Ruda on the ultrastructural organization may be found in Chapter 7.

The ultrastructure of norepinephrine terminals has been identified with the glyoxylic acid–$KMnO_4$ method (Satoh *et al.*, 1982). Noradrenergic terminals contain small granular round vesicles and appose mostly small-caliber dendrites and spines, rarely large shafts. Occasionally, NE terminals appose other unlabeled terminals containing small round vesicles; however, the direction of the synapse was unclear. These unlabeled terminals do not degenerate following dorsal rhizotomy. As discusses by Hammond (Chapter 15), both iontophoresis of NA and locus coeruleus stimulation suppress responses of dorsal horn neurons to noxious stimuli (Enberg and Ryall, 1966; Belcher *et al.*, 1978).

FIGURE 4. A: A schematic diagram illustrating some possible relationships among peptidergic primary afferents, dorsal horn projection neurons [e.g., spinothalamic tract (STT) neurons], local peptidergic interneurons (e.g., ENK neurons), and descending modulating systems (e.g., 5-HT neurons). The 5-HT raphe neurons receive a significant projection from the PAG. These systems have all been implicated as basic elements of spinal nociceptive circuits. Small-diameter primary afferents may contain SP, SS, CCK, and VIP and form contacts onto both projection neurons and interneurons in the superficial dorsal horn and lateral region of lamina V. Local ENK neurons may form axodendritic contacts onto dorsal horn cells and axoaxonic contacts onto terminals that resemble those of primary afferents. Serotoninergic terminals also form similar axodendritic and axoaxonic contacts onto dorsal horn neurons. B: A schematic diagram illustrating several types of SPLI, ELI, and SLI profiles and their possible interactions and relationships to neurons in the lamina I–II_O region of the monkey dorsal horn (LaMotte and de Lanerolle, 1983b). All terminals are represented as impinging on a single hypothetical neuron, but this is for convenience and does not imply that they actually do so. Most SPLI terminals (shaded) have large granular vesicles. Some form simple axodendritic asymmetric synapses with large (SP-2), medium (SP-3), and small (SP-1) dendrites. A few form symmetric synapses with neuronal somata (SP-4), and others form the central terminal of glomeruli with spines, small dendrites, and dendrites containing vesicles (SP-5). Congregate SPLI terminal formations consist of various combinations of LGV, LGV-C, and R terminals (SP-6,7). A small number of SPLI terminals are R terminals and form asymmetric axodendritic synapses (SP-8). Light microscopic observations of SPLI processes suggest the possibility that many terminals, *boutons en passant,* and varicosities (SP-9) may be part of the same SPLI axon(SP-10). The MELI terminals containing small round vesicles and a few large granular vesicles form asymmetric synapses onto large (ENK-1) and small (ENK-2) dendrites and commonly onto spines (ENK-3,4). Some terminals that contact spines also contact dendritic shafts (ENK-4). Rare axosomatic MELI terminals form symmetric junctions (ENK-5). The SLI terminals contain small round vesicles and a few large granular vesicles. They form symmetric synapses onto large (5HT-1) and small (5HT-2,3) dendrites, a few dendritic spines (5HT-4), and cell bodies (5HT-5). Appositions between terminals are also represented, with the suggestion that SPLE terminals (SP-2,3) may on occasion be postsynaptic in possible axoaxonic contacts and that MELI terminals (ENK-6,7,8) and SLI terminals (5HT-6) may be presynaptic in possible axoaxonic contacts. Both MELI (ENK-6) and SLI profiles (5HT-6) are often found in contact with LGV terminals. These LGV terminals are usually presynaptic to dendrites and resemble terminals immunoreactive for SP and terminals that arise from primary afferents. Other MELI terminals ((ENK-7,8) contact R terminals that form axodendritic or axospinous junctions and that may possibly arise from primary afferents.

D. Summary

Although the hypothesis that different functional populations of small-diameter primary afferents may be represented by different peptidergic fibers remains viable, it is now clear that a single transmitter cannot be associated with a single terminal type. Similarities of the primary afferent peptidergic fibers include partial overlap of terminal fields, sensitivity to capsaicin, and morphological resemblance of terminal ultrastructure. Differences are expressed in relative density of the peptides in each lamina, and differences are likely to be found in the frequency of each terminal type, in the type of target neurons (e.g., local, spinothalamic, or spinoreticular neruon), and in the distribution of the terminals along the proximal and distal dendritic fields of target neurons. The additional occurrence of most of these same peptides in the terminals of local neurons and descending fibers further emphasizes the importance of these target features.

Comparisons can also be drawn among some of the local interneuron systems. Particularly, there are several resemblances among the ENK, GABA, and NT systems in the superficial dorsal horn (LaMotte and de Lanerolle, 1983a; DiFiglia *et al.*, 1984). As described above, all three cell types are located manily in laminae II and III, with a smaller number in I or along the I–II border. Islet cells have been included in the cell types described for all three of these neurochemicals, and some ENK and GABA neurons have been identified as stalked cells also. Enkephalin, GABA, and NT neurons primarily form axodendritic contacts on dorsal horn cells; correspondingly, GABA and ENK neurons produce postsynaptic inhibition of dorsal horn neurons, as is sometimes the case for NT. For ENK and GABA, some target dendrites have been shown also to be postsynaptic to a primary afferent. GABA and ENK also produce presynaptic inhibition of dorsal horn cells, and axoaxonal contacts have been observed for both. (Neurotensin axoaxonic contacts have not been reported.) Enkephalin terminals are presynaptic to simple LGV and to R terminals and are most common in apical and lateral lamina I, where a likely target of the ENK terminals may be nociceptive primary afferents. GABA terminals are more frequently presynaptic to C-glomerular terminals and R terminals and are found mostly in laminae II and III, where the target is more likely to be a nonnociceptive afferent.

The descending 5-HT and NA systems, like the local ENK, GABA, and NT systems, make mostly axodendritic contacts. However, ENK and NE terminals are thought to occur more often on small dendrites and spines, whereas 5-HT terminals may occur more on dendritic shafts, although small dendrite innervation is also frequent. Of the axoaxonic contacts observed, it may be significant that the C glomerulus in laminae I and II is not a target of ENK, 5-HT, or NE terminals; rather, it is the simple LGV or R terminal that is postsynaptic. Only in the case of the deeper laminae II and III C terminals is there presynaptic contact, by GABA terminals. Thus, the tight coupling of the glomerulus and its family of dendrites in laminae I and II_O appears to be unaffected directly by presynaptic inhibition. Instead, the laminae I and II_O intrinsic and descending systems that modulate nociception must affect that circuitry either by direct contact onto target neurons or by presynaptic inhibition of simple terminals, possibly of primary afferent origin. (Figure 4). Further, the restriction of these axoaxonic contacts to the apical region suggests that although the presynaptic contacts may be neither widespread nor numerous their location may be strategic. It is possible that either the dendritic target of the triplet complex at the apical site may be of unique origin or a presynaptic mechanism at the outlet of Lissauer's tract, through which all the peptidergic primary afferents must pass, may be particularly effective. That is, because this point is located at the beginning of a chain of synaptic varicosities that will distribute throughout the superficial dorsal horn, inhibition here might possibly also affect activity at more distal points along the varicose axon.

References

ANAUD, P., GIBSON, S. J., MCGGREGOR, G. P., BLANK, M. A., GHATEI, M. A., BACARESE-HAMILTON, A. J., POLAR, J. M., AND BLOOM, S. R. A VIP-containing system concentrated in the lumbosacral region of human spinal cord. *Nature* 305:143–145, 1983.

ANDEN, N.E., JUKES, M. G. M., LUNDBERG, A, AND VYKLICKY, L. The effect of DOPA on the spinal cord. I. Influence on transmission from primary afferents. *Acta Physiol Scand.* 67:373–386, 1966.

APRISON, M. H., SHANK, R. P., AND DAVIDOFF, R. A. Glycine: A transmitter suspect in different areas of the brain and spinal cord in seven different vertebrates. *Comp. Biochem. Physiol.* 28:1345–1355, 1969.

ARONIN, N., DIFIGLIA M., LIOTLA, A. S., AND MARTIN, J. B. Ultrastructural localization and biochemical features of immunoreactive leu-enkephalin in monkey dorsal horn. *J. Neurosci.* 1:561–577, 1981.

BARBER, R. P., VAUGHN, J. E., SAITO, K., MCLAUGHLIN, B. J., AND ROBERT, E. GABAergic terminals are presynaptic to primary afferent terminals in the substantia gelatinosa of the rat spinal cord. *Brain Res. 141:35–55, 1978.*

BARBER, R. P., VAUGHAN, J. E., SLEMMON, J. R., SALVATERRA, R. M., ROBERTS, E, AND LEEMAN, S. E. The orgin, distribution and synaptic relationships of substance P axons in rat spinal cord. *J. Comp. Neurol.* 184:331–352, 1979.

BARBER, R. P., VAUGHN, J. E., AND ROBERTS, E. The cytoarchitecture of GABAergic neurons in rat spinal cord.*Brain Res. 238:305–328, 1982.*

BASBAUM, A. L., AND FIELDS, H. L. The origin of descending pathways in the dorsolateral funiculus of the spinal cord of the cat and rat: Further studies on the anatomy of pain modulation. *J. Comp. Neurol.* 187:513–532, 1979.

BASBAUM, A. I., AND GLAZER, E. J. Immunoreactive vasoactive intestinal polypeptide is concentrated in the sacral spinal cord: A possible marker for pelvic visceral afferent fibers. *Somatosen. Res.* 1:69–82, 1983.

BASBAUM, A. I., CLANTON, C. H., AND FIELDS, H. L. Three bulbospinal pathways from the rostral medulla of the cat: An autoradiographic study of pain modulating systems. *J. Comp. Neurol.* 178:209–224, 1978.

BELCHER, G., RYALL, R. W., AND SCHAFFNER, R. The differential effect of 5-hydroxytryptamine, noradrenaline and raphe stimulation on nociceptive and non-nociceptive dorsal horn interneurons in the cat. *Brain Res.* 151:307–321, 1978.

BENNETT, G. J., RUDA, M., GOBEL, S., AND DUBNER, S. Enkephalin immunoreactive stalked cells and lamina IIb islet cell in the cat substantia gelatinose. *Brain Res.* 240:162–165, 1982.

BJORKLUND, A., AND SKAGERBERG, G. Evidence for a major spinal cord projection from diencephalic A11 dopamine cell group in the rat using transmitter-specific fluorescent retrograde tracing. *Brain Res.* 177:170–175, 1979.

BOWKER, R.M., STEINBUSCH, H. W. M., AND COULTER, J. D. Serotonin and peptidergic projections to the spinal cord demonstrated by a combined retrograde HRP histochemical staining method. *Brain Res.* 211:412–417, 1981.

BURNWEIT, C., AND FORSSMANN, W. G. Somatostatinergic nerves in the cervical spinal cord of the monkey. *Cell Tissue Res.* 200:83–90, 1979.

CARSTENS, E., KLUMPP, D., RANDIC, M., AND ZIMMERMAN, M. Effect of iontophoretically applied 5-hydroxytryptamine on the excitability of single primary afferent C- and A-fibers in the cat spinal cord. *Brain Res.* 220:151–158, 1981

CHARNAY, Y., PAULIN, C., DRAY, F., AND DUBOIS, P. Distribution of enkephalin in human fetus and infant spinal cord: An immunofluorescence study. *J. Comp. Neurol.* 223:415–423, 1984.

CLINESCHMIDT, B. V., MCGUFFIN, J. C., AND BUNTING, P. B. Neurotensin: Antinociceptive action in rodents. *Eur. J. Pharmacol.* 54:129–139, 1979.

DALSGAARD, C. J., HÖKFELT, T., JOHNSSON, O., AND ELDE, R. Somatostatin immunoreactive cell bodies in the dorsal horn and the parasympathetic intermediolateral nucleus of the rat spinal cord. *Neurosci. Lett.* 27:335–339, 1981.

DALSGAARD, C. J., VINCENT, S. R., HÖKFELT, T., LUNDBERG, J. M., DAHLSTROM, A., SCHULTZBERG, M. DOLKRAL, G. J. AND CVELLO, A. C. Coexistence of cholecystokinin- and substance P-like peptides in neurons of the dorsal root ganglia of the rat. *Neurosci. Lett.* 33:159–164, 1982.

DAVIDOFF, R. A. Handbook of the Spinal Cord, Vol. 1: Pharmacology, Marcel Dekker, New York, 1983.

DAVIES, J., AND DRAY, A. Depression and facilitation of synaptic responses in cat dorsal horn by substance P administered into substantia gelatinosa. *Life Sci.* 27:2037–2042, 1980.

DAVIES, J. E., AND ROBERTS, H. M. T. 5-Hydroxytryptamine reduces substance P responses on dorsal horn interneurons: A possible interaction of neurotransmitters. *Brain Res.* 217:399–404,1981.

DE LANEROLLE, N. C., AND LAMOTTE, C. C. The human spinal cord: Substance P and methionine-enkephalin immunoreactivity. *J. Neurosci.* 2:1369–1386, 1982.

DE LANEROLLE, N. C., AND LAMOTTE, C. C. Ultrastructure of chemically defined neuron systems in the dorsal horn of the monkey. I. Substance P immunoreactivity. *Brain Res.* 274:31–49, 1983a.

DE LANEROLLE, N. C., AND LAMOTTE, C. C. Laminar organization of five neuropeptides and serotonin in the monkey dorsal horn. *Neurosci.Soc. Abstr.* 9:256, 1983b.

DIFIGLIA, M., ARONIN, N., AND LEEMAN, S. E. Light microscopic and ultrastructural localization of immunoreactive substance P in the dorsal horn of monkey spinal cord. *Neuroscience* 7:1127–1139, 1982.

DIFIGLIA, M., ARONIN, M., AND LEEMAN, S. E. Ultrastructural localization of innumoreactive neurotensin in the monkey superficial dorsal horn. *J. Comp. Neurol.* 225:1–12, 1984.

DITIRRO, F. J., HO, R. N., AND MARTIN, G. F. Immunohistochemical localization of substance P, somatostatin, and methionine-enkephalin in the spinal cord and dorsal root ganglia of the North American opossum, *Didelphis virginiana. J. Comp. Neurol.* 198:351–363, 1981.

DITIRRO, F. J., MARTIN, G. F., AND HO, R. H. A developmental study of substance P, somatostatin, enkephalin, and serotonin immunoreactive elements in the spinal cord of the North American opossum. *J. Comp. Neurol.* 213:241–261, 1983.

DUGGAN, A. W., HALL, J., AND HEADLY, P. Enkephalins and dorsal horn neurones of the cat: Effects on responses to noxious and innocuous skin stimuli. *Br. J. Pharmacol.* 61:399–408, 1977.

ENBERG, I., AND RYALL, R. W. The inhibitory action of noradrenaline and other monoamines on spinal neurones. *J. Physiol. (Lond.)* 185:298–322, 1966.

FIELDS, H. L., BASBAUM, A. I., CLANTON, C. H., AND ANDERSON, S. D. Nucleus raphe magnus inhibition of spinal cord dorsal horn neurons. *Brain Res.* 126:441–454, 1977.

FUXE, K. Evidence for the existence of monoamine neurons in the central nervous system. *Acta Physiol. Scand. [Suppl.]* 247:39–85, 1965.

GERHART, K. T., WILCOX, T. K., CHUNG, J. M., AND WILLIS, W. D. Inhibition of nociceptive and non-nociceptive responses of primate spinothalamic cells by stimulation in medial brainstem. *J. Neurophysiol.* 45:121–136, 1981.

GIBSON, S. J., POLAK, J. M., BLOOM, S. R., AND WALL, P. D. The distribution of nine peptides in rat spinal cord with special emphasis on the substantia gelatinosa and on the area around the central canal (lamina X). *J. Comp. Neurol.* 201:65–79, 1981.

GLAZER, E. J., AND BASBAUM, A. I. Immunohistochemical localization of leucine-enkephalin in the spinal cord of the rat: Enkephalin containing marginal neurons and pain modulation. *J. Comp. Neurol.* 196:377–389, 1981.

GLAZER, E. J., AND BASBAUM, A. I. Opioid neurons and pain modulation: An ultrastructural analysis of enkephalin in cat superficial dorsal horn. *Neuroscience* 10:357–376, 1983.

GOBEL, S. Golgi studies of the neurons in layer I of the dorsal horn of the medulla (trigeminal nucleu caudalis). *J. Comp. Neurol.* 180:375–394, 1978a.

GOBEL, S. Golgi studies of the neurons in layer II of the dorsal horn of the medulla (trigeminal nucleus caudalis). *J. Comp. Neurol.* 180:395–414, 1978b.

GOBEL, S., FALLS, W. M., AND HUMPHREY, E. Morphology and synaptic connections of ultrafine primary axons in lamina I of the spinal dorsal horn: Candidates for the terminal arbors of primary neurons with unmyelinated (C) axons. *J. Neurosci.* 1:1163–1179, 1981.

HANCOCK, M. B. Cells of origin of hypothalamo-spinal projection in the rat. *Neurosci. Lett.* 3:179–184, 1976.

HAYES, A. G., AND TYERS, M. B. Effects of capsaicin on nociceptive heat, pressure, and chemical thresholds and on substance P levels in the rat. *Brain Res.* 189:561–564, 1980.

HENRY, J. L. Effects of substance P on functionally identified units in cat spinal cord. *Brain Res.* 114:439–451, 1976.

HENRY, J. L. Electrophysiological studies on the neuroactive properties of neurotensin. *Ann. N.Y. Acad. Sci.* 400:216–217, 1982.

HOFFERT, M. J., MILETIC, V., RUDA, M. A. AND DUBNER, R. Immunocytochemical identification of serotonin axonal contacts on characterized neurons in laminae I and II of the cat dorsal horn. *Brain Res.* 267:361–364, 1983.

HÖKFELT, T., ELDE, R., JOHANSSON, O, LUFT, AND ARIMURA A. Immunohistochemical evidence for the presence of somatostatin, a powerful inhibitory peptide, in some primary sensory neurons. *Neurosci. Lett.* 1:231–235, 1975a.

HÖKFELT, T., KELLERETH, J. O., NILSSON, G., AND PERNOW, B. Experimental immunohistochemical studies on the localization and distribution of substance P in the cat primary sensory neurons. *Brain Res.* 100:235–252, 1975b.

HÖKFELT, T., TERENIUS, L., KUYPERS, H. G. J. M., AND DANN, O. Evidence for enkephalin immunoreactive neurons in the medulla oblongata projecting to the spinal cord. *Neurosci. Lett.* 14:55–60, 1979.

HONDA, C. N., RETHELYI, M., AND PETRUSZ, P. Preferential immunohistochemical localization of vasoactive intestinal polypeptide (VIP) in the sacral spinal cord of the cat: Light and electron microscopic observations. *J. Neurosci.* 3:2183–2196, 1983.

HUNT, S. P., KELLY, J. S., EMSON, P. C., KIMMEL, J. R., MILLER, R. J., AND WU, Y. An immunohistochemical study of neuronal populations containing neuropeptides or γ-aminobutyrate within the superficial layers of the rat dorsal horn. *Neuroscience* 6:1883–1898, 1981.

JANSCO, G., HÖKFELT, T., LUNDBERG, J. M., KIRALY, E., HALASZ, N., NILSSON, G., TERENIUS, L., REHFELD, J., STEINBUSCH, H., VEREHOFSTAD, A., ELDE, R., SAID, S., AND BROWN, M. Immunohistochemical studies on the effect of capsaicin on spinal and medullary peptide and monoamine neurons using antisera to substance P, gastrin/CCK, somatostatin, VIP, enkephalin, neurotensin, and 5-hydroxytryptamine. *J. Neurocytol.* 10:963–980, 1981.

JEFTINIJA, S., MILETIC, V., AND RANDIC, M. Cholecystokinin octapeptide excites dorsal horn neurons both *in vivo* and *in vitro*. *Brain Res.* 213:231–236, 1981.

JEFTINIJA, S., MURASE, K., NEDELJKOV, V., AND RANDIC, M. Vasoactive intestinal polypeptide excites mammalian dorsal horn neurons both *in vivo* and *in vitro*. *Brain Res.* 243:158–164, 1982.

JESSELL, T. M., AND IVERSEN, L. L. Opiate analgesics inhibit substance P release from rat trigeminal nucleus. *Nature* 268:549–551, 1977.

JORDAN, L. M., KENSHALO, D. R., JR., MARTIN, R. F., HABER, L. A., AND WILLIS, W. D. Two populations of spinothalamic tract neurons with opposite responses to 5-hydroxytryptamine. *Brain Res.* 164:343–346, 1979.

KNYIHAR-CSILLIK, E., CSILLIK, B., AND RAKIC, P. Ultrastructure of normal and degenerating glomerular terminals of dorsal root axons in the substantia gelatinosa of the rhesus monkey. *J. Comp. Neurol.* 210:357–375, 1982.

LAMOTTE, C. C. Distribution of the tract of Lissauer and dorsal root fibers in the primate spinal cord. *J. Comp. Neurol.* 172:529–561, 1977.

LAMOTTE, C. C., AND DE LANEROLLE, N. C. Ultrastructure of chemically defined neuron systems in the dorsal horn of the monkey. II. Met-enkephalin immunoreactivity. *Brain Res.* 274:51–63, 1983a.

LAMOTTE, C. C., AND DE LANEROLLE, N. C. Ultrastructure of chemically defined neuron systems in the dorsal horn of the monkey. III. Serotonin immunoreactivity. *Brain Res.* 274:65–77, 1983b.

LAMOTTE, C. C., AND DE LANEROLLE, N. C. Vasoactive intestinal polypeptide (VIP): Distribution throughout the length of primate spinal cord. *Neurosci. Soc. Abstr.* 9:256, 1983c.

LAMOTTE, C. C., PERT, C. B., AND SNYDER, S. H. Opiate receptor binding in primate spinal cord: Distribution and changes after dorsal root section. *Brain Res.* 112:407–412, 1976.

LAMOTTE, C. C., JOHNS, D. R., AND DE LANEROLLE, N. C. Immunohistochemical evidence of indolamine neurons in monkey spinal cord. *J. Comp. Neurol.* 206:359–370, 1982.

LIGHT, A. R., AND PERL, E. R. Spinal termination of functionaly identified primary afferent neurons with slowly conducting myelinated fibers. *J. Comp. Neurol.* 186:133–150, 1979.

LIGHT, A. R., KAVOOKJIAN, A. M., AND PETRUSZ, P. The ultrastructure and synaptic connections of serotonin-immunoreactive terminals in spinal laminae I and II. *Somatosens. Res.*1:33–50, 1983.

LUNDBERG, J. M., HÖKFELT, T., NILSSON, G., TERENIUS, L., REHFELD, J., ELDE, R., AND SAID, S. Peptide neurons in the vagus, splanchnic and sciatic nerves. *Acta Physiol. Scand.* 104:499–501, 1978.

MACDONALD, R. L., AND NOWAK, L. M. Substance P and somatostatin actions on spinal cord neurons in primary dissociated cell culture. *Adv. Biochem Psychopharmacol.* 28:159–173, 1981.

MACIEWICZ, R., PHIPPS, B. S., GRENIER, J., AND POLETTI, C. E. Edinger–Westphal nucleus: Cholecystokinin immunohistochemistry and projections to the spinal cord and trigeminal nucleus in the cat. *Brain Res.* 299:139–145, 1984.

MARTIN, R. F., HABER, L. H., AND WILLIS, W. D. Primary afferent depolarization of identified cutaneous fibers following stimulation in medial brainstem. *J. Neurophysiol.* 42: 779–790, 1979.

MCLAUGHLIN, B. J., BARBER, R., SAITO, K., ROBERTS, E., AND WU, J. Y. Immunocytochemical localization of glutamate decarboxylase in rat spinal cord. *J. Comp. Neurol.* 164:305–322, 1975.

MESSING, R. B., AND LYTLE, L. D. Serotonin containing neurons: Their possible role in pain and analgesia. *Pain* 4:1–21, 1977.

MILETIC, V., AND RANDIC, M. Neurotensin excites cat spinal neurons located in laminae I–III. *Brain Res.* 169:600–604, 1979.

NAGY, J. I., HUNT, S. P., IVERSEN, L. L., AND EMSON, P. C. Biochemical and anatomical observations on the degenertion of peptide-containing primary afferent neurons after neonatal capsaicin. *Neuroscience* 6:1923–1934, 1981.

NINKOVIC, M. C., HUNT, S. P., AND KELLY, J. S. Effect of dorsal rhizotomy on the autoradiographic distribution of opiate and neurotensin receptors and neurotensin-like immunoreactivity within the rat spinal cord. *Brain Res.* 230:111–119, 1981.

NYGREN, L. G., AND OLSON, L. A new major projection from locus coeruleus: The main source of noradrenergic nerve terminals in the ventral and dorsal columns of the spinal cord. *Brain Res.* 132:85–93, 1977.

OLGART, L., HÖKFELT, T., NILSSON, G., AND PERNOW, B. Localization of substance P-like immunoreactivity in nerves in the tooth-pulp. *Pain* 4:153–160, 1977.

PITTMAN, Q. J., RIPHAGEN, C. L.,AND LEPERIS, K. Release of immunoassayable neurohypophyseal peptides from the rat spinal cord, *in vivo*. *Brain Res.* 300:321–326, 1984.

RALSTON, H. J., AND RALSTON, D. D. The distribution of dorsal root axons in laminae I, II and III of the macaque spinal cord: A quantitative electron microscopic study. *J. Comp. Neurol.* 184:643–684, 1979.

RANDIC, M. AND MILETIC, V. Effect on substance P in cat dorsal horn neurons activated by noxious stimuli. *Brain Res.* 128:164–169, 1977.

RANDIC, M., AND MILETIC, V. Depressant actions of met-enkephalin and somatostatin in cat dorsal horn neurons activated by noxious stimuli. *Brain Res.* 152:196–202, 1978.

RANDIC, M., AND YU, H. H. Effects of 5-hydroxytryptamine and bradykinin in cat dorsal horn neurones activated by noxious stimuli. *Brain Res.* 111:197–203, 1976.

RETHELYI, M., LIGHT, A. R., AND PERL, E. R. Synaptic complexes formed by functionally defined primary afferent units with fine myelinated fibers. *J. Comp. Neurol.* 207:381–393, 1982.

RITCHIE, T. C., ROOS, L. J., WILLIAMS, B. J., AND LEONARD, R. B. The descending and intrinsic serotonergic innervation of an elasmobranch spinal cord. *J. Comp. Neurol.* 224:395–406, 1984.

RUDA, M. A. Opiates and pain pathways: Demonstration of enkephalin synapses on dorsal horn projection neurons. *Science* 215:1523–1524, 1982.

RUDA, M. A., COFFIELD, J., AND STEINBUSCH, H. W. M. Immunocytochemical analysis of serotonergic axons in laminae I and II of the lumbar spinal cord of the cat. *J. Neurosci.* 2:1660–1671, 1982.

SALT, T. E., AND HILL, R. G. Neurotransmitter candidates of somatosensory primary afferent fibres. *Neuroscience* 10:1083–1103, 1983.

SATOH, K., KASHIBA, A., KIMURA, H., AND MAEDA, T. Noradrenergic axon terminals in the substantia gelatinosa of the rat spinal cord. *Cell Tissue Res.* 222:359–378, 1982.

SCHRØDER, H. D. Localization of cholecystokinin-like immunoreactivity in the rat spinal cord, with particular reference to the autonomic innervation of the pelvic organs. *J. Comp. Neurol.* 217:176–186, 1983.

SCHRØDER, H. D. Somatostatin in the caudal spinal cord: An immunohistochemical study of the spinal centers involved in the innervation of pelvic organs. *J. Comp. Neurol.* 223:400–414, 1984.

SEYBOLD, V. S., AND ELDE, R. P. Neurotensin immunoreactivity in the superficial laminae of the dorsal horn of the rat: I. Light microscopic studies of cell bodies and proximal dendrites. *J. Comp. Neurol.* 204:89–100, 1982.

SUMAL, K. K., PICKEL, V. M., MILLER, R. J., AND REIS, D. J. Enkephalin-containing neurons in substantia gelatinosa of spinal trigeminal complex: Ultrastructure and synaptic interaction with primary sensory afferents. *Brain Res.* 248:223–236, 1982.

SWANSON, L. W., AND MCKELLAR, S. The distribution of oxytocin and neurophysin stained fibers in the spinal cord of the rat and monkey. *J. Comp. Neurol.* 188:87–106, 1979.

WOOLF, C. J., AND FITZGERALD, M. Do opioid peptides mediate a presynaptic control of C-fiber transmission in the rat spinal cord? *Neurosci. Lett.* 29:67–72, 1982.

YAKSH, T. L. Direct evidence that spinal serotonin and noradrenaline terminals mediate the spinal nociceptive effects of morphine in the periaqueductal gray. *Brain Res.* 160:180–185, 1979.

YAKSH, T. L., FARB, D. H., LEEMAN, S. E., AND JESSELL, T. M. Intrathecal capsaicin depletes substance P in the rat spinal cord and produces prolonged thermal analgesi. *Science* 206:481–483, 1979.

YAKSH, T. L., JESSELL, T. M., GAMSE, R., MUDGE, A. W., AND LEEMAN S. E. Intrathecal morphine inhibits substance P release from mammalian spinal cord in vivo. *Nature* 286:155–157, 1980.

YAKSH, T. L., ABAY, E. O., AND GO, V. L. W. Studies on the location and release of cholecystokinin and vasoactive intestinal polypeptide in rat and cat spinal cord. *Brain Res.* 242:272–290, 1982a.

YAKSH, T. L., SCHMAUSS, C., MICEVYCH, P. E., ANAY, E. O., AND GO, V. L. W. Pharmacological studies on the application, disposition and release of neurotensin in the spinal cord. *Ann. N.Y. Acad. Sci.* 400:228–243, 1982b.

ZIEGLGANSBERGER, W., AND TULLOCH, I. F. The effects of methionine- and leucine-enkephalin on spinal neurons of the cat. *Brain Res.* 167:53–64, 1979.

6 Neurotransmitter Receptor Sites in the Spinal Cord

VIRGINIA S. SEYBOLD

A. *Introduction*

Since the studies discussed in this chapter concern the distribution of receptors for neurotransmitters, it is important to specify that the term "receptor" implies a physiologically functional unit. Binding of a transmitter molecule to its binding site on the neuronal membrane surface initiates a physical change in the receptor unit that results in a physiological change, i.e., a change in membrane ion permeability (nicotinic cholinergic receptor) or activation of an enzyme resulting in a change in the level of a biochemical intermediate within the cell (β-adrenergic receptors and many peptide hormone receptors). Binding studies and autoradiograms, however, reflect just the binding site portion of the receptor unit, and such data must be described in terms of binding sites. However, the radiolabeled ligands used to prepare the autoradiograms are pharmacologically active compounds whose physiological effects on the system may be well characterized. Therefore, in this discussion of the biological significance of binding sites, I refer to them as receptors.

A significant portion of the data this chapter discusses concerns the distribution of receptors for putative neurotransmitters in the dorsal horn of the spinal cord. The diversity of these putative neurotransmitter systems and the complexity of the elements of these dorsal horn systems are discussed elsewhere in this volume (see LaMotte, Chapter 5; Ruda, Chapter 7; Cervero, Chapter 9).

VIRGINIA S. SEYBOLD • Department of Anatomy, University of Minnesota, Minneapolis, Minnesota 55455.

Although the superficial laminae of the dorsal horn are generally considered to be most important in synaptic transmission of nociception through the spinal cord, the region around the central canal (lamina X) is also emerging as a site involved in spinal transmission of nociceptive stimuli. Electrophysiological studies in this region have characterized neurons that respond to noxious peripheral stimuli (Fields *et al.*, 1975; Honda and Perl, 1981; Nahin *et al.*, 1983). The peripheral input to these cells may be direct, since the termination of A-δ nociceptors has been described in lamina X in the cat (Light and Perl, 1979) and substance-P-containing fibers are also dense in this region (Barber *et al.*, 1979; Gibson *et al.*, 1981; Ljungdahl *et al.*, 1978). Therefore, descriptive data on this region are included, since such information may form the basis of new hypotheses concerning transmission of nociception in the spinal cord.

B. Biochemical Surveys of Regional Levels of Neurotransmitter Binding Sites in Spinal Cord

Biochemical analyses of neurotransmitter binding sites in the spinal cord have generally utilized homogenates of whole spinal cord segments so that sufficient tissue would be available for analysis. Two different approaches to measurement of binding sites *in vitro* allow for different comparisons of ligand binding sites of the spinal cord. By using several concentrations of radiolabeled ligand to generate a Scatchard plot, one can determine the dissociation constant (K_D) and the maximum number of binding sites in the spinal cord (B_{max}) for each ligand. These data allow one to compare the number of receptors within the spinal cord for different ligands. In addition, the K_D for each ligand can be compared to its K_D within other regions of the central nervous system to determine whether there are unique biochemical or biophysical characteristics of the binding sites within the spinal cord. The second approach is to look for differences in receptor densities by comparing the binding of one nonsaturating concentration of ligand among homogenates of microdissected brain regions. Since the concentration of ligand directly affects the amount of ligand bound per gram of protein and has varied among ligands, data obtained with this approach are not useful for comparison of the number of binding sites among ligands and therefore are not included here.

Data generated from Scatchard analyses of ligand binding in rat spinal cord homogenates are summarized in Table I. Comparison of B_{max} values in rat indicates that the high-affinity binding sites with the greatest density in the spinal cord are muscarinic, with an excess of 1000 fmol of ligand bound per milligram of protein (Kayaalp and Neff, 1980). The high-affinity GABA binding site, as revealed by muscimol binding, ranks second in density, followed by opiate binding sites, which have been reported in the range of 100–200 fmol/mg protein. The catecholaminergic binding sites rank fourth as a group, with very similar densities of α_1, α_2, and dopamine binding sites.

TABLE I
Summary of Neurotransmitter Binding Sites in Rat Spinal Cord[a]

Receptor	Ligand	Subregion	K_D (nM)	B_{max} (fmol/mg protein)	Temp (°C)	Reference
Opiate	Etorphine	l+s	0.21	133	37	Gouarderes *et al.* (1982)
μ	DAGO		0.51	7.8[b]	31	Traynor *et al.* (1982)
	Sufentanil	d	0.24	192	31	Leysen *et al.* (1983)
		v	0.44	178		
δ	D-Ala-D-Leu-Enk		0.33	4.4[b]	31	Traynor *et al.* (1982)
κ	Ethylketocyclazocine	l+s	2.2	98	37	Gouarderes *et al.* (1982)
			1.27	22.3[b]	31	Traynor *et al.* (1982)
			1.8	101	25	Harris and Sethy (1980)
Cholinergic muscarinic	QNB	c	0.055	1250	37	Kayaalp and Neff (1980)
		t	0.057	1100		
		l	0.074	1600		
		s	0.067	1750		
GABA	Muscimol	c+l, d horn	—	502	4	Singer and Placheta (1980)
			5.6	250	4	Frere *et al.* (1982)
	GABA		340	9880	4	Frere *et al.* (1982)
Glycine	Strychnine	c+l,d horn	—	1250	4	Singer and Placheta (1980)
Catecholamine						
β	Dihydroalprenolol		0.21	10.2	27	Jones *et al.* (1982)
α_1	Prazosin		0.38	44	25	Astrachan *et al.* (1983)
	WB4101		0.22	66.5	27	Jones *et al.* (1982)
α_2	Clonidine		2.1	20	27	Jones *et al.* (1982)
Dopamine	Haloperidol	d horn	0.99–1.23	5.6[b]	37	Demenge *et al.* (1980)
		l horn		34		
		v horn		31		
		d horn	0.99	5.6[b]	37	Demenge *et al.* (1980)
Serotonin						
5-HT_1	LSD		7.2	8[b]	37	Blackshear *et al.* (1981)

[a] Unless indicated under the heading of subregion, assays were performed on homogenates of whole spinal cord segments and pooled levels of spinal cord. All ligands were used in a tritiated form. Abbreviations: c, cervical; t, thoracic; l, lumbar; s, sacral; d, dorsal; l, lateral; v, ventral; QNB, quinuclidinyl benzilate; DAGO, D-Ala[2],MePhe[4],Glyol[5]-enkephalin.
[b] B_{max} determined in picomoles per gram of wet tissue.

Binding sites for the ligands used to characterize spinal cord receptors are likely to be similar to sites in other regions of the brain since no differences in K_D were reported.

In spinal cord homogenates, opiate receptor binding sites have been studied most widely. However, lack of selectivity of ligands in conjunction with differences in experimental design and reporting of data make comparisons between studies difficult. Using one tissue pool, Fields and co-workers (1980) report μ receptors about equal to δ receptors in density, with 8.1 fmol [^{3}H]morphine and 4.9 fmol [^{3}H]D-Ala-D-Leu-enkephalin bound per milligram protein, respectively. The data of Traynor and co-workers (1982, Table I) are consistent with this relationship. However, there is a 20-fold difference in the reports of the density of μ receptors in rat spinal cord by Fields *et al.* (1980) and Leysen *et al.* (1983). Differences in experimental design and radiolabeled ligand affinities may contribute to this discrepancy.

The relative density of κ binding sites with respect to μ and δ binding sites is unclear, as a selective κ-receptor radiolabeled ligand has not been available. The number of [^{3}H]ethylketocyclazocine binding sites in rat spinal cord exceeds twice the number of μ or δ sites (Traynor *et al.*, 1982), but an apparent affinity of ethylketocyclazocine for μ and δ binding sites indicates that the actual number is smaller. Since the availability of highly selective receptor ligands (i.e., ligands approaching 100 : 1 ratios of multiple receptor affinities) is currently increasing with substances such as D-Ala^2,MePhe^4,Gly-ol^5-enkephalin (DAGO, μ receptor ligand) and D-Ser^2,Thr^6,Leu-enkephalin (DSLET, δ receptor ligand), the distribution of opiate receptor substypes in spinal cord will be reevaluated.

Although the binding density in the spinal cord of most ligands is estimated to be low in comparison to other brain levels or microdissected regions, it is important to keep in mind that whole spinal cord segments were generally selected for analyses. High densities of receptors may occur in small regions of the cord, but this density would be diluted out and obscured in an analysis of homogenate of the whole spinal cord. It is for this reason that autoradiographic analysis of ligand binding within a tissue becomes important. The autoradiogram not only documents what ligands are bound, but its resolution in exposing where the binding occurs exceeds that of microdissection techniques at the present time.

C. Receptor Autoradiography

The advantage of autoradiography, then, is that it can document the anatomic distribution of neurotransmitter binding sites within selected neuroanatomic regions of the central nervous system. The extent to which the distribution of these binding sites overlaps with that of identified, endogenous putative transmitters in varicosities and nerve terminals provides supportive evidence for specific chemically coded synapses. Information about the cellular site of the binding sites (e.g., perikarya, axons, and terminals) may be inferred from the grain pattern, experimental manipulations (e.g., denervation), and ultrastructural studies of synaptology of chemically identified nerve terminals.

1. Considerations of Procedure

Several limitations to the technique, however, must be pointed out. As with any quantitative approach, there is a limit to the sensitivity of the technique, and negative results (in this case, low grain densities) must be interpreted with caution. It is important to consider that the lack of a difference in density of silver grains between a specific region and the gray matter in general does not necessarily mean that receptors are absent. Specific binding (the difference in the number of silver grains between the total and nonspecific binding slides) may be present but low and uniform. Although these binding sites may be sufficient to mediate physiological effects, one may question the functional significance of such an effect in the system. In fact, low, diffuse grain densities may have more association with nonneuronal receptor sites such as glia or vascular elements. Finally, recent evidence has indicated that myelin may impair tritium exposure of autoradiographic emulsions (Alexander *et al.,* 1981; Herkenham and Sokoloff, 1983), thereby obscuring binding of radiolabeled ligands to axons or to receptors in regions of high myelin content.

Table II summarizes reports to date of dense distributions of neurotransmitter binding sites in substantia gelatinosa (lamina II) of the spinal cord. The list parallels that for imunohistochemical localization of endogenous ligands (see LaMotte, Chapter 5) except in a few instances. The localization of benzodiazepam, histaminergic, and kainate receptors in substantia gelatinosa precedes the localization of the endogenous ligand in this region either because the endogenous substance is unknown (benzodiazepam, kainate) or because morphological techniques have been unable to detect the substance (histamine).

Each of the reports listed in Table II notes that the density of binding sites is higher in substantia gelatinosa (lamina II) than over other regions of the spinal cord. Autoradiograms of some of the ligand-binding sites in cat spinal cord appear in Figure 1. In rat, the narrowness of lamina I makes it difficult to specifically compare grain densities between laminae I and II. However, when monkey or cat spinal cord is used, the wider dimensions of the superficial laminae offer some resolution of laminae, and differences are noted below in the discussion of each class of ligands. In considering the data in Table II and Figure 1, it is not prudent to compare the density of grains among published autoradiograms. Such a comparison requires controlling or correcting for differences in ligand specific activity, binding constants, experimental conditions with respect to saturation of the receptors, and exposure times.

TABLE II
Neurotransmitter Binding Sites Present in Substantia Gelatinosa as Determined by Receptor Autoradiography[a]

Receptor type	[^{3}H] Ligand	Reference	Species
Opiate	Etorphine	Ninkovic *et al.* (1982)	Monkey
μ	Diprenorphine	Wamsley *et al.* (1982)	Monkey
		Pert *et al.* (1975, 1976)	Rat
		Atweh and Kuhar (1977)	Rat
		Pearson *et al.* (1980)	Rat
	Dihydromorphine	Seybold and Elde (1984)	Rat
δ	Enkephalin[b]	Goodman *et al.* (1980)	Rat
κ	Bremazocine	Slater and Patel (1983)	Rat
Catecholamine		Young and Kuhar (1979c)	Rat
α_2	*p*-Aminoclonidine	Seybold and Elde (1984)	Rat
Serotonin	Serotonin	Young and Kuhar (1980b)	Rat
	LSD	Young and Kuhar (1980b)	Rat
	LSD	Seybold and Elde (1984)	Rat
Cholinergic			
Muscarinic	QNB	Wamsley *et al.* (1981a,b)	Rat
		Seybold and Elde (1984)	Rat
	Pirenzepine	Yamamura *et al.* (1983)	Rat
Nicotinic	α-Bungarotoxin	Polz-Tejera *et al.* (1980)	Rat
Histmine (H_1)	Mepyramine	Ninkovic *et al.* (1982)	Monkey
Peptide			
Cholecystokinin	CCK[b]	Zarbin *et al.* (1983)	Rat Guinea pig
Neurotensin	Neurotensin	Young and Kuhar (1979b, 1981)	Rat
Substance P	Substance P	Maurin, *et al.* (1984)	Rat
Glycine	Strychnine	Zarbin *et al.* (1981)	
GABA	GABA	Price *et al.* (1984)	Rat
	Muscimol	Palacios *et al.* (1981)	Rat
Adenosine	Cyclohexyladenosine	Goodman and Snyder (1982)	Rat
Benzodiazepine	Flunitrazepam	Young and Kuhar (1980a)	Rat
Kainate	Kainic acid	Monaghan and Cotman (1982)	Rat

[a] In each case, the density of autoradiographic grains over substantia gelatinosa is greater than that over the gray matter in general. Abbreviations: CCK, cholecystokinin; LSD, lysergic acid diethylamide; QNB, quinuclidinyl benzilate.
[b] [^{125}I]-labeled ligand used.

2. *Opiate Receptors*

Opiate receptors in the spinal cord have the distinction of being the first spinal receptors to be visualized in autoradiograms (Pert *et al.*, 1975), and the distribution of μ, δ, and κ binding sites has been described to date. *In vivo* and *in vitro* binding of various radiolabeled μ ligands in the spinal cord have consistently demonstrated a high density of grains in substantia gelatinosa of rat (Atweh and Kuhar, 1977; Goodman *et al.*, 1980; Pearson *et al.*, 1980; Pert *et al.*, 1975, 1976), monkey (Ninkovic *et al.*, 1982; Wamsley *et al.*, 1982), and cat (Figure 1C), and data from monkey suggest that receptor density in lamina

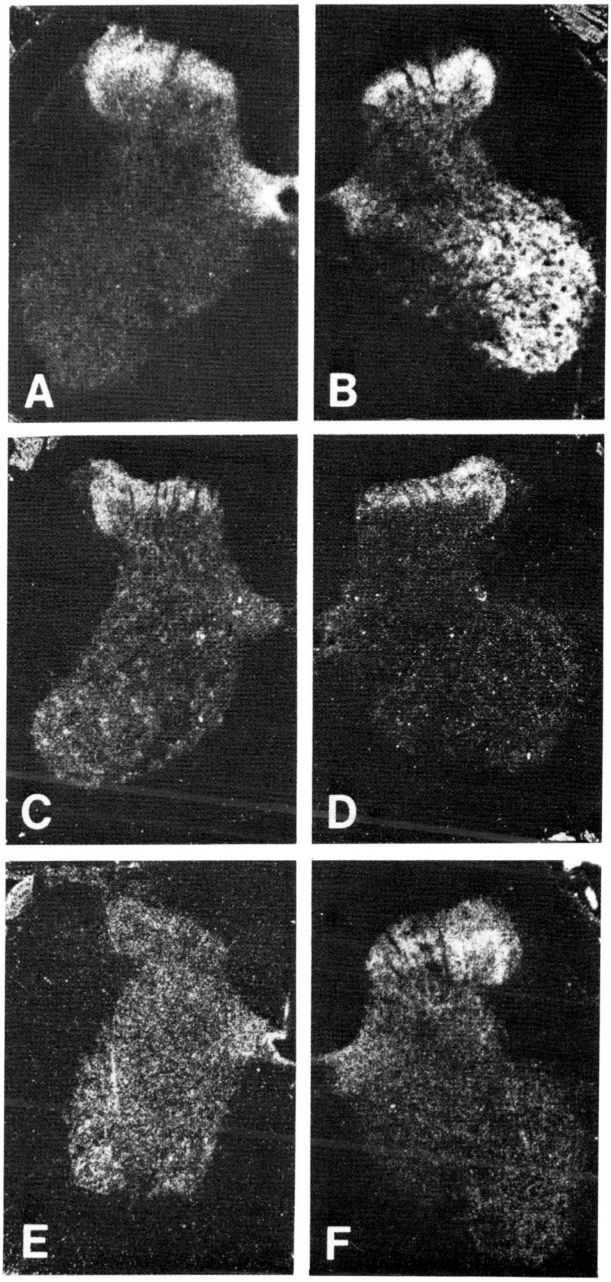

FIGURE 1. Neurotransmitter binding sites in cat spinal cord as revealed by receptor autoradiography. Specific binding sites were labeled with (A) mepyramine (H_1 histaminergic), (B) quinuclidinyl benzilate (QNB, muscarinic cholineregic), (C) dihyromorphine (μ opioid), (D) D-Ala,D-Leu-enkephalin (DADL, δ opioid), (E) prazosin (α_1 catecholaminergic), and (F) lysergic acid diethylamide (LSD, serotonergic). Tritiated ligands were incubated with slide-mounted 10-μm cryostat sections of cat spinal cord, lumbar level, fixed with 0.1% paraformaldehyde. Radiolabeled ligands were used in the following concentratons: 3 nM mepyramine, 0.5 nM QNB, 5 nM dihydromorphine, 5 nM DADL, 1.5 nM prazosin, and 6 nM LSD. Autoradiograms were prepared according to the technique of Young and Kuhar (1979a).

II may be greater than that in lamina I (Ninkovic *et al.*, 1982). Similarly, Leu-enkephalin binding sites, believed to be consistent with δ receptors (Lord *et al.*, 1977), are more concentrated in substantia gelatinosa than over any other part of the spinal cord (Goodman *et al.*, 1980; Figure 1D), as are κ receptors (Slater and Patel, 1983).

Several points of interest have emerged concerning the location of opiate receptors in the spinal cord. First, a species difference has appeared in comparison of autoradiograms prepared from rat and monkey spinal cords. Autoradiograms of [^{3}H]diprenorphine or [^{3}H]etorphine binding sites prepared from brain after intravenous administration of the drugs consistently show a single, distinct band of grains in the substantia gelatinosa region of rat spinal cord (Atweh and Kuhar, 1977; Pearson *et al.*, 1980; Pert *et al.*, 1976). In contrast, autoradiograms of monkey spinal cord (diprenorphine, i.v.) show a gradual decrease in density of binding sites from lamina II to the ventral aspect of lamina IV (Wamsley *et al.*, 1982). Since experimental conditions were essentially the same, these data indicate that opiate peptides may participate more generally in modulation of sensory stimuli in monkey than in rat.

Secondly, there is not a one-to-one correlation in the distribution of high densities of opioid peptides and opiate receptors in spinal cord. Although substantia gelatinosa and lamina X both exhibit moderate densities of enkephalin (Gibson *et al.*, 1981; Hökfelt *et al.*, 1977) and dynorphin peptides (Sasek *et al.*, 1984), μ, δ, and κ receptors in significant densities appear limited to substantia gelatinosa. A high density of opioid binding sites around the central canal has not been noted to date. Pearson and co-workers (1980) noted that [^{3}H]diprenorphine binding sites in this region were not different from the gray matter in general. Whether the lack of a significant density is real for other ligands or an oversight needs to be addressed more carefully. Since other inhibitory transmitters and their binding sites are distributed in both substantia gelatinosa and lamina X (α_2-adrenergic and serotonergic, see below), a differential distribution of opiate receptors may indicate fundamental biochemical differences by which sensory information is processed in the two regions.

Finally, there is a discrepency between experimental evidence for a location of opiate receptors on primary afferent fibers and what can be resolved at the ultrastructural level. LaMotte and co-workers (1976) were the first to provide evidence that opiates may modulate nociception in part by a presynaptic mechanism. In biochemical studies of microdissected monkey spinal cords, these investigators demonstrated that dorsal rhizotomy produced a significant decrease in [^{3}H]naloxone binding sites in the ipsilateral superficial dorsal horn. Similar results were subsequently observed autoradiographically with [^{3}H]etorphine by Ninkovic and co-workers (1982). Their autoradiograms excluded the possibility that transsynaptic degeneration after rhizotomy accounts for receptor loss, since grain densities decreased over Lissauer's tract as well as the dorsal horn. Direct evidence that the binding sites are associated with primary afferent neurons is observed in autoradiograms of opiate binding to rat (Young *et al.*, 1980) and monkey (Ninkovic *et al.*, 1982) dorsal root ganglia where clusters of silver grains are distributed over perikarya. In addition, opiate binding sites have been quantitated biochemically in dorsal roots (Fields *et al.*, 1980) and in neuritic outgrowths of fetal mouse dorsal root ganglion cells (Hiller *et al.*, 1978), the processes of primary afferent neurons.

Additionally, morphological and biochemical data indicate that the μ and δ opiate receptors are preferentially associated with small-diameter primary afferent neurons. Autoradiograms of [^{3}H]etorphine binding to monkey dorsal root ganglia show silver grains limited in distribution to a pool of small (35–45 μm) cells (Ninkovic *et al.*, 1982). Biochemical analyses of receptor numbers in the dorsal root after selective destruction of small-diameter fibers by lesion of sciatic nerve (Fields *et al.*, 1980) and in the dorsal horn after neonatal capsaicin treatment (Gamse *et al.*, 1979; Nagy *et al.*, 1980) show significant decreases in opiate binding. The relationship with small-diameter fibers is further substantiated in physiological studies measuring substance P release. Substance P has been localized to small-diameter neurons (Barber *et al.*, 1978; Jessell *et al.*, 1978, 1979; Nagy *et al.*, 1980), and opiates are inhibitory to the efflux of substance P from spinal cord *in vivo* (Yaksh *et al.*, 1980) and the spinal nucleus of V *in vitro* (Jessell and Iversen, 1977; Mudge *et al.*, 1979).

The dilemma that exists concerning opiate receptors on terminals of primary afferent neurons is that a morphological correlate cannot be identified ultrastructurally. Examination with the electron microscope of spinal cord immunostained for enkephalin reveals dendrites as the predominant synaptic target for enkephalin-containing terminals in rat (Hunt *et al.*, 1980; Sumal *et al.*, 1982), cat (Glazer and Basbaum, 1983), and monkey (Aronin *et al.*, 1981) and spinothalamic tract cells as targets of axosomatic contacts (Ruda, 1982). In an effort to reconcile the ultrastructural data with the data in support of receptors on primary afferent terminals, a nonsynaptic effect of opiate peptides on afferent terminals is postulated. A similar explanation has been given for the lack of synaptic specializations associated with monoamine varicosities (Descarries *et al.*, 1975; Descarries and Lapierre, 1973) and for the far-reaching effects of the LHRH-like peptide in frog sympathetic ganglia (Jan *et al.*, 1980). Glazer and Basbaum (1983) propose that the high incidence of enkephalin-containing profiles in apposition to unlabeled axons observed in their material is evidence of a nonsynaptic functional relationship. Alternatively, dynorphin or an unidentified endogenous opiate substance may be the relavent component in terminals presynaptic to primary afferent fibers in the spinal cord. Colocalizaton of the endogenous opiate and its binding site at the ultrastructural level may be necessary to resolve the issue.

Assuming that both pre- and postsynaptic opiate receptors exist, an interesting biochemical aspect of the neuronal circuitry in the dorsal horn concerns the differential distribution of these receptor subtypes. Two laboratories (Fields *et al.*, 1980; Traynor *et al.*, 1982) report comparable μ and δ opiate receptor densities in the dorsal horn, but Fields and co-workers report that the ratio of $\mu : \delta$ receptors is greater than 2 in dorsal roots. Together, these data sugget that there are more δ than μ receptors on spinal neurons.

3. Catecholamine Receptors

Autoradiographic studies of spinal cord sections and cultures have been used to determine the sites of spinal catecholamine receptors. Of the adrenergic receptor sites that have been studied autoradiographically, the α_2 receptors seem to be the most relevant to spinal transmission of nociception. Young and Kuhar (1979c) were first to document a dense distribution of $[^3H]$*p*-aminoclonidine binding sites in lamina II of the rat spinal cord. We have confirmed their observations in rat (Seybold and Elde, 1984) and have also noted a density of α_2 binding sites adjacent to the central canal and in the intermediolateral cell column. Therefore, the distribution of α_2 binding sites parallels that of catecholamine-containing varicosities in the spinal cord (Carlsson *et al.*, 1964; Westlund and Coulter, 1980; Zivin *et al.*, 1975).

As with opiate receptors, the cellular site of α_2 receptors has important implications for the neuronal circuitry underlying catecholamine-mediated analgesia in the spinal cord. Although some α_2 receptors may be presynaptic on catecholamine-containing terminals and fulfill the role of autoreceptors, a significant population mediate analgesia at a postsynaptic site. In behavioral studies, Howe and Yaksh (1982) reported development of supersensitivity to analgesic effects of α_2 agonists in rat spinal cord after denervation with 6-hydroxydopamine. Whether these postsynaptic receptors occur on dendrites and cell bodies and/or terminals of primary afferent neurons has not been fully explored experimentally. Since spinally administered clonidine is analgetic in a behavioral assay that uses intrathecal substance P as the noxious stimulus (Hylden and Wilcox, 1983c), an effective population of α_2 receptors occurs on spinal neurons. This relationship is supported morphologically. Ultrastructural examination of catecholamine-containing terminals labeled with $KMnO_4$ found few synaptic contacts, but most of these contained axodendritic relationships (Satoh *et al.*, 1982).

Support of α_2 receptors on primary afferent neurons is only indirect but worthy of future investigation. The most interesting circumstantial evidence is the high degree of overlap between the distribution of α_2 and μ opiate binding sites noted by Kuhar (1981). This overlap has functional significance in that α_2 agonists have been shown to attenuate opiate withdrawal (Fielding *et al.*, 1978; Sparber and Meyer, 1978). Since several lines of evidence support a significant population of μ receptors on primary afferent terminals (see above), this possibility for α_2 receptors deserves further experimentation. Furthermore, autoradiograms of dissociated spinal neurons prepared by Hosli and Hosli (1982) resulted in little labeling over perikarya with α_2 ligands in comparison to a β-receptor ligand. Since α_2 binding sites may be denser in substantia gelatinosa than β-adrenergic binding sites, these data together support a location of α_2 receptors on primary afferent fibers. Howe and Yaksh (1984) observed that dorsal or spinal ganglionectomy resulted in a small but significant reduction in the density of $[^3H]$rauwolscine binding sites in the spinal cord, and measurable levels of binding were found in dorsal root ganglia. This supports the idea that a portion of the dorsal horn α_2 receptors may be on primary afferent neurons.

There are some data linking α_1 receptors with analgesia but no data linking β receptors with sensory transmission in the spinal cord (see Hammond, Chapter 15). Alpha$_1$ antagonists are reported to block some catecholamine analgesia at the level of the spinal cord but are less potent than α_2 antagonists (Howe *et al.*, 1983; Hylden and Wilcox, 1983c). Autoradiograms we have prepared of rat and cat spinal cords show a low density of prazosin (α_1) binding sites over substania gelatinosa and lamina X (Figure 1E) and a low homogeneous grain density over the gray matter for the β-receptor antagonist dihydroalprenolol (DHA; unpublished observation).

4. *Serotonin Receptors*

Several lines of evidence (reviewed by Hammond, Chapter 15, and Ruda, Chapter 7) have documented that a descending serotonergic system has an important inhibitory effect on nociceptive processing at the spinal level. Immunohistochemical studies at the light and ultrastructural levels have identified varicose serotonin-containing fibers throughout the dorsal horn of the spinal cord with relatively dense accumulations in laminae I and II and around the central canal (Dahlstrom and Fuxe, 1965; Ruda and Gobel, 1980; Segu and Calas, 1978; Steinbusch, 1981). That these regions are the morphologically important sites of serotonin action in the spinal cord is corroborated by autoradiograms of the binding of tritiated serotonergic ligands. Two studies (Young and Kuhar, 1980b; Seybold and Elde, 1984) document high densities of serotonin binding sites in the superficial laminae of rat spinal cord and also note a moderate density around the central canal. A comparable distribution appears in cat spinal cord (Figure 1F); however, the binding in substantia gelatinosa appears particularly dense in the inner portion of lamina II. Recently, biochemical data have emerged that support two subtypes of serotonin receptors: 5-HT$_1$ and 5-HT$_2$ (Peroutka *et al.*, 1981). Biochemical studies of membrane homogenates from rat spinal cord indicate that the 5-HT$_1$ receptor type is the predominant one in this region (Blackshear *et al.*, 1981).

The postsynaptic sites of these receptors can be inferred from morphological and behavioral studies. Ultrastructural studies of radiolabeled serotonin uptake (Ruda and Gobel, 1980) and immunohistochemically stained material (Light *et al.*, 1983) have identified serotonin-containing terminals in axodendritic relationships only. Evidence that spinally administered serotonin is analgesic in the behavioral intrathecal substance P assay supports a postsynaptic site on spinal neurons (Hylden and Wilcox, 1983b). Therefore, it is unlikely that serotonin receptors are located presynaptic to other axon terminals.

5. *Cholinergic Receptors*

Although there is no clear physiological correlate for a cholinergic modulation of nociception at the present time, the basic elements of a neuronal circuit are present in the superficial laminae of the spinal cord. Histochemical and immunohistochemical studies have documented high densities of acetylcholinesterase enzyme (Paxinos and Watson, 1982) and choline-acetyltransferase-containing elements (Kimura *et al.*, 1981) in substantia gelatinosa and adjacent to the central canal, thus providing evidence for the existence of cholinergic synapses. Autoradiograms prepared with the muscarinic antagonist quinuclidinyl benzilate (QNB; Wamsley *et al.*, 1981a,b; Seybold and Elde, 1984; Figure 1B) document high densities of muscarinic cholinergic binding sites in the same regions, with lamina IV having the fewest of binding sites. Within substantia gelatinosa, some of these binding sites may be on primary afferent terminals. Autoradiograms of dorsal root ganglia show clusters of grains over perikarya (Wamsley *et al.*, 1981b; Figure 2), and ligation experiments demonstrated that these receptors are also transported peripherally on somatic nerves. Biochemical studies by Kayaalp and Neff (1980) argue against the posibility that the receptors are located on terminals of descending fibers on the basis that transections of the spinal cord changed neither the K_D nor the B_{max} for the muscarinic ligand.

Interestingly, the nonclassical muscarinic antagonist pirenzepine differentially labels muscarinic binding sites in the spinal cord. By comparing autoradiograms prepared with [^{3}H]pirenzepine to those prepared with [^{3}H]QNB, Yamamura and co-workers (1983) determined that the muscarininc sites in substantia gelatinosa are labeled by pirenzepine, whereas those in the ventral horn are not. Investigation of the physiological effects of these muscarinic receptor subtypes may facilitate documentation of modulation of somatosensation by muscarinic cholinergic mechanisms.

There is also the possibility that nicotinic cholinergic receptors play some role in the modulation of the transmission of sensory stimuli in the spinal cord. In autoradiograms of [^{125}I]α-bungarotoxin binding sites in dorsal root ganglia, silver grains were clustered over medium to large perikarya, with about 20% of the total population of cells labeled (Polz-Tejera *et al.*, 1980). A recent electrophysiological investigation of cholinergic receptors in frog dorsal root ganglia determined differential responses of primary afferent neurons to nicotinic and muscarinic agonists (Morita and Katayama, 1984). In the absence of evidence for synapses in dorsal root ganglia, nicotinic and muscarinic effects would most likely occur peripherally or centrally on processes of primary afferent fibers.

6. *Histamine Receptors*

Experimentally, there is almost as much information concerning the location of histamine binding sites in the dorsal horn as there is concerning

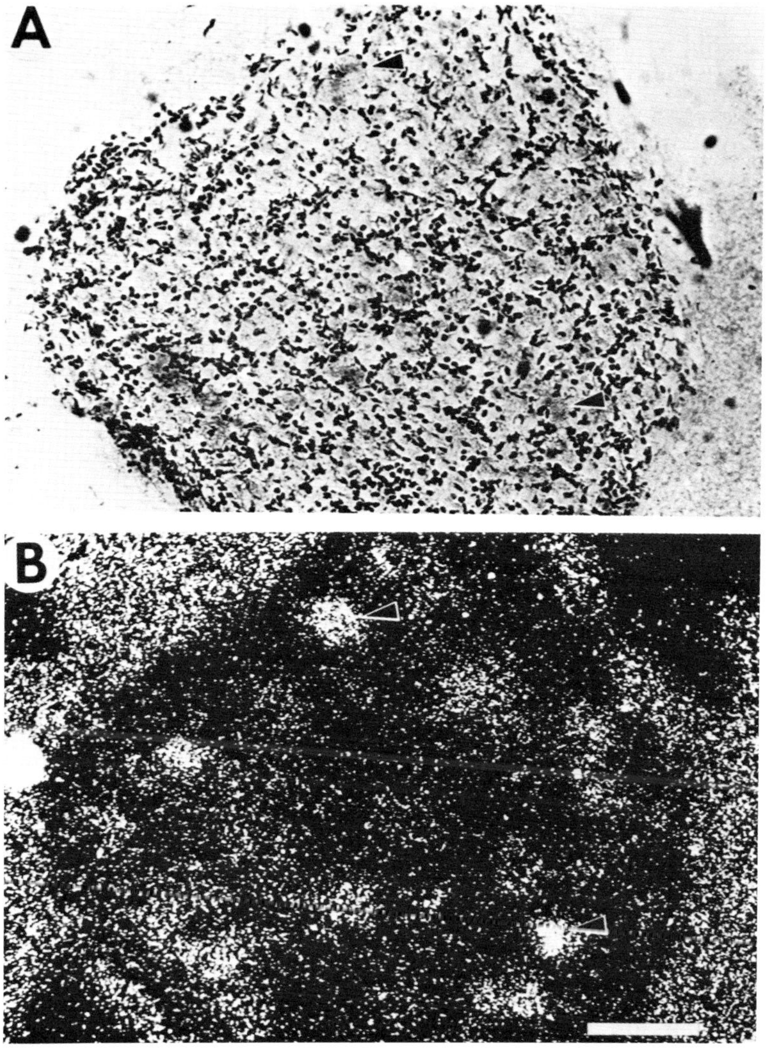

FIGURE 2. Muscarinic cholinergic binding sites associated with rat dorsal root ganglion cells. Bright-field photomicrograph of the tissue (A) and dark-field photomicrograph of the autoradiogram of the same section (B) showing densities of silver grains associated with some of the ganglion cells (arrows). Tissue section was incubated in 1 nM [^{3}H]QNB. Bar = 500 μm. (From Wamsley *et al.*, 1981b, reprinted with permission of the authors.)

μ opiate binding sites, but we know very little about the physiological consequences of histamine receptor binding in the spinal cord. Taylor *et al.* (1982) studied the binding sites biochemically in cat spinal cord and determined that receptor density in homogenates of the dorsal gray was among the lowest of the areas surveyed in the brain. Although two histamine receptor subtypes have been described biochemically for other brain regions (a high- and a low-affinity binding site), it has been possible to study only the high-affinity site autoradiographically with [^{3}H]mepyramine (pyrilamine). Ninkovic and coworkers (1982) have reported that in monkey spinal cord, these H_1 binding sites are confined to lamina II in the dorsal horn and are also associated with large motor neurons in the ventral horn. A putative inhibitory action of histamine in the ventral horn may confound effects to document the action of histamine at the spinal level in behavioral studies for analgesia. In cat spinal cord, a high density of H_1 binding sites in the region adjacent to the central canal was also noted (Figure 1A). Interestingly, the region of highest density in lamina X occurs where [^{3}H]QNB binding sites were sparse (compare Figures 1A and 1B), indicating a differential distribution of receptor types in lamina X and, therefore, an underlying functional organization of the region.

The histamine binding sites in the substantia gelatinosa of the dorsal horn may be proven to have a modulatory effect on spinal transmission of nociception. Dorsal rhizotomy in monkey results in a decrease in binding sites only in the dorsal horn, indicating a population of receptors on primary afferent neurons. That these receptors may be located on nociceptors is suggested by autoradiograms of dorsal root ganglia in which silver grains are found in clusters over small perikarya ranging from 35 to 45 μm, the same population that bound μ opiate ligands (Ninkovic *et al.*, 1982).

7. *Peptide Receptors*

Autoradiographic studies of the distribution of radiolabeled peptides in spinal cord have been done for neurotensin, cholecystokinin (CCK)-33, substance P, and enkephalin (see above) to date. Radiolabeled ligands involved tritiated derivatives of neurotensin, substance P, and enkephalin analogues as well as iodinated derivatives of CCK and enkephalin. Iodinated peptides have been prepared for a wide variety of radioimmunoassays using straightforward physical or enzymatic reactions, yet this technology is largely untapped for studies of peptidergic binding sites. Although the iodine isotope offers no barriers to the technique of autoradiography, the use of iodinated peptides in binding assays will depend on whether the relatively large iodine atom (with respect to tritium) will cause steric hindrance and thus decrease the affinity of the ligand for the receptor.

The distribution of substance P binding sites in thoracic spinal cord parallels the distribution of substance-P-immunoreactive terminals. High densities of binding sites were noted in substantia gelatinosa, lamina X, and the intermediolateral cell column (Maurin *et al.*, 1984).

Both CCK (Zarbin *et al.*, 1983) and neurotensin (Ninkovic *et al.*, 1981; Young and Kuhar, 1979b, 1981) binding sites appear differentially distributed in autoradiograms of rat spinal cord, with their greatest density in the superficial laminae. The receptor density in this region is consistent with data indicating that substantia gelatinosa is the region in the spinal cord that contains the highest density of these peptidergic nerve terminals (see Yaksh, Chapter 8). Since there is some evidence that each of these substances mediates analgesia at the spinal level (neurotensin: Hylden and Wilcox, 1983a; Yaksh *et al.*, 1982; CCK: Jurna and Zetler, 1981), an important question concerns the postsynaptic sites of receptors mediating these effects.

The majority of evidence suggests that neurotensin receptors occur primarily on dendrites and cell bodies. Dorsal rhizotomy does not produce a decrease in neurotensin binding sites, as observed for opiate receptors (Ninkovic *et al.*, 1981); thus, there is no evidence for binding sites on terminals of primary afferent fibers. Furthermore, in ultrastructural studies of neurotensin immunoreactivity, only dendrites were found postsynaptic to terminals containing neurotensin immunoreactivity (DiFiglia *et al.*, 1984; Seybold and Maley, 1984). Interestingly, there is some behavioral evidence that opiate-containing neurons may bear these neurotensin receptors in that naloxone partially blocks the effects of intrathecal neurotensin in rat (Yaksh *et al.*, 1982) and mouse (Hylden and Wilcox, 1983a) spinal cord.

Autoradiograms of both rat and guinea pig spinal cord are reported to contain a moderately high density of CCK binding sites over laminae I and II of the dorsal horn (Zarbin *et al.*, 1983). There is questionable evidence that the physiological effect of this synapse may be analgesia. Some behavioral evidence indicates that CCK causes a decrease in nociception that is naloxone reversible (Jurna and Zetler, 1981), suggesting that analgesia is mediated via an opiatergic interneuron. However, biochemical evidence that CCK and enkephalins are metabolized by the same extracellular enzyme system (Deschodt-Lanckman *et al.*, 1981) raises the possibility that the behavioral analgesia results from an increase in the half life of endogenously released enkephalins. A nonopioid mechanism of CCK analgesia may be mediated via presynaptic receptors on primary afferent neurons. The localization of CCK binding sites to axonal pathways in other regions of the nervous system (Zarbin *et al.*, 1983) makes this possibility worthy of investigation.

The distribution of substance P and CCK receptors among neuronal elements in the dorsal horn has important implications for the functional significance of the colocalization of two peptides. Substance P and CCK have been determined to coexist in primary afferent neurons (Dalsgaard *et al.*, 1982; Tuchscherer and Seybold, 1985). Therefore, determination of different distributions of binding sites for these peptides among axonal, dendritic, and somatic elements in the neuropil will indicate whether either peptide is involved in an autoregulatory role or each has a postsynaptic effect on a different population of neurons intrinsic to the spinal cord. Such information would add a new dimension to our appreciation of the breadth of neuronal circuitry affected by sensory stimuli.

8. Glycine Receptors

Glycine receptors in the spinal cord have a unique distribution in rat for two reasons. First, autoradiograms of [^{3}H]glycine binding to rat tissue show that the highest densities in central nervous system occur in the spinal cord.

Second, a differential distribution by level was observed through the ventral and intermediate gray regions of the cord (Zarbin *et al.*, 1981). Within the dorsal horn, though, distributions of grain densities were consistent throughout all levels of the spinal cord examined (cervical, thoracic, lumbar). The lowest grain density was reported for lamina I, whereas the highest grain densities (60–70% of the total grains in the dorsal horn) were divided between laminae II and III and the lateral aspect of lamina V. This distribution of binding sites parallels the distribution of putative glycinergic nerve terminals visualized by uptake of radiolabeled glycine (Ribeiro-da-Silva and Coimbra, 1980). Thus, glycine receptors are in a position to modulate transmission of both noxious and innocuous stimuli through the spinal cord.

9. GABA Receptors

The amino acid derivative GABA has been shown to have an inhibitory role in somatosensation, and some of its receptors may be presynaptic. Using [^{3}H]muscimol as a selective ligand for the high-affinity GABA binding site, Palacios and co-workers (1981) visualized a low density of GABA receptors in lamina II of the rat cervical spinal cord and a similar concentration in the medial aspects of laminae III and IV. Using [^{3}H]GABA as the ligand in conjunction with isoguvacine to reveal $GABA_B$ (bicuculline-insensitive) receptors, Price and co-workers (1984) found high densities of binding sites in lamina II and outer lamina III and moderate densities in lamina I and around the central canal.

There are both biochemical and morphological data that some GABA receptors are on primary afferent terminals. Neonatal capsaicin treatment causes an approximately 25% decrease in muscimol binding in spinal cord homogenates (Singer and Placheta, 1980) and a 40–50% decrease in the $GABA_B$ sites in all laminae of the dorsal horn when determined autoradiographically (Price *et al.*, 1984). Additionally, there is ultrastructural evidence that GABA terminals are presynaptic to the central terminal (believed to be primary afferent) in glomeruli of the dorsal horn (Ribeiro-da-Silva and Coimbra, 1980; McLaughlin *et al.*, 1975; Barber *et al.*, 1978).

D. Future Directions

The field of receptor autoradiography is currently in a growth phase. It has recently undergone expansion with the development of more ligands with the high specific activity needed to reveal low numbers of binding sites and *in vitro* techniques that will utilize small quantities of these expensive materials. Although further descriptive data are needed on the distribution of receptors in the spinal cord, autoradiography can also be combined with other techniques to address more specific questions of neuronal circuitry.

In terms of descriptive data, there have been few quantitative studies comparing receptor densities in the spinal cord by laminae. In our experience it is difficult to appreciate small but significant (1.5-fold) variations in grain densities visually. Perhaps this is why significant concentrations of opiate receptors around the central canal have not been apparent to date. Quantification of grains may be necessary to recognize these more subtle distributions. Inclusion of tritiated standards during exposure of the emulsion in quantitative studies will be important to insure a linear relationship between densities of silver grains and radioisotope content of the tissue in areas that are quantified.

Furthermore, studies on differences in receptor densities with respect to cord levels are very few. No reports were found that addressed the distribution of neurotransmitter binding sites in sacral spinal cord, and few addressed thoracic cord segments. Since examples of the differential distribution of peptide-containing primary afferent neurons by cord segments have been noted (Basbaum and Glazer, 1983; Tuchscherer and Seybold, 1985), and autonomic nuclei have a restricted distribution in the cord, variations in receptor density may parallel these segmental differences in the distribution of chemically identified neurons and autonomic circuitry.

Receptor autoradiography may also be combined with other morphological techniques to address questions of neuronal circuitry more directly. The primary limitation to combined approaches is that the methodologies for two techniques are rarely optimum under the same conditions. The general usage of fresh frozen or lightly fixed (0.1% paraformaldehyde) tissue sections for *in vitro* receptor autoradiography (Young and Kuhar, 1979a) would be expected to preclude other histochemical techniques, but there are noteworthy exceptions. We have been able to study the distribution of several neurotransmitter binding sites associated with sympathoadrenal preganglionic neurons retrogradely labeled with the fluorescent dye fast blue (Seybold and Elde, 1984). No tissue processing is required to visualize fast blue in cryostat sections, but the marker is not retained during subsequent processing of the sections for ligand binding. Therefore, the distribution of labeled neurons needs to be documented before the tissues are exposed to aqueous solutions.

Autoradiography may also be combined with immunohistochemistry in two different systems. Questions concerning receptors on specific peptide-containing populations of dorsal root ganglion cells may be addressed by combining the two techniques on cultures of dorsal root ganglia. Insights into synaptic relationships *in vivo* may be obtained by combining receptor autoradiography with immunohistochemistry on adjacent sections. Although we have not been successful in revealing immunohistochemically labeled varicosities in cryostat sections fixed with paraformaldehde vapors or solutions after sectioning, several peptide-containing perikarya were visualized. What peptides may be visualized seems to depend on their size (e.g., neurophysin, 10,000 mol. wt.) or their physical properties (e.g., somatostatin, highly basic). Alternatively, stronger concentrations of fixative should not be assumed to impair the binding of all ligands to receptors. Individual exceptions to general conditions of immunohistochemistry and ligand binding occur that may be exploited to address specific relationships of binding sites with immunohistochemically identified neurons.

The development of ligands that irreversibly bind to receptor sites will be important in visualizing receptors at the ultrastructural level. Ligands modified for photoaffinity labeling after binding offer this possibility. Although statistical methods will be required to establish whether the radioactive sources are on pre- or postsynaptic membranes, studies on the distribution of receptors at the ultrastructural level will be important to address the distribution of nonsynaptic opiate receptors and will facilitate studies of the codistribution of receptors and peptides.

E. Concluding Remarks

The recent development of radiohistochemical techniques has resulted in many descriptive studies of ligand binding sites in the spinal cord, but there are two important issues concerning the neurobiology of sensory transmission that stem from the studies that have been done to date. One concerns the function of receptors on processes of primary afferent neurons. In addition to opioid receptors, muscarinic and histaminergic receptors have been correlated with small perikarya in dorsal root ganglia, and all receptor types are transported both centrally and peripherally. Although opiates are considered analgetic when administered in the region of the central process and acetylcholine and histamaine are considered noxious when applied to the peripheral process of small-diameter primary afferent neurons, the consequences of receptor activation in the opposite domains remain to be determined. The possibility of multiple presynaptic receptors on primary afferent terminals also has important implications for therapeutic approaches to the management of chronic pain. If the release of transmitter from nociceptors can be blocked at the level of the first synapse in the spinal cord, many secondary consequences of chronic pain may be alleviated.

The second issue concerns the apparent nonsynaptic distribution of opioid receptors. Although a neuromodulator role was originally ascribed to peptides that have been localized to neurons, it has generally been assumed that these effects are mediated via synaptic constructs. The lack of a correlation between immunostained enkephalin terminals in synaptic contact with primary afferent terminals and experimental data indicating presynaptic opioid receptors suggests that some substances released from neurons may have physiological effects over greater distances than have been appreciated in the past. The consequences of these paracrine influences remain to be determined.

Finally, many parallels have been noted in the distribution of neurotransmitter binding sites between substantia gelatinosa and lamina X of the spinal cord. Since similar parallels exist for the distribution of peptidergic and monoaminergic nerve terminals, these two areas may share a common functional role. Further investigation of the connections and neuronal circuitry of lamina X will be important in establishing its relationship to sensory systems.

References

ALEXANDER, G. M., SCHWARTZMAN, R. J., BELL, R. D., YU, J., AND RENTHAL, A. Quantitative measurement of local cerebral metabolic rate for glucose utilizing tritiated 2-deoxyglucose. *Brain Res.* 223:59–67, 1981.

ARONIN, N., DIFIGLIA, M., LIOTTA, A. S., AND MARTIN, J. S. Ultrastructural localization and biochemical features of immunoreactive leu-enkephalin in monkey dorsal horn. *J. Neurosci.* 1:561–577, 1981.

ASTRACHAN, D. I., DAVIS, M., AND GALLAGER, D. W. Behaviour and binding: Correlations between alpha-1 adrenergic stimulation of acoustic startle and alpha-1 adrenoceptor occupancy and number in rat lumbar spinal cord. *Brain Res.* 260:81–90, 1983.

ATWEH, S. F., AND KUHAR, M. J., Autoradiographic localization of opiate receptors in rat brain. I. Spinal cord and lower medulla. *Brain Res.* 124:53–67, 1977.

BARBER, R. P., VAUGHN, J. E., SAITO, K., MC LAUGHLIN, S. J., AND ROBERTS, E. GABAergic terminals are presynaptic to primary afferent terminals in the substantia gelatinosa of the rat spinal cord. *Brain Res.* 141:35–55, 1978.

BARBER, R. P., VAUGHN, J. E., SLEMMON, J. R., SALVATERRA, P. M., ROBERTS, E., AND LEEMAN, S. E. The origin, distribution and synaptic relationships of substance P axons in rat spinal cord. *J. Comp. Neurol.* 184:331–352, 1979.

BASBAUM, A. I., AND GLAZER, E. J. Immunoreactive vasoactive intestinal polypeptide is concentrated in the sacral spinal cord: A possible marker for pelvic visceral afferent fibers. *Somatosens. Res.* 1:69–82, 1983.

BLACKSHEAR, M. A., STERANKA, L. R., AND SANDERS-BUSH, E. Multiple serotonin receptors: Regional distribution and effect of raphe lesions. *Eur. J. Pharmacol.* 76:325–334, 1981.

CARLSSON, J., FALK, B., FUXE, K., AND HILLARY, N. J., Cellular localization of monoamines in the spinal cord. *Acta. Physiol. Scand.* 60:112–119, 1964.

DAHLSTROM, A., AND FUXE, K. Evidence for the existence of monoamine containing neurons in the central nervous system. II. Experimentally induced changes in the intraneuronal amine levels of bulbospinal neuron systems. *Acta Physiol. Scand. [Suppl.]* 247:1–36, 1965.

DALSGAARD, C.-J., VINCENT, S. R., HÖKFELT, T., LUNDBERG, J. M., DAHLSTROM, A., SCHULTZBERG, M., DOCKRAY, G. J., AND CUELLO, A. C. Coexistence of cholecystokinin- and substance P-like peptides in neurons of the dorsal root ganglia of the rat. *Neurosci. Lett.* 33:159–163, 1982.

DEMENGE, P., FEUERSTEIN, C., MOUCHET, P., AND GUERIN, B. Stereospecific binding of [^{3}H]-haloperidol in rat dorsal spinal cord. *Eur. J. Pharmacol.* 66:117–120, 1980.

DEMENGE, P., MOUCHET, P., GUERIN, B., AND FEUERSTEIN, C. Identification and distribution of neuroleptic binding sites in the rat spinal cord. *J. Neurochem.* 37:53–59, 1981.

DESCARRIES, L., AND LAPIERRE, Y. Noradrenergic axon terminals in the cerebral cortex of the rat. I. Radioautographic visualization after topical application of DL-[^{3}H]-norepinephrine. *Brain Res.* 51:141–160, 1973.

DESCARRIES, L., BEAUDET, A., AND WATKIN, K. C. Serotonin nerve terminals in adult rat neocortex. *Brain Res.* 100:563–588, 1975.

DESCHODT-LANCKMAN, M., BUI, N.D., AND CHRISTOPHE, J. Cholecystokinin octa- and tetrapeptide degradation by synaptic membranes. Evidence for competition with enkephalins for common degradation pathways. *Neurosci. Lett. [Suppl.]* 7:S321, 1981.

DIFIGLIA, M., ARONIN, N., AND LEEMAN, S. E. Ultrastructural localization of immunoreactive neurotensin in monkey superficial dorsal horn. *J. Comp. Neurol.* 225:1–12, 1984.

FIELDING, S., WILBUR, J., HYNER, M., SZEWCZAK, M., NOVICK, W. J., JR. AND HARBANS, L. A comparison of clonidine with morphine for antinociceptive and withdrawal actions. *J. Pharmacol. Exp. Ther.* 207:899–905, 1978.

FIELDS, H. L., WAGNER, G. M., AND ANDERSON, S. D. Some properties of spinal neurons projecting to the medial brain-stem reticular formation. *Exp. Neurol.* 47:118–134, 1975.

FIELDS, H. L., EMSON, P. C., LEIGH, B. K., GILBERT, R. F. T., AND IVERSEN, L. L. Multiple opiate receptor sites on primary afferent fibres. *Nature* 284:351–353, 1980.

FRERE, R. C., MAC DONALD, R. L., AND YOUNG, A. B. GABA binding and bicuculline in spinal cord and cortical membranes from adult rat and from mouse neurons in cell culture. *Brain Res.* 244:145–153, 1982.

GAMSE, R., HOLZER, P., AND LEMBECK, F. Indirect evidence for presynaptic location of opiate receptors on chemosensitive primary sensory neurones. *Naunyn Schmiedebergs Arch. Pharmacol.* 308:281–285, 1979.

GIBSON, S. J., POLAK, J. M., BLOOM, S. R., AND WALL, P. D. The distribution of nine peptides in rat spinal cord with special emphasis on the area around the central canal (lamina X). *J. Comp. Neurol.* 201:65–79, 1981.

GLAZER, E. J., AND BASBAUM, A. I. Opioid neurons and pain modulation: An ultrastructural analysis of enkephalin in cat superficial dorsal horn. *Neurosci.* 10:357–376, 1983.

GOODMAN, R. R., AND SNYDER, S. H. Autoradiographic localization of adenosine receptors in rat brain using [^{3}H]cyclohexyladenosine. *J. Neurosci.* 2:1230–1241.

GOODMAN, R. R., SYNDER, S. H., KUHAR, M. J., AND YOUNG, W. S. III. Differentiation of delta and mu opiate receptor localizations by light microscopic autoradiography. *Proc. Natl. Acad. Sci. U.S.A.* 77:6239–6243, 1980.

GOUARDERES, C., AUDIGIER, Y., AND CROS, J. Benzomorphan binding sites in rat lumbo-sacral spinal cord. *Eur. J. Pharmacol.* 78:483–486, 1982.

HARRIS, D. W., AND SETHY, V. H. High affinity binding of [^{3}H]cthylketocyclazocine to rat brain homogenate. *Eur. J. Pharmacol.* 66:121–123, 1980.

HERKENHAM, M., AND SOKOLOFF, L. Quantification of receptor densities by autoradiography: Tissue defatting minimizes differential absorbance of tritium by gray and white matter. *Soc. Neurosci. Abstr.* 9:329, 1983.

HILLER, J. M., SIMON, E. J., CRAIN, S. M., AND PETERSEN, E. R. Opiate receptors in cultures of fetal mouse dorsal root ganglia (DRG) and spinal cord: Predominance in DRG neurites. *Brain Res.* 145:396–400, 1978.

HÖKFELT, T., ELDE, R., JOHANSSON, O., TERENIUS, L., AND STEIN, L. The distribution of enkephalin-immunoractive cell bodies in the rat central nervous system. *Neurosci Lett.* 5:25–31, 1977.

HONDA, C. N., AND PERL, E. R. Properties of neurons in lamina X and the midline dorsal horn of the sacrococcygeal spinal cord of the cat. *Soc. Neurosci. Abstr.* 7:610, 1981.

HOSLI, E., AND HOSLI, L. Evidence for the existence of alpha- and beta-adrenoceptors on neurones and glial cells of cultured rat central nervous system—an autoradiographic study. *Neuroscience* 7:2873–2881, 1982.

HOWE, J., AND YAKSH, T. Changes in sensitivity to intrathecal norepinephrine and serotonin after 6-hydroxydopamine (6-OHDA), 5,6-dihyroxytryptamine (5,6-DHT) or repeated monoamine administration. *J. Pharmacol. Exp. Ther.* 220:311–321, 1982.

HOWE, J., AND YAKSH, T. Alpha$_2$-adrenoceptor binding and monoamine content in the cat lumbar spinal cord after intrathecal 6-hydroxydopamine on cervical hemisection. *Soc. Neurosci. Abstr.* 10:489, 1984.

HOWE, J. R., WANG J.-Y., AND YAKSH, T. L. Selective antagonism of the antinociceptive effect of intrathecally applied α-adrenergic agonists by intrathecal prazosin and intrathecal yohimbine. *J. Pharmacol. Exp. Ther.* 224:552–558, 1983.

HUNT, S. P., KELLY, J. S., AND EMSON, P. C. The electron microscopic localization of methionine enkephalin within the superficial layers (I and II) of the spinal cord. *Neuroscience* 5:1871–1890, 1980.

HYLDEN J. L. K., AND WILCOX G. L. Antinociceptive action of intrathecal neurotensin in mice. *Peptides* 4:517–520, 1983a.

HYLDEN, J. L. K., WILCOX, G. L. Intrathecal serotonin in mice: Analgesia and inhibition of a spinal action of substance P. *Life Sci.* 33:789–795, 1983b.

HYLDEN, J. L. K., AND WILCOX, G. L. Pharmacological characterization of substance P-induced nociception in mice: Modulation by opioid and noradrenergic agonists at the spinal level. *J. Pharmacol. Exp. Ther.* 226:398–404, 1983c.

JAN, L. Y., JAN, Y. N., AND BROWNFIELD, M. S. Peptidergic transmitters in synaptic boutons of sympathetic ganglia. *Nature* 288:380–382, 1980

JESSELL, T. M., AND IVERSEN, L. L. Opiate analgesics inhibit substance P release from rat trigeminal nucleus. *Nature* 268:549–551, 1977.

JESSELL, T. M., IVERSEN, L. L., AND CUELLO, A. C. Capsaicin-induced depletion of substance P from primary sensory neurones. *Brain Res.* 152:183–188, 1978.

JESSELL, T., TSUNOO, A., KANAZAWA, I., AND OTSUKA, M. Substance P: Depletion in the dorsal horn of rat spinal cord after section of the peripheral processes of primary sensory neurons. *Brain Res.* 168:247–259, 1979.

JONES, D. J., KENDALL, D. E., AND ENNA, S. J. Adrenergic receptors in rat spinal cord. *Neuropharmacology* 21:191–195, 1982.

JURNA, I. AND ZETLER, G. Antinociceptive effect of centrally administered caerulein and cholecystokinin octapeptide (CCK-8). *Eur. J. Pharmacol.* 73:321, 1981.

KAYAALP, S. O., AND NEFF, N. H. Regional distribution of cholinergic muscarinic receptors in spinal cord. *Brain Res.* 196:429–436, 1980.

KIMURA, H., MCGEER, P. L., PENG, J. H., AND MCGEER, E. G. The central cholinergic system studied by choline acetyltransferase immunohistochemistry in the cat. *J. Comp. Neurol.* 200:151–201, 1981.

KUHAR, M. J. Autoradiographic localization of drug and neurotransmitter receptors in the brain. *Trends Neurosci.* 4:60–64, 1981.

LAMOTTE, C., PERT, C. B., AND SNYDER, S. H. Opiate receptor binding in primate spinal cord: Distribution and changes after dorsal root section. *Brain Res.* 112:407–412, 1976.

LEYSON, J. E., GOMMEREN, W., AND NIEMEGEERS, C. J. E. [^{3}H]Sufentanil, a superior ligand for μ-opiate receptors: Binding properties and regional distribution in rat brain and spinal cord. *Eur. J. Pharmacol.* 87:209–225, 1983.

LIGHT A. R., AND PERL, E. R. Spinal termination of functionally identified primary afferent neurons with slowly conducting myelinated fibers. *J. Comp. Neurol.* 186:133–150, 1979.

LIGHT, A. R., KAVOOKJIAN, A. M., AND PETRUSZ, P. The ultrastructure and synaptic connections of serotonin-immunoreactive terminals in spinal laminae I and II. *Somatosens. Res.* 1:33–50, 1983.

LJUNGDAHL, A., HÖKFELT, T., AND NILSSON, G. Distribution of substance P-like immunoreactivity in the central nervous system of the rat. I. Cell bodies and nerve terminals. *Neuroscience* 3:861–943, 1978.

LORD, J. A. H., WATERFIELD, A. A., HUGHES, J., AND KOSTERLITZ, H. W. Endogenous opioid peptides: Multiple agonists and receptors. *Nature* 267:495–499, 1977.

MAURIN, Y., BUCK, S. H., WAMSLEY, J. K., BURKS, T. F., AND YAMAMURA, H. I. Light microscopic autoradiographic localization of [^{3}H]substance P binding sites in rat thoracic spinal cord. *Life Sci.* 34:1713–1716, 1984.

MCLAUGHLIN, B. J., BARBER, R., SAITO, K., ROBERTS, E., AND WU, J. Y. Immunohistochemical localization of glutamate decarboxylase in rat spinal cord. *J. Comp. Neurol.* 164:305–322, 1975.

MONAGHAN, D. T., AND COTMAN, C. W. The distribution of [^{3}H]kainic acid binding sites in rat CNS as determined by autoradiography. *Brain Res.* 252:91–100, 1982.

MORITA, K., AND KATAYAMA, Y. Two types of acetylcholine receptors on the soma of primary afferent neurons. *Brain Res.* 290:348–352, 1984.

MUDGE, A. W., LEEMAN, S. E., AND FISCHBACH, G. D. Enkephalin inhibits release of substance P from sensory neurons in culture and decreases action potential duration. *Proc. Natl. Acad. Sci. U.S.A.* 76:526–530, 1979.

NAGY, J. I., VINCENT, S. R., STAINES, W. M. A., FIBIGER, H. C., REISINE, T. D., AND YAMAMURA, H. I. Neurotoxic action of capsaicin on spinal substance P neurons. *Brain Res* 186:435–444, 1980

NAHIN, R. L., MADSEN, A. M., AND GIESLER, G. J., JR. Anatomical and physiological studies of the gray matter surrounding the spinal cord central canal. *J. Comp. Neurol.* 220:321–335, 1983.

NINKOVIC, M., HUNT, S. P., AND KELLY, J. S. Effect of dorsal rhizotomy on autoradiographic distribution of opiate and neurotensin receptors and neurotensin-like immunoreactivity within the rat spinal cord. *Brain Res.* 230:111–119, 1981.

NINKOVIC, M., HUNT, S. P., AND GLEAVE, J. R. W. Localization of opiate and histamine H1-receptors in the primate sensory ganglia and spinal cord. *Brain Res.* 241:197–206, 1982.

PALACIOS, J. M., WAMSLEY, J. K., AND KUHAR, M. J. High affinity GABA receptors—autoradiographic localization. *Brain Res.* 222:285–307, 1981.

PAXINOS, G., AND WATSON, C. *The Rat Brain in Stereotaxic Coordinates,* Academic Press, Sydney, 1982.

PEARSON, J., BRANDEIS, L., SIMON, E., AND HILLER, J. Radioautography of binding of tritiated diprenorphine to opiate receptors in the rat. *Life Sci.* 26:1047–1052, 1980.

PEROUTKA, S. J., LEBOVITZ, R. M., AND SNYDER, S. H. Two distinct central serotonin receptors with different physiological functions. *Science* 212:828–829, 1981.

PERT, C. B., KUHAR, M. J., AND SNYDER, S. H. Autoradiographic localization of the opiate receptor in rat brain. *Life Sci.* 16:1849–1854, 1975.

PERT, C. B., KUHAR, M. J., AND SNYDER, S. H. Opiate receptor: Autoradiographic localization in rat brain. *Proc. Natl. Acad. Sci. U.S.A.* 73:3729–3733, 1976.

POLZ-TEJERA, G., HUNT, S. P., AND SCHMIDT, J. Nicotinic receptors in sensory ganglia. *Brain Res.* 195:223–230, 1980.

PRICE, G. W., WILKIN, G. P., TURNBULL, M. J., AND BOWERY, N. G. Are baclofen-sensitive $GABA_{\beta}$ receptors present on primary afferent terminals of the spinal cord? *Nature* 307:71–74, 1984.

RIBEIRO-DA-SILVA, A., AND COIMBRA, A. Neuronal uptake of [^{3}H]GABA and [^{3}H]glycine in laminae I–III(substantia gelatinosa Rolandi) of the rat spinal cord. An autoradiographic study. *Brain Res.* 188:449–464, 1980.

RUDA, M. A. Opiates and pain pathways: Demonstration of enkephalin synapses on dorsal projection neurons. *Science* 215:1523–1525, 1982.

RUDA, M. A., AND GOBEL, S. Ultrastructural characteriation of axonal endings in the substantia gelatinosa which take up [^{3}H]serotonin. *Brain Res.* 184:57–83, 1980 .

SASEK, C. A., SEYBOLD, V. S., AND ELDE, R. P. The immunohistochemical localization of nine peptides in the sacral parasympathetic nucleus and the dorsal gray commissure in rat spinal cord. *Neuroscience* 12:855–873, 1984.

SATOH, K., KASHIBA, A., KIMURA, H., AND MAEDA, T. Noradrenergic axon terminals in the substantia gelatinosa of the rat spinal cord. *Cell Tissue Res.* 222:359–378, 1982.

SEGU L., AND CALAS, A. The topographical distribution of serotoninergic terminals in the spinal cord of the cat: Quantitative radioautographic studies. *Brain Res.* 153:449–464, 1978.

SEYBOLD, V., AND ELDE, R. Receptor autoradiography in thoracic spinal cord: Correlation of neurotransmitter binding sites with sympathoadrenal neurons. *J. Neurosci.* 10:2533–2542, 1984.

SEYBOLD, V., AND MALEY, B. Ultrastructural localization of neurotensin-like immunoreactivity in the superficial laminae of the rat dorsal horn. *Peptides* 5:1179–1189, 1984.

SINGER E., AND PLACHETA, P. Reduction of [^{3}H]muscimol binding sites in rat dorsal spinal cord after neonatal capsaicin treatment. *Brain Res.* 202:484–487, 1980.

SLATER, P., AND PATEL, S. Autoradiographic localization of opiate kappa receptors in the rat spinal cord. *Eur. J. Pharmacol.* 92:159–160, 1983.

SPARBER, S. B., AND MEYER, D. R. Clonidine antagonizes naloxone-induced suppression of conditioned behavior and body weight loss in morphine-dependent rats. *Pharmacol. Biochem. Behav.* 9:319–325, 1978.

STEINBUSCH, H. W. M. Distribution of serotonin-immunoreactivity in the central nervous system of the rat—cell bodies and terminals. *Neuroscience* 6:557–618, 1981.

SUMAL, K. K., PICKEL, V. M., MILLER, R. J., AND REIS, D. J. Enkephalin-containing neurons in substantia gelatinosa of spinal trigeminal complex: Ultrastructure and synaptic interaction with primary sensory afferents. *Brain Res.* 248:223–236, 1982.

TAYLOR, J. E., YAKSH, T. L., AND RICHELSON, E. Histamine H_1 receptors in the brain and spinal cord of the cat. *Brain Res.* 243:391–394, 1982.

TRAYNOR, J. R., KELLY, P. D., AND RANCE, M. J. Multiple opiate binding sites in rat spinal cord. *Life Sci.* 31:1377–1380, 1982.

TUSCHSCHERER, M. M., AND SEYBOLD, V. Immunohistochemical studies of substance P, cholecystokinin-betapeptide and somatostatin in dorsal root ganglia of the rat. *Neuroscience* 14:593–605, 1985.

WAMSLEY, J. K., LEWIS, M. S., YOUNG, W. S. III, AND KUHAR, M. J. Autoradiographic localization of muscarinic cholinergic receptors in rat brainstem. *J. Neurosci.* 1:176–191, 1981a.

WAMSLEY, J. K., ZARBIN, M. A., AND KUHAR, M. J. Muscarinic cholinergic receptors flow in the sciatic nerve. *Brain Res.* 217:155–161, 1981b.

WAMSLEY, J. K., ZARBIN, M. A., YOUNG, W. S. III, AND KUHAR, M. J. Distribution of opiate receptors in the monkey brain: An autoradiographic study. *Neuroscience* 7:595–613, 1982.

WESTLUND, K. N., AND COULTER, J. D. Descending projections of the locus coeruleus and subcoeruleus/medial parabrachial nuclei in monkey: Axonal transport studies and dopamine-B-hydroxylase immunohistochemistry. *Brain Res. Rev.* 2:235–264, 1980.

YAKSH, T. L., JESSELL, T. M., GAMSE, R., MUDGE, A. W., AND LEEMAN, S. E. Intrathecal morphine inhibits substance P release from mammalian spinal cord *in vivo. Nature* 286:155–157, 1980.

YAKSH, T. L., SCHMAUSS, C., MICEVYCH, P. E., ABAY, E. O., AND GO, V. L. W. Pharmacological studies on the application, disposition and release of neurotensin in the spinal cord. *Ann. N.Y. Acad. Sci.* 400:228–247, 1982.

YAMAMURA, H. I., WAMSLEY, J. K., DESHMUKH, P., AND ROESKE, W. R. Differential light microscopic autoradiographic localization of muscarinic cholinergic receptors in the brainstem and spinal cord of the rat using [^{3}h]pirenzepine. *Eur. J. Pharmacol.* 91:147–149, 1983.

YOUNG, W. S. III, AND KUHAR, M. J. A new method for receptor autoradiography: [^{3}H]Opioid receptors in rat brain. *Brain Res.* 179:255–270, 1979a.

YOUNG, W. S. III, AND KUHAR, M. J. Neurotensin receptors: Autoradiographic localization in rat CNS. *Eur. J. Pharmacol.* 59:161–163, 1979b.

YOUNG, W. S. III, AND KUHAR, M. J. Noradrenergic alpha-1 and alpha-2 receptors: Autoradiographic visualization. *Eur. J. Pharmacol.* 59:317–319, 1979c.

YOUNG, W. S. III, AND KUHAR, M. J. Radiohistochemical localization of benzodiazepine receptors in rat brain. *J. Pharmacol. Exp. Ther.* 212:337–346, 1980a.

YOUNG, W. S. III, AND KUHAR, M. J. Serotonin receptor localization in rat brain by light microscopic autoradiography. *Eur. J. Pharmacol.* 62:237–239, 1980b.

YOUNG, W. S. III, AND KUHAR, M. J. Neurotensin receptor localization by light microscopic autoradiography in rat brain. *Brain Res.* 206:273–285, 1981.

YOUNG, W. S. III, WAMSLEY, J. K., ZARBIN, M. A., AND KUHAR, M. J. Opioid receptors undergo axonal flow. *Science* 210:76–77, 1980.

ZARBIN, M. A., WAMSLEY, J. K., AND KUHAR, M. J. Glycine receptor: Light microscopic autoradiographic localization with [^{3}H]strychnine. *J. Neurosci.* 1:532–547, 1981.

ZARBIN, M. A., INNIS, R. B., WAMSLEY, J. K., SNYDER, S. H., AND KUHAR, M. J. Autoradiograpahic localization of cholecystokinin receptors in rodent brain. *J. Neurosci.* 3:877–906, 1983.

ZIVIN, J. A., REID, J. L., SAAVEDRA, J. M., AND KOPIN, I. J. Quantitative localization of biogenic amines in the spinal cord. *Brain Res.* 99:293–301, 1975.

7
The Pattern and Place of Nociceptive Modulation in the Dorsal Horn
A Discussion of the Anatomically Characterized Neural Circuitry of Enkephalin, Serotonin, and Substance P

M. A. RUDA

A. *Introduction*

Recent technical innovations have advanced the study of the mechanisms of pain and analgesia. These advances have resulted in an increased understanding of the anatomical organization of the dorsal horn at the medullary and spinal levels. Studies employing immunocytochemical labeling of neurotransmitters, retrograde transport of HRP, and intracellular HRP techniques have been at the forefront. The greatest strides, however, have been made when two of these approaches were combined in a single experiment to identify relationships between two labeled elements simultaneously. Many of the multiple-label experiments that were first accomplished in the dorsal horn are applicable throughout the nervous system. The observations are useful from the perspective of basic concepts of neural circuitry as well as a characterization of the pathways involved in pain and analgesia. Study of the spinal cord dorsal horn offers a unique advantage in that it contains many of the identified

M. A. RUDA • Neurobiology and Anesthesiology Branch, National Institute of Dental Research, National Institutes of Health, Bethesda, Maryland 20892.

substances in the nervous system that act as neurotransmitters or neuromodulators (Table I). These neurochemicals include both classical neurotransmitters such as the monoamines and amino acids as well as recently discovered families of neuropeptides. This chapter seeks to address some of the fundamental observations on the anatomical and neurochemical organization of the dorsal horn and to apply the findings to basic issues of integration in the nervous system as well as to the study of pain and analgesia.

B. Structural and Functional Diversity within the Dorsal Horn

The medullary and spinal dorsal horns are laminated structures that contain distinctive neuronal components within each lamina. The diversity includes the chemistry, morphology, and function of the neurons and afferent axons that occur within each lamina. The variety of neuronal organization in the dorsal horn is indicative of the complexity of the underlying neural circuitry of pain and analgesia.

The dorsal horn can be thought of as having three basic component parts: intrinsic neurons, primary afferent axons, and axons that descend from higher centers of the neuraxis. The unique characteristics of each of these components have recently been reviewed (Dubner and Bennett, 1983). Briefly, the intrinsic dorsal horn neurons may be either projection neurons, which transfer their message rostrally to higher centers of the brain, or interneurons, which are involved in local circuit interactions within the dorsal horn. Different classes of projection neurons are concentrated in laminae I, IV, V, and VI (see discussion by Willis, Chapter 11), whereas a variable number of interneurons occur in all laminae.

Physiologically, dorsal horn neurons represent a diverse population that

TABLE I
Neurochemicals Found in the Dorsal Horn

Monamines	Amino acids
Serotonin	GABA
Norepinephrine	Glycine
Dopamine	Glutamate
	Taurine
Neuropeptides	
Leu-Enkephalin	Substance P
Met-Enkephalin	Substance K
Dynorphin	Bombesin
Adrenocorticotropin	Cholecystokinin
Kyotorphin	Somatostatin
β-Endorphin	Vasoactive intestinal polypeptide
α-MSH	Corticotropin-releasing factor
Neuropeptide Y	Oxytocin
FMRFamide	Vasopressin
Neurotensin	Thryotropin-releasing hormone

includes nociceptive specific neurons (responding only to noxious forms of stimulation), wide-dynamic-range neurons (responding maximally to noxious stimulation but also to low-threshold stimulation), and low-threshold neurons (responding only to innocuous forms of stimulation) (see comments by Cervero, Chapter 9; Price, Chapter 18; and Le Bars and colleagues, Chapter 19). Primary afferent axons carry nociceptive and nonnociceptive information from the periphery to the spinal cord. Nociceptors include both unmyelinated and finely myelinated axons, subpopulations of which terminate in laminae I, IIa, and V. As discussed by Hammond (Chapter 15), descending afferent axons originate from several brainstem nuclei as well as the cerebral cortex. The descending axons distribute differentially to the various laminae of the spinal cord. The diversity of their termination involves variations in location as well as density.

In addition to the anatomical complexity of the dorsal gray, advances in immunohistochemistry have demonstrated that these systems may be characterized by a variety of neurotransmitter elements. The broad diversity of such systems in the dorsal gray have been discussed by La Motte (Chapter 5). In this discussion I focus on the distribution of three neurochemicals in the dorsal horn, enkephalin, serotonin, and substance P, which appear to represent the receptor-active agents for spinal systems involved in the transmission and processing of nociceptive information.

C. *Enkephalin, Serotonin, and Substance P at the Light Microscopic Level*

Enkephalin is an opioid peptide that is a natural ligand for opiate receptors. In the dorsal horn, most of the enkephalin originates from a subpopulation of dorsal horn neurons (Sar *et al.*, 1978; Seybold and Elde, 1980; Glazer and Basbaum, 1981; Hunt *et al.*, 1981; Bennett *et al.*, 1982; Sumal *et al.*, 1982; Ruda *et al.*, 1983). Serotonin is a monoamine neurotransmitter originating from brainstem raphe cell groups involved in descending control of nociception (Dahlström and Fuxe, 1964, 1965; Basbaum *et al.*, 1978; Bowker *et al.*, 1981a,b). Dorsal horn substance P is a neurochemical originating mainly from primary afferent axons (Hökfelt *et al.*, 1975a,b; Cuello *et al.*, 1978; Takahashi and Otsuka, 1975; Jessell *et al.*, 1979; Barber *et al.*, 1979; Massari *et al.*, 1983). Observations on these three neurotransmitters can be used to illustrate fundamental principles of dorsal horn neural circuitry.

Enkephalin-immunoreactive varicosities are concentrated in laminae I and II of the dorsal horn (Hökfelt *et al.*, 1977; Sar *et al.*, 1978; Hunt *et al.*, 1981; Glazer and Basbaum, 1981; Bennett *et al.*, 1982). Their density is greatest in laminae I and IIb, decreasing somewhat in lamina IIA (Figure 1A). A second concentration of enkephalin terminals occurs in the neck of the dorsal horn, in laminae V and VI. These two areas of high concentration of enkephalin terminals correspond to the dorsal horn laminae most involved with nociception (Dubner *et al.*, 1984). Dorsal horn enkephalin has been shown to

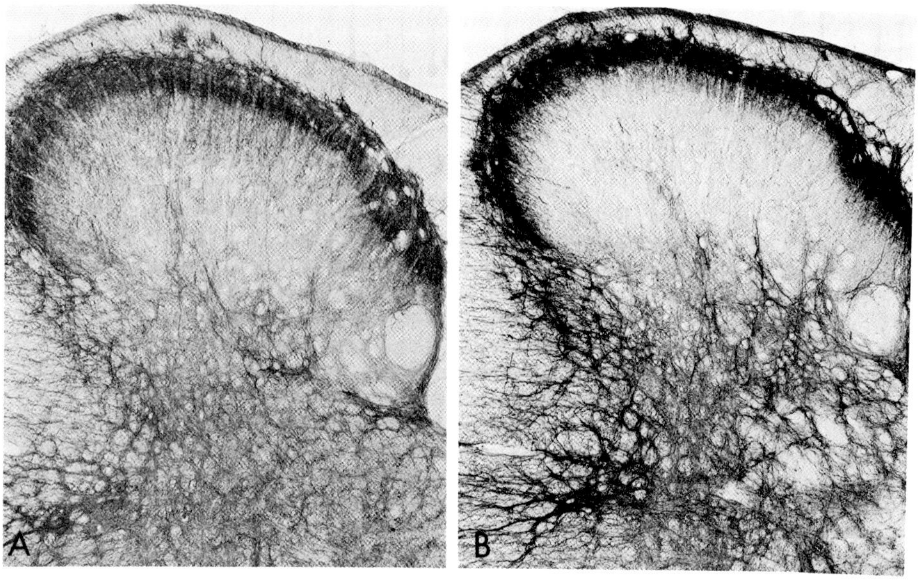

FIGURE 1. Comparison of immunocytochemical staining for enkephalin (A) and substance P (B) from neighboring sections of the medullary dorsal horn of the cat. Although both of these peptides are found in the same dorsal horn laminae, the relative density of immunoreactive axons for each peptide is different. The superficial, dense enkephalin-staining band is thicker than that of substance P, encompassing laminae I, IIa, and IIb. The substance P band is densest in laminae I and IIa. Lamina IIb contains a dense network of enkephalin axons but few substance P axons. In laminae V and VI, the density of substance P axons is typically greater than that of enkephalin. ×38. (Reproduced at 83%.)

originate mainly from intrinsic dorsal horn neurons, since transection of the thoracic spinal cord results in a negligible loss of lumbar enkephalin assayed by immunocytochemistry (Seybold and Elde, 1980; Ruda *et al.*, 1983) or radioimmunoassay (Hunt *et al.*, 1981). The contribution of descending enkephalin axons to dorsal horn neural circuitry is unclear, since double-label studies have failed to differentiate between afferents to the dorsal and ventral horns (Hökfelt *et al.*, 1979; Bowker *et al.*, 1981a).

Enkephalin-containing neurons are found in varying numbers in all laminae of the dorsal horn (Figure 2A) (Hunt *et al.*, 1980, 1981; Glazer and Basbaum, 1981; Bennett *et al.*, 1982), where they represent different morphological types of neurons. Most enkephalin neurons are likely to be interneurons rather than long-distance projection neurons. In lamina I, thalamic projection neurons do not appear to contain enkephalin (Basbaum, 1982). Lamina I neurons with a local axonal arbor (Bennett *et al.*, 1981a) may represent a subpopulation of enkephalin neurons. Two types of enkephalin interneurons in lamina II have been identified as stalked cells and IIb islet cells on the basis of their morphology (Bennett *et al.*, 1982). Some small enkephalin lamina III cells resemble intracellularly HRP-filled neurons that receive only low-threshold mechanoreceptor input (Bennett *et al.*, 1981b). The identity of Enkephalin neurons in other laminae is unknown. Thus, in the dorsal horn,

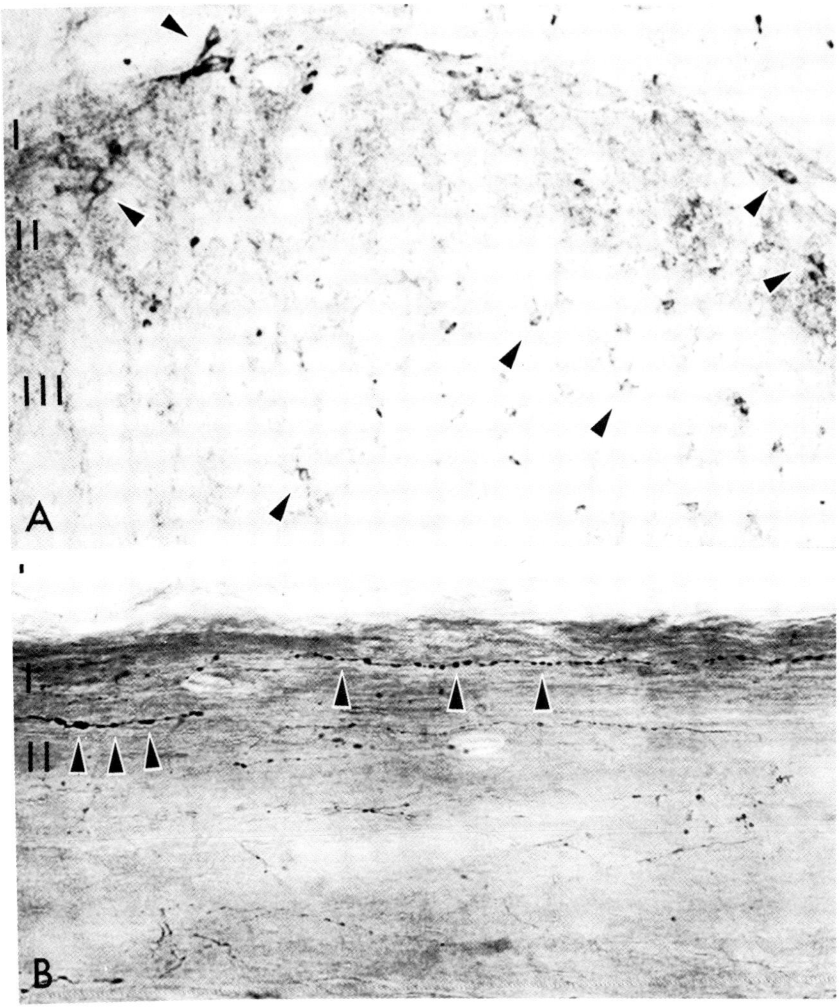

FIGURE 2. (A) Immunocytochemically stained enkephalin neurons are found in all laminae of the cat medullary dorsal horn. In colchicine-treated animals, numerous enkephalin cell bodies (arrows) are visible in laminae I, II, and III. They represent different morphological types of neurons that contain the same neurotransmitter. ×164. (B) Sagittal section of the lumbar spinal cord of the cat immunocytochemically stained (without penetrating agents) for serotonin. A few axonal strands are visible on the surface of the section. In laminae I and II, the serotonin axons tend to orient rostrocaudally. An individual axonal strand may contain different-size varicosities along its length (arrowheads). ×462.

different morphological and functional types of neurons may contain the same neurotransmitter. However, since enkephalin neurons of each type appear to be less numerous than all cells of that type seen in Golgi studies, it is likely that in the dorsal horn, a distinct morphological type of neuron is neurochemically diverse.

Serotonin axonal endings are found in all laminae of the dorsal horn and are densest in lamina I and the outer portion of lamina II, lamina IIa (Figure 3) (Steinbusch, 1981; Ruda *et al.*, 1982; Light *et al.*, 1983; LaMotte and DeLanerolle, 1983). The inner part of lamina II, lamina IIb, contains noticeably fewer serotonin axons. The pattern of termination of serotonin axons as seen at the light microscopic level is readily distinguished from that of enkephalin or substance P by both density and laminar specificity. The density of serotonin axons in laminae I and II is not as great as either enkephalin or substance P axons, whereas in laminae III and IV, serotonin axons outnumber both enkephalin and substance P axons (Compare Figures 1 and 3). The decrease in serotonin axons in lamina IIb parallels somewhat a decrease in substance P axons in that lamina, whereas enkephalin axons are dense in lamina IIb. The primary orientation of the serotonin axons is rostrocaudal. The serotonin-immunoreactive axonal strands display some variety with respect to the size and shape of their varicosities. The varicosities range in length from 0.8 to 3.0 μm. An individual axon can exhibit considerable variety with respect to the size of varicosities along its length (Figure 2B). Many enkephalin and substance P terminal arbors and axonal varicosities are morphologically similar to those that contain serotonin, suggesting that axons containing different neurotransmitters do not demonstrate a distinct morphology at the light microscopic level.

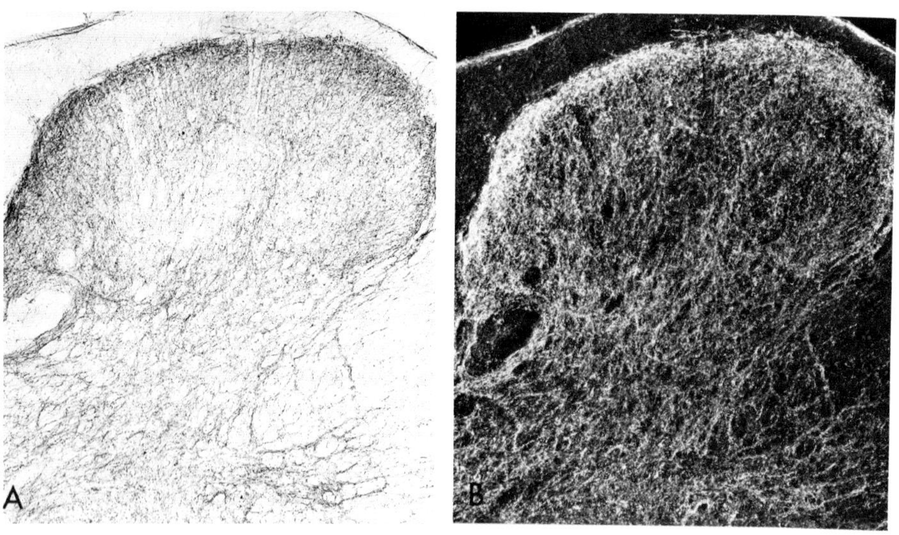

FIGURE 3. Immunocytochemical labeling of serotonin axons in the medullary dorsal horn. The tissue is taken from the same cat as Figure 1. The bright-field photomicrograph (A) allows direct comparison of the density of serotonin versus enkephalin and substance P axons shown in Figure 1. Serotonin-immunoreactive axons are noticeably fewer in laminae I and II by comparison. Dark-field optics (B) of the same section provides a dramatic demonstration of the serotonin-immunoreactive terminal plexus throughout all laminae of the dorsal horn. ×38. (Reproduced at 77%.)

Dorsal horn substance P is concentrated superficially in laminae I and IIa and in the neck of the dorsal horn in laminae V and VI (Figure 1B) (Cuello *et al.*, 1978; Barber *et al.*, 1979; Hökfelt *et al.*, 1975a,b, 1977; Gibson *et al.*, 1981; DiFiglia *et al.*, 1982; deLanerolle and LaMotte, 1983). Following rhizotomy, there is a substantial decrease in the density of substance P in the superficial layers, suggesting that primary afferent axons are a major source of dorsal horn substance P (Hökfelt *et al.*, 1975a,b; Cuello *et al.*, 1978; Takahashi and Otsuka, 1975; Jessel *et al.*, 1979; Massari *et al.*, 1983). The dense superficial banding pattern of substance P axons is distinct from that of enkephalin and serotonin (compare Figures 1A, 1B, and 3A). Substance P axons are densest in laminae I and IIa, decreasing substantially to few axons in lamina IIb. The distinctive pattern of termination may reflect differential involvement of each peptide in nociceptive neural circuits. Nociceptive substance P primary afferent axons may be absent from lamina IIb, since neurons in lamina IIb respond exclusively to low-threshold primary afferent input (Bennett *et al.*, 1980; Light *et al.*, 1979; Price *et al.*, 1979).

The assignment of function to substance P terminals is confounded by the disparate origin of substance P afferents. Although it is clear that primary afferent axons are the major source of dorsal horn substance P, some part of the staining pattern can be attributed to the axons of intrinsic dorsal horn substance-P-containing neurons, which are found in laminae I and II (Ljungdahl *et al.*, 1978; Gibson *et al.*, 1981; Tessler *et al.*, 1981; Hunt *et al.*, 1981). Designation of a morphological type of substance P neuron is speculative (Hunt *et al.*, 1981), although, as with enkephalin, it is likely that substance P neurons represent different morphological types.

Substance-P-containing neurons in the raphe nuclei have been shown to project to the spinal cord (Bowker *et al.*, 1981b). A small number of the substance P axons in the dorsal horn may originate from this descending system, since a slight decrease in the amount of dorsal horn substance P can be detected following spinal cord transection. Some descending substance P in the dorsal horn may coexist in the same axon terminal as serotonin, since the serotonin neurotoxin 5,7-dihydroxytryptamine causes a slight loss in assayable substance P (Gilbert *et al.*, 1982).

Substance-P-containing axons in the dorsal horn are an example of a neurotransmitter system with diverse origin that includes primary afferent axons, axons of intrinsic neurons, and axons of descending modulatory systems. The diverse origin implies different functions in the modulation of dorsal horn output by the same neurotransmitter system.

D. Ultrastructure of Enkephalin-, Serotonin-, and Substance-P-Containing Dorsal Horn Elements

Immunocytochemistry provides a definitive method for identifying the neurotransmitter contained in an axon at the ultrastructural level. Historically, the shape of an axonal ending, the types of vesicles it contains, and the type of synapse it forms were used as criteria for neurochemical identification. Although perhaps useful in a general sense, each criterion has not proved valid in all systems. Immunocytochemistry has allowed anatomy to go beyond these criteria with a distinctive ultrastructural marker to indicate neurochemical function. Using this tool, we have been able to demonstrate that axons that contain different neurotransmitters exhibit the same morphology when examined at the ultrastructural level. Conversely, axons that contain the same neurotransmitter can display different morphologies at the electron microscopic level. The ultrastructure of enkephalin, serotonin, and substance P axons in the dorsal horn can be used to illustrate these points. Description of their ultrastructural morphology in different species has been made by several investigators (Pickel *et al.*, 1977; Barber *et al.*, 1979; Hunt *et al.*, 1980; Aronin *et al.*, 1981; DiFiglia *et al.*, 1982; Glazer and Basbaum, 1982; Priestley *et al.*, 1982; Ruda, 1982; Ruda *et al.*, 1982, 1984; Sumal *et al.*, 1982; deLanerolle and LaMotte, 1983; LaMotte and deLanerolle, 1983a,b; Light *et al.*, 1983).

Most enkephalin-, serotonin-, and substance-P-immunoreactive axonal endings in the superficial dorsal horn are dome-shaped and measure 1.0 to 3.5 μm in length (compare Figures 4, 5, and 6). They typically form a single synapse with an adjacent neuronal profile. The synaptic specialization is small (0.25 to 0.6 μm in length) and occupies only a small portion of the varicosities' perimeter (Figure 4). The diminutive size of the synaptic site of some enkephalin axonal endings may even be less than 0.1 μm in length (Glazer and Basbaum, 1983), requiring extensive serial section analysis to identify the postsynaptic target. The synapse may be either symmetrical (Figure 5A), slightly asymmetrical, or display a prominent asymmetrical subsynaptic density (Figure 6). Although some enkephalin, serotonin, and substance P endings fall into each of these categories of synaptic types, there appears to be a differential number of endings of each type. Enkephalin axonal endings are more likely to form an asymmetrical type of synapse (Figure 4A), often with a prominent subsynaptic density. Serotonin axonal endings most frequently form symmetrical synapses, although several examples of asymmetrical synapses can also be found. Substance P axonal endings tend to be slightly asymmetrical.

Substance P varicosities in the superficial dorsal horn are an example of different morphological types of axonal endings that contain the same neurotransmitter. In addition to dome-shaped endings (Figure 5B), a large population of substance P endings are the central endings of a glomerulus (Figure 6). The central ending is surrounded by several different neuronal profiles, which are impressed into its surface, imparting a characteristic scalloped shape. The central ending forms asymmetrical synapses with several different dendritic profiles. The heterogeneous morphology of substance P endings in the superficial dorsal horn may in part reflect their diverse origin. It is tempting to speculate that the central substance P endings originate from primary afferents, whereas the dome-shaped endings originate from descending fibers or intrinsic dorsal horn neurons. However, this characterization may be an oversimplification, since autoradiographic studies at the ultrastructural level

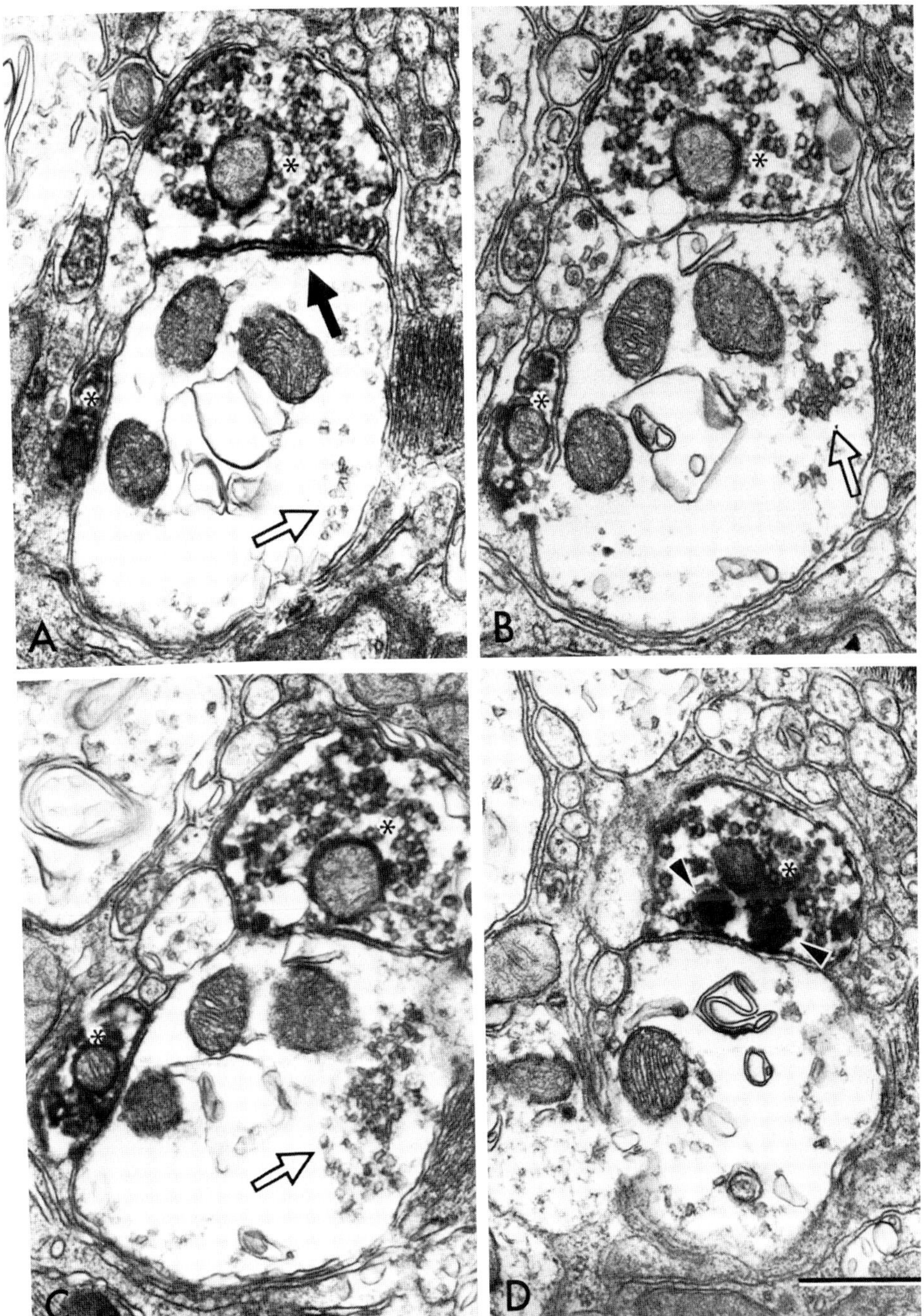

FIGURE 4. Semiserial sections through two enkephalin-immunoreactive axonal endings (asterisks) that contact a dendrite in lamina I of cat medullary dorsal horn. In section A, one of the labeled endings forms an asymmetrical synapse (arrow) with a dendrite. In sections B and C, an aggregation of vesicles (open arrows) is present in the dendritic shaft. The PAP reaction product coats the mostly round or oval agranular vesicles and the outer mitochondrial membrane of the enkephalin-immunoreactive axonal ending. Two dense-core vesicles in section D are also associated with reaction product (arrowheads). ×32,400. Scale bar represents 0.5 μm.

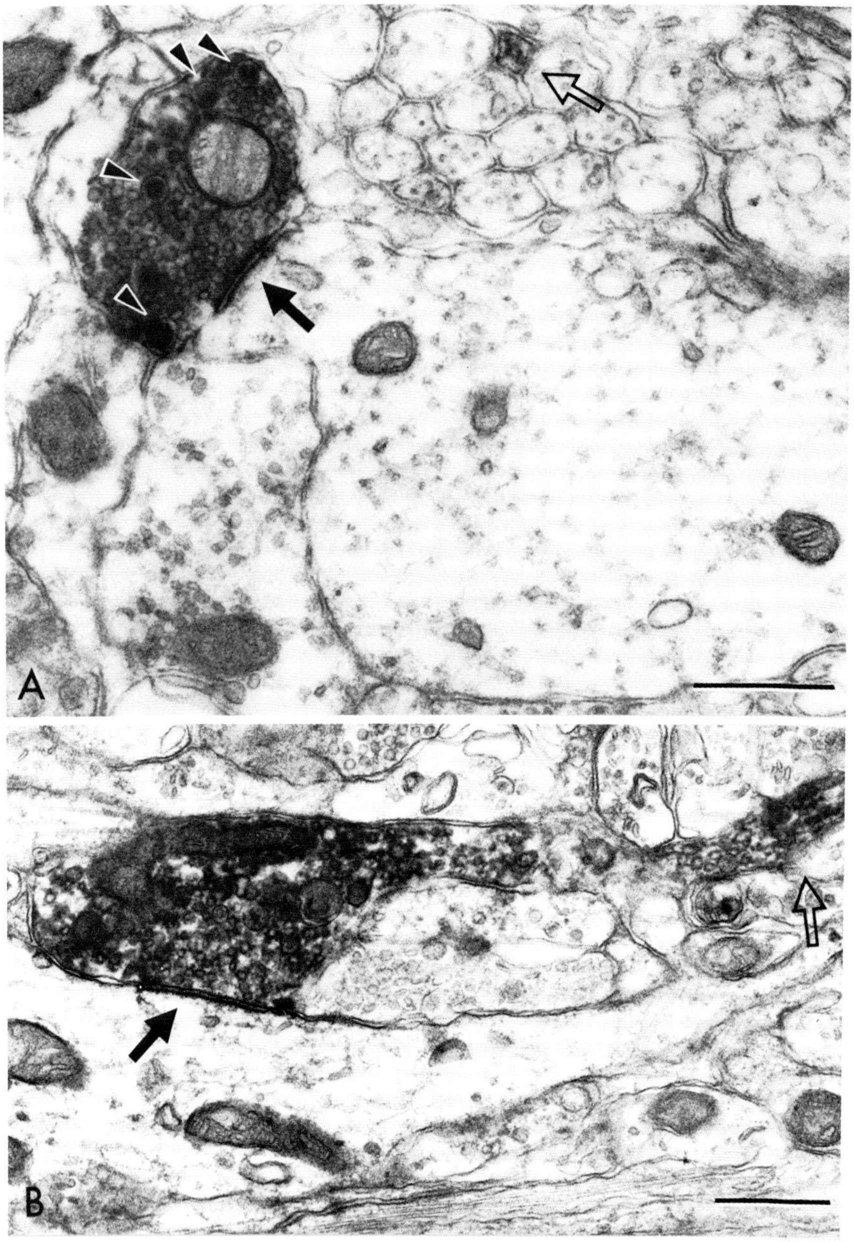

FIGURE 5. (A) An immunocytochemically stained dome-shaped serotonin axonal varicosity synapses (arrow) on a spinelike dendritic protrusion in cat lumbar superficial dorsal horn. The serotonin varicosity contains mainly round or oval agranular synaptic vesicles and a few dense-core vesicles (arrowheads). An immunoreactive intervaricose portion of an unmyelinated axon is nearby (open arrow). ×38,400. Scale bar represents 0.5 μm. (B) An immunocytochemically stained dome-shaped substance P axonal varicosity synapses (arrow) on a dendrite in cat lumbar superficial dorsal horn. The ending contains a mixture of round, oval, and flattened agranular vesicles. The continuation of the intervaricose portion of the axon is also visible (open arrow). Magnification × 31,650. Scale bar represents 0.5 μm.

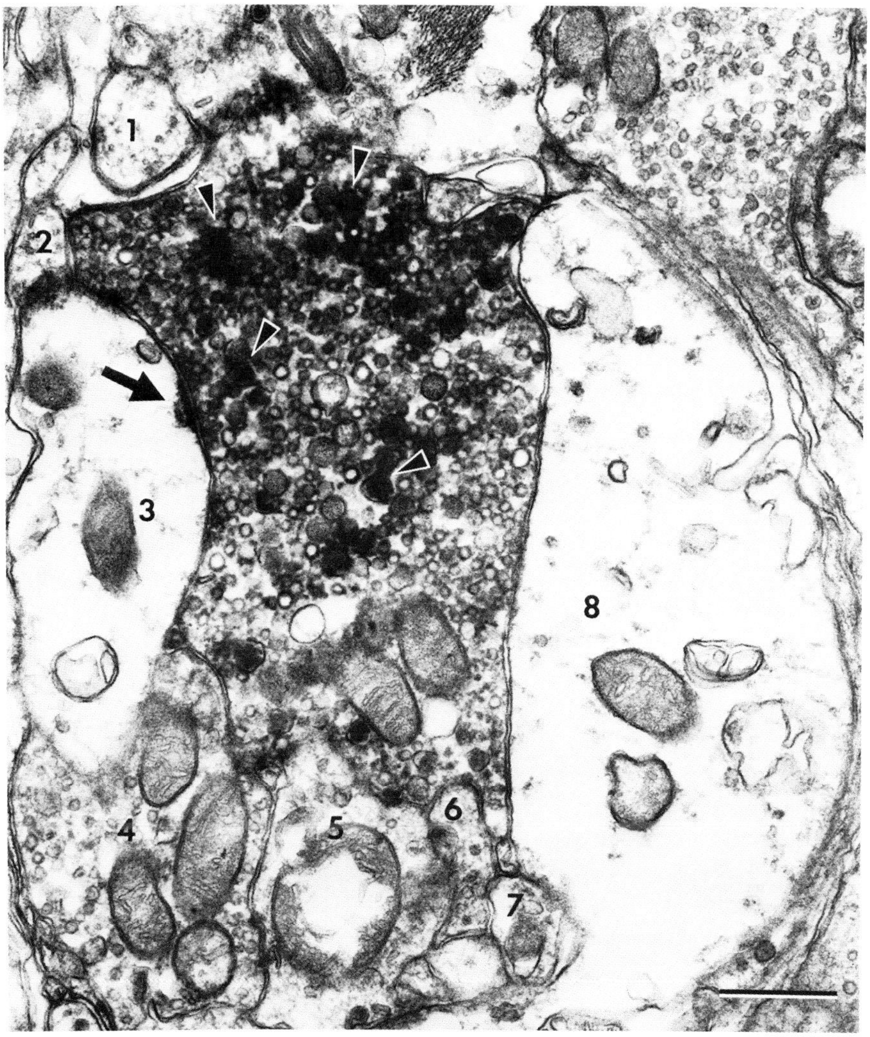

FIGURE 6. A scalloped central ending in the cat lumbar dorsal horn is immunocytochemically stained for substance P. Eight different profiles surround the ending. Dendrite number 3 receives an asymmetrical synapse with a prominent subsynaptic density (arrow). Dendrite number 8 was seen in serial sections to likewise receive a synapse from the substance P ending. Numerous dense-core vesicles are associated with the PAP reaction product (arrowheads). ×31,650. Scale bar represents 0.5 μm.

have demonstrated a population of dome-shaped primary afferent axon terminals in the superficial layers of the dorsal horn (Ralston, 1979).

Enkephalin, serotonin, and substance P varicosities contain mainly round or oval agranular vesicles and a variable number of dense-core vesicles. The largest varicosities are more likely to contain numerous dense-core vesicles (Figure 6), whereas the more common smaller varicosities often contain few, requiring serial section analysis to demonstrate their presence (Figure 4). A few enkephalin, serotonin, and substance P axonal varicosities contain pleomorphic agranular vesicles, which range in shape from highly flattened to round. In each case, axonal varicosities with pleomorphic vesicles represent a minority of the population.

At the ultrastructural level, enkephalin, serotonin, and substance P have been shown predominantly to act postsynaptically on intrinsic dorsal horn neurons (Barber *et al.*, 1979; Hunt *et al.*, 1980; Aronin *et al.*, 1981; DiFiglia *et al.*, 1982; Glazer and Basbaum, 1982; Priestley *et al.*, 1982; Ruda, 1982; Ruda *et al.*, 1982, 1984; deLanerolle and LaMotte, 1983; LaMotte and deLanerolle, 1983a,b; Light *et al.*, 1983). Most enkephalin and serotonin synapses occur on dendritic shafts. A few are also found on dendritic spines. Substance P synapses occur largely on spines. Axosomatic synaptic contacts are few in number compared to the total number of axodendritic synaptic contacts. The paucity of synaptic contacts on this important synaptic modulation site may reflect, in part, the fact that the surface area of a neuron is largely dendritic, providing a greater number of potential contact sites on dendrites.

Narotsky and Kerr (1978) have shown that superficial dorsal horn neuronal cell bodies receive a differential number of axonal contacts. Subpopulations of thalamic projection neurons in lamina I also receive varying numbers of somatic contacts. The axonal endings that form axosomatic synapses on these projection neurons may contain enkephalin (Ruda *et al.*, 1984), serotonin (Ruda and Coffield, 1983), and many unidentified neurotransmitters as well. Some thalamic projection neurons, often those with large cell bodies, exhibit a dense somatic innervation pattern, whereas the smaller thalamic projection neurons receive few somatic contacts (Figure 7). Laminae I and II enkephalin-containing neurons also display variety with respect to their somatic innervation pattern. Some enkephalin neurons receive numerous somatic synaptic contacts (Glazer and Basbaum, 1983), whereas others receive few (Figure 8). Neurons with few somatic contacts are often encompassed by glial cells.

E. Afferents That Project to Identified Dorsal Horn Neurons

The preponderance of postsynaptic target sites in the dorsal horn prompts the question of which types of dorsal horn neurons receive aminergic and peptidergic input. Multiple-label techniques help to answer this question, since the synaptic interaction can be identified by a definitive marker rather than arbitrary morphological criteria. Neurochemically identified afferents to different types of dorsal horn neurons are listed in Table II. The combination

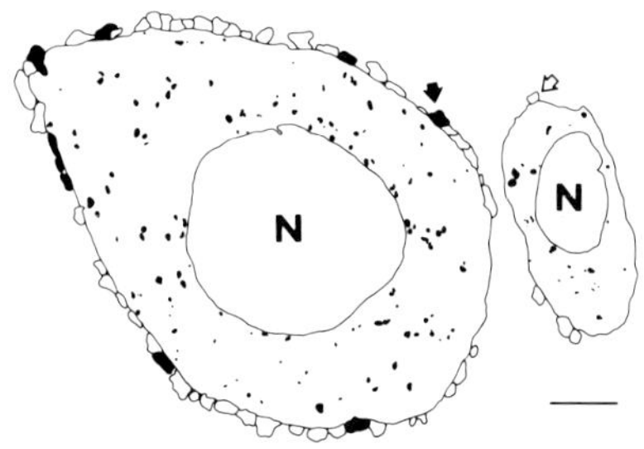

FIGURE 7. Pattern of somatic innervation of two different neurons in lamina I of the cat medullary dorsal horn. Retrogradely transported HRP granules dispersed in the cell's cytoplasm identify these neurons as projecting to the thalamus. The drawings were made from a photomontage reconstruction of each neuron photographed with the electron microscope. Enkephalin-immunoreactive varicosities are blackened (arrow), whereas unlabeled varicosities (open arrow) are drawn in outline. Enkephalin input represents only a small portion of the somatic innervation. Although both neurons transfer information from the dorsal horn to the thalamus, each has a different density of afferent input on its somata. Scale bar represents 10 μm. (From Ruda *et al.*, 1984.)

of immunocytochemistry to label axons with either retrograde or intracellular HRP to label neurons has provided most of the observations.

1. Interneurons

Afferent input to dorsal horn local-circuit neurons in laminae I and II have been studied with the intracellular HRP technique at the light microscopic level (Hoffert *et al.*, 1983; Miletic *et al.*, 1984). This approach renders a Golgi-like staining of the full extent of the neuron's dendritic arbor, offering the unique advantage of examining contact distribution of immunocytochemically labeled afferents on a neuron's soma, proximal and distal dendrites, and spines. Lamina I neurons, some of which may be projection neurons, and stalked cells, interneurons in lamina II, were observed to receive numerous serotonin-labeled contacts (Hoffert *et al.*, 1983; Miletic *et al.*, 1984). Islet cells, Golgi type II interneurons in lamina II, received few serotonin contacts (Miletic *et al.*, 1984). Substance-P-labeled varicosities contacted both spiny and aspiny lamina I neurons (Hoffert *et al.*, 1982). In general, the serotonin-immunoreactive contacts preferentially occurred on dendritic shafts, whereas substance P contacts tended to be located on spines (Hoffert *et al.*, 1982).

The neurotransmitters of two types of afferents to enkephalin neurons have been identified. Enkephalin-containing neurons were immunocytochemically identified at the ultrastructural level, and enkephalin-immunoreactive axonal endings were found synapsing on the dendrites of some enkephalin-immunoreactive neurons (Aronin *et al.*, 1981; Glazer and Basbaum, 1982). In another study, autoradiographically labeled axonal endings that took up [^{3}H]5-HT were found synapsing on enkephalin-immunoreactive neurons (Glazer and Basbaum, 1984).

The observations gained from these multiple-label experiments illustrate

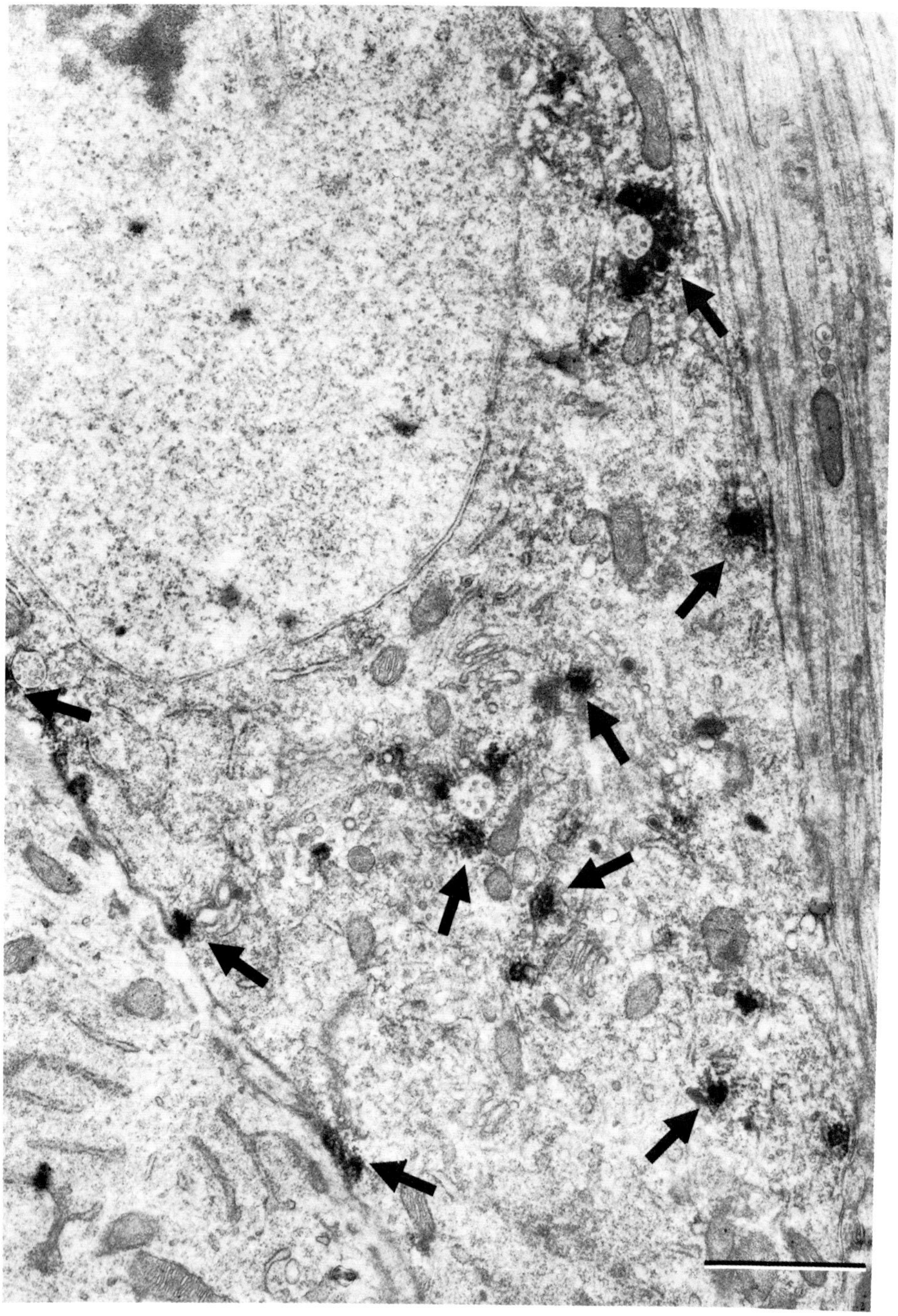

FIGURE 8. Ultrastructure of a portion of the cell soma of an enkephalin-immunoreactive neuron in lamina II of the dorsal horn. No axonal endings contact this part of the neuron, which, when examined in serial sections, rarely received somatic input. The immunocytochemical reaction product is localized to discrete areas within the cytoplasm (arrows). This enkephalin-immunoreactive neuron is taken from tissue that was not treated with colchicine. ×21,330. Scale bar represents 1.0 μm.

TABLE II
Neurotransmitters of Afferents to Identified Dorsal Horn Neurons[a]

Histochemically characterized afferents	Projection neurons			Physiologically and morphologically characterized neurons				Histochemically characterized neurons:
	LI TPN	LV TPN	DCPS	Marginal neurons	Stalked cells	LIIa islet cells	LIIb islet cells	Enkephalin neurons
5-HT	C[1]M[1,2]	C[1]M[1,2]	(CM)[3]	C[4,5]	C[4,5]	C[4,5b]	C[4,5b]	C[6]
SP	R[7]	—	—	C[8]	—	—	—	—
ENK	(CM)[9]	C[9,10]M[9]	—	—	—	—	—	C[11]M[12]

[a] Abbreviations used: LI, lamina I; LII, lamina II; LV, lamina V; TPN, thalamic projection neurons; DCPS, dorsal column postsynaptic neurons; C, cat; M, monkey; R, rat. The superscript numbers refer to references as follows: [1]Ruda *et al.*, 1983; [2]Ruda and Coffield, 1983; [3]Nishikawa *et al.*, 1984; [4]Hoffert *et al.*, 1983; [5]Miletic *et al.*, 1984; [6]Glazer and Basbaum, 1984b; [7]Preistley and Cuello, 1983; [8]Hoffert *et al.*, 1983; [9]Ruda *et al.*, 1984; [10]Ruda, 1981; [11]Glazer and Basbaum, 1984a; [12]Aronin *et al.*, 1981.
[b] Islet cells receive significantly fewer contacts than either marginal or stalked cells.

key points in the pattern of connectivity in the dorsal horn. First, different types of neurons receive input from the same neurotransmitters, and, conversely, different neurotransmitters access the same types of neurons. Second, the density of afferent input varies within a cell type as well as across cell types. Third, some form of preferential location of afferent input may occur. Each of these points has been extensively demonstrated in the thalamic projection neuron system (Ruda, 1982; Ruda *et al.*, 1984).

2. *Thalamic Projection Neurons*

The spinothalamic and trigeminothalamic tracts are major output systems of the dorsal horn that transmit nociceptive information from the spinal cord to higher levels of the neuraxis. The neurons that send their axons to the thalamus are concentrated in laminae I and V (Carstens and Trevino, 1978; Hockfield and Gobel, 1978; Giesler *et al.*, 1979; Willis *et al.*, 1979; Burton and Craig, 1979; see Willis, Chapter 11). Physiologically, they are diverse, responding either exclusively to noxious stimuli or to stimuli in both the noxious and nonnoxious range (Trevino *et al.*, 1972; Willis *et al.*, 1974; Price *et al.*, 1976, 1979; Giesler *et al.*, 1981; Kenshalo *et al.*, 1979). Because of their role in the cephalad transmission of information from the periphery, modulation of the responses of thalamic projection neurons critically affects the conscious appreciation of nociceptive information.

The examination of retrogradely labeled thalamic projection neurons demonstrates that they represent different morphological types with respect to the shape and size of their somata. In lamina I, they appear to be predominantly bipolar in shape and occasionally multipolar. The short diameter of the cell soma ranges from 10 to 30 μm with most cells measuring around 15 μm. Lamina V thalamic projection neurons are typically larger, mainly multipolar in shape, with a short diameter often greater than 20 μm.

Some thalamic projection neurons in lamina V have branched axons (Figure 9A). The branch occurs in the vicinity of the somatic origin of the axon, after a long initial segment and prior to myelination. The ultimate terminations of the different branches are unknown. It is tempting to speculate that in addition to the main axon terminus in the thalamus, some thalamic projection neurons have a local axonal arbor that functions in local dorsal horn neural circuits.

At the EM level, we examined the axon hillock and initial segment of a thalamic projection neuron in lamina V of the cat medullary dorsal horn. Several axonal endings contacted the axon hillock at its origin on the cell soma. As illustrated in Figure 9B, the synaptic contacts were mainly asymmetrical, with the varicosities replete with flattened agranular synaptic vesicles. Synaptic contacts were not found on the initial segment of this axon, which was readily identified by a layer of dense material beneath the axolemma

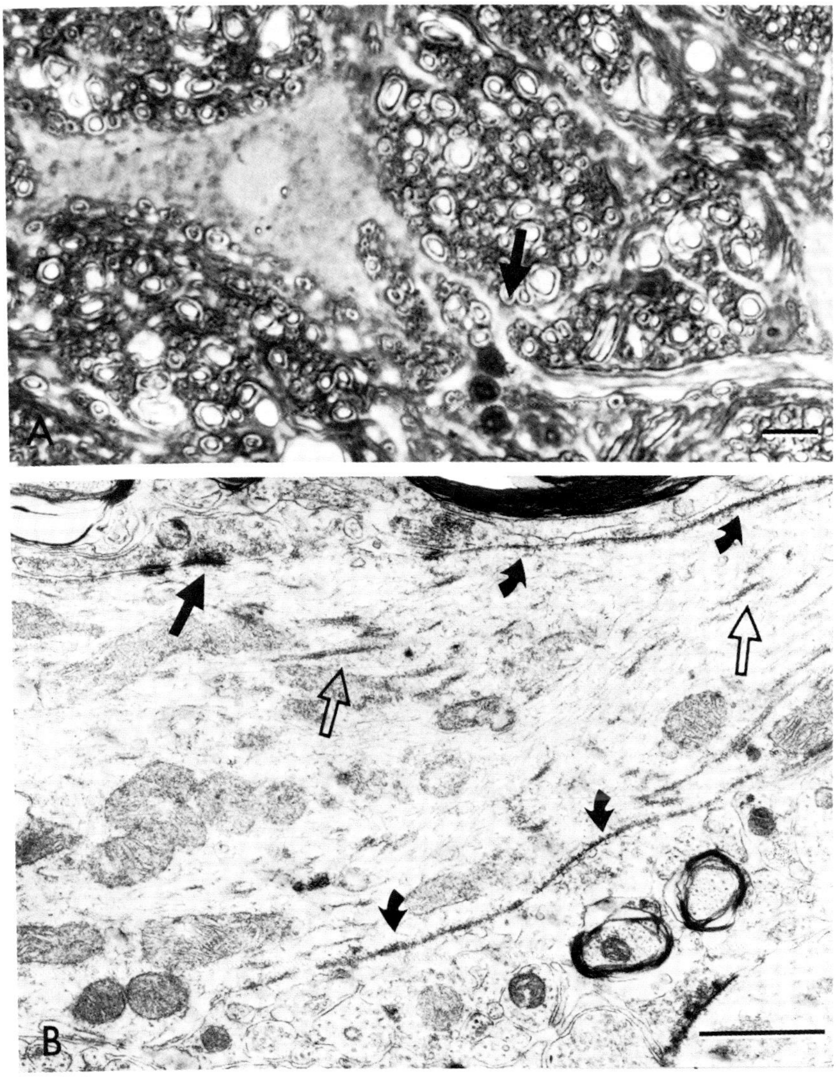

FIGURE 9. (A) Example of a thalamic projection neuron in lamina V of the medullary dorsal horn that exhibits local branching of its axon (arrow) prior to myelination. This illustration is from a 1-μm plastic section counterstained with toluidine blue. Phase-contrast microscopy accentuates the retrograde HRP granules that identify the neuron as a projection neuron. A few HRP granules are visible at this focal plane. ×650. Scale bar represents 10 μm. (B) Electron microscopic photomicrograph of a portion of the axon hillock and initial segment of the same neuron shown in A. The axon hillock and initial segment contain fascicles of microtubules (open arrows). The initial segment of the axon also exhibits a characteristic layer of dense material (curved arrows). A single flattened vesicle containing axonal varicosity forms an asymmetric synapse (arrow) with the axon hillock. ×17,240. Scale bar represents 1.0 μm.

(Figure 9B). The presence of synapses at this important site on projection neurons argues for strong postsynaptic control of the output of some thalamic projection neurons.

Ultrastructural analysis of thalamic projection neurons revealed variability in the number of axonal endings that synapsed on their somata and proximal dendrites. In lamina I, the larger projection neurons were typically contacted by a greater number of axonal endings than were the smaller projection neurons (Figure 7). The axonal endings contained either oval or pleomorphic agranular synaptic vesicles. Both asymmetrical and symmetrical synapses were present. Immunocytochemical studies have identified the neurotransmitters of three afferents to thalamic projection neurons as enkephalin (Ruda, 1982; Ruda *et al.*, 1984), serotonin (Ruda and Coffield, 1983; Ruda *et al.*, 1983), and substance P (Priestley and Cuello, 1983). Enkephalin and serotonin inputs to thalamic projection neurons are of particular interest since iontophoresis of these neurochemicals produces a profound inhibition of the projection neurons responses to noxious stimulation (Willcockson *et al.*, 1984a,b).

Examination of the enkephalin input onto thalamic projection neurons demonstrates that some variety is evident with respect to the density of afferent input onto this functionally defined class of neurons. At least 30% of the thalamic projection neurons in lamina I received enkephalin contacts, whereas in lamina V, approximately 50% of the projection neurons exhibited contacts. The number of enkephalin contacts varied from a dense innervation of greater than 100 contacts on the retrogradely labeled soma and proximal dendrites to no apparent contacts at the light microscopic level. The limit of retrograde labeling to only the proximal portion of a neuron excludes identification of contacts on the more distal portion of the dendritic arbor. At the ultrastructural level, enkephalin-immunoreactive contacts were observed to form asymmetrical synaptic contacts (Figure 10A). The origin of the enkephalin input onto thalamic projection neurons is unknown, but it is likely that the projection neurons receive input from intrinsic dorsal horn enkephalin interneurons, which may lie in their respective laminae.

Serotonin innervation of projection neurons exhibited a differential pattern of input from that of enkephalin. Serotonin contacts were generally less dense than enkephalin contacts, with most occurring on the proximal dendrites rather than on the cell soma. At the ultrastructural level, serotonin-immunoreactive synaptic contacts were mainly symmetrical (Figure 10B) in contrast to the predominantly asymmetrical enkephalin immunoreactive contacts. Greater than 50% of the retrogradely labeled thalamic projection neurons received contacts from serotonin-immunoreactive axonal endings. These observations suggest that a subset of thalamic projection neurons in laminae I and V can be postsynaptically modulated directly by descending serotonin afferent input. Since greater than 50% of the retrogradely identified thalamic projection neurons received input from either enkephalin or serotonin afferents, it is likely that some receive input from each pharmacologically distinct

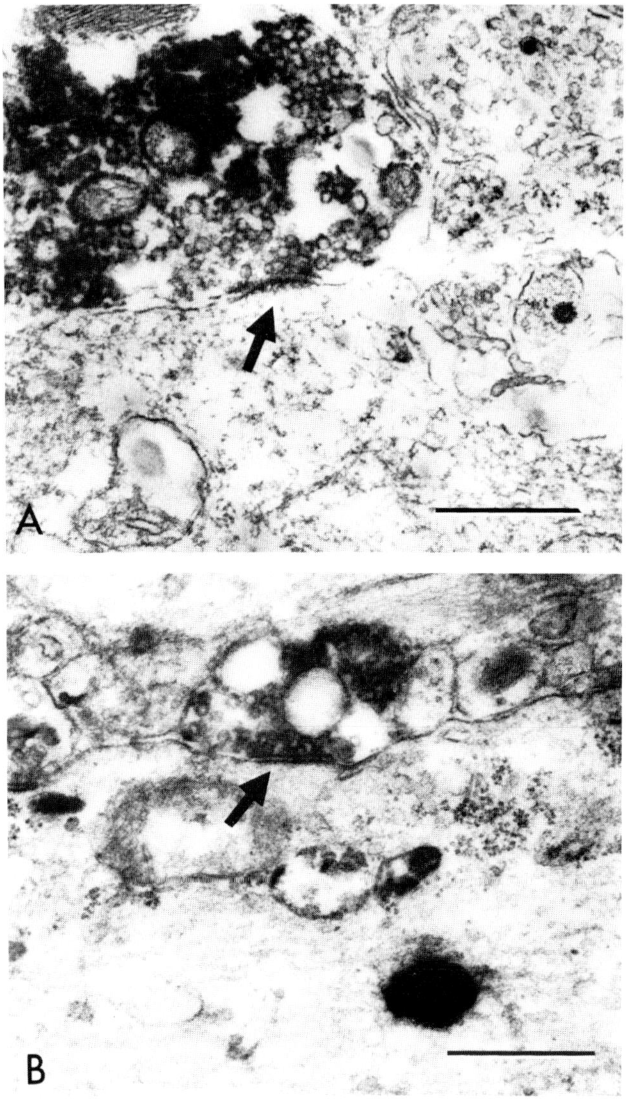

FIGURE 10. Ultrastructure of immunocytochemically identified afferents to a retrogradely labeled thalamic projection neuron. In A, an enkephalin-immunoreactive axonal ending forms an asymmetrical synapse (arrow) on a thalamic projection neuron in lamina V of the cat medullary dorsal horn. In B, a serotonin-immunoreactive axonal ending forms a symmetrical (arrow) synapse on the proximal portion of a dendrite of a thalamic projection neuron in lamina I of monkey cervical spinal cord. A granule of retrogradely transported HRP is nearby (curved arrow). ×38,400. Scale bar represents 0.5 μm.

system. Ultrastructural studies have also shown synaptic contacts from numerous axonal endings containing unidentified neurotransmitters. Thus, enkephalin and serotonin inputs represent only a small part of the chemical modulation of the output of thalamic projection neurons. The striking observation is not so much that a thalamic projection neuron's output is modulated by both a monoamine and a peptide neurotransmitter but rather that a subclass of these neurons is modulated by numerous as yet unidentified neurotransmitters as well (Figure 7).

Projection neurons in laminae III and IV (dorsal column postsynaptic neurons) of the cat and monkey, retrogradely labeled via their axons in the dorsal columns, have also been shown to receive input from serotonin-immunoreactive axonal endings (Nishikawa *et al.*, 1984). This clearly suggests that the descending serotonin system may play a role in modulating systems having a diversity of functions.

Studies of retrogradely labeled neurons are limited to identification of afferent input onto the soma and proximal dendrites. The location of input onto a neuron may reflect the efficacy of the synaptic drive for which it is responsible. Conductance changes occurring on the dendrites, soma, axon hillock, and axon of a neuron may carry variable weight with respect to the summation of the neuron's resulting output. Future studies in which the full extent of the neuron's dendritic arbor is intracellularly filled with horseradish peroxidase can help identify sites of preferential afferent input on the complete projection neuron.

Based on the above observations, it appears that although thalamic projection neurons represent a single functional type in that they are responsible for the cephalad transmission of noxious information from the spinal cord, they represent different morphological and physiological types of neurons. In addition, subpopulations of thalamic projection neurons clearly display differential patterns of innervation by both primary afferents and intrinsic and supraspinal elements with respect to both the density of a given neurochemical input and the location of that input on the neuron.

F. Conclusion

The advent of multiple-label techniques has lead to a substantial increase in our understanding of the neuronal organization of the nervous system. The site of action of enkephalin, serotonin, and substance P in the dorsal horn has been elucidated by immunocytochemical labeling at the light and electron microscopic levels. Each of these neurotransmitters acts through conventional synapses on dorsal horn neurons. The location of the synaptic input suggests that they act in large part through postsynaptic mechanisms via receptors located on dorsal horn neurons. Enkephalin, serotonin, and substance P act at multiple sites located on different morphological and functional classes of neurons, including projection neurons and interneurons. These observations suggest that enkephalin, serotonin, and substance P exert a complex synaptic modulation of noxious information in the dorsal horn. Both the intrinsic opioid system and the descending monoaminergic system act, in part, on the same neuron rather than exclusively through separate neural circuits. Because of the widespread distribution of peptides and monoamines in the dorsal horn, it is likely that they also act at other neural circuits in addition to those involved in pain and analgesia. Future investigation of the pattern and place of neurochemical modulation of dorsal horn neurons will aid in our understanding of the general organization of the nervous system and how relevent sensory cues are extracted from the environment.

ACKNOWLEDGMENT. I would like to thank Drs. Ronald Dubner and Gary Bennett for their careful reading of this chapter, Julie Coffield, Emma Humphrey, and Barbara Allen for their technical assistance, and Edie Welty for typing.

References

ARONIN, N., DIFIGLIA, M., LIOTTA, A. S., AND MARTIN, J. B. Ultrastructural localization and biochemical features of immunoreactive leu-enkephalin in monkey dorsal horn. *J. Neurosci.* 1:561–577, 1981.

BARBER, R. P., VAUGHN, J. E., SHERMAN, J. R., SALVATERRA, P. M., ROBERTS, E., AND LEEMAN, S. E. The origin, distribution and synaptic relationships of substance P axons in rat spinal cord. *J. Comp. Neurol.* 184:331–352, 1979.

BASBAUM, A. I. Anatomical substrates for the descending control of nociception, in: *Brain Stem Control of Spinal Mechanisms* (B. Sjöland and A. Björklund, eds.), Elsevier, Amsterdam, 1982, pp. 119–133.

BASBAUM, A. I., CLANTON, C. H., AND FIELDS, H. L. Three bulbospinal pathways from the rostral medulla of the cat: An autoradiographic study of pain modulating systems. *J. Comp. Neurol.* 1:209–224, 1978.

BENNETT, G. J., ABDELMOUMENE, M., HAYASHI, H., AND DUBNER, R. Physiology and morphology of substantia gelatinosa neurons intracellularly stained with horseradish peroxidase. *J. Comp. Neurol.* 194:809–827, 1980.

BENNETT, G. J., ABDELMOUMENE, M., HAYASHI, H., HOFFERT, M. J., AND DUBNER, R. Spinal cord layer I neurons with axon collaterals that generate local arbors. *Brain Res.* 209:421–426, 1981a.

BENNETT, G. J., ABDELMOUMENE, M., HAYASHI, H., HOFFERT, M. J., RUDA, M. A., AND DUBNER, R. Physiology, morphology and immunocytology of dorsal horn layer III neurons. *Pain* [*Suppl.*] 1:S240, 1981b.

BENNETT, G. J., RUDA, M. A., GOBEL, S., AND DUBNER, R. Enkephalin immunoreactive stalked cells and lamina IIb islet cells in cat substantia gelatinosa. *Brain Res.* 240:162–166, 1982.

BOWKER, R. M., STEINBUSCH, H. W. M., AND COULTER, J. D. Serotonergic and peptidergic projections to the spinal cord demonstrated by a combined retrograde HRP histochemical and immunocytochemical staining method. *Brain Res.* 211:412–417, 1981a.

BOWKER, R. M., WESTLUND, K. N., AND COULTER, J. D. Origins of serotonergic projections to the spinal cord in rat: An immunocytochemical–retrograde transport study. *Brain Res.* 226:187–199, 1981b.

BURTON, H., AND CRAIG, A. D., JR. Distribution of trigeminothalamic projection cells in cat and monkey. *Brain Res.* 161:515–521, 1979.

CARSTENS, E., AND TREVINO, D. L. Laminar origins of spinothalamic projections in the cat as determined by the retrograde transport of horseradish peroxidase. *J. Comp. Neurol.* 182:151–166, 1978.

CUELLO, A. C., DEL FIACCO, M., AND PAXINOS, G. The central and peripheral ends of the substance P-containing sensory neurones in the rat trigeminal system. *Brain Res.* 152:499–509, 1978.

DAHLSTRÖM, A., AND FUXE, K. Evidence for the existence of monoamine-containing neurons in the central nervous system. I. Demonstration of monoamines in the cell bodies of brain stem neurons. *Acta Physiol. Scand.* [*Suppl.*] 232:1–55, 1964.

DAHLSTRÖM, A., AND FUXE, K. Evidence for the existence of monoamine-containing neurons in the central nervous sytem. II. Experimentally induced changes in the intraneuronal amine levels of bulbospinal neuron systems. *Acta Physiol. Scand.* [*Suppl.*] 247:7–36, 1965.

DELANEROLLE, N. C., AND LAMOTTE, C. C. Ultrastructure of chemically defined neuron systems in the dorsal horn of the monkey. I. Substance P immunoreactivity. *Brain Res.* 274:31–49, 1983.

DIFIGLIA, M., ARONIN, N., AND LEEMAN, S. E. Light microscopic and ultrastructural localization of immunoreactive substance P in the dorsal horn of monkey spinal cord. *Neuroscience* 7:1127–1139, 1982.

DUBNER, R., AND BENNETT, G. J. Spinal and trigeminal mechanisms of nociception. *Annu. Rev. Neurosci.* 6:381–418, 1983.

DUBNER, R., RUDA, M. A., MILETIC, V., HOFFERT, M. J., BENNETT, G. J., NISHIKAWA, N., AND COFFIELD, J. Neural circuitry mediating nociception in the medullary and spinal dorsal horns, in: *Advances in Pain Research and Therapy,* Vol. 6 (L. KRUGER AND J. C. LIEBESKIND, eds.), Raven Press, New York, 1984, pp. 151–166.

GIBSON, S. J., POLAK, J. M., BLOOM, S. R., AND WALL, P. D. The distribution of nine peptides in rat spinal cord with special emphasis on the substantia gelatinosa and on the area around the central canal (lamina X). *J. Comp. Neurol.* 201:65–79, 1981.

GIESLER, G. J., JR., MENETREY, D., AND BASBAUM, A. I. Differential origins of spinothalamic tract projections to medial and lateral thalamus in the rat. *J. Comp. Neurol.* 184:107–126, 1979.

GIESLER, G. J., JR., YEZIERSKI, R. P., GERHART, K. D., AND WILLIS, W. D. Spinothalamic tract neurons that project to medial and/or lateral thalamic nuclei: Evidence for a physiologically novel population of spinal cord neurons. *J. Neurophysiol.* 46:1285–1308, 1981.

GILBERT, R. F. T., EMSON, P. C., HUNT , S. P., BENNETT, G. W., MARSDEN, C. A., SANDBERG, B. E. B., STEINBUSCH, H. W. M., AND VERHOFSTAD, A. A. J. Effects of monoamine neurotoxins on peptides in the rat spinal cord. *Neuroscience* 7:69–87, 1982.

GLAZER, E. J., AND BASBAUM, A. I. Immunohistochemical localization of leucine-enkephalin in the spinal cord of the cat. Enkephalin-containing marginal neurons and pain modulation. *J. Comp. Neurol.* 196:377–389, 1981.

GLAZER, E. J., AND BASBAUM, A. I. Opiate neurons and pain modulation: An ultrastructural analysis of enkephalin in cat superficial dorsal horn. *Neuroscience* 10:357–376, 1982.

GLAZER, E. J., AND BASBAUM, A. I. Axons which take up [^{3}H]serotonin are presynaptic to enkephalin immunoreactive neuron in cat dorsal horn. *Brain Res.* 298:386–391, 1984.

HOCKFIELD, S., AND GOBEL, S. Neurons in and near nucleus caudalis with long ascending projection axons demonstrated by retrograde labeling with horseradish peroxidase. *Brain Res.* 139:333–339, 1978.

HOFFERT, M. J., MILETIC, V., RUDA, M. A., AND DUBNER, R. A comparison of substance P and serotonin axonal contacts on identified neurons in cat spinal dorsal horn. *Soc. Neurosci. Abstr.* 8:805, 1982.

HOFFERT, M. J., MILETIC, V., RUDA, M. A., AND DUBNER, R. Immunocytochemical identification of serotonin axonal contacts on characterized neurons in laminae I and II of the cat dorsal horn. *Brain Res.* 267:361–264, 1983.

HÖKFELT, T., KELLERTH, J. O., NILSSON, G., AND PERNOW, B. Substance P localization in the central nervous system and in some primary sensory neurons. *Science* 190:889–890, 1975a.

HÖKFELT, T., KELLERTH, J. O., NILSSON, G., AND PERNOW, B. Experimental immunohistochemical studies on the localization and distribution of substance P in the cat primary sensory neurons. *Brain Res.* 100:235–252, 1975b.

HÖKFELT, T., LJUNGDAHL, A., TERENIUS, L., ELDE, R., AND NILSSON, G., Immunohistochemical analysis of peptide pathways possibly related to pain and analgesia: Enkephalin and substance P. *Proc. Natl. Acad. Sci. U.S.A.* 74:3081–3085, 1977.

HÖKFELT, T., TERENIUS, L., KUYPERS, H. G. J. M., AND DANN, O. Evidence for enkephalin immunoreactive neurons in the medulla oblongata projecting to the spinal cord. *Neurosci. Lett.* 14:55–60, 1979.

HUNT, S. P., KELLY, J. S., AND EMSON, P. C. The electron microscopic localization of methionine-enkephalin within the superficial layers (I and II) of the spinal cord. *Neuroscience* 5:1871–1890, 1980.

HUNT, S. P., KELLY, J. S., EMSON, P. C., KIMMEL, J. R., MILLER, R. J., AND WU, J. Y. An immunohistochemical study of neuronal populations containing neuropeptides or gamma-aminobutyrate within the superficial layers of the rat dorsal horn. *Neuroscience* 6:1883–1898, 1981.

JESSELL, T., TSUNOO, A., KANAZAWA, I., AND OTSUKA, M. Substance P: Depletion in the dorsal horn of rat spinal cord after section of the peripheral processes of primary sensory neurons. *Brain Res.* 168:247–259, 1979.

KENSHALO, D. R., JR., LEONARD, R. B., CHUNG, J. M., AND WILLIS, W. D. Responses of primate spinothalamic neurons to graded and to repeated noxious heat stimuli *J. Neurophysiol.* 42:1370–1389, 1979.

LAMOTTE, C. C., AND DELANEROLLE, N. C. Ultrastructure of chemically defined neuron systems in the dorsal horn of the monkey. II. Methionine-enkephalin immunoreactivity. *Brain Res.* 274:51–63, 1983a.

LAMOTTE, C. C., AND DELANEROLLE, N. C. Ultrastructure of chemically defined neuron systems in the dorsal horn of the monkey. III. Serotonin immunoreactivity. *Brain Res.* 274:65–77, 1983b.

LIGHT, A. R., TREVINO, D. L., AND PERL, E. R. Morphological features of functionally defined neurons in the marginal zone and substantia gelatinosa of the spinal dorsal horn. *J. Comp. Neurol.* 186:151–171, 1979.

LIGHT, A. R., KAVOOKJIAN, A. M., AND PETRUSZ, P. The ultrastructure and synaptic connections of serotonin-immunoreactive terminals in spinal laminae I and II. *Somatosens. Res.* 1:33–50, 1983.

LJUNGDAHL, A., HÖKFELT, T., AND NILSSON, G. Distribution of substance P-immunoreactivity in the central nervous system of the rat. I. Cell bodies and nerve terminals. *Neuroscience* 3:861–943, 1978.

MASSARI, V. J., TIZABI, Y., PARK, C. H., MOODY, T. W., HELKE, C. J., AND O'DONOHUE, T. L. Distribution and origin of bombesin, substance P and somatostatin in cat spinal cord. *Peptides* 4:673–681, 1983.

MILETIC, V., HOFFERT, M. J., RUDA, M. A., DUBNER, R., AND SHIGENAGA, Y. Serotonergic axonal contacts on identified cat spinal dorsal horn neurons and their correlation with nucleus raphe magnus stimulation. *J. Comp. Neurol.* 228:129–141, 1984.

NAROTSKY, R. A., AND KERR, F. W. L. Marginal neurons of the spinal cord: Types, afferent synaptology and functional considerations. *Brain Res.* 139:1–20, 1978.

NISHIKAWA, N., BENNETT, G. J., RUDA, M. A., LU, G.-W., AND DUBNER, R. Immunocytochemical evidence for a serotonergic innervation of dorsal column postsynaptic neurons in cat and monkey. *Neuroscience* 10:1333–1340, 1983.

PICKEL, V. M., REIS, D. J., AND LEEMAN, S. E. Ultrastructure of substance P in neurons of rat spinal cord. *Brain Res.* 122:534–540, 1977.

PRICE, D. D., DUBNER, R., AND HU, J. W. Trigeminothalamic neurons in nucleus caudalis responsive to tactile, thermal, and nociceptive stimulation of monkey's face. *J. Neurophysiol.* 39:936–953, 1976.

PRICE, D. D., HAYASHI, H., DUBNER, R., AND RUDA, M. A. Functional relationships between neurons of marginal and substantia gelatinosa layers of primate dorsal horn. *J. Neurophysiol.* 42:1590–1608, 1979.

PRIESTLEY, J. V., SOMOGYI, P., AND CUELLO, A. C. Immunocytochemical localization of substance P in the trigeminal nucleus of the rat: A light and electron microscopic study. *J. Comp. Neurol.* 211:31–49, 1982.

PRIESTLEY, J. V., AND CUELLO, A. C. Substance P immunoreactive terminals in the spinal trigeminal nucleus synapse with lamina I neurons projecting to the thalamus, in: *Substance P* (P. Skraborek and D. Powell, eds.), Book Press, Dublin, 1983, pp. 251–252.

RALSTON, H. J. III, AND RALSTON, D. D. The distribution of dorsal root axons in laminae I, II and III of the macaque spinal cord: A quantitative electron microscope study. *J. Comp. Neurol.* 184:643–684, 1979.

RUDA, M. A. Opiates and pain pathways: Demonstration of enkephalin synapses on dorsal horn projection neurons. *Science* 215:1523–1525, 1982.

RUDA, M. A., COFFIELD, J., AND STEINBUSCH, H. W. M. Immunocytochemical analysis of serotonergic axons in laminae I and II of the lumbar spinal cord of the cat. *J. Neurosci.* 2:1660–1671, 1982.

RUDA, M. A., COFFIELD, J., BENNETT, G. J., AND DUBNER, R. Role of serotonin (5-HT) and enkephalin (ENK) in trigeminal and spinal pain pathways. *J. Dent. Res.* 62:691, 1983.

RUDA, M. A., AND COFFIELD, J., Light and ultrastructural immunocytochemical localization of serotonin synapses on primate spinothalamic tract neurons. *Soc. Neurosci. Abstr.* 9:1, 1983.

RUDA, M. A., COFFIELD, J., AND DUBNER, R. Demonstration of postsynaptic opioid modulation of thalamic projection neurons by the combined techniques of retrograde horseradish peroxidase and enkephalin immunocytochemistry. *J. Neurosci.* 4:2117–2132, 1984.

SAR, M., STUMPF, W. E., MILLER, R. J., CHANG, K. J., AND CUATRECASAS, P. Immunohistochemical localization of enkephalin in rat brain and spinal cord. *J. Comp. Neurol.* 182:17–38, 1978.

SEYBOLD, V., AND ELDE, R. Immunohistochemical studies of peptidergic neurons in the dorsal horn of the spinal cord. *J. Histochem. Cytochem.* 28:367–370, 1980.

STEINBUSCH, H. W. M. Distribution of serotonin-immunoreactivity in the central nervous system of the rat—cell bodies and terminals. *Neuroscience* 6:557–618, 1981.

SUMAL, K., K., PICKEL, V. M., MILLER, R. J., AND REIS, D. J. Enkephalin-containing neurons in substantia gelatinosa of spinal trigeminal complex: Ultrastructure and synaptic interaction with primary sensory afferents. *Brain Res.* 248:223–236, 1982.

TAKAHASHI, T., AND OTSUKA, M. Regional distribution of substance P in the spinal cord and nerve roots of the cat and the effect of dorsal root section. *Brain Res.* 87:1–11, 1975.

TESSLER, A., HIMES, B. T., ARTMYSHYN, R., MURRAY, M., AND GOLDBERGER, M. E.. Spinal neurons mediate return of substance P following deafferentation of cat spinal cord. *Brain Res.* 230:263–281, 1981.

TREVINO, D. L., MAUNZ, R. A., BRYAN, R. N., AND WILLIS, W. D. Location of cells of origin of the spinothalamic tract in the lumbar enlargement of cat. *Exp. Neurol.* 34:64–77, 1972.

UHL, G. R., GOODMAN, R. R., KUHAR, M. J., CHILDREN, S. R., AND SNYDER, S. H. Immunohistochemical mapping of enkephalin containing cell bodies, fibers and nerve terminals in the brain stem of the rat. *Brain Res.* 166:75–94, 1979.

WILLCOCKSON, W. S., CHUNG, J. M., HORI, Y., LEE, K. H., AND WILLIS, W. D. Effects of iontophoretically released amino acids and amines on primate spinothalamic tract cells. *J. Neurosci.* 4:732–740, 1984a.

WILLCOCKSON, W. S., CHUNG, J. M., HORI, Y., LEE, K. H., AND WILLIS, W. D. Effects of iontophoretically released peptides on primate spinothalamic tract cells. *J. Neurosci.* 4:741–750, 1984b.

WILLIS, W. D., KENSHALO, D. R., JR, AND LEONARD, R. B. The cells of origin of the primate spinothalamic tract. *J. Comp. Neurol.* 188:543–574, 1979.

WILLIS, W. D., TREVINO, D. L., COULTER, J. D., AND MAUNZ, R. A. Responses to primate spinothalamic tract neurons to natural stimulation of hindlimb. *J. Neurophysiol.* 37:358–372, 1974.

8
The Central Pharmacology of Primary Afferents with Emphasis on the Disposition and Role of Primary Afferent Substance P

TONY L. YAKSH

A. *Introduction*

Apart from the cranial nerves, all somatic and visceral information enters the nervous system by the primary afferents, which largely have their first-order synapses in discrete regions of the dorsal gray matter of the spinal cord. Morphological (synaptic vesicles, end-plate thickening, synaptic cleft) and electrophysiological properties (presence of monosynaptic EPSPs but not monosynaptic IPSPs, synaptic delay) provide support for the premise that the afferent exerts its effect on the second-order neuron by the release of excitatory neurotransmitter(s).

B. *Identification of Primary Afferent Neurotransmitters*

Considerable efforts have been directed at establishing the identity of these neuroactive substances in the primary afferent. Several criteria have classically been accepted as minimum requirements in the establishment of the correspondence between the endogenous material and a given substance: (1) the material must be found in the terminals of the afferent population in

TONY L. YAKSH • Departments of Neurosurgery and Pharmacology, Mayo Clinic, Rochester, Minnesota 55905.

question (and it or its precursor in the respective dorsal root ganglion cell); (2) the material must be present in a fraction that is released when the appropriate afferents undergo depolarization; (3) the postsynaptic effects of the exogenously applied materials must mimic the effects resulting when the endogenous afferent systems are physiologically activated; and (4) those physiological effects resulting from the actions of the endogenously released and exogenously administered agents must possess an identical pharmacology (i.e., the characteristics of the receptor acted on by the endogenous and exogenous agents must be indistinguishable.

1. Localization

Currently, excitatory amino acids such as glutamate and aspartate (see Curtis and Johnson, 1974) and a growing list of peptides including substance P (sP), vasoactive intestinal peptide (VIP), somatostatin, a VIP homologue (PHI), cholecystokinin (CCK), somatostatin, angiotensin II, bombesin, and related peptides have been observed to possess the following characteristics: (1) they have been found in the dorsal horn of the spinal cord (where the majority of primary afferent terminals are found); (2) the levels in dorsal horn are reduced by rhizotomy and/or ganglionectomy; and (3) these peptides have been shown to exist within subpopulations of small dorsal root ganglion cells (type B cells of Anders) (see Table I). Immunohistochemical studies directed at the dorsal horn have revealed discriminable differences in the discrete distribution of the several peptides in the dorsal laminae. As discussed elsewhere in this volume (see comments by LaMotte, Chapter 5, and Ruda,

TABLE I
Summary of Evidence Suggesting the Presence of Certain Peptides in Spinal Primary Afferent Terminals[a]

Peptide	Dorsal horn > ventral horn: Immunohisto-chemistry	Dorsal horn > ventral horn: Radioim-munoassay	DRG/roots	Effect of rhizotomy on dorsal horn levels
sP	Yes (1)	Yes (2)	Yes (1)	(3)
Somatostatin	Yes (4)	Yes (2)	Yes (4)	(5)
VIP	Yes (6)	Yes (7)	Yes (8)	(7)
PHI	—	Yes (9)	Yes (9)	—
Cholecystokinin	Yes (10)	Yes (7)	Yes (10)	(7)
Angiotensin II	Yes (11)	—	Yes (11)	—
Bombesin	Yes (12)	—	Yes (13)	—

[a] Numbers in parentheses refer to references as follows: (1) Hökfelt *et al.*, 1975; (2) Gamse *et al.*, 1981; (3) Takahashi and Otsuka, 1975; (4) Hökfelt *et al.*, 1976; (5) P. E. Micevych and T. L. Yaksh, unpublished observations; (6) Kawatani *et al.*, 1983; (7) Yaksh *et al.*, 1982; (8) Luundberg *et al.*, 1978; (9) T. L. Yaksh, S. Michener, and V. L. W. Go, unpublished observations; (10) Dalsgaard *et al.*, 1982; (11) Hökfelt *et al.*, 1980; (12) Panula *et al.*, 1982; (13) Panula *et al.*, 1983.

Chapter 7), sP is predominantly located in Rexed lamina I and the outer layer of II, VIP is principally found in lamina I, and somatostatin is found in the outer layer of II. Fluoride-resistant acid phosphatase, found in small ganglion cells separate from those containing sP or somatostatin (Nagy and Hunt, 1982), is primarily distributed in the inner layer of lamina II in regions distinct from those to which sP, VIP, or somatostatin project (see Nagy and Hunt, 1983).

As has become considered characteristic, the synthetic cycle of the peptides uniformly appears to involve the synthesis by ribosomes in the cell body (Koenig, 1965) of large precursor prohormones, which are cleaved and transported in a particulate form to the terminal, where the material is stored (see Hökfelt *et al.,* 1980). Ligation or local cooling of the dorsal root or nerve or the application of an axon transport blocker such as vinblastine results in a significant accumulation of peptides such as somatostatin, sP, and VIP proximal to the cell body (Brimijoin *et al.,* 1980; Lundberg *et al.,* 1985). Such systematic studies have further revealed that as in the case of protein, more peptide (such as sP) is transported peripherally than centrally (*vide supra*).

The subcellular localization in vesicular fractions and/or their localization by EM immunohistochemistry (see comments by LaMotte, Chapter 5, and Ruda, Chapter 7), in vesicle profiles of several peptides, including sP, VIP, and somatostatin, provides suggestive evidence that these peptides are stored as neurotransmitters.

2. *Releasability*

An important consideration is whether the materials present in afferent terminals exist within a releasable fraction. In dorsal root ganglion cell culture, sP release has been demonstrated (Mudge *et al.,* 1979). From spinal cord slices, sP and somatostatin levels in the extracellular fluid have been shown to be elevated by depolarization (Otsuka and Konishi, 1976a,b; Jessell and Iversen, 1977; Sheppard *et al.,* 1979; Akagi *et al.,* 1980; Sawynok *et al.,* 1982). Importantly, in these cases, the enhanced efflux produced by depolarization is blocked by the depletion of Ca^{2+} or the substitution of other polyvalent cations such as cobalt or lanthanum. Such Ca^{2+} dependence is an important characteristic of the exocytotic process. *In vivo* release using a spinal superfusion model (Yaksh and Tyce, 1980) has similarly been used to demonstrate the release of materials from primary afferents including sP (Yaksh *et al.,* 1980; Kuraishi *et al.,* 1983), VIP, and CCK (Yaksh *et al.,* 1982). This is discussed further below.

The removal of the neuroactive agent from the vicinity of any receptors may occur by reuptake, diffusion, dilution in the extracellular volume, and/or by enzymatic alteration to an inactive form. To date no evidence of a significant reuptake of peptides has been reported. The amino acids, however, are subject to a powerful active transport into cells (Bennett *et al.,* 1973). Intuitively, diffusion alone represents a generally applicable and surprisingly efficient method of clearance, with focal concentration being inversely proportional to the cube of the distance diffused.

Enzymatic cleavage clearly plays a role in the loss of activity of a variety of neuroactive peptides. Loss of the carboxy terminus of sP will, in general, result in a profound reduction in biological activity and/or reduction in the measured affinity of binding in brain homogenates (see Iversen *et al.*, 1982). Changes in the length of the peptide chain by endopeptidases will also result in a reduction in biological activity. Thus, with sP, for example, in terms of neuronal depolarizing activity, fragments shorter than the sP_{6-11} sequence were considerably less active than sP_{1-11} (Otsuka and Konishi, 1976a,b; Piercey and Einspahr, 1980; Jones and Olpe, 1982). Although these changes may be achieved by a variety of generally distributed enzymes, such as trypsin, considerable effort has been directed at determining whether the relevant changes are brought about by specific enzyme systems. Thus, for example, a dipeptidylcarboxypeptidase has been identified that appears to have considerable selectivity for cleaving the enkephalin pentapeptides (Malfroy *et al.*, 1979).

3. *Postsynaptic Actions*

The postsynaptic effects of these materials have been studied at the electrophysiological level. Glutamate and aspartate applied to dorsal horn neurons result in a powerful reversible depolarization with rapid onset accompanied by an increase in membrane conductance (see, for example, Zieglgänsberger and Puil, 1973) that is unaffected by the intracellular injection of K^+ or Cl^-. Examination of the subclasses of neurons excited by glutamate or aspartate, however, reveals no functional selectivity. Thus, motor horn cells and/or dorsal horn neurons excited by A-β, A-δ, and C fibers show a characteristic excitatory response to glutamate administration (Besson *et al.*, 1974; Zieglgänsberger and Puil, 1973).

Iontophoretic application onto the dorsal horn of several peptides found in primary afferents has been shown to produce excitatory effects. The focal administration of sP onto spinal neurons results in a progressive depolarization of the cell (Henry, 1976; Zieglgänsberger and Tulloch, 1979; Murase and Randic, 1984). Characteristically, in contrast to the effects of the excitatory amino acids, the effects of sP, whether applied iontophoretically or in a bath, are slow in onset. In spinal neurons, the depolarization is accompanied by a decrease in conductance (Murase and Randic, 1984; but see Zieglgänsberger and Tulloch, 1979). Blockade of voltage-dependent calcium channels obtunded the sP-evoked depolarization (Murase and Randic, 1984). In dorsal horn cell culture, sP-evoked depolarization was attenuated by the intracellular injection of tetraethylammonium but not by alterations in the Cl^- equilibrium potential, suggesting that the depolarization is secondary to a reduced K^+ conductance (Nowak and MacDonald, 1982).

Both VIP and CCK have similarly been shown to evoke excitation of dorsal horn neurons (Jeftinija *et al.*, 1981a, 1982). Somatostatin has been shown to produce an inhibition of the activity of dorsal horn neurons after iontophoretic administration (Randic and Miletic, 1978). This finding is somewhat surprising, as a monosynaptic inhibition by primary afferents on second-order neurons has not been described.

Functionally, iontophoretic studies carried out in the dorsal horn have demonstrated that sP will excite cells that were naturally activated by noxious radiant heat (Henry, 1976), strong mechanical stimuli (Randic and Miletic, 1977), or the intraarterial injection of bradykinin (Wright and Roberts, 1980; Piercey *et al.*, 1980) and facilitate the response of cells activated by noxious cutaneous stimuli. Other agents such as glutamate, CCK, and VIP appear somewhat less selective, as they have been shown to produce excitatory and facilitatory effects on neurons that respond to a wide variety of innocuous stimuli (see above). Thus, there appears to be a significant correlation between the ability of sP to evoke a progessive depolarization in a dorsal horn neuron and the existence of an afferent drive from small fibers (but see Wright and Roberts, 1980).

It has become increasingly likely that some populations of afferents, particularly those of small diameter, may have more than one releasable material in their terminals. Electron microscopy has long indicated the presence of several morphologically distinct vesicle populations in primary afferent terminals, notably those that are dense core and now thought to contain peptides and smaller clear vesicles, which may contain amino acids (see Narotzky and Kerr, 1978). Urban and Randic (1984), recording intracellularly in rat spinal cord slices, observed that reptitive stimulation of the dorsal roots resulted in an initial burst of monosynaptically driven spikes followed by a prolonged slow hypopolarization. As is discussed below, several lines of evidence suggest that the two distinct places of depolarization may be attributable to the release of an excitatory amino acid and a peptide, respectively.

4. *Afferent Terminal Pharmacology*

The above observations indicate that certain iontophoretically applied peptides, including sP, VIP, or CCK, or an excitatory amino acid can evoke activity in the postsynaptic neuron. What evidence can be marshaled to suggest that the effects of the physiological stimulus reflect occupation of the same receptors acted on by exogenously administered agents? In the work of Urban and Randic (1984), two observations are relevant. First, they noted that the slow depolarization of dorsal horn neurons evoked by afferent stimulation or focally applied sP (but not VIP) was blocked by coadministration of a putative sP receptor antagonist such as D-Pro^{2}-D-Try^{7,9}-sP. Second, the administration of capsaicin—a neurotoxin that results in the depletion of afferent stores of sP and CCK but not VIP, destroys small afferents marked by the cytosol enzyme fluoride-resistant acid phosphatase, and has no effect on large-diameter afferents (see Section D.1, below)—blocked the slow depolarization but not the early spike activity evoked by afferent stimulation.

It should be noted that the effects of physiological stimulation could be mediated by sP release but need not necessarily reflect the release of this peptide from primary afferents. Excitation of an intrinsic sP neuron by a non-sP-containing small afferent might provide comparable results. As discussed by LaMotte (Chapter 5) and Ruda (Chapter 7), sP immunoreactivity is found in three populations of spinal terminalis, those deriving from afferents, descending pathways, and intrinsic neurons. However, capsaicin appears to have no effect on these nonafferent sP-containing spinal systems (see Section D.1, below). Indirect evidence of a direct postsynaptic effect of afferent-derived sP is provided by Wright and Roberts (1977). They observed after rhizotomy that dorsal horn neurons were rendered more responsive to eledoisin (a sP analogue). This was interpreted as a likely postsynaptic supersensitivity resulting from a loss of afferent input.

These observations suggest that for this particular neuronal population in neonatal rat spinal cord, sP may be released by afferent stimulation to facilitate the depolarization evoked by a more rapidly acting excitatory agent. Jahr and Jessell (1983), in a mixed spinal cell culture in which dorsal root ganglion (DRG) cells could be visually observed to make contact with spinal cord cells, observed that depolarization of the DRG cell results in an EPSP in the spinal cord neuron, the properties of which are mimicked by glutamate and ATP.

In summary, the above discussions, focusing at the cellular level, point to a potential role of several peptides in primary afferent function and to the likelihood that several receptor-selective agents with different effects on membrane permeability may be coreleased. Though limited, the pharmacological manipulations carried out to date suggest that for one population of afferent terminals, sP and an excitatory amino acid (glutamate) may be the putative neurotransmitters. Importantly, these observations suggest that the release of sP in contrast to glutamate in this situation is highly dependent on repetitive terminal activation. It is interesting to note that these characteristics resemble those of certain wide-dynamic-range neurons in which repetitive stimulation results in a continuous bursting of the cell referred to as "wind-up" (Mendell, 1966). Significantly, Cervero and colleagues (1984) reported that rats treated neonatally with capsaicin showed a significantly attentuated wind-up (but see Wall *et al.*, 1981).

C. In Vivo Studies on Spinal Neurotransmitter Release

During the past several years, we have sought to place emphasis on the functional correlates of these putative primary afferent neurotransmitter systems. By using a spinal superfusion procedure in the rat and cat, it is possible to determine whether a particular stimulus will result in a measurable increase in the extravascular–extracellular levels of a given peptide and whether this release possesses the characteristics thought to define exocytotic release, e.g., calcium dependence, and whether the measured level of peptide covaries with the characteristics of afferent stimulation. If such release can be demonstrated, it is then plausible to query whether the measured levels thought to reflect terminal activity of neurons containing the particular material can be altered by pharmacological interventions that alter terminal excitability through a receptor interaction. Such strategies, in conjunction with the examination of the effects of manipulating the levels of the peptide on various physiological and behavioral endpoints, can be used to shed insights into the possible role played by the afferent system for which the material is a putative neurotransmitter. Recently, such release of materials thought to be contained in primary afferents has been demonstrated for sP (Yaksh *et al.*, 1980; Bergström *et al.*, 1983; Jhamandas *et al.*, 1984; Kuraishi *et al.*, 1983), VIP, and CCK (Yaksh *et al.*, 1982; Blank *et al.*, 1984). In the following sections I should, however, like to focus in more detail on recent studies on the disposition of primary afferent stores of sP and the effects of altering its disposition on behavior.

1. Studies on the Spinal Release of Substance P in Vivo

The administration of depolarizing concentrations of K^+ into the spinal superfusate results in a dose-dependent increase in the levels of sP immunoreactivity (sPLI). As indicated in Table II, increasing concentrations of the K^+ result in a marked increase in sPLI levels. The addition of cobalt alone had no statistically significant effect on resting release but produced a highly significant attenuation of the release otherwise evoked by K^+.

TABLE II
Effect of K^+ on the Levels of sPLI in Rat Spinal Perfusate[a] in the Presence of Normal Calcium or in the Absence of Calcium with Cobalt

$[K^+]$ (mM)	[Cobalt] (mM)	[Calcium] (mM)	*N*	Percent (±S.E.) of control[b]
10	0	2.5	5	71 ± 33[c]
40	0	2.5	6	371 ± 42[c,d]
40	10	0	4	98 ± 36[c]
0	10	0	3	−12 ± 16

[a] Chloralose–urethane.
[b] Data from T. L. Yaksh and V. L. W. Go, unpublished observations.
[c] $P < 0.05$ as compared to control.
[d] $P < 0.05$ as compared to cobalt containing sample.

Electrical stimulation of the sciatic nerve in cats will result in a highly significant increase in the levels of sPLI in spinal superfusate when the intensity of the stimulus is adequate to evoke A-β and A-δ/C fiber compound action potentials (1-s train/2 s; 50 Hz; 0.05 ms; 40–50 V). As shown in Figure 1, stimulation of the A-β fibers alone results in no significant increase in the collected levels of sP over base line (Yaksh *et al.*, 1980).

An important question is whether the amount of material collected is proportional to the frequency of stimulation. Table III presents the percentage change from base line of the levels of sPLI over a stimulation range of 2–100 Hz. Between 2 and 20 Hz there is a stimulus-dependent increase in the collectable levels of sPLI. At the highest frequency (100 Hz), there was a remarkable decline in the amount of material collected; using a Newman–Keuls multiple-means analysis ($P < 0.05$), the relative levels of release are 20 Hz > 10 Hz ≥ 100 Hz > 2 Hz. These observations suggest that over a frequency range of 2–20 Hz, the amount of sPLI in the spinal superfusate reflects the degree of terminal activity. Examination of the compound action potential at 100 Hz reveals a significant fallout of all but the most rapidly conducting component in recordings made distally on the sural nerve.

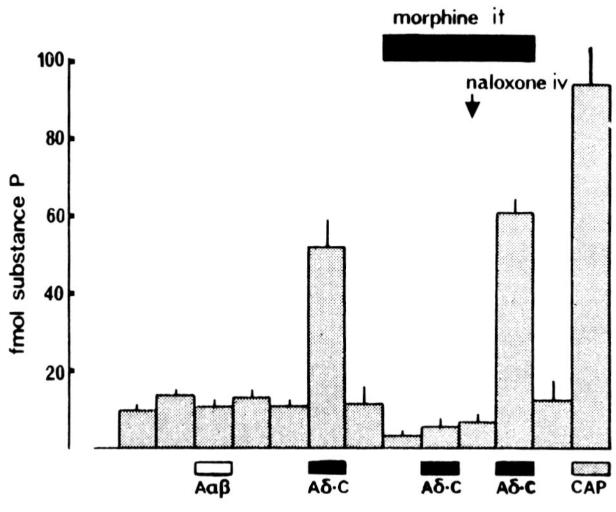

FIGURE 1. Release of substance P from superfused cat spinal cord in response to sciatic nerve stimulation and capsaicin (CAP). The nerve was stimulated with rectangular pulses (3–4 V, 0.05 ms, 50 Hz for activation of A-α and A-β fibers and 40–50 V, 0.05 ms, 50 Hz for recruitment of A-δ and C fibers). Perfusion samples (3 ml) were collected into glacial acetic acid (final concentration of 2 M) and immediately frozen and lyophilized. Samples were reconstituted in 1.0 ml assay buffer and neutralized and aliquots of each fraction were used to determine the content of substance P by radioimmunoassay. Each value is the mean ± S.E.M. of four separate experiments. (From Yaksh *et al.*, 1980.)

TABLE III
Effect of Stimulation Frequency on the Release of Substance P from the Spinal Cord of the Decerebrate Spinal Cat[a]

Stimulation frequency[b] (Hz)	N	Change from control (%)
2	8	21 ± 16%
10	6	126 ± 26%
20	6	218 ± 36%
100	5	98 ± 48%

[a] Data from T. L. Yaksh and V. L. W. Go (unpublished observations).
[b] Stimulus was delivered in 1-s bursts every 2 s to either sciatic nerve for a period of 30 min at intensities that generated compound action potentials conducting velocities corresponding to A-β/a-δ/C-fiber components.

2. *Characterization of the Spinal Systems from Which Substance P Is Released*

More recently, we have attempted to specify the characteristics of the relevant fiber tracts by employing the double-pulse procedure to determine the refractory period of the fibers from which the sPLI originates.

Figure 2 shows the release evoked by high-intensity stimulation of the sciatic nerve (1-s trains/2 s; 20 Hz; 0.5-ms pulse; 40–50 V). On the first stimulation interval, the pulses are presented such that every second pulse occurs 2 ms after the preceding one. At 20 Hz, all normal interpulse intervals are 50 ms. As the pulse pair interval decreases, those smaller fibers with longer refractory periods will cease to follow. As indicated, there is a significant reduction in the amount of sPLI collected at the shorter interpulse interval. In systematic studies, release was examined with trains of pulse pairs having intrapair intervals of 50 ms (i.e., 20 Hz), 10, 2 or 0 ms (i.e., 10 Hz). It is clear that there is a significant reduction in the percentage increase of sP (260% to 180%) released at an interpulse interval of 10 ms as compared to that observed with a 50-ms interpulse pair. Examination of the area under the compound action potential measured at the dorsal root evoked by the second pulse given on the sciatic nerve indicates that the fiber population with velocities of 2 m/s or less (C fibers) was diminished by 86% with a 10-ms pulse interval and was essentially occluded at the 2-ms interval. The A-δ component (2 m/s $< X <$ 30 m/s) was not diminished at the 10-ms interval. These observations strongly suggest that the evoked changes in sPLI in spinal superfusates result from the activation of fibers with a relatively long refractory period, possibly correlating with a C-fiber population.

Though it appears likely that spinal afferent terminals that contain sP are activated by the nerve stimulation, one may ask whether the collected

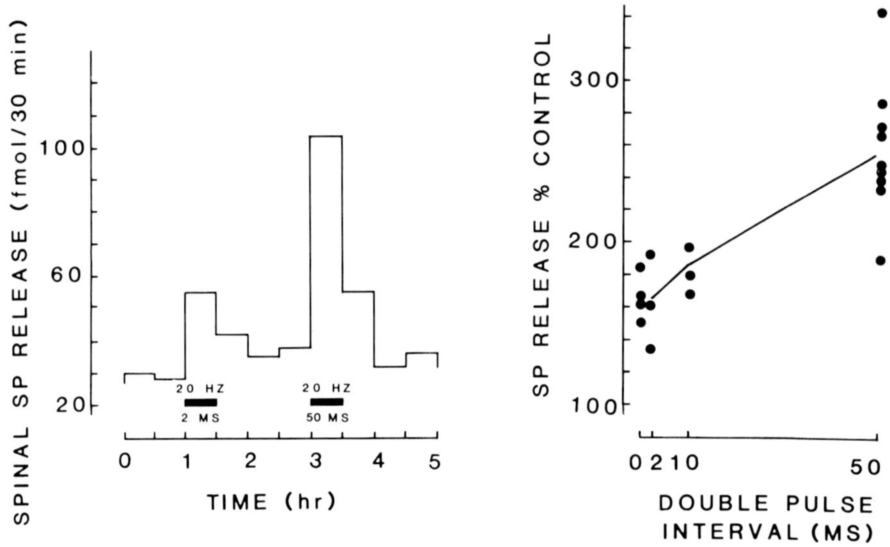

FIGURE 2. (A) Results showing the release of substance P from spinal cord in a single animal. At black bar animal received bilateral stimulation of the sciatic nerves at 20 Hz. In the first stimulation sequence, the interval between pulse pairs was 2 ms, whereas in the second stimulation sequence, the interpulse intervals were all equal (i.e., 50 ms). (B) Percentage increase in substance P levels in spinal superfusates observed during double-pulse stimulation at intervals of 0, 2, 10, and 50 ms. As can be seen, maximum increases were observed at the 50-ms pulse interval. The stimulation paradigm is as presented in the figure on the left.

sPLI indeed originated from afferent terminals. Since sPLI is found in descending serotonergic pathways and intrinsic spinal neurons (see Ruda, Chapter 7), it is important to query to what extent the K^+ or electrical stimulation of sPLI in these nonafferent systems may contribute to measured release. In rats, intrathecal treatment with 5,6-dihydroxytryptamine will produce a significant reduction in the measured levels of spinal 5-HT and sPLI (see Figure 3 and Micevych *et al.,* 1983). In rats pretreated with capsaicin but not 5,6-DHT, both K^+- and capsaicin-evoked sPLI release was remarkably attenuated.

In cats several lines of evidence also suggest that the sPLI release derives from local afferent terminal systems. We have demonstrated that spinopetal serotonergic pathways (some of which contain colocated sP) are activated by afferent input with stimulus characteristics comparable to those that increase sPLI in the superfusate (Tyce and Yaksh, 1981). The spinal 5-HT release is reduced by cold block of the cervical cord. Yet, as shown in Table IV, sP release evoked by afferent stimulation is, if anything,. higher in the cold-blocked spinal cords. This actually suggests a possible descending modulation that is concurrently evoked by high-intensity afferent input. In addition to the failure of cold block to reduce afferent-evoked increases in sP release,

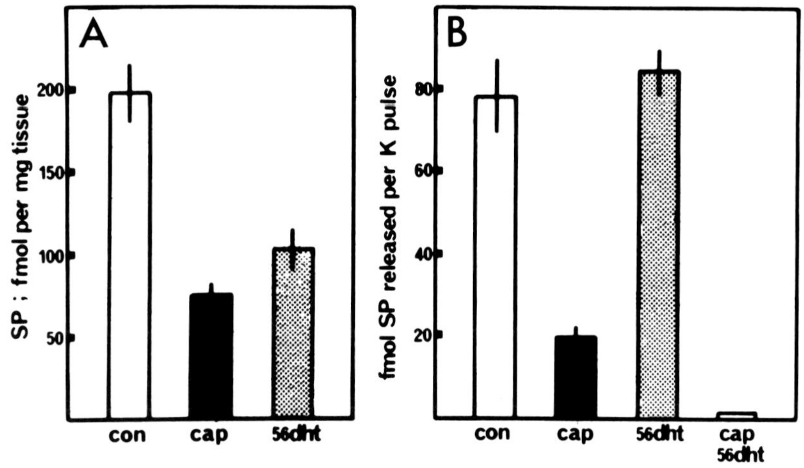

FIGURE 3. Effect of intrathecal capsaicin (cap) and 5,6-dihydroxytryptamine (56dht) on substance P content and release from rat spinal cord. (A) Immunoreactive substance P content in rat lumbar spinal cord 7 days after intrathecal capsaicin or 5,6-dihydroxytryptamine. (From Yaksh *et al.*, 1979.) (B) Release of immunoreactive substance P from rat spinal cord in response to 40 mM KCl (10 min). Each column represents the mean ± S.E.M. of at least four animals. con, controls. (From Jessell, 1982, with permission.)

treatment with intrathecal capsaicin, as shown in Figure 4, resulted in a significant attenuation in the collected levels of sPLI otherwise evoked by high-intensity afferent stimulation.

As capsaicin does not appear to alter the levels of sPLI in descending pathways or interneuronal systems (see Fitzgerald, 1983) or to deplete sPLI in the ventral horn, it appears likely that the above studies provide evidence that a significant proportion of the levels of sPLI found in the spinal superfusate derives fromm a depolarization-dependent, exocytotic movement from primary afferent terminals.

3. Pharmacological Manipulations of Primary Afferent Terminals

From the preceding comments, it appears that the levels of sPLI in the spinal superfusate reflect the movement of material from afferent terminals, with the amount of material released being proportional to neuronal activity. Under these circumstances, it is plausible to consider the effect of pharmacological manipulations of spinal receptors that are thought to alter afferent excitability either directly or indirectly. Several such pharmacologically defined systems are known to exist, including those that originate at the brainstem level to project to the spinal cord to release norepinephrine or serotonin

TABLE IV
Effect of Cervical Cold Block[a] in the Cat on sPLI Levels Measured in Spinal Superfusates of Chloralose–Urethane Anesthetized Cats[b]

	N	Levels of sP release during stimulation (% control)
Control	4	193 ± 28[c]
Cold block	4	233 ± 34[c]

[a] Cold block achieved at the level of a C1–C2 laminectomy.
[b] Data from T. L. Yaksh and V. L. W. Go (unpublished data).
[c] $P < 0.05$ as compared to control.

(see Hammond, Chapter 15; Ruda, Chapter 7) and those that are intrinsic to the spinal cord and act, for example, on opioid and GABA receptors (see LaMotte, Chapter 5). Receptors for such putative neurotransmitters have been identified in the dorsal horn, perhaps in some cases presynaptic to primary afferents (see Seybold, Chapter 6).

a. Spinopetal Systems

As noted above, descending aminergic pathways have been shown to modulate spinal function. Norepinephrine will decrease primary afferent excitability (Jeftinija *et al.*, 1981b). Figure 5 presents the effects of an α_2-adrenergic agonist on the release of spinal sPLI. In this experiment, ST-91 (10^{-4}

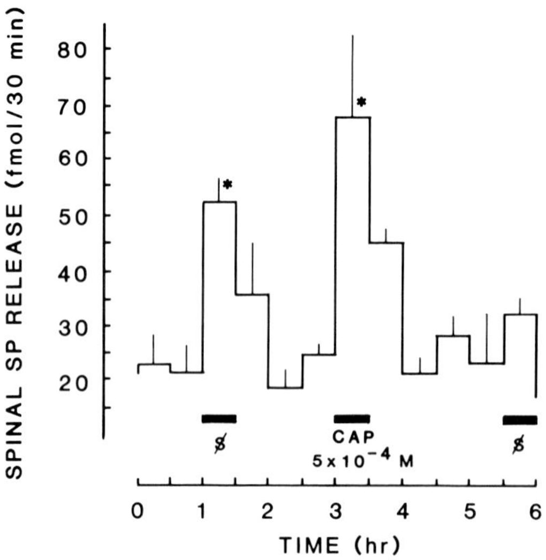

FIGURE 4. Mean ± S.E. ($N = 6$) of the levels of sPLI measured in spinal superfusates during stimulation ($, same parameters as in Figure 1) or during the administration of capsaicin (cap: 5×10^{-4} M) into the spinal perfusate. *$P < 0.05$ compared to control. As shown, after capsaicin-evoked release, sciatic stimulation was ineffective.

M) in the perfusate resulted in a significant diminution of the levels of sPLI evoked by somatic stimuli. The concurrent spinal administration of an equimolar concentration of phentolamine clearly attenuated the inhibition observed with ST-91 alone. In contrast to the powerful effect of the adrenergic receptor agonists, serotonin in concentrations of 10^{-4} M or administered in conjunction with fluoxetine (a serotonin uptake antagonist) did not significantly alter the evoked release (see Table V).

b. Intrinsic Spinal Systems

Considerable evidence has pointed to the role of intrinsic spinal opioid receptor systems in the modulation of spinal afferent excitability. Thus, morphine will decrease the excitability of afferent terminals. In the pioneering work in this field, Jessell and Iversen (1977) observed that opioid alkaloids and peptides would attenuate the *in vitro* K^+-evoked release from spinal cord but not substantia nigra slices. Subsequently, it was shown that morphine would suppress the release of sPLI evoked by somatic stimulation. Currently, considerable emphasis has been placed on the types of opioid receptors that potentially modulate spinal activity, including the μ, δ, and κ receptors. Binding studies have demonstrated the existence of such sites in dorsal roots/ganglion cells and a partial loss of such binding in the dorsal horn after rhizotomy or ganglionectomy (see Seybold, Chapter 6). In experiments comparable to those presented in Figure 5 for ST-91, the effect of μ (morphine), δ (D-Ala²-D-Leu⁵-enkephalin), or κ (U50488H) ligands given into the spinal superfusate on

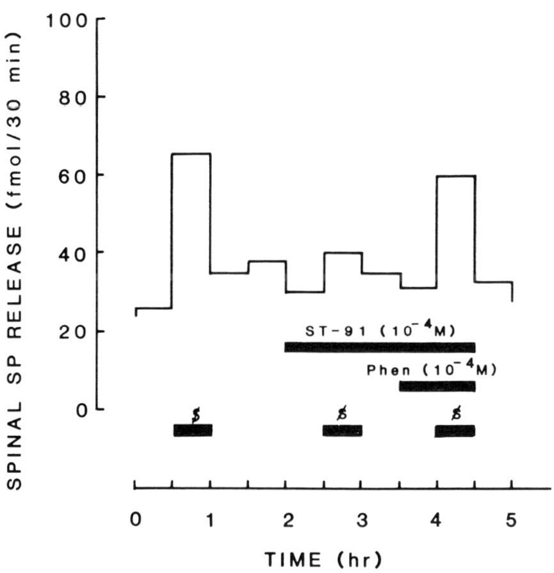

FIGURE 5. Effect of intrathecal ST-91 (10^{-4} M) on the release otherwise evoked by bilateral stimulation of the sciatic nerves (stimulation parameters same as in Figure 1). Phentolamine (Phen: 10^{-4} M) was added prior to the third stimulus and was able to reverse the apparent inhibition produced by ST-91.

TABLE V
Percentage Inhibition by Receptor-Selective Agonists of the Release of sPLI in Spinal Superfusates Evoked by Sciatic Nerve Stimulation in Chloralose–Urethanized Cats[a]

Perfused agent	Concentration	N	Percent of control release
CSF alone	—	4	106 ± 9
ST-91	10^{-4} M	5	44 ± 12[c]
ST-91 + phentolamine	10^{-8} M	3	76 ± 13
Serotonin[b]	10^{-4} M	3	106 ± 21
Morphine	10^{-4} M	4	23 ± 14[c]
Morphine + naloxone	10^{-4} M	3	121 ± 12
DADL	10^{-5} M	3	35 ± 19[c]
DADL + naloxone	10^{-4} M	3	131 ± 22
U50488H	10^{-3} M	3	82 ± 31
Naloxone	10^{-4} M	5	146 ± 18[c]
GABA	10^{-4} M	4	74 ± 18[d]
Phentolamine	10^{-4} M	4	163 ± 28[c]

[a] Table summarizes the effects of the highest concentration of drug thus far examined. Data from T. L. Yaksh and V. L. W. Go (unpublished data).
[b] Fluoxetine (10^{-4} M) added.
[c] $P < 0.05$ compared to control stimulation (100%).
[d] $P < 0.10$ compared to control stimulation.

somatic evoked release of sPLI into the cat spinal superfusate have been examined. As shown in the preliminary studies summarized in Table V, morphine and DADL produce a powerful suppression of sPLI evoked release. The κ ligand (U50488H) in doses used herein resulted in no statistically significant effect on sPLI levels. Importantly, the suppressive effects of morphine and DADL were antagonized by coadministration of equimolar concentrations of naloxone.

GABA is thought to act presynaptically on afferent systems (Game and Lodge, 1975). In the present studies, a small but statistically significant reduction in the levels of sPLI was observed.

It should be stressed that failure to see a major effect, as with GABA or serotonin, may occur because the dose is inadequate, because inactivation occurs too rapidly, or because the receptor plays no role in modulating the observed endpoint.

D. The Effects of Manipulating the Levels of Substance P in Spinal Cord

If sP serves as a neurotransmitter, indications as to its function should be considered in the context of the behavioral effects produced by manipulations that alter the disposition of primary afferent pools of sP in spinal cord.

1. Capsaicin-Evoked Depletion of Substance P

The observation that capsaicin, a homovanillic derivative, would selectively deplete fluoride-resistant acid phosphatase (FRAP) in the dorsal horn of the spinal cord was the first piece of biochemical evidence that this agent was a neurotoxin whose action was directed largely at small fibers (see Knyihar-Csillik and Csillik, 1981, for review). Subsequent observations indicated that the systemic administration of this compound would indeed produce a significant depletion of sP immunoreactivity in the dorsal horn of the spinal cord (Jessell *et al.*, 1978). Topical and systemic administration of this agent had been observed to produce a peripheral desensitization to chemical and thermal noxious stimuli (see Fitzgerald, 1983; Knyihar-Csillik and Csillik, 1981, for review).

With regard to the central action of this agent, it was observed that the intrathecal administration of capsaicin at doses that were systemically inactive would produce a prolonged desensitization of the animal's response to thermal and chemical algogenic stimuli (Yaksh *et al.*, 1979; Nagy *et al.*, 1981, 1983; Gamse, 1982).

Examination of the spinal cord after intrathecal or systemic treatment indicates that the effects of capsaicin are not uniquely limited to sP. Thus, significant reductions in the levels of somatostatin and perhaps CCK were also observed (Yaksh *et al.*, 1979; Jancso *et al.*, 1981; Nagy *et al.*, 1981; Micevych *et al.*, 1983; Jhamandas *et al.*, 1984). Moreover, as indicated in the beginning, FRAP appears to represent a marker for a population of small afferent terminals that do not contain any of the abovementioned peptides, and this marker was also diminished by capsaicin. In spite of this activity, it cannot be said that capsaicinoid neurotoxins are nonspecific. Thus, intrathecal or systemic administration of doses of capsaicin in excess of those required to significantly diminish sP in spinal cord has no effect on the assayed spinal levels of 5-HT, norepinephrine, neurotensin, Met-enkephalin, and VIP (or CCK as measured by RIA) (Jhamandas *et al.*, 1984; Micevych *et al.*, 1983; T. L. Yaksh, V. L. W. Go, and G. M. Tyce, unpublished observations; Singer *et al.*, 1982). Similarly, systematic examination revealed that capsaicin in doses that deplete dorsal horn sP had no effect on the levels of a variety of spinal amino acids including glutamic acid, aspartic acid, glycine, and GABA as well as a number of enzyme systems (choline acetyltransferase, GAD) and glutamic acid uptake (*vide supra*; Singer *et al.*, 1982). Moreover, histochemical examinations of sP immunoreactivity following intrathecal capsaicin reveal that the majority of the depletion is limited to those systems that lie in the dorsal gray matter.

Figure 6 presents the immunohistochemistry from three rats with intrathecal catheters: one of them received intrathecal capsaicin; the second received 5,6-dihydroxytryptamine, the serotonin neurotoxin; the third received saline. As can be seen, following intrathecal capsaicin, there was a profound depletion of the levels of sP in the dorsal gray matter. The punctate immunoreactivity found throughout the spinal cord, however, was not affected. In contrast, 5,6-dihydroxytryptamine, which also results in a significant reduction in radioimmunoassayable levels of sP (see Figure 6), failed to reduce the levels of sP immunoreactivity in the dorsal gray matter. Thus, it appears that the neurotoxin directs its effects largely at the stores of sP that are in populations of primary afferent terminals. Evidence for such anatomic selectivity is also supported by the observation that opiate and GABA binding, thought to be partly located on primary afferents, is significantly reduced (Singer and Placheta, 1980).

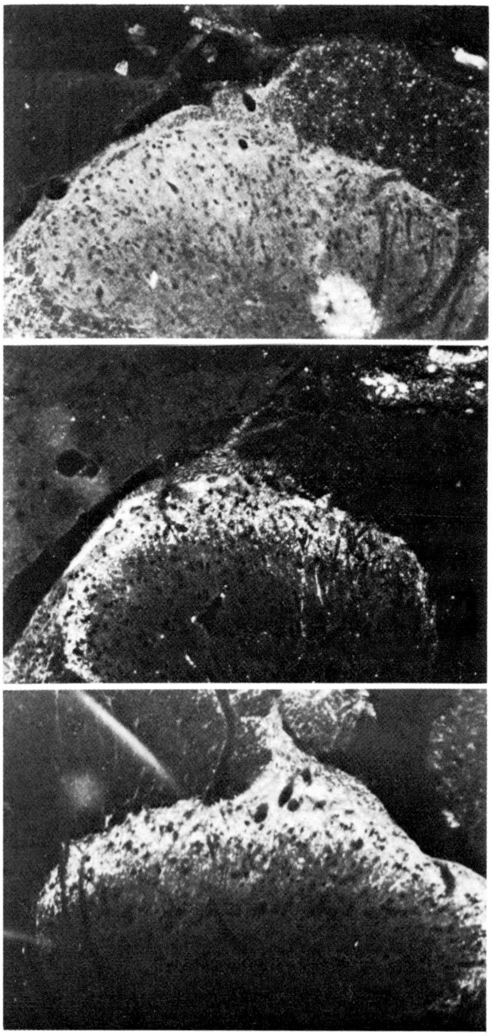

FIGURE 6. Photomicrograph showing the effect in rats on sP immunofluorescence in dorsal horn of intrathecal capsaicin (30 μg; top), 5,6-dihydroxytryptamine (20 μg, middle), or vehicle (bottom) injected in a volume of 15 μl 7 days before sacrifice. (From Yaksh *et al.*, 1984.)

With regard to mechanisms, the present results are consistent with the observation that capsaicin results in a prolonged depolarization of small primary afferent ganglion cells (Williams and Zieglgänsberger, 1982). This likely accounts for the releasing effect of capsaicin and the acute desensitization observed with these agents. With regard to cellular toxicity, it appears probable that elevated intracellular calcium fluxes secondary to the chronic depolarization produced by capsaicin may be toxic to cell function (see Siesjö, 1981). Alternatively, capsaicin will diminish transport in small afferents (Gamse *et al.*, 1982). This may indeed account in some as yet undetermined way for the long-term toxicity observed with capsaicin, although it appears unlikely that this itself may represent the underlying cause for the acute desensitization observed when the drugs are applied directly to the peripheral or central terminal.

2. *Effect of Intrathecal Capsaicin on Behavior*

After the intrathecal administration of capsaicinoid compounds in the unanesthetized animal, there is a profound agitation response followed by a period of quiesence. Measurement of the responsiveness of the animal to cutaneous thermal stimuli reveals a significant increase in the response latency in the absence of any significant effects on motor function (Yaksh *et al.*, 1979).

To determine whether there was a correlation between the levels of reduction in sP immunoreactivity and the effects on the cutaneous thermal nociceptive response, we examined the effect of capsaicin and a number of capsaicinoid analogues for their ability to (1) cause agitation response, (2) produce a blockade of the thermal nociceptive reflex, and (3) deplete several of the dorsal horn peptides including sP, VIP, and CCK. Figure 7 shows the effects of 75 μg of these several analogues on the tail flick response and on the levels of these three peptides in the spinal cord. As can be seen, capsaicin produced a significant powerful depletion, as did L-nonanoylvanillamide. Significantly, there was a clear correlation between the ability to deplete sP and the amount of sP depletion. Examination of the effects of piperine (a pungent agent unrelated to capsaicin) and kainic acid (a neurotoxin of the glutamate receptor) revealed that these agents also produced a significant depletion of sP immunoreactivity, but in neither case was this effect associated with a significant increase in the hot-plate or tail-flick response latency.

Further studies on the effects of capsaicin were carried out in which the ability of these agents to release sP from spinal cord *in vivo* was examined. In these experiments, rats anesthetized with chloralose–urethane underwent spinal superfusion, and the several agents were administered intrathecally in the perfusate. As shown in Figure 8, agents that produced a significant depletion of sP from the dorsal horn, and produced a significant decrease in the levels of sP immunoreactivity in the spinal superfusates were those agents

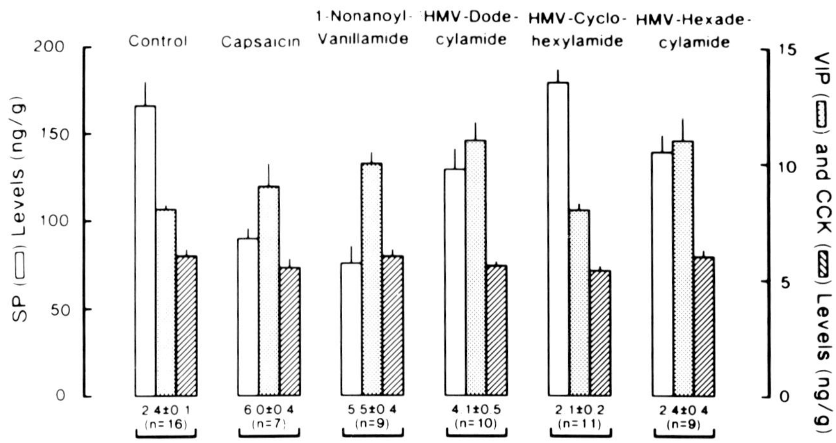

FIGURE 7. Effect of intrathecal injection of capsaicin and four structurally related analogues on the content of substance P (SP), cholecystokinin (CCK), and vasoactive intestinal peptide (VIP) in the rat lumbar spinal cord and on the tail-flick latency. The tail-flick latencies given below each set of histograms were measured 7 days after a single injection (75 μg) of capsaicin or its derivatives. n = the number of animals used. Note the difference between the vertical scales on the left and right sides. (From Jhamandas *et al.*, 1984.)

that produced the most profound effects on thermal response latency. Neither piperine nor kainic acid was active. These results suggest that the ability of the capsaicinoid agents to evoke the release of sP from the spinal cord, presumably by depolarization, and the ability of these agents to deplete sP are closely correlated, the principal exception being piperine. That these several capsaicinoid agents act on the same site in the cell membrane is suggested by the observation of cross desensitization. Thus, the exposure of the spinal cord to agents that were able to release sP resulted in a blockade of the ability of subsequent applications of another agent such as capsaicin to evoke comparable release. In contrast, agents that did not release sP did not result in subsequent cross desensitization for an active agent (Jhamandas *et al.*, 1984).

E. Effects of Blockade of the Spinal Substance P Receptor

Folkers, Rosell, and their colleagues (Folkers *et al.*, 1981) reported that sP analogues, synthesized with a variety of D-amino-acid substitutions, displayed the ability to antagonize the effects of sP applied *in vitro* in a variety of smooth muscle preparations. Given the possibility that sP is a transmitter in small primary afferents, it is reasonable to query whether or not the intrathecal administration of these agents will produce any change in the animal's response to a strong stimulus. Early studies indicated that intrathecal

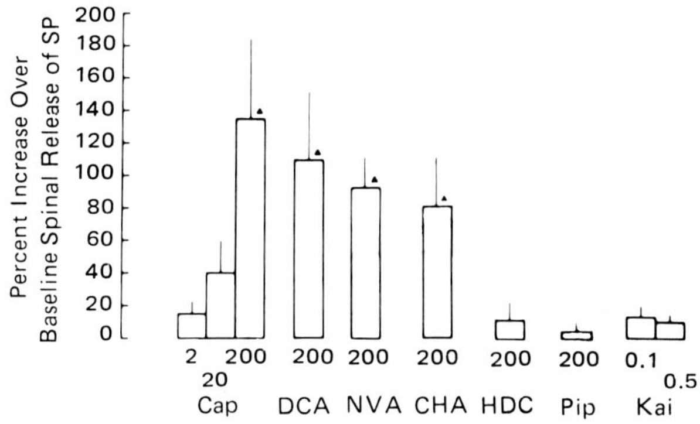

FIGURE 8. Comparative effects of capsaicin (Cap), HMV-dodecylamide (DCA), 1-nonenoylvanillylamide (NVA), HMV-cyclohexylamide (CHA), HMV-hexadecylamide (HDC), piperine (Pip), and kainic acid (Kai) on the release of SP-like immunoreactivity from the superfused rat spinal cord *in vivo*. Concentrations below each histogram are given in micromoles per liter. The release values have been standardized by expressing release in the presence of the drug as a percentage of release measured in the sample immediately preceding the drug application. Each value shown represents the mean ± S.E.M., n = 4–6 experiments. Triangle, $P < 0.05$. (From Jhamandas *et al.*, 1984.)

administration of these putative sP antagonists would indeed produce an elevation in the nociceptive threshold as measured in several nociceptive measures (Akerman *et al.*, 1982; Piercey *et al.*, 1981b).

Table VI presents the effects of two putative sP antagonists administered intrathecally on the pinch vocalization threshold, the tail-flick latency, and the loss of hindlimb responsiveness. As can be seen, the ability to block pinch vocalization and the tail flick appears to occur with the evident onset of hindlimb

TABLE VI
Effects of Intrathecal Substance P Analogues on the Tail-Flick and Hot-Plate Responses and the Development of Hindlimb Flaccidity[a]

		ED_{50} value (μg)				
Agent	N	Pinch vocalization	Tail flick	Hind-paw flaccidity	Acetic acid writhing	Died[b]
D-Pro²-D-Try⁷·⁹-sP	32	8.3 ± 1.5	7.9 ± 2.1	11 ± 5	5.8 ± 2.0[c]	25
D-Pro²-D-Phe⁷-D-Try⁹-sP	18	1.9 ± 0.3	2.1 ± 0.3	1.8 ± 0.3	1.1 ± 0.3	5

[a] Data from T. L. Yaksh, G. Harty, and M. Randic (unpublished observations).
[b] Dose at which 50% of rats or more died as a result of respiratory paralysis.
[c] Writhing carried out as described by Schmauss and Yaksh (1983).

flaccidity. It should be stressed that the agent likely produced an effect on "pain" transmission inasmuch as the pinch-induced vocalization, an endpoint that is not influenced, as was the tail flick, by the flaccidity-producing effects of this agent, was clearly abolished. So profound is the flaccidity, however, that it represents one of the overriding observations made with these classes of agents. Toxicity with these drugs appeared related to a potent muscle paralysis that spread over a 30-min period to encompass levels at or above the brachial plexus. Breathing became diaphragmatic and then ceased. As indicated, there was a close covariance between the ability of the agents to block the pinch vocalization and tail flick and the ability to produce flaccidity and subsequent death. It is interesting to note that the ability to inhibit the writhing response was considerably greater than for any of the other measures.

F. Effects of the Intrathecal Administration of Substance P on Behavior in the Unanesthetized Rat

An important question is what effect sP has on behavior when administered into the spinal space, presumably mimicking the effects of activating spinal afferents. A variety of observations have been made ranging from analgesia to signs of agitation. The intrathecal administration of sP will produce scratching in rats and mice (Hylden and Wilcox, 1981; Rackham *et al.*, 1981). It should be noted that other peptides such as somatostatin will also produce a similar effect (Seybold *et al.*, 1982). In comparable experiments in this laboratory, we have examined the effects of sP on the ability of rats to produce escape behavior as judged by an observer blind to the agent received (T. L. Yaksh and G. J. Harty, unpublished observations). As shown in Table VII, out of 20 rats, 15% of the animals showed escape behavior after 1 μg and 55% after 5 μg. Glutamate, a powerful neuronal excitant, produced minimal escape behavior at 0.1 μg intrathecally, but nearly one-third of the animals showed a response of 0.5 μg.

Given the observations noted above that sP might be coreleasing an excitatory transmitter, we considered what would happen if these agents were coadministered. As shown, the intrathecal administration of 0.1 μg of sP along with 0.1 μg of glutamate resulted in a highly significant increase in the proportion of animals showing escape behavior (90%). These data, though limited, suggest a powerful synergy between the effects of excitatory amino acid and the peptide sP. In subsequent experiments, we sought to determine whether a dose of the putative sP antagonist D-Pro^{2}-D-Try^{7,9}-sP at intrathecal doses that did not produce any detectable signs of flaccidity would have an effect on the response. As noted, the administration of these three agents resulted in a significant reduction in the proportion of animals in which the administration of the peptide and amino acid resulted in escape behavior.

TABLE VII
Percentage of Rats Showing Escape Behavior after Intrathecal Administration of Glutamate, Substance P, and D-Pro[2]-D-Try[7,9]-sP[a]

Intrathecal drugs	Escape response/total	Percent
Saline	2/20	10
Substance P 1.0 μg	3/20	15
5.0 μg	11/20	55
Glutamate 0.1 μg	2/22	9
Substance P 0.1 μg + glutamate 0.1 μg	18/20	90[b]
0.5 μg + glutamate 0.1 μg	6/18	33
Substance P 1 μg + glutamate 0.1 μg + D-Pro[2]-D-Try[7,9]-sP 1 μg	3/21	14[c]

[a] All drugs or combinations were injected in a final volume of 10 μl and were delivered in a random fashion, with each rat being injected and judged by an observer blind to the drug.
[b] $P < 0.05$ compared to control.
[c] $P < 0.05$ compared to substance P and glutamate dose group.

G. General Discussion

1. Manipulations of Spinal Substance P

The current line of investigation directed at assaying the extravascular–extracellular levels of sP in spinal cord appears to support the concept that a significant fraction of this sPLI is released in a conventional (Ca^{2+}-dependent) manner from the spinal terminals of primary afferents. Thus, the release remains after destruction of descending pathways and disappears when the system is treated with capsaicin, a neurotoxin that does not affect nonafferent stores of sP. The double-pulse stimulation studies and the sensitivity to capsaicin suggest that the primary afferent terminals from which this sP arises are unmyelinated, or at most lightly myelinated, fibers.

These spinal terminals releasing sP appear to be under the modulating control of several spinal receptor systems. Thus, it appears that the local activation of spinal opioid (including μ and δ) and α_2-adrenergic and perhaps GABAergic receptor systems will result in a dose-dependent suppression of the physiologically evoked release of spinal sP. At doses employed, the κ opioid ligands and serotonin do not appear directly to influence the releasability of sP. As extensive pharmacological studies have not been carried out with the several agonists, one must be careful not to ascribe without reservation the effect of these agents to their unique interaction with their associated receptor (i.e., morphine with μ and DADL with δ).

These observations suggest the likelihood that these respective receptor systems may exert a presynaptic action on terminals that contain sP. As discussed by Seybold (Chapter 6), radioligand binding studies have demonstrated the presence of μ, δ, κ, and adrenergic binding sites in the dorsal spinal gray. The presence of μ and δ binding in dorsal root ganglion and the loss of μ/δ and α_2 binding sites after ganglionectomy or rhizotomy (see Yaksh, Chapter 20) suggest that a proportion of these binding sites are indeed located on primary afferents. Capsaicin, a treatment that will destroy unmyelinated fibers, further results in a reduction in opioid binding and suggests that a proportion of the binding sites are on the terminals of small primary afferents (see Section D1). Both opiates and adrenergic agonists have been shown to diminish primary afferent excitability (Carstens *et al.*, 1979; Sastry, 1980; Jeftinija *et al.*, 1981b) and thereby reduce the releasability of the respective neurotransmitters.

The failure of GABA to produce a major effect on sPLI release is surprising in view of the powerful presynaptic effects of GABA receptors on dorsal and ventral horn functions (Game and Lodge, 1975). Nevertheless, these effects, consistent with those previously reported by Sawynok and colleagues (1982) with baclofen, suggest that such receptor systems are not preponderantly localized on small afferent terminals from which the release of spinal sP is derived.

2. *What Role Do the Central Terminals of the Substance-P-Containing Primary Afferent Terminals Play?*

As indicated initially, the complexity of the information coded by afferents makes it reasonable that several neurotransmitters are involved in afferent transmission. The likelihood of multiple neurotransmitters in the same terminals suggests that different postsynaptic events may be evoked by different stimulation parameters.

What evidence if any may be drawn to associate the function of primary afferents within which sP is contained with a particular modality?

The following points supported by data presented in the present work and reported by other laboratories can briefly be summarized.

1. Substance P appears to be largely located in small primary afferents. This evidence is supported by immunohistochemistry showing sP in dorsal root type B ganglion cells and the loss of sP in the dorsal gray matter secondary to treatment with capsaicin, a neurotoxin that appears largely to limit its effects to small afferent fiber systems.
2. The sP that is released in the extracellular fluid secondary to neural stimulation appears to derive from these small primary afferents, as the release of sP is unaffected by manipulations that inactivate descending pathways (5,6-dihydroxytryptamine) but is diminished by

manipulations that destroy small primary afferent terminals (capsaicin). Substance P is released primarily by electrical stimuli that activate autonomic responses in the anesthetized animal and generate an A-β/A-δ/C-fiber compound action potential. Moreover, the electrophysiology as evidenced by the double-pulse stimulation studies suggests that small and not large fibers may be involved.

3. The release of sP from these small fibers is influenced by agents that, when administered into the spinal cord, act on a receptor (opioid α_2) to yield a relatively selective blockade of single-unit activity evoked by high-intensity stimulation and produces analgesia when applied into the intrathecal space of the unanesthetized animal (see Yaksh, Chapter 20).
4. The direct spinal administration of agents with an apparent affinity for the receptor site acted on by sP but without efficacy at that site (e.g., antagonists) results in a significant increase in the nociceptive threshold, but this effect, as noted, is also clearly associated with changes in motor function.
5. The direct administration of capsaicin into the intrathecal space results in initial signs of agitation and subsequent densensitization. These phenomena appear related to the activation of small fibers and to a subsequent prolonged depolarization of these fiber systems, which either directly or indirectly results in their degeneration and a long-term loss of sP immunoreactivity of the dorsal gray matter.
6. The direct application of sP into the dorsal horn of the spinal cord results in mild scratching behavior, but this effect is translated into a profound increase in behavioral signs of irritation when the peptide is coadministered with the excitatory amino acid glutamate. Importantly, the potentiating effect appears to be reduced when this is coadministered with low doses of putative sP receptor antagonists.

The above data appear to provide compelling support for the speculation that sP may play a particular role in a population of fibers through which certain classes of nociceptive information may travel, although sP itself is unlikely to be the only element in the coding process.

The potentiating effects of sP on the nociceptive effects of intrathecal glutamate are in accord with the observations by Urban and Randic (1984) that high repetitive stimulation results in a prolonged depolarization that is sensitive to a putative sP antagonist. The characteristic phenomenon of "wind-up" observed in wide-dynamic-range neurons is attributed to C-fiber input (Mendell, 1966) and could be accounted for by such a prolonged depolarization. Significantly, wind-up, as is the sP antagonist-sensitive depolarization, is most readily evoked by repetitive and not single-pulse stimulation. It should be stressed, however, that this hypothesis is an interpretation of the data that is at best controversial. For every set of experiments, there are points of contention, and indeed, not all of the findings in the various laboratories are compatible. Wall and Fitzgerald (1982), in a detailed examination of this problem, have emphasized these discrepancies. It should be stressed that even though sP may be an important element in coding certain aspects of nociception, it does not appear likely that this is the only function subserved by afferents in which it is contained.

As noted, one of the most evident effects of the putative sP antagonists is a profound flaccidity. In preliminary experiments in cats, Abay (1982) has observed that high doses of capsaicin produced profound, long-lasting motor weakness reminiscent of the effects produced by sP antagonists. These observations stress the likelihood that sP-releasing systems are important in providing a tonic influence on motor horn cells. Rats rendered nonresponsive to thermal and chemical nociceptive stimuli show abolition of bladder function. These phenomena do not likely reflect systems uniquely related to the afferent processing of pain information.

At this point, with the given discrepancies and controversy, one might despair that we have progressed little in our understanding of the afferent systems in the spinal cord. On the contrary, I think the very fact that the above questions can now be raised reflects how far the field has advanced since the early 1950s when sP was proposed as a potential afferent transmitter because of the high levels of bioassayable activity in dorsal column nuclei (which, curiously, do not receive small afferent terminals; see McLennon, 1970).

3. *Role of Receptor Systems That Modulate Spinal Substance P Release*

The presence of these several classes of receptors, which are postsynaptic to the terminals of several anatomically and pharmacologically well-defined systems, leads one to query under what conditions these several classes of receptors, which appear to affect the release of stores of primary afferent sP, are physiologically activated.

With regard to this question, we have demonstrated that afferent stimuli similar to those that activate sPLI release from spinal cord will markedly increase the release of spinal 5-HT and norepinephrine (see Hammond, Chapter 15) as well as a variety of endorphins (Yaksh *et al.*, 1983). The evoked release from spinal cord of monoamine, but not endorphin release, is attenuated by cervical cold block (Yaksh and Elde, 1981). In the absence of stimulation, the collectable levels of these agents are at or near the level of absolute sensitivity of the several assays. It is significant, as noted above, that spinal block will have little effect on the resting levels of sPLI observed in the spinal superfusate. Yet such a cold block results in a facilitation of the physiologically evoked release of spinal sPLI. Neither naloxone nor phentolamine alone had any measurable effect on the resting release of spinal sPLI but commonly facilitated the increase in sPLI release evoked by high-intensity afferent stimulation.

It thus appears that the afferent terminals from which sP is released are subject to a modulation by segmentally (opioid) and suprasegmentally (noradrenergic) organized systems that are not tonically active but are reflexly activated by a high-intensity afferent input. Tang *et al.* (1983) have indeed observed that an extended enkephalin (Met-Enk-Arg^6,Phe^7) may be released from spinal cord by the addition of sP into the perfusate. In recent work we have observed that glutamate (10^{-5} M) or a stable analgesic, kainic acid (10^{-6} M), will also increase the levels of Met-enkephalinlike immunoreactivity in spinal superfusates (T. L. Yaksh, G. J. Harty, and V. L. W. Go, unpublished observations). Importantly, there appears to be evidence that the enkephalin-releasing effects of glutamate are enhanced by the addition of sP. It is intriguing to speculate that these observations reflect a correlate of the long depolarizing effects of sP on dorsal horn neurons and that the activation of spinal enkephalinergic neurons that produces enkephalin release may require a prolonged depolarization optimally achieved by glutamate in the presence of a sP-like agent.

These data therefore appear to provide a unique insight into the organization of the pharmacology of the neurotransmitter systems that influence the terminals of primary afferents from which sP originates.

4. Other Afferent Peptide Neurotransmitters

Although the emphasis in the present chapter is directed at sP, it also appears that comparable studies can and will be carried out with other putative neurotransmitters. We have observed that VIP- and CCK-like immunoreactivity is also released from the dorsal horn of the spinal cord by high- but not low-intensity stimulation but that this release is not evoked by capsaicinlike drugs, and in our hands the levels of these materials in spinal cord as measured by radioimmunoassay are not reduced by capsaicin (Yaksh *et al.*, 1982). Kawatani *et al.* (1983) observed that VIP levels, which are relatively low in the lumbar cord, are exceedingly high in the sacral cord.

In recent studies, Blank and colleagues (1984) observed that stimulation of the pelvic nerve resulted in highly significant increases in the level of collectable VIP in spinal superfusates. These elevated levels contrast remarkably with the rather meager release that we have observed following sciatic nerve stimulation. This correlation between degree of release produced by afferent input and content is an important observation suggesting validation of the superfusion procedures. Studies comparable to those described for sP-like immunoreactivity should be performed for VIP released by pelvic nerve stimulation to determine the pharmacology of its release. As noted, such studies permit us not only to examine the phenomenon of release but also to determine the characteristics of the receptors that govern the excitability of the primary afferent terminals from which the putative neurotransmitter is released.

5. *Considerations of the Nonclassical Aspects of Primary Afferent Neurotransmitter Function*

Finally, I would like to note that the emphasis has been directed at the pharmacology of central terminals. Substance P is found, however, also in peripheral terminals such as in cortical blood vessels (Moskowitz *et al.*, 1979; Mayberg *et al.*, 1981), tooth pulp (Olgart *et al.*, 1977), and eye (Bill *et al.*, 1979). Nearly four times as much sP is transported peripherally as centrally (Brimijoin *et al.*, 1980). Stimulation of the trigeminal nerve has been shown to release sP from tooth pulp (Broden *et al.*, 1981). Such stimulation, as does exogenously administered sP, produces an increase in local blood flow and capillary permeability. The effects of either manipulation are reversed by putative sP antagonists (Rosell *et al.*, 1981; Couture and Cuello, 1983). These observations appear to reflect mechanisms that may be quite common. Thus, the axon flare reflex secondary to injury and the extravasation that occurs in the distribution of the peripheral nerve after proximal electrical stimulation clearly reflect local dilatation and changes in vascular permeability (see comments by Campbell and Meyer, Chapter 3). Moskowitz and colleagues (1979) have indeed argued that the sP in plexi surrounding cerebral vessels and originating in the trigeminal ganglion may be released and occasion the vascular syndrome of migraine.

It should be stressed that antidromic nerve activity in dorsal roots secondary to afferent input in an adjacent root is readily demonstrated and is commonly seen in the early phases of primary afferent depolarization (Barron and Matthews, 1939; Eccles *et al.*, 1961, 1962). In elegant work, Selzer and Spencer (1969) indeed described the ability of visceral and somatic afferent terminals to mutually produce primary afferent depolarization and dorsal root reflexes in the other. Thus, given that visceral and autonomic terminals possess stores of sP that are associated with primary afferents (see Cuello *et al.*, 1982), one might propose a very credible mechanism whereby somatic input may directly interact with autonomic/visceral systems and *vice versa*. Moreover, it raises the intriguing possibility that as the activity of central terminals is governed by selected receptor populations, so might the peripheral terminals also be governed. Indeed, the characteristics of the effects of neurotoxins (such as capsaicin) after topical application to the skin or to the cord are identical (Jhamandas *et al.*, 1984). These observations together thus suggest that the primary afferent neurotransmitter systems may play a pervasive role far beyond their coding of afferent information by also influencing peripheral vascular and autonomic systems.

In short, it appears that we are just beginning to shed light on the field of primary afferent pharmacology, and to our surprise, we find that we are only beginning to see the complexity of the role played by this first-order link.

ACKNOWLEDGMENTS. I should like to thank my collaborators, Dr. V. L. W. Go, Ms. Gail Harty, Ms. Sandra Michener, and Ms. Ann Rockafellow, without whom much of the work described herein would not have been possible. Work described in this paper was supported in part by funds from NS16541 and the Mayo Foundation.

References

ABAY, E. O. *Studies in Intrathecal Capsaicin in the Cat,* Masters Degree Thesis, Mayo Medical School, 1982.

AKAGI, H., OTSUKA, M., AND YANAGISAWA, M. Identification by high-performance liquid chromatography of immunoreactive substance P released from isolated rat spinal cord. *Neurosci. Lett.* 20:259–263, 1980.

AKERMAN, B., ROSELL, S., AND FOLKERS, K. Intrathecal (D-PRO^2, D-TRP^{7,9})-SP elicits hypoalgesia and motor blockade in the rat and antagonizes noxious responses induced by substance P. *Acta Physiol. Scand.* 114:631–633, 1982.

BARRON, D. H., AND MATTHEWS, B. H. C. Dorsal root reflexes. *J. Physiol. (Lond.)* 94:26P–27P, 1939.

BENNETT, J. P., JR., LOGAN, W. J., AND SNYDER, S. H. Amino acids as central nervous transmitters: The influence of ions, amino acid analogues, and ontogeny on transport systems for L-glutamic and L-aspartic acids and glycine into central nervous synaptosomes of the rat. *J. Neurochem.* 21:1533–1550, 1973.

BERGSTRÖM, L., HAMMOND, D. L., GO, V. L. W., AND YAKSH, T. L. Concurrent measurement of substance P and serotonin in spinal superfusates: Failure of capsaicin and *p*-chloroamphetamine to co-release. *Brain Res.* 270:181–184, 1983.

BESSON, J. M., CATCHLOVE, R. F. H., FELTZ, P., AND LE BARS, D. Further evidence for postsynaptic inhibitions on lamina V dorsal horn interneurons. *Brain Res.* 66:531–536, 1974.

BILL, A., STJERNSCHANTZ, J., MANDAHL, A., BRODIN, E., AND NILSSON, G. Substance P: Release on trigeminal nerve stimulation, effects in the eye. *Acta Physiol. Scand.* 106:371–373, 1979.

BLANK, M. A., ANARD, P., LUMB, B. M., MORRISON, J., AND BLOOM, S. R. Release of vasoactive intestinal polypeptide-like immunoreactivity (VIP) from cat urinary bladder and sacral spinal cord during pelvic nerve stimulation. *Dig. Dis. Sci.* 27:11S, 1984.

BRIMIJOIN, S., LUNDBERG, J. M., BRODIN, E., HÖKFELT, T., AND NILSSON, G. Axonal transport of substance P in the vagus and sciatic nerves of the guinea pig. *Brain Res.* 191:443–457, 1980.

BRODIN, E., GAZELIUS, B., OLGART, L., AND NILSSON, G. Tissue concentration and release of substance P-like immunoreactivity in the dental pulp. *Acta Physiol. Scand.* 111:141–149, 1981.

CARSTENS, E., TULLOCH, I., ZIEGLGÄNSBERGER, W., AND ZIMMERMAN, M. Presynaptic excitability changes induced by morphine in single cutaneous afferent C- and A-fibers. *Pflugers Arch.* 379:143–147, 1979.

CERVERO, F., SHOUENBORG, J., SJÖLUND, B. H., AND WADDELL, P. J. Cutaneous inputs to dorsal horn neurones in adult rats treated at birth with capsaicin. *J. Physiol. (Lond.)* 301:47–57, 1984.

COUTURE, R., AND CUELLO, A. C. Substance P antagonists and the antidromic stimulation of peripheral sensory branches of the trigeminal nerve, in: *Substance P* (P. SKRABANEK AND D. POWELL, eds.) Boole Press, Dublin, 1983, pp. 192–193.

CUELLO, C. A., PRIESTLEY, J. V., AND MATTHEWS, M. R. Localization of substance P in neuronal pathways. *Ciba Found. Symp.* 91:55–83, 1982.

CURTIS, D. R., AND JOHNSTON, G. A. R. Amino acid transmitters in the mammalian central nervous system. *Rev. Physiol.* 69:98–188, 1974.

DALSGAARD, C.-J., VINCENT, S. R., HÖKFELT, T., LUNDBERG, J. M., DAHLSTRÖM, A., SCHULTZBERG, M., DOCKRAY, G. J., AND CUELLO, A. C. Coexistence of cholecystokinin- and substance P-like peptides in neurons of the dorsal root ganglia of the rat. *Neurosci. Lett.* 33:159–163, 1982.

ECCLES, J. C., ECCLES, R. M., AND MAGNI, F. Central inhibitory action attributable to presynaptic depolarization produced by muscle afferent volleys. *J. Physiol. (Lond.)* 159:147–166, 1961.

ECCLES, J. C., KOSTYUK, P. G., AND SCHMIDT, R. F. Central pathways responsible for depolarization of primary afferent fibers. *J. Physiol. (Lond.)* 161:237–257, 1962.

FITZGERALD, M. Capsaicin and sensory neurones—a review. *Pain* 15:109–130, 1983.

FOLKERS, K., HÖRIG, J., ROSELL, S., AND BJÖRKROTH, U. Chemical design of antagonists of substance P. *Acta Physiol. Scand.* 111:505–506, 1981.

GAME, C. J. A., AND LODGE, D. The pharmacology of the inhibition of dorsal horn neurones by impulses in myelinated cutaneous afferents in the cat. *Exp. Brain Res.* 23:75–84, 1975.

GAMSE, R. Capsaicin and nociception in the rat and mouse. *Naunyn Schmiedebergs Arch. Pharmacol.* 320:205–216, 1982.

GAMSE, R., LEEMAN, S., HOLZER, P., AND LEMBECK, F. Differential effects of capsaicin on the content of somatostatin, substance P, and neurotensin in the nervous system of the rat. *Naunyn Schmiedebergs Arch. Pharmacol.* 317:140–148, 1981.

GAMSE, R., PETSCHE, U., LEMBECK, F., AND JANSCO, G. Capsaicin applied to peripheral nerve inhibits axoplasmic transport of substance P and somatostatin. *Brain Res.* 239:447–462, 1982.

HENRY, J. L. Effects of substance P on functionally identified units in cat spinal cord. *Brain Res.* 114:439–451, 1976.

HÖKFELT, T., KELLERTH, J. O., NILSSON, G., AND PERNOW, B. Experimental immunohistochemical studies on the localization and distribution of substance P in cat primary sensory neurons. *Brain Res.* 100:235–252, 1975.

HÖKFELT, T., ELDE, R., JOHANSSON, O., LUFT, R., NILSSON, G., AND ARIMURA, A. Immunohistochemical evidence for separate populations of somatostatin-containing and substance P-containing primary afferent neurons in the rat. *Neuroscience* 1:131–136, 1976.

HÖKFELT, T., JOHANSSON, O., LJUNGDAHL, A., LUNDBERG, J. M., AND SCHULTZBERG, M. Peptidergic neurones. *Nature* 284:515–521, 1980.

HYLDEN, J., AND WILCOX, G. L. Intrathecal substance P elicits a caudally-directed biting and scratching behavior. *Brain Res.* 217:212–215, 1981.

IVERSEN, L. L., HANLEY, M. R., SANDBERG, B. E. B., LEE, C.-M., PINNOCK, R. D., AND WATSON, S. P. Substance P receptors in the nervous system and possible receptor subtypes. *Ciba* 91:186–205, 1982.

JAHR, C. E., AND JESSELL, T. M. ATP excites a subpopulation of rat dorsal horn neurons. *Nature* 304:730–732, 1983.

JANCSO, H., HÖKFELT, T., LUNDBERG, J. M., KIRALY, E., HALÁSZ, N., NILSSON, G., TERENIUS, L., REHFELD, J., STEINBUSCH, H., VERHOFSTAD, A., ELDE, R., SAID, S., AND BROWN, M. Immunohistochemical studies on the effect of capsaicin on spinal and medullary peptide and monoamine neurons using antisera to substance P, gastrin/CCK, somatostatin, VIP, enkephalin, neurotensin, and 5-hydroxytryptamine. *J. Neurocytol.* 10:963–980, 1981.

JEFTINIJA, S., MILETIC, V., AND RANDIC, M. Cholecystokinin octapeptide excites dorsal horn neurons both *in vivo* and *in vitro*. *Brain Res.* 213:231–236, 1981a.

JEFTINIJA, S., SEMBA, K., AND RANDIC, M. Norepinephrine reduces excitability of single cutaneous primary afferent C-fibers in the cat spinal cord. *Brain Res.* 219:456–463, 1981b.

JEFTINIJA, S., MURASE, K., NEDELJKOV, V., AND RANDIC, M. Vasoactive intestinal polypeptide excites mammalian dorsal horn neurons both *in vivo* and *in vitro*. *Brain Res.* 243:158–164, 1982.

JESSELL, T. M. Substance P in nociceptive sensory neurons in: *Substance P in the Nervous System.* Ciba Foundation Symposium 91, Pittman, London, 1982, pp. 225–248.

JESSELL, T. M., AND IVERSEN, L. L. Opiate analgesics inhibit substance P release from rat trigeminal nucleus. *Nature* 268:549–551, 1977.

JESSELL, T. M., IVERSEN, L. L., AND CUELLO, A. C. Capsaicin induced depletion of substance P from primary sensory neurones. *Brain Res.* 152:183–188, 1978.

JHAMANDAS, K., YAKSH, T. L., HARTY, G., SZOLCSANYI, J., AND GO, V. L. W. Action of intrathecal capsaicin and its structural analogues on the content and release of spinal substance P: Selectivity of action and relationship to analgesia. *Brain Res.* 306:215–225, 1984.

JONES, R. S. G., AND OLPE, H.-R. A structure–activity profile of substance P and some of its fragments on supraspinal neurones in the rat. *Neurosci. Lett.* 33:67–71, 1982.

KAWATANI, M., LOWE, I. P., NADELHAFT, I., MORGAN, C., AND DE GROAT, W. C. Vasoactive intestinal polypeptide in visceral afferent pathways to the sacral spinal cord of the cat. *Neurosci. Lett.* 42:311–316, 1983.

KNYIHAR-CSILLIK, E., AND CSILLIK, B. FRAP: Histochemistry of the primary nociceptive neuron. *Prog. Histochem. Cytochem.* 14:1–137, 1981.

KOENIG, E. Synthesis mechanisms in the axon. II. RNA in myelin-free axons of the cat. *J. Neurochem.* 12:357–361, 1965.

KURAISHI, Y., HIROTA, N., SUGIMOTO, M., SATOH, M., AND TAKAGI, H. Effects of morphine on noxious stimuli-induced release of substance P from rabbit dorsal horn *in vivo*. *Life Sci.* 33:693–696, 1983.

LUNDBERG, J. M., HÖKFELT, T., NILSSON, G., TERENIUS, L., REHFELD, J., ELDE, R., AND SAID, S. Peptide neurons in the vagus splanchnic and sciatic nerves. *Acta Physiol. Scand.* 104:499–501, 1978.

LUNDBERG, J. M., FAHRENKRUG, J., AND BRIMIJOIN, S. Characteristics of the axonal transport of vasoactive intestinal polypeptide in nerves of the cat. *Acta Physiol. Scand.* (in press), 1985.

LYNN, B., AND HUNT, S. P. Afferent C-fibres: Physiological and biochemical correlations. *Trends Neurosci.* 7:186–188, 1984.

MALFROY, B., SWERTS, J. P., LLORENS, C., AND SCHWARTZ, J. C. Regional distribution of a high-affinity enkephalin-degrading peptidase ('enkephalinase') and effects of lesions suggest localization in the vicinity of opiate receptors in brain. *Neurosci. Lett.* 11:329–334, 1979.

MAYBERG, M., LANGER, R. S., ZERVAS, N. T., AND MOSKOWITZ, M. A. Perivascular meningeal projections from cat trigeminal ganglia: Possible pathway for vascular headaches in man. *Science* 213:228–230, 1981.

MCLENNON, H. *Synaptic Transmission*, W. B. Saunders, Philadelphia, 1970.

MENDELL, L. M. Physiological properties of unmyelinated fiber projection to the spinal cord. *Exp. Neurol.* 16:316–332, 1966.

MICEVYCH, P. E., YAKSH, T. L., AND SZOLCSANYI, J. Effect of intrathecal capsaicin analogues on the immunofluorescence peptides and serotonin in the dorsal horn in rats. *Neuroscience* 8:123–131, 1983.

MOSKOWITZ, M. A., REINHARD, J. F., JR., ROMERO, J., MELAMED, E., AND PETTIBONE, D. J. Neurotransmitters and the fifth cranial nerve: Is there a relation to the headache phase of migrane? *Lancet* 1:883–885, 1979.

MUDGE, A. W., LEEMAN, S. E., AND FISCHBACH, G. D. Enkephalin inhibits release of substance P from sensory neurons in culture and decreases action potential duration. *Proc. Natl. Acad. Sci. U.S.A.* 76:526–530, 1979.

MURASE, K., AND RANDIC, M. Actions of substance P on rat spinal dorsal horn neurones. *J. Physiol. (Lond.)* 346:203–217, 1984.

NAGY, J. J. AND HUNT, S. P. Fluoride-resistant acid phosphatase-containing neurones in dorsal root ganglia are separate from those containing substance P or somatostatin. *Neuroscience* 7:89–97, 1982.

NAGY, J. J. AND HUNT, S. P. The termination of primary afferents within the rat dorsal horn: Evidence for rearrangement following capsaicin treatment. *J. Comp. Neurol.* 218:145–158, 1983.

NAGY, J. J., EMSON, P. C. AND IVERSON, L. L. A re-evaluation of the neurochemical and antinociceptive effects of intrathecal capsaicin in the rat. *Brain Res.* 211:497–502, 1981.

NAGY, J. J., IVERSEN, L. L. GOEDERT, M., CHAPMAN, D., AND HUNT, S. P. Dose-dependent effects of capsaicin on primary sensory neurons in the neonatal rat. *J. Neurosci.* 3:399–406, 1983.

NAROTZKY, R. A., AND KERR, F. W. L. Marginal neurons of the spinal cord: Types, afferent synaptology and functional considerations. *Brain Res.* 139:1–20, 1978.

NOWAK, L. M., AND MACDONALD, R. L. Substance P: Ionic basis for depolarizing responses of mouse spinal cord neurons in cell culture. *J. Neurosci.* 2:1119–1128, 1982.

OLGART, L., HÖKFELT, T., NILSSON, G., AND PERNOW, B. Localization of substance P-like immunoreactivity in nerves in the tooth pulp. *Pain* 4:153–159, 1977.

OTSUKA, K., AND KONISHI, S. Substance P, an excitatory transmitter of primary sensory neurones. *Cold Spring Harbor Symp. Quant. Biol.* 40:135–143, 1976a.

OTSUKA, M., AND KONISHI, S. Release of substance P-like immunoreactivity from isolated spinal cord of newborn rat. *Nature* 264:83–84, 1976b.

PANULA, P., YANG, H. Y., AND COSTA, E. Neurohumoral localization of bombesin-like immunoreactivity in the CNS of the rat. *Regul. Peptides* 4:275–283, 1982.

PANULA, P., HADJICONSTANTINOU, M., YANG, H. Y., AND COSTA, E. Immunohistochemical localization of bombesin, substance P and gastrin-releasing peptide in primary sensory neurons. *J. Neurosci.* 3:2021–2029, 1983.

PIERCEY, M. F., AND EINSPAHR, F. J. Use of substance P partial fragments to characterize substance P receptors of cat dorsal horn neurons. *Brain Res.* 187:481–486, 1980.

PIERCEY, M. F., DOBRY, P. J. K., SCHROEDER, L. A., AND EINSPAHR, F. J. Behavioral evidence that substance P may be a spinal cord sensory neurotransmitter. *Brain Res.* 210:407–412, 1981a.

PIERCEY, M. F., SCHROEDER, L. A., FOLKERS, K., XU, J. C., AND HORIG, J. Sensory and motor functions of spinal cord substance P. *Science* 14:60–65, 1981b.

RACKHAM, A., THERRIAULT, M., AND WOOD, P. L. Substance P: Evidence for spinal mediation of some behavioural effects. *Neuropharmacology* 20:753–755, 1981.

RANDIC, M., AND MILETIC, V. Effect of substance P in cat dorsal horn neurones activated by noxious stimuli. *Brain Res.* 128:164–169, 1977.

RANDIC, M., AND MILETIC, V. Depressant actions of methionine–enkephalin and somatostatin in cat dorsal horn neurones activated by noxious stimuli. *Brain Res.* 152:196–202, 1978.

ROSELL, S., OLGART, L., GAZELIUS, B., PANOPOULOS, P., FOLKERS, K., AND HÖRIG, J. Inhibition of antidromic and substance P-induced vasodilatation by a substance P-antagonist. *Acta Physiol. Scand.* 111:381–382, 1981.

SASTRY, B. R. Potentiation of presynaptic inhibition of nociceptive pathways as a mechanism for analgesia. *Can. J. Physiol. Pharmacol.* 58:97–100, 1980.

SAWYNOK, J., KATO, N., HAVLICEK, V., AND LABELLA, F. S. Lack of effect of baclofen on substance P and somatostatin release from the spinal cord *in vitro*. *Naunyn Schmiedeberg's Arch. Pharmacol.* 319:78–81, 1982.

SCHMAUSS, C. AND YAKSH, T. L. *In vivo* studies on spinal opiate receptor systems mediating antinoreception. II. Pharmacological profiles suggesting a differential association of mu, delta, and kappa receptors with visceral, chemical, and cutaneous thermal stimuli in the rat. *J. Pharmacol. Exp. Ther.* 228:1–12, 1984.

SELZER, M., AND SENCER, W. A. Interactions between visceral and cutaneous afferents in the spinal cord: Reciprocal primary afferent fiber depolarization. *Brain Res.* 14:349–366, 1969.

SEYBOLD, V. S., HYLDEN, J. L. K., AND WILCOX, G. L. Intrathecal substance P and somatostatin in rats: Behaviors indicative of sensation. *Peptides* 3:49–54, 1982.

SHEPPARD, M., KHRONHEIM, S., ADAMS, C., AND PIMSTONE, B. Immunoreactive somatostatin release from rat spinal cord *in vitro*. *Neurosci. Lett.* 15:65–70, 1979.

SIESJÖ, B. K. Cell damage in the brain: A speculative synthesis. *J. Cereb. Blood Flow Metab.* 1:155–185, 1981.

SINGER, E., AND PLACHETA, P. Reduction of [^{3}H]muscimol binding sites in rat dorsal spinal cord after neonatal capsaicin treatment. *Brain Res.* 202:484–487, 1980.

SINGER, E. A., SPERK, G., AND SCHMID, R. Capsaicin does not change tissue levels of glutamic acid, its uptake, or release in the rat spinal cord. *J. Neurochem.* 38:1383–1386, 1982.

TAKAHASHI, T., AND OTSUKA, M. Regional distribution of substance P in the spinal cord and nerve roots of the cat and the effect of dorsal root section. *Brain Res.* 87:1–11, 1975.

TANG, J., CHOU, J., YANG, H.-Y. T., AND COSTA, E. The effect of peptidase inhibitors on the release of met^5-enk-arg^6-phe^7 (YGGFMRF) and met^5-enkephalin (YGGFM) from spinal cord induced by substance P *in vivo*. *Life Sci.* 33:121–124, 1983.

TYCE, G. M., AND YAKSH, T. L. Monoamine release from cat spinal cord by somatic stimuli: An intrinsic modulatory system. *J. Physiol. (Lond.)* 314:513–529, 1981.

URBAN, L., AND RANDIC, M. Slow excitatory transmission in rat dorsal horn: Possible mediation by peptides. *Brain Res.* 290:336–341, 1984.

WALL, P. D., AND FITZGERALD, M. If substance P fails to fulfil the criteria as a neurotransmitter in somatosensory afferents, what might be its function? *Ciba Found. Symp.* 91:249–266, 1982.

WALL, P. D., FITZGERALD, M., AND GIBSON, S. J. The response of rat spinal cord cells to unmyelinated afferents after peripheral nerve section and after changes in substance P levels. *Neuroscience* 6:2205–2215, 1981.

WILLIAMS, J. T., AND ZIEGLGÄNSBERGER, W. The acute effects of capsaicin on rat primary afferents and spinal neurons. *Brain Res.* 253:125–131, 1982.

WRIGHT, D. M., AND ROBERTS, M. H. T. Supersensitivity to a substance P analogue following dorsal root section. *Life Sci.* 22:19–24, 1977.

WRIGHT, D. M., AND ROBERTS, M. H. T. Responses of spinal neurones to a substance P analogue, noxious pinch and bradykinin. *Eur. J. Pharmacol.* 64:165–167, 1980.

YAKSH, T. L., AND ELDE, R. P. Factors governing release of methionine enkephalin-like immunoreactivity from mesencephalon and spinal cord of the cat *in vivo. J. Neurophysiol.* 46:1056–1075, 1981.

YAKSH, T. L., AND TYCE, G. M. Resting and K^+ evoked release of serotonin and norepinephrine *in vivo* from the cat and rat spinal cord. *Brain Res.* 192:133–146, 1980.

YAKSH, T. L., FARB, D., LEEMAN, S., AND JESSELL, T. Intrathecal capsaicin depletes substance P in the rat spinal cord and produces prolonged thermal analgesia. *Science* 206:481–483, 1979.

YAKSH, T. L., JESSELL, T. M., GAMSE, R., MUDGE, A. W., AND LEEMAN, S. E. Intrathecal morphine inhibits substance P release from mammalian spinal cord *in vivo. Nature* 286:155–156, 1980.

YAKSH, T. L., ABAY, E. O., AND GO, V. L. W. Studies on the location and release of cholecystokinin and vasoactive intestinal peptide in rat and cat spinal cord. *Brain Res.* 242:279–290, 1982.

YAKSH, T. L., TERENIUS, L., NYBERG, F., JHAMANDAS, K., AND WANG, J.-Y. Studies on the release by somatic stimulation from rat and cat spinal cord of active materials which displace dihydromorphine in an opiate-binding assay. *Brain Res.* 268:119–128, 1983.

YAKSH, T. L., MICEVYCH, P. E., ELDE, R. P., AND GO, V. L. W. Spinal neurotransmitter systems associated with activity in the rostrad transmission systems by pain-evoking stimuli. *Adv. Pain Res. Ther.* 7:27–42, 1984.

ZIEGLGÄNSBERGER, W. AND PUIL, E. A. Actions of glutamic acid on spinal neurons. *Exp. Brain Res.* 17:35–49, 1973.

ZIEGLGÄNSBERGER, W., AND TULLOCH, I. F. Effects of substance P on neurones in the dorsal horn of the spinal cord of the cat. *Brain Res.* 166:273–282, 1979.

9
Dorsal Horn Neurons and Their Sensory Inputs

FERNANDO CERVERO

A. *Introduction*

The mammalian skin is innervated by a variety of afferent nerve fibers connected to highly specialized sensory detectors whose adequate stimulation leads to the experience of tactile, thermal, or painful sensations. Microneurographic studies of human sensory nerves have demonstrated a direct correlation between the functional properties of a given sensory detector and the elementary sensory experience evoked by its stimulation (Ochoa and Torebjörk, 1983). Under normal circumstances, this elementary specificity of cutaneous sensory receptors (see Winkelmann, Chapter 2, and Campbell and Meyer, Chapter 3) is subjected to the integrative and modulatory influences of the central nervous system. Therefore, complex sensory perceptions are the consequence of the activation of specific sensory channels whose output can be profoundly modified by the activity of other pathways within the central nervous system.

Sensory processing can occur at every level of synaptic relay in the somatosensory pathway. The link between the terminals of primary afferent fibers in the spinal cord and the second-order neurons of the dorsal horn provides the first opportunity for interactive modulations between sensory channels or for the action of descending systems from supraspinal areas. Discussion of such modulating substrates may be found in Chapters 8, 10, and 15. Indeed, the concept of modulation plays an important role in the spinal systems that encode the vast amount of afferent input (see Chapter 18

FERNANDO CERVERO • Department of Physiology, The Medical School, University of Bristol, Bristol BS8 1TD, England.

and 19). In this discussion, the properties of the dorsal horn neurons that receive the afferent inflow are reviewed in relation to the contributions that this relay system makes to somatosensory processing.

Our current knowledge of dorsal horn structure and function comes from a variety of sources and has been gathered by scientists whose particular interests in research were also varied. A major contribution to this field has been made by scientists interested in somatosensory mechanisms, but many key observations on dorsal horn physiology come from studies on motor control, spinal organization of reflex activity, development of sensory systems, degeneration and regeneration in the central nervous system, altered sensory perception after peripheral nerve injury, and, more recently, on neurochemical and neuropharmacological aspects of synaptic transmission in sensory pathways.

Most of these lines of research are based on the 150-year-old "Law of Bell and Magendie," which proposed the dorsoventral separation of sensory and motor organization in the spinal cord (see Coggeshall, Chapter 4). It is to some extent surprising that this rigid separation has been questioned only very recently. For many years, sensory physiologists did not cross the dividing line between the dorsal and the ventral horn of the spinal cord, whereas those interested in the organization of spinal reflexes studied the relevant neuronal circuitry entirely within the ventral horn. A close examination of the common paths for sensory and motor function within the spinal gray matter is still lacking, but it is very likely that many dorsal horn neurons contribute to both sensory processing and reflex activity. It is also well known that some somatosensory pathways originate from neurons whose cell bodies are located in the ventral horn. The traditional close association between sensory mechanisms in the spinal cord and the functional organization of the dorsal horn should be reexamined and a less rigid distinction established between sensory and motor functions of the spinal cord. This also applies to the analysis of nociception and pain, an area of research responsible for many studies on the anatomy and physiology of dorsal horn sensory systems. Transmission of nociceptive information through the spinal cord is often regarded as the interactive work of a relay station in or around the superficial layers of the dorsal horn. But, on the other hand, nociceptive thresholds are not uncommonly measured as variations in latency and intensity of spinal reflexes (i.e., the tail-flick test).

Although the study of peripheral inputs to dorsal horn neurons can be a useful tool to analyze the organization of the afferent projection to the central nervous system, a full understanding of the way in which the spinal cord integrates incoming sensory information requires a more comprehensive view of the whole system. Account has to be taken of the contributions made to the integrated message by motor and reflex activity as well as by the immediate sensory relay. Therefore, the data reviewed here on the electrophysiology of dorsal horn neurons should be linked to other pieces of information on spinal cord structure and function before models for the organization of spinal sensory systems can be proposed.

B. Dorsal Horn Nomenclature

Having gone through the looking glass, Alice finally came face to face with Humpty Dumpty, who confused her with his strange use of words. But when Alice objected, Humpty Dumpty replied in rather a scornful tone: "When *I* use a word it means just what *I* choose it to mean—neither more nor less." "The question is," insisted Alice, "whether you can make words mean so many different things." "The question is," replied Humpty Dumpty, "which is to be master, that's all" (Carroll, 1872).

The lack of a common and meaningful nomenclature has been, and still is, one of the greatest obstacles for the understanding of the anatomy and physiology of the dorsal horn. This lack of uniformity applies to the nomenclature used for the topography of the dorsal horn, for the anatomic descriptions of the different cell types, for the names used to designate functional categories of neuronal response and even for the type of incoming signals to dorsal horn neurons produced by a given form of peripheral stimulation. Dorsal horn nomenclature is a beginner's nightmare and a continuous scource of conflict between individual scientists. There have been several attempts to agree on a common nomenclature and, more important than that, on a common meaning of concepts and hypotheses. So far these attempts have had little success. "The question is"—one should remember—"which is to be master, that's all."

It is not the intention of this chapter to make matters worse by supporting one or another nomenclature, or even worse still by suggesting a new classification. Rather, the following paragraphs give the equivalences between different nomenclatures with a short comment on their use. An excellent account of the various classifications and a comprehensive table of dorsal horn nomenclature was published by Willis and Coggeshall (1978).

1. Dorsal Horn Topography

Nomenclature of dorsal horn topography has gone through two distinct historical eras: before Rexed and after Rexed. In 1952, Rexed proposed the anatomic division of the spinal cord gray matter into ten regions or laminae oriented along the dorsoventral axis of the cord and designated by Roman numerals I to X (Figure 1). Before Rexed, the nomenclature of dorsal horn topography was a lot more colorful and a lot less precise, largely but loosely based on Latin terms from the *Nomina Anatomica.* Rexed's proposal met with some criticism, particularly on the grounds of the somewhat artificial boundaries between some of the laminae. However, its simplicity and the chance to replace a complicated set of long Latin words with a list of ten Roman numerals have made Rexed's lamination a universally accepted nomenclature, extrapolated without objections from the cat, where it was originally proposed, to practically every mammal studied.

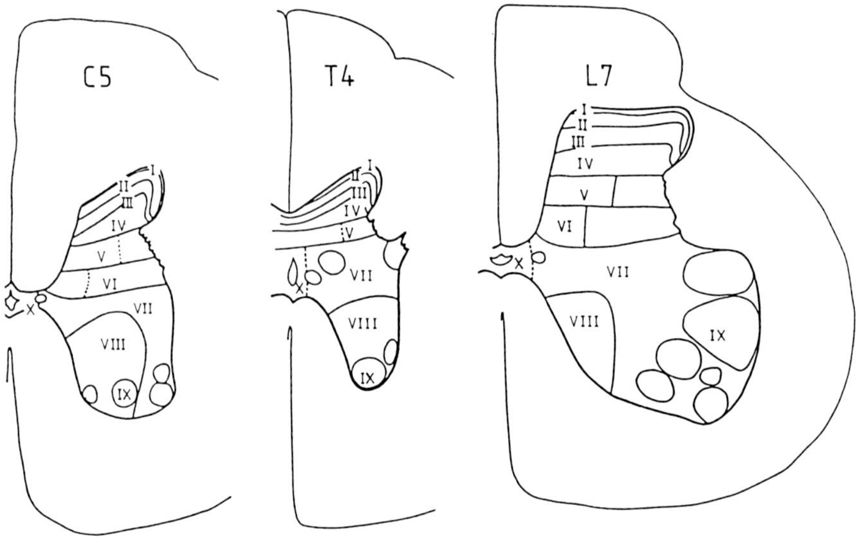

FIGURE 1. Schematic diagram indicating the locations of Rexed's laminae in the segments C5, T4, and L7 of the adult cat's spinal cord. The dorsal horn is generally considered to correspond to laminae I to VI. (From Rexed, 1952.)

A certain amount of confusion was created as a consequence of the different equivalence assumed by a number of authors between some of Rexed's laminae and those dorsal horn regions that retained pre-Rexed names, such as the substantia gelatinosa and the marginal zone. This particular dispute is now over—or nearly over—and the interested reader is therefore referred to a review article in which the matter was discussed at some length (Cervero and Iggo, 1980). It is now generally accepted that the marginal zone corresponds to Rexed's lamina I and the substantia gelatinosa to Rexed's lamina II. In the past, the substantia gelatinosa was referred to by some as Rexed's laminae II and III together.

2. *Histology of Dorsal Horn Neurons*

Current reports on the anatomy and physiology of the substantia gelatinosa (lamina II) tend to use the nomenclature of histological cell types proposed recently by Gobel, who has conducted comprehensive anatomic examinations of the superficial layers of the trigeminal nucleus caudalis and of the dorsal horn (Gobel, 1976, 1978a,b; Falls and Gobel, 1979). Other reports still maintain the nomenclature for cell types in the substantia gelatinosa that has been available since Cajal's histological examinations of the spinal cord (Ramon y Cajal, 1891, 1909). Cajal described two main cell types in the substantia gelatinosa: central cells and limiting cells, renamed islet cells and stalked cells by Gobel. Cajal's terms are topographical; Gobel's relate to the appearance of the cells. Both are perfectly adequate, although users of Cajal's or of Gobel's nomenclature seem to have different perceptions of historical time scales. However, a recent report by Bicknell and Beal (1984) suggests that islet, stalked, central and limiting cells of the substantia gelatinosa may be four anatomically different kinds of neurons. Further discussion of the histochemistry and anatomy of the dorsal gray can be found in Chapters 5 and 7.

3. *Functional Classification of Dorsal Horn Neurons*

The need to classify dorsal horn neurons according to their peripheral inputs has stimulated the imagination of sensory neurophysiologists. Several classifications coexist in the literature so that the same kind of functional response can be described by three or four different names depending on individual preferences. Wall (1967, 1973) calls "lamina 4-type neurons" those that are driven only by innocuous stimulation of the skin and "lamina 5-type neurons" those that are driven by noxious and by innocuous stimulation. This arose from the now outdated concept of a "cascade" of neurons in the dorsal horn in which neurons of one lamina projected onto cells located in the immediately ventral lamina. As it is possible to find "lamina 4-type neurons" outside lamina IV and "lamina 5-type neurons" outside lamina V, this nomenclature is not widely used.

Iggo and co-workers (Iggo, 1974; Handwerker *et al.*, 1975; Cervero *et al.*, 1976) have used a numerical system of classification: class 1 neurons are those driven only by low-threshold mechanoreceptors from the skin; class 2 neurons are driven by low-threshold mechanoreceptors and by nociceptors; and class 3 neurons are driven only by nociceptors, either mechanonociceptors (class 3a) or mechano- and thermal nociceptors (class 3b).

A nomenclature first proposed by Mendell (1966) and used now by many laboratories describes those dorsal horn neurons driven by noxious and by innocuous stimuli as "wide dynamic range (WDR)" and those with only one kind of peripheral input as either "low threshold (LT)" or "nociceptive specific (NS)." Other names found in current reports include "convergent neurons" for those with noxious and innocuous inputs (Le Bars and Chitour, 1983), "deep neurons" for those with inputs from subcutaneous structures (Willis *et al.*, 1974), "cold units" for those with an input from cold thermoreceptors (Iggo and Ramsey, 1976), and so on (see Willis and Coggeshall, 1978, for further details).

An attempt was made in 1980, on the occasion of an international symposium on dorsal horn sensory mechanisms (Brown and Rethelyi, 1981), to establish a common and universally acceptable nomenclature for the different functional types of dorsal horn neuron. The recommendations are contained in the symposium proceedings and suggest a new set of terms: mechanoreceptive neurons if they have inputs exclusively from skin mechanoreceptors, nocireceptive neurons if they are driven only by nociceptors, and multireceptive neurons if they are driven by both types of cutaneous receptor. In addition, the new proposal suggests that the denomination of a neuron should include information on the location of the cell body, destination of the axon, and nature of the peripheral drive. One of the examples used to illustrate this proposal is "hair-mechano-noci-multireceptive lamina V postsynaptic dorsal column neuron," or HNM-V-PSDC for short. This is a high-precision nomenclature but one unlikely to be received with a great deal of enthusiasm by authors and editors alike.

C. Receptive Fields of Dorsal Horn Neurons

Somatosensory functions of dorsal horn neurons are commonly analyzed in terms of their cutaneous receptive fields. Properties of peripheral receptive fields such as their location, size, type of afferent input, and strength of excitatory drives are usually interpreted as powerful indicators of the role played by central neurons in the processing of sensory information.

A cutaneous receptive field is generally defined as the area of skin from which the activity of a neuron can be influenced. This definition needs to be qualified when applied to the analysis of cutaneous receptive fields of dorsal horn neurons. Caveats to take into account include the following:

1. Cutaneous stimulation can influence the activity of a dorsal horn neuron through either excitation or inhibition. Many dorsal horn neurons have an excitatory and an inhibitory receptive field, either adjacent to each other or far apart (ipsi- or contralaterally). In some cases, excitatory and inhibitory drives coexist within the same skin area.
2. The development of neural connectivity between a cutaneous region and the dorsal horn and the long-term maintenance of such linkage are influenced by chemical as well as by electrical signals traveling back and forth between the spinal cord and the periphery. Rigorous studies of this long-term trophic relationship are much needed.
3. Mapping cutaneous receptive fields of dorsal horn neurons is usually carried out in acute electrophysiological experiments on decerebrate, spinalized, or anesthetized preparations. Under these conditions, peripheral inputs to the spinal cord may be subjected to central influences that are not necessarily present in the intact animal. Neurons may be described as having (or not having) a particular peripheral input when in fact that input is only active (or inactive) under the experimental procedure. This obstacle can be negotiated by careful use of combined electrical and natural stimulation of the peripheral input so that the hard-wired connectivity can be established as well as the functional linkage under the particular experimental circumstances.
4. The final caveat, and perhaps the most important of all, points to the

lack of direct evidence to link neuronal responses obtained in acute electrophysiological experiments with the sensory experiences of intact animals. It is assumed that a dorsal horn neuron that receives excitatory drives from the skin and sends this information to the brain must be involved in the processing of cutaneous sensory experiences. However, it is also likely that many of these neurons play a role in the control of reflex activity, in the triggering of autonomic reactions, or in the mechanisms of arousal. Resolving this ambiguity does indeed offer a considerable challenge to sensory physiologists.

D. *Afferent Input to Dorsal Horn Neurons*

Aside from the organization of the receptive fields, one can distinguish dorsal horn neurons on the basis of the particular physical stimulus that gives rise to their excitation. As noted above, and as is discussed further in a later section, many neurons in the spinal cord may be concurrently driven by several different stimulus modalities.

1. *Cutaneous Mechanoreceptors*

The mechanoreceptive input to the dorsal horn originates in the low-threshold, sensitive mechanoreceptors of the skin and is mediated by large and small myelinated afferent fibers (A fibers) (Brown and Iggo, 1967). Most species, with the apparent exception of man, have, in addition, a low-threshold mechanoreceptive input to the dorsal horn mediated by unmyelinated afferent fibers (C fibers) (Iggo, 1960).

Intracellular filling of primary afferent terminals with horseradish peroxidase (HRP) has demonstrated the existence of a close association among the functional type of peripheral mechanoreceptors, the morphology of their spinal cord terminals, and the area of projection of their afferent collaterals within the dorsal horn (Brown, 1981). The large A-β afferent fibers connected to sensitive mechanoreceptors distribute their axons to some or all of laminae III, IV, V, and the dorsal part of VI. Hair-follicle afferent fibers have dorsal horn collaterals that form the "flame-shaped arbors" described by Ramon y Cajal (1909). Synaptic buttons from these terminals are confined to lamina III, but occasionally a few buttons may be seen in the inner portion of lamina II or in the dorsal part of lamina IV. Hair-follicle mechanoreceptors connected to thin A-δ fibers distribute their dorsal horn collaterals in the same way as and with a similar morphology to the hair-follicle mechanoreceptors connected to thicker A-β fibers (Light and Perl, 1979b). Axons from other cutaneous mechanoreceptors have collaterals that terminate in a wider area of the dorsal horn, including the innermost part of lamina II and laminae III, IV, V, and dorsal VI (Brown, 1981). There is no projection from low-threshold mechanoreceptors with myelinated axons to laminae I and outer II. Figure 2 shows, in schematic form, some features of the distribution of primary afferent collaterals within the dorsal horn.

It has not been possible to inject markers into single, functionally identified C-fiber terminals, and therefore there is no direct evidence on the mode of termination within the spinal cord of single C-mechanoreceptive afferents. However, the type of cutaneous drive to neurons in the inner substantia gelatinosa (inner lamina II) and the general belief that most cutaneous C fibers terminate within lamina II point to the inner lamina II as a likely projection area for C-mechanoreceptive afferents (Light and Perl, 1979a,b).

Two types of dorsal horn neurons can be distinguished according to their mechanoreceptive input: (1) neurons with an exclusive mechanoreceptive drive from the skin (mechanoreceptive/class 1/low threshold/lamina 4-type) and (2) neurons with excitatory inputs from other types of cutaneous receptor (multireceptive/class 2/wide dynamic range/lamina 5-type). The properties of this second type of neuron are discussed below under a separate heading.

Mechanoreceptive neurons tend to be located in laminae III and IV. Some have long ascending axons that project through the spinocervical tract or the postsynaptic dorsal column pathway. Mechanoreceptive neurons have

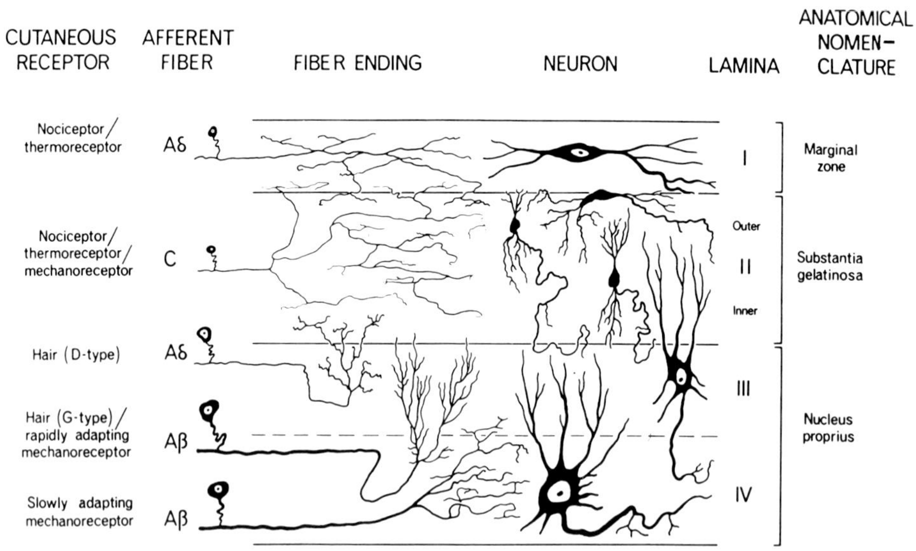

FIGURE 2. Schematic diagram of the neuronal organization of and afferent input to the superficial dorsal horn. To the left of the diagram, the types of afferent fiber and relevant receptor groups associated with them are listed. Fiber endings in the dorsal horn are schematized diagrams taken from published morphological studies. Neurons in the diagram represent standard neuron types in the superficial dorsal horn. Indicated at the right of the diagram are the laminar divisions of the superficial dorsal horn and corresponding anatomic nomenclature. (From Cervero and Iggo, 1980.)

also been found with axons in the spinoreticular or spinothalamic tracts. It is assumed that mechanoreceptive neurons encode tactile information by maintaining peripheral specificity (Willis and Coggeshall, 1978).

The responses of some neurons in the substantia gelatinosa to cutaneous stimulation suggest that their input is dominated by drives from C-mechanoreceptors. These are the neurons described as "slow-brush" (Light *et al.*, 1979) by reference to the type of cutaneous stimulation that activates them. Their functional role is obscure.

2. *Cutaneous Nociceptors*

Nociceptive information from the skin reaches the spinal cord via small A-δ fibers (mechanonociceptors) and C fibers (polymodal nociceptors). The former distribute their terminal arborizations within lamina I (the marginal zone) and send further collaterals to lamina V (Light and Perl, 1979b). The latter probably terminate within the substantia gelatinosa (lamina II), especially in the outer portions of this dorsal horn region (Light and Perl, 1979a) (Figure 2).

As with the mechanoreceptive input, two groups of neurons can be distinguished according to their responses to noxious stimulation of the skin: (1) neurons with an exclusive drive from cutaneous nociceptors (nocireceptive/class 3 (a and b)/nociceptor specific) and (2) neurons with excitatory inputs from other types of cutaneous receptor (multireceptive/class 2/wide dynamic range/lamina 5-type). Nocireceptive neurons can have an input from either mechanonociceptors only (class 3a) or from both mechano- and polymodal nociceptors (class 3b) (Cervero *et al.*, 1976). They are preferentially, but not exclusively, located in or around the marginal zone (lamina I), and it is generally acknowledged that most of the flat and relatively large marginal cells (Waldeyer cells) in this region are nocireceptive (Molony *et al.*, 1981). A proportion of nocireceptive lamina I neurons send their axons to supraspinal regions (Cervero *et al*, 1979a), notably through the spinoreticular and spinothalamic tracts (Willis and Coggeshall, 1978). For this reason, and in view of their responses to cutaneous noxious stimulation, nocireceptive cells are believed to play a key role in the transmission of sensory information that will eventually lead to the experience of cutaneous pain.

3. *Cutaneous Thermoreceptors*

Cutaneous thermoreceptors (cold and warm receptors) are connected to small A-δ and C fibers (Iggo, 1969). Little is known about the pattern of termination within the dorsal horn of identified cutaneous thermoreceptors. Some of the neurons in the superficial dorsal horn appear to be exclusively driven by thermoreceptors, particularly cold receptors ("cold units"), whereas other neurons in these regions show convergence from thermo- and nociceptors (Christensen and Perl, 1970; Hellon and Misra, 1973). There seem to be great differences in the processing of thermoreceptive information between different animal species and between different somatosensory relay areas within the same species. Thermoreceptive neurons are more numerous in the dorsal horn of primates and in the trigeminal region of cats and rats (Iggo and Ramsey, 1976; Dickenson *et al.*, 1979). Thermoreception is an area of sensory neurophysiology that requires further and detailed examination.

4. *Muscle Receptors*

Muscle afferent fibers that convey proprioceptive information to the spinal cord include a group Ia axons (A-α) from the primary endings in muscle spindles, group II axons (A-β) from secondary endings in muscle spindles, and group Ib axons (A-α) from Golgi tendon organs. Group Ia axon collaterals terminate in laminae VI and VII and in lamina IX (the motoneuronal pool); group II axon collaterals are found in laminae IV, V, VI, VII, and IX, and group Ib axon collaterals terminate in a wide region between laminae V and VII (Brown, 1981). Dorsal horn neurons with proprioceptive inputs are generally found in or around lamina VI, and those with long ascending projections join pathways such as the spinocerebellar tracts (Willis and Coggeshall, 1978).

The spinal cord projections of small myelinated afferent fibers from muscle (A-δ or group III) have also been traced by intracellular HRP injections (Mense *et al.*, 1981). These fibers, connected to muscle nociceptors, provide afferent terminals to laminae I and V with a similar pattern of projection to that of the cutaneous mechanonociceptors connected to Aδ afferents. However, the pattern of termination of muscle C-fibers (group IV) appears to differ from that of their cutaneous counterparts. Craig and Mense (1983) have shown that fine afferent fibers from muscle terminate within laminae I and V of the dorsal horn but do not send projections to the substantia gelatinosa (lamina II). Dorsal horn neurons activated by fine muscle afferents are located in laminae I and V and include some cells whose long ascending axons join pathways such as the spino thalamic tract (Willis and Coggeshall, 1978). These neurons are supposed to be involved in the signaling and integration of muscle pain.

5. *Visceral Receptors*

Another source of afferent inputs to dorsal horn neurons is provided by the central endings of visceral afferent fibers, particularly in those spinal cord regions—thoracic and sacral segments—that receive a projection from sympathetic and parasympathetic nerves. These visceral afferents represent a very small proportion of the total afferent inflow to the spinal cord (Cervero *et al.*,

1984a) but can activate a large number of neurons in the spinal cord through extensive functional divergence (Cervero, 1983b). Anatomic studies have shown that visceral afferent fibers terminate in laminae I and V of the dorsal horn with little or no projection to the substantia gelatinosa or to laminae III and IV of the dorsal horn (Morgan *et al.*, 1981; Cervero and Connell, 1984).

Dorsal horn and other spinal cord neurons can be classified into two groups depending on the presence or absence of an excitatory visceral input. Some neurons are not driven by visceral afferent fibers and can only be excited from their somatic receptive fields (somatic neurons). Other cells have, in addition to their somatic input, an excitatory visceral drive (viscerosomatic neurons) (Pomeranz *et al.*, 1968; Gokin, 1970; Guilbaud *et al.*, 1977; Foreman and Ohata, 1980; Cervero, 1982, 1983a,b). Thus, visceral sensation can only be mediated through convergent signals via somatosensory pathways. No evidence has been found for the presence of a sensory pathway exclusively concerned with the transmission of visceral sensory signals.

In agreement with the anatomic data on the mode of termination of somatic and visceral afferent fibers within the spinal cord, the locations of the recording sites of somatic and of viscerosomatic neurons show a differential distribution in the gray matter. Somatic neurons are mainly located in laminae II, III, and IV of the dorsal horn, whereas viscerosomatic cells are located in lamina I, lamina V, and in the ventral horn. The majority of somatic cells are mechanoreceptive, whereas viscerosomatic neurons are driven by nociceptors either specifically (nocireceptive) or in addition to their low-threshold inputs (multireceptive). As for the nature of the visceral input to viscerosomatic neurons, no evidence has so far been produced for a spinal cord projection of the larger A-β fibers in visceral nerves. These fibers, connected to mesenteric Pacinian corpuscles, are known to project to other areas of the central nervous system via the dorsal columns, but the available evidence indicates that they do not send collaterals to the dorsal horn.

Viscerosomatic neurons are driven by the fine A-δ and C afferent fibers of visceral nerves (see comments by Foreman in Chapter 10). When natural stimulation of viscera was used to ascertain the nature of the visceral input, it was found that noxious intensities of visceral stimulation were necessary to drive viscerosomatic neurons (Foreman and Ohata, 1980; Cervero, 1982, 1983a; Milne *et al.*, 1981). Not all somatosensory spinal cord pathways contain axons of viscerosomatic cells. In fact, a clear segregation exists between pathways of projection of somatic and of viscerosomatic neurons. The latter have been found to project through pathways in the ventrolateral funiculus of the cord, including the spinothalamic and spinoreticular tracts (Hancock *et al.*, 1975; Foreman and Weber, 1980; Cervero, 1983b). On the other hand, pathways such as the spinocervicothalamic tract and the postsynaptic dorsal column pathway appear to contain exclusively somatic neurons (Cervero and Iggo, 1978; Cervero, 1983b).

The observations that visceral afferent fibers converge onto somatosensory spinal cord neurons, that most of these neurons have a somatic nociceptive input, that the visceral input to these cells is also of nociceptive nature, and that some of these viscerosomatic neurons project through nociceptive pathways provide strong experimental support for all the main postulates of the "convergence–projection" theory of referred visceral pain (Ruch, 1947). The referral of the visceral sensation is therefore the consequence of the activation of pathways normally concerned with the integration of somatic nociceptive signals. These pathways will be activated by their visceral inputs with a different spatial and temporal pattern than that normally generated by their cutaneous drives. Therefore, the sensation produced by visceral stimulation is that of a vaguely localized pain referred to the somatic structures whose afferent fibers project to the same spinal cord area. Further discussion of the characteristics of the spinal processing of visceral input is given by Foreman in Chapter 10.

E. *Multireceptive Neurons in the Dorsal Horn*

As described above, many neurons in the dorsal horn can be activated by several qualities of cutaneous sensory stimulation. These are the neurons termed class 2, convergent, lamina 5-type, wide dynamic range, or multireceptive (Figure 3). They have been the object of many electrophysiological studies, partly because it is not very difficult to record from them and partly because their lack of specificity poses some interesting questions regarding the mechanisms of sensory processing in the dorsal horn. It is indeed true that multireceptive neurons are abundant in the dorsal horn, but it is also a fact that sensory-specific neurons, particularly nocireceptive cells, are considerably smaller than most multireceptive units and consequently more difficult to record from. These technical difficulties play a part in the protagonism given to multireceptive neurons in dorsal horn function.

Multireceptive neurons receive convergent inputs from several categories of cutaneous receptor (i.e., mechanoreceptors and nociceptors) and in some cases from several peripheral organs (i.e., skin, muscle, and viscera). They tend to be located in or around lamina V, but their presence has also been described in other dorsal horn laminae. Some multireceptive neurons have long ascending axons that join somatosensory pathways. All ascending pathways from the spinal cord contain a proportion of axons from multireceptive neurons (Willis and Coggeshall, 1978).

The role of multireceptive neurons in the mechanisms of sensory processing in the dorsal horn has been the object of a certain amount of speculation. Some authors have suggested that supraspinal centers, which are known to exert a modulatory influence over dorsal horn function (see Hammond, Chapter 15), are able to decode the original source of input to a multireceptive neuron by contrast-enhancing mechanisms and selective inhibitions of one or another of their multiple drives (Le Bars and Chitour,

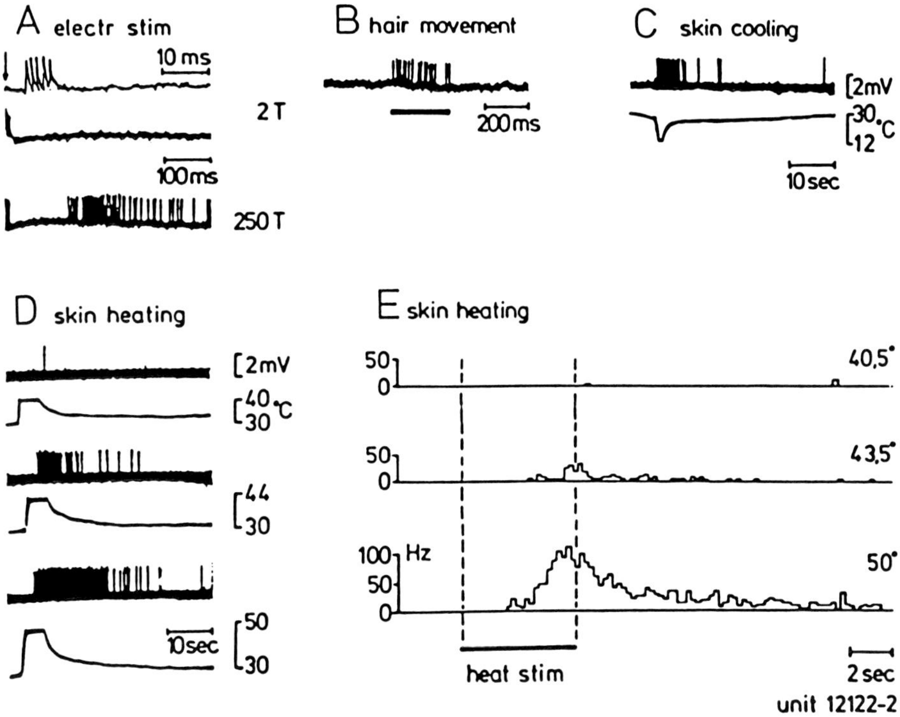

FIGURE 3. Responses of a multireceptive neuron in the dorsal horn to various kinds of stimuli. A: Electrical stimulation of the plantar nerves at $2T$ (upper two traces) and at $250T$ (lowermost trace). B: Hair movement on the plantar surface of the foot. C: Skin cooling; the skin surface temperature is shown below. D: Heating the skin of the footpad by radiation to 40°, 44°, and 50°C, respectively. E: Time course of discharge frequencies plotted as histograms during and after heating the footpad to various temperatures. (From Handwerker *et al.*, 1975.)

1983). This proposal is based on the observation that the nociceptive input to multireceptive neurons can be modified by noxious volleys from other parts of the body. This concept, described as DNIC (diffuse noxious inhibitory controls) is discussed further in the contribution by Le Bars and colleagues (see Chapter 19).

An alternative interpretation of multireceptive neuronal function could be proposed in which the presence within the dorsal horn of both specific and nonspecific sensory channels takes a central role. Every cutaneous sensation has two elementary components: the nature of the sensation and its origin, location, intensity, and relationship with the sensory state of surrounding tissue. It could be suggested that the specific sensory channel carries information about the first component and the nonspecific multireceptive channel deals with the processing of the second component. Sensory discrimination is a function that requires considerably more central integration than the simple transmission of a signal through a labeled line; therefore, the larger population of multireceptive neurons could be a reflection of their more sophisticated sensory role. Other conceptualizations on the "coding" of dorsal horn afferent input are presented by Price in Chapter 18.

F. Neurons in the Substantia Gelatinosa

Over the last few years a number of laboratories have published accounts of the electrophysiological responses of neurons in the substantia gelatinosa (lamina II). Initially, some of the descriptions appeared to be in conflict (see Cervero and Iggo, 1980, for a review), but the continuous use of intracellular HRP labeling by some of the groups and the exchange of information between laboratories have produced a more uniform picture. Three broad categories based on functional response characteristics have been identified in the substantia gelatinosa:

1. Nocireceptive neurons. These are located mainly in the marginal zone (lamina I) and identified as either Waldeyer cells or limiting (stalked) cells.
2. Inverse neurons. These neurons have a variable amount of background activity and are more readily inhibited than excited by cutaneous stimulation (Figure 4). Many also have an excitatory drive from concentric, overlapping, or distant, but not remote, receptive fields. These neurons are both central (islet) and limiting (stalked) cells.
3. Neurons with an input dominated by drives from peripheral C-mechanoreceptors. These cells tend to be located in the inner substantia gelatinosa and are described as "slow brush." Morphologically they are of the central (islet) type.

It is possible that the same unit response could have been classified in a different category depending on the functional classification used in a particular laboratory, since the proportions of the three different response groups vary widely from laboratory to laboratory. Nevertheless, the variety of functional responses found in the substantia gelatinosa strengthens the view that this region of the spinal cord contains cells with a diversity of roles including the relay of afferent signals from the skin and their sensory integration (Cervero and Iggo, 1980).

An interesting development regarding the functional significance of the substantia gelatinosa has been the finding that fine muscle and visceral afferent fibers do not terminate in this area of the dorsal horn. This would indicate that neurons of this region are only concerned with the processing of cutaneous sensory signals and not, as was thought, with the relay of all afferent information mediated by C fibers.

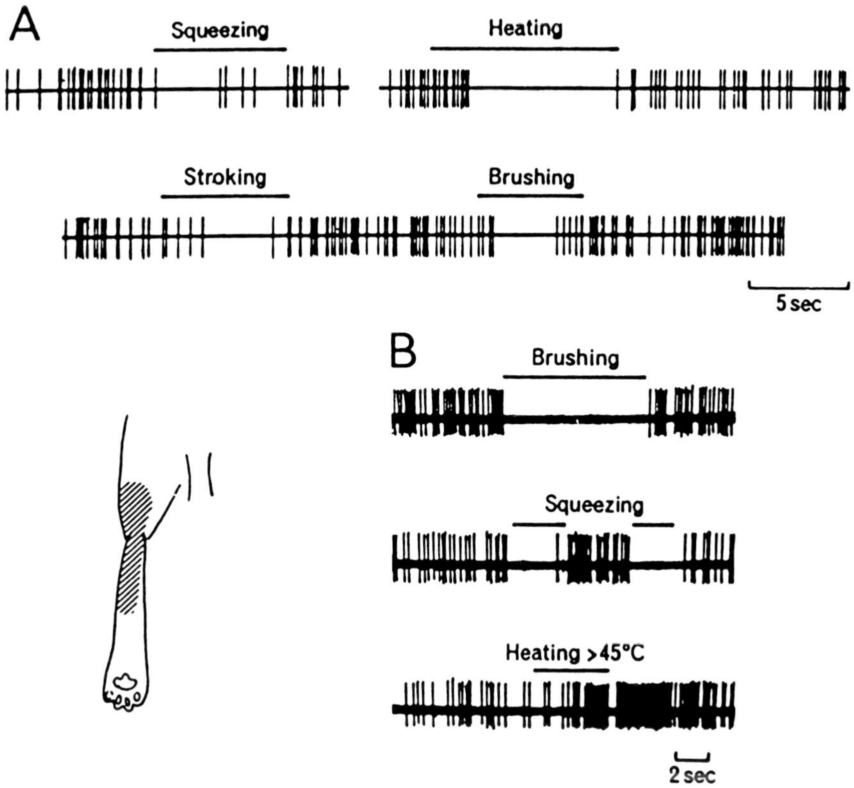

FIGURE 4. A: Responses of a substantia gelatinosa "inverse" neuron to natural stimulation of its cutaneous receptive field (also shown in the figure). B: Responses of a similar kind of neuron, which in this case was excited by noxious heating of the receptive field. (From Cervero *et al.*, 1979b.)

G. Special Consideration of C-Fiber Input to Dorsal Horn Neurons

It has now become clear that the input to the dorsal horn mediated by C fibers has enough anatomic and functional peculiarities to warrant the proposal of a fundamental difference in the roles played by A and C fibers in sensory function. Special properties of the C-fiber input to dorsal horn neurons include the following:

1. Anatomic distribution. Afferent C fibers can activate dorsal horn neurons in a diffuse manner. Yet, destruction of up to 95% of afferent C fibers with the neurotoxin capsaicin reduces the number of dorsal horn neurons driven by the surviving C fibers by only 50% (Cervero *et al.*, 1984b) with no evidence of sprouting of the central terminals

of the remaining C fibers (Ribeiro da Silva and Coimbra, 1984). This indicates a great deal of divergence and a lack of precision in the anatomic distribution of afferent C fibers to the spinal cord.

2. Functional properties. Many of the dorsal horn neurons driven by afferent C fibers increase their responses and their levels of background activity on continuous and repetitive C fiber stimulation. This "wind-up" phenomenon is interpreted as a sign of neuronal arousal and of a general increase in excitability following the activation of a C-fiber input (Figure 5).
3. C-fiber neurochemistry. Many biologically active peptides whose presence has been detected in the spinal cord are concentrated in the terminals of afferent C fibers (Hunt *et al.,* 1981) but not on those of myelinated afferent fibers. Enzymes such as flouride-resistant acid phosphatase (FRAP) (Coimbra *et al.,* 1974) are also exclusive to afferent C fibers. The functional significance of these compounds is far from clear, but their differential distribution according to the type of afferent fiber points to a further diversity between the two sets of afferent fibers. Further discussion of the potential neurotransmitters associated with primary afferents and the second-order systems that they drive is given in Chapters 5, 7, and 11.

Animals with severe reductions in the number of afferent C fibers as a consequence of neonatal injections of the neurotoxin capsaicin show profound changes in the organization of the dorsal horn. These changes include alterations of somatotopic maps and decreased responses to stimulation of the surviving C fibers (Wall *et al.,* 1982; Cervero *et al.,* 1984b). In addition, many

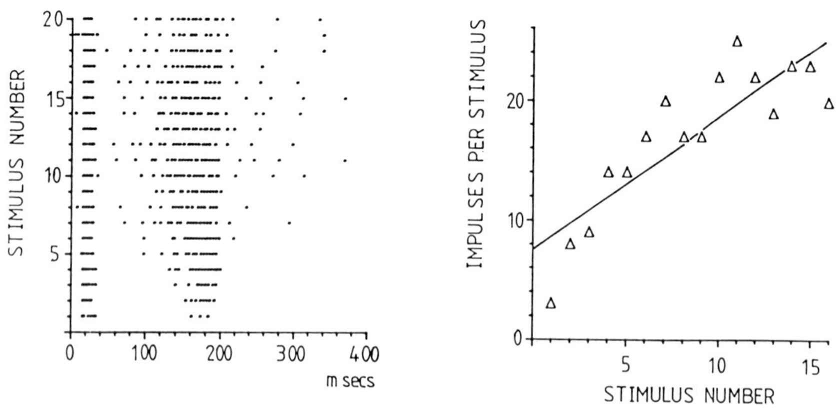

FIGURE 5. Dot-raster display and "wind-up" analysis of the responses of a dorsal horn neuron recorded in the rat's spinal cord to electrical stimulation of C fibers in the sural nerve at 1 Hz. Responses to 20 consecutive stimuli are displayed as dot rasters (left) or as the number of impulses counted in the C fiber evoked response of the neuron in each stimulus (right). (From Cervero *et al.,* 1984b.)

central inhibitory mechanisms appear depressed after a life-long absence of afferent C fibers (Cervero *et al.*, 1984b). These results strongly suggest that the lack of a normal afferent C-fiber input prevents the development of adequate central inhibitory controls, which are normally needed to regulate the powerful excitation mediated by afferent C fibers. The role of the C-fiber input to the dorsal horn could be that of a general alerting and arousing drive that evokes the perception of an unpleasant experience as part of the whole-body response to its peripheral activiation.

H. The Sensory Spinal Cord

The perception of a sensory experience is a complex and coordinated phenomenon that cannot be explained with a simplistic neural circuit placed at the first synaptic relay in the dorsal horn. The greatest advance made in the last few years in the field of somatosensory physiology has been the realization that the afferent input to the spinal cord can activate a variety of systems, not all of which will immediately be concerned with the perception of one or another sensory experience. Peripheral receptor specificity is preserved in the spinal cord by second-order systems likely to transmit sensory information related to the nature of the stimulus. Nonspecific systems in the dorsal horn may help the discrimination of the sensory experience or may be concerned with general mechanisms of arousal and with the triggering of reflex activity and autonomic reactions. The chemistry of the afferent fiber terminals may play an important role in the immediate synaptic modulation or in the long-term maintenance of the sensory channel.

It will not be long before some of the obstacles that still prevent a full understanding of the sensory spinal cord can be effectively removed.

References

BICKNELL, H. R., AND BEAL J. S. Axonal and dendritic development of substantia gelatinosa neurons in the lumbosacral spinal cord of the rat. *J. Comp. Neurol.* 226:508–522, 1984.

BROWN, A. G. *Organisation in the Spinal Cord.* Springer Verlag, Heidelberg, 1981.

BROWN, A. G., AND IGGO, A. A quantitative study of cutaneous receptors and afferent fibres in the cat and rabbit. *J. Physiol. (Lond.)* 193:707–733, 1967.

BROWN, A. G., AND RETHELYI, M. *Spinal Cord Sensation.* Scottish Academic Press, Edinburgh, 1981.

CARROLL, L. *Through the Looking Glass,* Puffin Books, 1872, reprinted 1962.

CERVERO, F. Noxious intensities of visceral stimulation are required to activate viscero-somatic multireceptive neurones in the thoracic spinal cord of the cat. *Brain Res.* 240:350–352, 1982.

CERVERO, F. Somatic and visceral inputs to the thoracic spinal cord of the cat: Effects of noxious stimulation of the biliary system. *J. Physiol. (Lond.)* 337:51–67, 1983a.

CERVERO, F. Supraspinal connections of neurons in the thoracic spinal cord of the cat: Ascending projections and effects of descending impulses. *Brain Res.* 275:251–261, 1983b.

CERVERO, F., AND CONNELL, L. A. Fine afferent fibres from viscera do not terminate in the substantia gelatinosa of the thoracic spinal cord. *Brain Res.* 294:370–374, 1984.

CERVERO, F., AND IGGO, A. Natural stimulation of urinary bladder afferents does not affect transmission through lumbrosacral spinocervical tract neurones in the cat. *Brain Res.* 156:375–379, 1978.

CERVERO, F., AND IGGO, A. The substantia gelatinosa of the spinal cord: A critical review. *Brain* 103:717–772, 1980.

CERVERO, F., IGGO, A., AND OGAWA, H. Nociceptor-driven dorsal horn neurones in the lumbar spinal cord of the cat. *Pain* 1:5–24, 1976.

CERVERO, F., IGGO, A., AND MOLONY, V. Ascending projections of nociceptor-driven lamina I neurones in the cat. *Exp. Brain Res.* 35:135–149, 1979a.

CERVERO, F., IGGO, A., AND MOLONY, V. An electrophysiological study of neurones in the substantia gelatinosa Rolandi of the cat's spinal cord. *Q. J. Exp. Physiol.* 64:297–314, 1979b.

CERVERO, F., CONNELL, L. A., AND LAWSON, S. N. Somatic and visceral primary afferents in the lower thoracic dorsal root ganglia of the cat. *J. Comp. Neurol.* 228:422–431, 1984a.

CERVERO, F., SCHOUENBORG, J., SJÖLUND, B. H. AND WADDELL, P. J. Cutaneous inputs to dorsal horn neurons in adult rats treated at birth with capsaicin. *Brain Res.* 301:47–57, 1984b.

CHRISTENSEN, B. N., AND PERL, E. R. Spinal neurones specifically excited by noxious or thermal stimuli: Marginal zone of the dorsal horn. *J. Neurophysiol.* 33:293–307, 1970.

COIMBRA, A., SODRE-BORGES, B. P., AND MAGALHAES, M. M. The substantia gelatinosa Rolandi of the rat. Fine structure, cytochemistry (acid phosphatase) and changes after dorsal root section. *J. Neurocytol.* 3:199–217, 1974.

CRAIG, A. D., AND MENSE, S. The distribution of afferent fibres from the gastrocnemius-soleus muscle in the dorsal horn of the cat, as revealed by the transport of HRP. *Neurosci. Lett.* 41:233–238, 1983.

DICKENSON, A. H., HELLON, R. F., AND TAYLOR, D. C. M. Facial thermal input to the trigeminal spinal nucleus of rabbits and rats. *J. Comp. Neurol.* 185:203–210, 1979.

FALLS, W., AND GOBEL, S. Golgi and EM studies of the formation of dendritic and axonal arbors: The interneurones of the substantia gelatinosa of Rolando in newborn kittens. *J. Comp. Neurol.* 187:1–18, 1979.

FOREMAN, R. D., AND OHATA, C. A. Effects of coronary artery occlusion on thoracic spinal neurones receiving viscero-somatic inputs. *Am. J. Physiol.* 238:H667–H674, 1980.

FOREMAN, R. D., AND WEBER, R. N. Responses from neurones of the primate spinothalamic tract to electrical stimulation of afferents from the cardiopulmonary region and somatic structures. *Brain Res.* 186:463–468, 1980.

GOBEL, S. Dendroaxonic synapses in the substantia gelatinosa glomeruli of the spinal trigeminal nucleus of the cat. *J. Comp. Neurol.* 167:165–176, 1976.

GOBEL, S. Golgi studies of the neurones in layer I of the dorsal horn of the medulla (trigeminal nucleus caudalis). *J. Comp. Neurol.* 180:375–394, 1978a.

GOBEL, S. Golgi studies of the neurones in layer II of the dorsal horn of the medula (trigeminal nucleus caudalis). *J. Comp. Neurol.* 180:395–414, 1978b.

GOKIN, A. P. Synaptic activation of interneurones in the thoracic spinal cord by cutaneous muscle and visceral afferents. *Neurofiziologiia (Moscow)* 2:563–572, 1970.

GUILBAUD, G., BENELLI, G., AND BESSON, S. M. Response of thoracic dorsal horn interneurones to cutaneous stimulation and to the administration of algogenic substances into the mesenteric artery in the spinal cat. *Brain Res.* 124:437–448, 1977.

HANCOCK, M. B. FOREMAN, R. D., AND WILLIS, W. D. Convergence of visceral and cutaneous input onto spinothalamic tract cells in the thoracic spinal cord of the cat. *Exp. Neurol.* 47:240–248, 1975.

HANDWERKER, H. O., IGGO, A., AND ZIMMERMANN, M. Segmental and supraspinal actions on dorsal horn neurones responding to noxious and nonnoxious skin stimuli. *Pain* 1:147–166, 1975.

HELLON, R. F., AND MISRA, N. K. Neurones in the dorsal horn of the rat responding to scrotal skin temperature changes. *J. Physiol. (Lond.)* 232:375–388, 1973.

HUNT, S. P., KELLY, J. S., EMSON, P. C., KIMMEL, J. R., MILLER, R. J., AND WU, J. Y. An immunohistochemical study of neuronal populations containing neuropeptides of γ-aminobutyrate within the superficial clayers of the rat dorsal horn. *Neuroscience* 6:1883–1898, 1981.

IGGO, A. Cutaneous mechanoreceptors with afferent C fibres. *J. Physiol. (Lond.)* 152:337–353, 1960.

IGGO, A. Cutaneous thermoreceptors in primates and sub-primates. *J. Physiol. (Lond.)* 200:403–430, 1969.

IGGO, A. Activation of cutaneous nociceptors and their actions on dorsal horn neurones. *Adv. Neurol.* 4:1–9, 1974.

IGGO, A., AND RAMSEY, R. L. Thermosensory mechanisms in the spinal cord of monkeys, in: *Sensory Functions of the Skin* (Y. ZOTTERMAN, ed.), Pergammon Press, New York, 1976, pp. 285–304.

LE BARS, D., AND CHITOUR, D. Do convergent neurones in the spinal dorsal horn discriminate nociceptive from non-nociceptive information? *Pain* 17:1–19, 1983.

LIGHT, A. R., AND PERL, E. R. Reexamination of the dorsal root projection to the spinal dorsal horn including observations on the differential termination of coarse and fine fibres. *J. Comp. Neurol.* 186:117–132, 1979a.

LIGHT, A. R., AND PERL, E. R. Spinal termination of functionally identified primary afferent neurones with slowly conducting myelinated fibers. *J. Comp. Neurol.* 186:133–150, 1979b.

LIGHT, A. R., TREVINO, D. L., AND PERL, E. R. Morphological features of functionally defined neurones in the marginal zone and substantia gelatinosa of the spinal dorsal horn. *J. Comp. Neurol.* 186:151–172, 1979.

MENDELL, L. M. Physiological properties of unmyelinated fiber projection to the spinal cord. *Exp. Neurol.* 16:316–332, 1966.

MENSE, A., LIGHT, A. R., AND PERL, E. F. Spinal terminations of subcutaneous high-threshold mechanoreceptors, in: *Spinal Cord Sensation* (A. G. BROWN and M. RETHELYI, eds.), Scottish Academic Press, Edinburgh, 1981, pp. 79–86.

MILNE, R. J., FOREMAN, R. D., GIESLER, G. J., JR., AND WILLIS, W. D. Convergence of cutaneous and pelvic visceral nociceptive inputs onto primate spinothalamic neurones. *Pain* 11:153–184, 1981.

MOLONY, F., STEEDMAN, W. M., CERVERO, F., AND IGGO, A. Intracellular marking of identified neurons in the superficial dorsal horn of the cat spinal cord. *Q. J. Exp. Physiol.* 66:211–223, 1981.

MORGAN, C., NADELHAFT, I., AND DE GROAT, W. The distribution of visceral primary afferents from the pelvic nerve to Lissauer's tract and the spinal gray metter and its relationship to the sacral parasympathetic nucleus. *J. Comp. Neurol.* 201:415–440, 1981.

OCHOA, J., AND TOREBJÖRK, E. Sensations evoked by intraneural microstimulation of single mechanoreceptor units innervating the human hand. *J. Physiol. (Lond.)* 341:633–654, 1983.

POMERANZ, B., WALL, P. D., AND WEBER, W. V. Cord cells responding to fine myelinated afferents from viscera, muscle and skin. *J. Physiol. (Lond.)* 199:511–532, 1968.

RAMON Y CAJAL, S. La sustancia gelatinosa de Rolando, in: *Pequeñas Contribuciones al Conocimiento del Sistema Nervioso*, Casa Provincial de Caridad, Barcelona, 1891, pp. 50–53.

RAMON Y CAJAL, S. *Histologie du Systeme Nerveux de l'Homme et des Vertebres*, Vol. I, Maloine, Paris, 1909.

REXED, B. The cytoarchitectonic organisation of the spinal cord in the cat. *J. Comp. Neurol.* 96:415–495, 1952.

RIBEIRO DA SILVA, A., AND COIMBRA, A. Capsaicin causes selective damage to type I synaptic glomeruli in rat substantia gelatinosa. *Brain Res.* 290:380–383, 1984.

RUCH, T. C. Visceral sensation and referred pain, in: *Howell's Textbook of Physiology* (J. F. FULTON, ed.), W. B. Saunders, Philadelphia, 1947, pp. 385–401.

WALL, P. D. The laminar organisation of dorsal horn and effects of descending impulses. *J. Physiol. (Lond.)* 188:403–423, 1967.

WALL, P. D. Dorsal horn electrophysiology, in: *Handbook of Sensory Physiology*, Vol. 2 (A. IGGO, ed.), Springer Verlag, Berlin, Heidelberg, New York, 1973, pp. 253–270.

WALL, P. D., FITZGERALD, M., NUSSBAUMER, J. C., VAN DER LOOS H., AND DEVOR, M. Somatotopic maps are disorganised in adult rodents treated neonatally with capsaicin. *Nature* 295:691–693, 1982.

WILLIS, W. D., AND COGGESHALL, R. E. *Sensory Mechanisms of the Spinal Cord,* John Wiley & Sons, New York, 1978, p. 477.

WILLIS, W. D., TREVINO, D. L., COULTER, S. D., AND MAUNZ, R. A. Responses of primate spinothalamic tract neurones to natural stimulation of hindlimb. *J. Neurophysiol.* 37:358–372, 1974.

10
Spinal Substrates of Visceral Pain

ROBERT D. FOREMAN

A. *Introduction*

Visceral pain is a common finding of patients who require medical attention. Yet, neurophysiological mechanism underlying visceral pain, associated referred pain, and parietal pain have not been vigorously pursued (Cervero, 1983a). Several theories have been proposed to explain visceral pain, but only recently they have been reexamined using techniques that were developed to study the spinothalamic tract or dorsal horn cells with ascending projections. The spinothalamic tract (STT) in anesthetized monkeys has provided new insights to the mechanisms of visceral pain and referred pain.

Electrophysiological and behavioral studies have been used extensively to elucidate some of the neural mechanisms associated with external cutaneous pain, but the same approach for visceral pain is limited. At least three complicating factors make studies of visceral pain more difficult. One difficulty is choosing the appropriate stimulus to activate nociceptors of visceral organs. Often simple distention or localized pinch is insufficient to produce a pain response (Lewis, 1942). Another difficulty is the type of sensation elicited with onset of visceral pain. The pain is usually dull, aching, and diffuse in origin. This sensation is different from the sharp, acute, well-localized pain noted during cutaneous stimulation. A third complicating factor in studying visceral pain is the associated referred pain.

In spite of the inherent difficulties, we have pursued studies on visceral pain for the past 9 years. Our studies have centered around neural mechanisms associated with angina pectoris. Only recently, we have begun to study the complicating factors of anginalike pain associated with gallbladder disease.

ROBERT D. FOREMAN • Department of Physiology and Biophysics, University of Oklahoma Health Sciences Center, College of Medicine, Oklahoma City, Oklahoma 73190.

The model used to study the neural mechanisms was the recording of electrical activity from single cells of origin of the STT in the monkey. The decision to use this model was based on evidence that the STT was the classical pathway of the transmission of noxious stimuli that would be perceived as pain in the conscious animal and human. The decision was substantially strengthened when investigators (Hoffman *et al.*, 1981) showed that the response characteristics of medullary dorsal horn cells to somatic manipulation in conscious monkeys were similar to the responses obtained in the anesthetized animal (Willis and Coggeshall, 1978). In addition, numerous studies in monkeys and humans have shown a correlation between nociceptor activity and behavior related to noxious stimuli (Dubner *et al.*, 1977; Gybels *et al.*, 1979; LaMotte and Campbell, 1978; Torebjörk and Hallin, 1974; Van Hees and Gybels, 1981).

This chapter focuses on the central organization of ascending pathways transmitting afferent activity from the heart and gallbladder. Part of the chapter is directed to the organization of sympathetic afferent fibers and, in particular, the cardiopulmonary fibers. Discussion of the central organization includes the types of stimuli from the heart and gallbladder that produce activity in STT cells, the convergence of visceral and somatic input, and the inputs of two visceral organs on the same STT cell. Finally, it is shown that electrical stimulation of vagal afferent fibers and of the nucleus raphe magnus inhibits visceral input. After the discussion of the neural mechanisms, explanations for visceral pain and, in particular, angina pectoris are considered.

B. Sympathetic Afferent Fibers

Terminology for afferent fibers traveling within nerves of the sympathetic nervous system has remained controversial because this system was originally defined as being only motor in function (Langley, 1903). Langley (1903) based this conclusion on the fact that afferent fibers in sympathetic nerves did not elicit reflexes similar to those produced by stimulating depressor nerves; therefore, he felt that sympathetic reflexes were of little significance in the intact animal. In spite of this, Langley used the term "afferent sympathetic fiber." Over the past 20 years many studies have demonstrated that sympathetic afferent fibers do elicit reflex responses (Malliani, 1982); thus, because these fibers are important for reflex adjustments, the term sympathetic afferent should be used to describe those fibers that enter the spinal cord via the white rami communicantes.

This chapter focuses on sympathetic afferent fibers arising from the heart and from the gallbladder. Other visceral organs also have sympathetic afferent input, but the majority of work related to referred pain and the STT has been done on the heart, and initial studies have now begun on the gallbladder; the urinary bladder is the only other organ examined for neural mechanisms of referred pain that involved STT cells (Milne *et al.*, 1981). Another reason for focusing on the heart and gallbladder is that angina pectoris or anginalike pain is used as the basic model for explaining mechanisms of referred pain associated with visceral and somatic inputs.

1. Myelinated and Unmyelinated Fibers

Sympathetic afferent fibers in the cardiopulmonary regions are sensitive to mechanical deformation and to chemicals. Myelinated afferent fibers originate from the ventricles and atria (Malliani *et al.*, 1972; Ueda *et al.*, 1969), superior and inferior vena cava (Ueda *et al.*, 1969), aorta (Malliani and Pagani, 1976; Uchida, 1975b), pulmonary vessels (Kostreva *et al.*, 1975; Lombardi *et al.*, 1976; Nishi *et al.*, 1974), and in or near the coronary vessels (Brown, 1967, 1979; Uchida and Murao, 1974a). These myelinated fibers display a spontaneously active discharge pattern that occurs in synchrony with cardiac rhythm (Brown, 1979). Sympathetic afferent activity increased when pressure changed within the chamber of the heart and blood vessels (Malliani *et al.*, 1973; Uchida, 1975a; Uchida and Murao, 1974a; Ueda *et al.*, 1969). Not every cardiac cycle elicits impulses, but when afferent fibers are activated, one to three impulses are observed and are entrained with the cardiac cycle.

Unmyelinated C-fiber afferents are also found within the sympathetic nervous system and originate from the heart and cardiopulmonary region (Seagard *et al.*, 1978). Unmyelinated fibers exhibit an irregular discharge pattern that generally does not occur with cardiac rhythm (Casati *et al.*, 1979). The receptors are sensitive to mechanical changes in the heart; therefore, they may provide tonic input to regions of the central nervous system involved in the neural control of cardiovascular system (Casati *et al.*, 1979; Malliani *et al.*, 1975).

2. Effective Stimuli

Pressure changes in the cardiopulmonary region have been used to explain the associated sympathetic afferent activity, but recent work in our laboratory demonstrates that, at least for the heart, left ventricular pressure may not be the stimulus producing activation of these afferent fibers. Sonomicrometers were used to measure three-dimensional changes of the length fields surrounding a receptor either for the myelinated or unmyelinated fiber. Afferent activity could readily be associated with the length changes but in most situations was not correlated with changes in left ventricular pressure (Holmes *et al.*, 1982, 1983). Therefore, the stimulus for the receptors of these sympathetic afferent fibers may be more complex than pressure change in the ventricle. For example, left ventricular pressure was not always correlated with length changes, particularly in some dimensions. So the exact stimulus activating these receptors remains to be determined.

Sympathetic afferent information associated with small to reasonably large changes in blood pressure may participate in local spinal reflexes or supraspinal reflexes and may also be involved in the transmission of innocuous information. Cervero (1983b) has suggested that visceral innervation may have afferent fibers that elicit reflexes but no perception of sensation (afferent innervation) as well as afferent fibers that contribute to a sensation (sensory innervation). He then further proposes that the sensory input is noxious, and innocuous information may not be transmitted. Indeed, he suggests that the afferent innervation that elicits cardiovascular reflexes would not necessarily produce a sensation. This concept is not completely supported on the basis of sensations associated with the heart. For example, when the heart produces a premature ventricular contraction, sensation is noted by the person who experienced it, but sensation is not always noxious and is quite clearly defined to the general area of the chest (Harrison and Reeves, 1968; Scherf and Boyd, 1958). Therefore, this is at least a small piece of evidence to demonstrate that this information may be innocuous in nature. Dorsal horn neurons, spinoreticular tract cells, and STT cells are excited when the heart produces a premature ventricular contraction (Blair *et al.,* 1981b, 1982a). Therefore, the possibility exists that the visceral organs do sense information that does not necessarily produce a sensation of discomfort or pain.

C. *Central Organization of the Spinothalamic Tract System*

In the following sections, I discuss the characteristics of the neurons we have identified that project into the spinothalamic system.

1. *Somatic Inputs*

Natural forms of mechanical stimuli were used to characterize the receptive field for each STT cell (Willis *et al.,* 1974). A given unit was classified according to the mildest mechanical stimulus that activated it. Cells were classified according to their responsiveness to somatic manipulation including hair movement, touching or pinching of the skin, or pinching of the skin and muscle (Blair *et al.,* 1981a). A higher percentage of cells were classified as high threshold because these cells responded to pinching of the skin or pinching of the skin and muscle (Figure 1A). Wide-dynamic-range cells responded with a low discharge rate to hair movement or touching of the skin but discharged vigorously when pinch was applied to the skin or the skin and muscle (Figrure 1B). A third category of cells responded vigorously to high-threshold stimulation, that is, pinching of the skin or skin and muscle, but was inhibited when hair was moved. These cells were classified as high-threshold inhibitory (Blair *et al.,* 1981a).

Since recordings were made from cells of the left dorsal horn, the re-

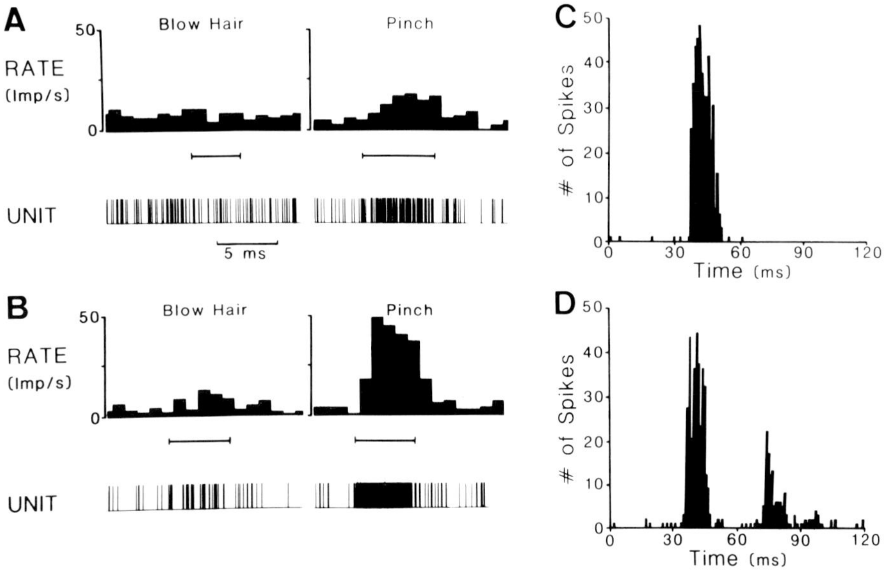

FIGURE 1. Viscerosomatic convergence onto STT cells. Responses of a high-threshold cell are shown in A. The cell did not respond to blowing hair but increased its discharge rate during a pinch applied to the left chest and triceps region. Cell activity of a wide-dynamic-range cell is shown in B. The histograms in C and D are responses of a STT cell to stimulation of sympathetic afferents at stimulus strengths sufficient to activate the A-δ fibers (C) and the A-δ and C fibers (D). The stimulus was applied at 30 ms.

ceptive fields were commonly found on the left side of the animal. Somatic receptive fields were located on the upper chest and left forelimb of the monkey. Receptive fields for wide-dynamic-range cells were generally larger than those for high-threshold cells. One of the common features of high-threshold cells was the fact that in many cases cells not only responded to skin input but also responded to muscle input (Figure 2). Muscle input provided an interesting insight into the characteristics of sensations associated with referred pain caused by visceral disease. Usually referred pain is described as a dull, aching sensation (Lewis, 1942). The same description is also used for pain associated with muscle, probably because so many cells receive muscle input. It may not be surprising that the common sensation is dull, aching pain and that cells that are being activated receive muscle input.

2. *Sympathetic Inputs: Electrical Stimulation*

Electrical stimulation of cardiopulmonary sympathetic afferent fibers (Figure 3, electrode pair A) indicated that all STT cells received visceral as well as somatic input (Blair *et al.,* 1981a). Separation of afferent input into

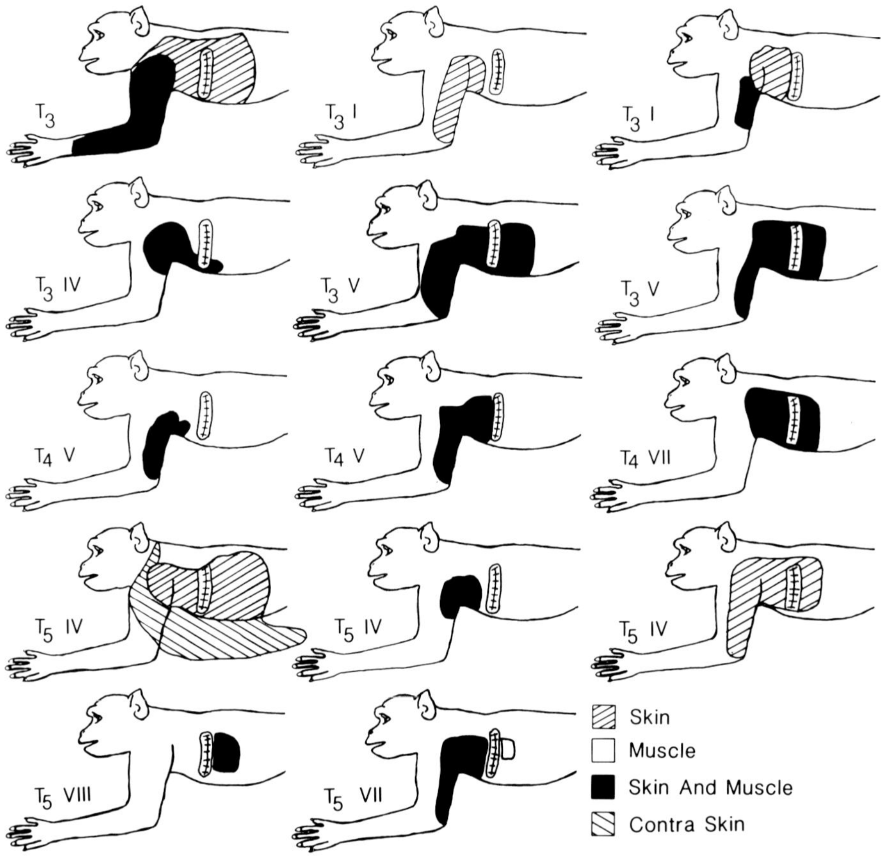

FIGURE 2. High-threshold receptive fields of STT cells that responded to intracardiac injections of bradykinin. Segmental and laminar locations of each cell are listed just above the left forelimb in each figurine.

A-δ- and C-fiber classes was determined from poststimulus time histograms and from stimulus strength data (Figure 1C,D). Stimulation of sympathetic afferent fibers produced either a single peak or two peaks of activity in STT cells. These peaks were separated by several milliseconds. Minimum afferent conduction velocity was calculated for each peak as the distance from the stimulating electrode to the location of the recording electrode in the spinal cord divided by the latency for the appearance of each peak. Minimum afferent conduction velocity was based on the assumption that cells were activated monosynaptically and that synaptic delay was 1 ms (Foreman *et al.*, 1975; Pomeranz *et al.*, 1968). At low stimulus strengths, only an A-δ-fiber volley was observed (Figure 1C), but when the intensity was increased with the same stimulus duration or duration was increased to 500 μs, C-fiber input was also observed (Figure 1D).

The STT cells could be separated into three categories based on the type

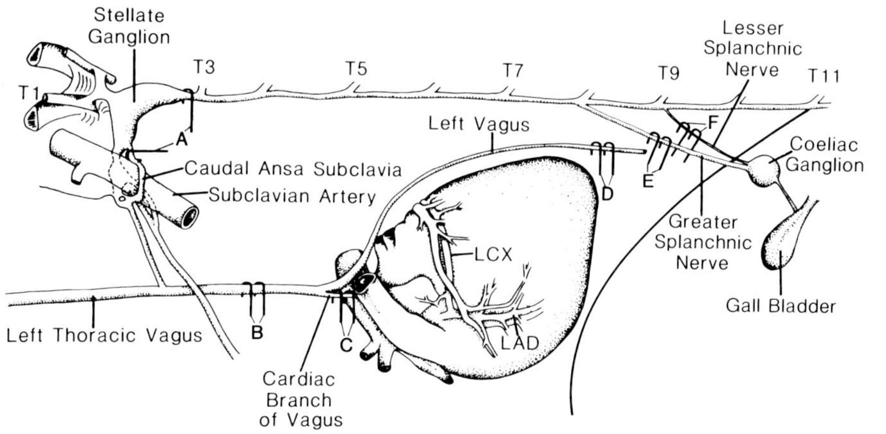

FIGURE 3. Schematic diagram of electrode placement on nerves originating from the heart and gallbladder. Pairs of electrodes were placed on the nerves to activate sympathetic afferent fibers. The following pairs of electrodes are placed: A, on the ansa subclavia and just caudal to the stellate ganglion; B, on the trunk of the left vagus nerve; C, on the cardiac branch of the vagus nerve; D, on the vagus midway between the heart and the diaphragm; E, on the greater splanchnic nerve; F, on the lesser splanchnic nerve. Abbreviations: LCX, left circumflex coronary artery; LAD, left anterior descending coronary artery.

of sympathetic afferent input they receive. Approximately 40% of the cells received both A-δ- and C-fiber input, 50% received only A-δ-fiber input, and 10% received only C-fiber input (Blair *et al.*, 1981a). The minimum afferent conduction velocity for the A-δ peak was approximately 9 m/s and for the C fiber peak was about 1.0 m/s.

3. Sympathetic Inputs: "Natural" Cardiac Stimuli

After viscerosomatic convergence was demonstrated for each STT cell, noxious stimuli such as coronary artery occlusion or injection of an algesic chemical, bradykinin, into the heart was used to determine whether the STT cell would change its activity to a stimulus that would activate cardiac receptors.

a. Bradykinin

This agent was chosen as the algesic chemical because it was found in increased amounts in effluent of the coronary sinus following coronary artery occlusion (Hashimoto *et al.*, 1977; Kimura *et al.*, 1973). Injections of bradykinin also produced pseudoaffective responses indicative of pain when injected into hearts of dogs (Guzman *et al.*, 1962). In addition, sympathetic afferent fibers are excited when bradykinin is injected into the heart or dripped on the epicardium (Baker *et al.*, 1980; Lombardi *et al.*, 1981; Nishi *et al.*, 1977).

Bradykinin injections were made in the left atrial appendage and in the aorta, near the aortic arch or the brachiocephalic artery. Bradykinin can either stimulate endocardial receptors of atria and ventricles directly or can stimulate receptors after entering the coronary circulation. Injections into the aorta were used as controls to insure that other areas of the peripheral circulation did not increase the discharge rate of STT cells. The usual dose of bradykinin was 2 μg/kg. Bradykinin excited approximately 75% of the STT cells tested (Blair *et al.*, 1982b). After a latency of approximately 15 s, the average change in cell activity increased about 14 impulses/s. (Figure 4A). In most experiments, three injections were made into the atrium at 10-min intervals. Activity changed very little when identical injections of bradykinin were made in the aorta. Since it was extremely important to determine if, in fact, receptors of the heart were activating these STT cells, lidocaine was administered into the pericardial sac to anesthetize sympathetic afferent fibers from the heart without affecting fibers in other regions of the thorax. Following a bradykinin injection, cell activity did not change compared to control. Therefore, our results indicate that bradykinin activates cardiac receptors transmitting their information to the spinal cord via sympathetic afferent fibers. Since bradykinin is a strong candidate for one of the substances being released during myocardial ischemia, it seems likely that STT cells become excited when insufficient blood is supplied during partial coronary artery occlusion or during vasospasm.

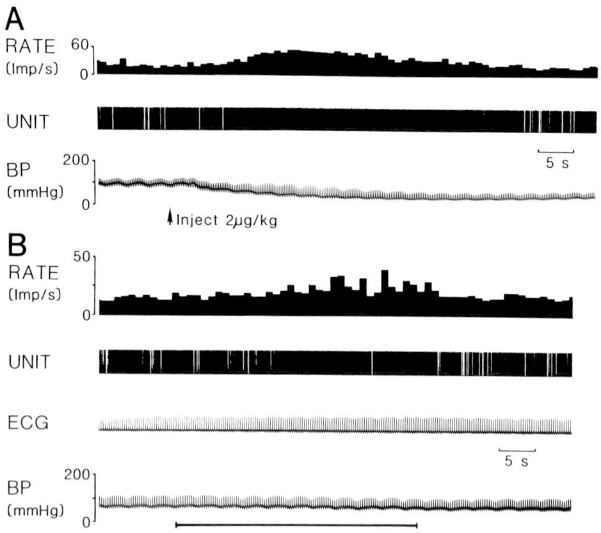

FIGURE 4. Effects on STT cell activity of injecting bradykinin (2 μg/kg) into the left atrium (A). Effects of occluding the left circumflex branch of the coronary artery are shown in panel B. The upper tracing is the rate the cell discharged in impulses/second; the middle tracing is individual action potentials after passing through a window discriminator (unit), and the bottom trace is blood pressure (BP) in millimeters of mercury. The arrow in A marks the time of injection of bradykinin. The black horizontal bar in B marks the period of coronary artery occlusion.

b. Coronary Artery Occlusion

Coronary artery occlusion is a logical way to compare the response of STT cells to that which would be anticipated during myocardial ischemia. Sympathetic afferent fibers are excited approximately 10–20 s following the onset of coronary artery occlusion (Brown, 1967; Brown and Malliani, 1971; Casati *et al.*, 1979; Uchida and Murao, 1974a). To test effects of coronary artery occlusion on spinothalamic cells, ischemia of the heart was produced by occluding the left main coronary artery or the left circumflex artery and left anterior descending artery with ligatures snared around each artery. Seven out of 14 cells (Figure 4B) responded to coronary artery occlusion (Blair *et al.*, 1984). The average latency following the onset of the occlusion was 13 s. The mean discharge rate increased from 19 to 27 spikes/s ($P < 0.01$). Five of the responding cells were activated by occlusion of the left main coronary artery, and left circumflex artery and left anterior descending artery occlusions each activated one cell. We noted that responding cells tended to have a higher spontaneous activity than did nonresponders (19 versus 7 spikes/s). These results demonstrate that coronary artery occlusion excites STT cells, and they lead to the suggestion that these cells convey information about cardiac pain during myocardial ischemia.

A comparison of responses to bradykinin (BK) and to coronary artery occlusion (CAO) pointed out several interesting differences. A cell responsive to BK did not always respond to CAO. In addition, cells responding to the injection of bradykinin discharged at a higher frequency than they did in response to coronary artery occlusion. Some explanations can be provided for why these differences occurred. First, the dose of bradykinin used in these studies may be higher than the amount of bradykinin released during coronary artery occlusion. If this is the case, then more cardiac afferent fibers will be excited during the bradykinin injection, resulting in excitation of more STT cells. Second, the volume of cardiac tissue affected by bradykinin is greater than the volume affected by coronary artery occlusion because bradykinin injected into the left atrium will probably affect the entire heart, whereas coronary occlusion will affect only that portion of the heart being perfused by the artery. As a result, bradykinin may stimulate more receptors than coronary artery occlusion, and this would increase the likelihood of increased cell activity. Third, activation of receptors during occlusion may result from an interaction of other endogenous substances in addition to bradykinin alone. Consequently, bradykinin and coronary artery occlusion are not equivalent stimuli to receptors.

Coronary artery occlusion simulates myocardial ischemia more effectively than does the injection of bradykinin. However, in these primate experiments, coronary arteries often went into vasospasm following the first occlusion, leading to fibrillation and death of the animal. Since this altered our ability to obtain several cells in each experiment, we chose to use bradykinin as a noxious stimulus to compare the results of these studies and make some statements about cardiac pain.

Although cells that were excited by ischemia may be important for cardiac pain, it should be pointed out that some neurons, including STT cells, also responded to the onset of occlusion (Foreman and Ohata, 1980). There is a good possiblity that some of these cells might be responding to mechanical deformations of the heart or to the coronary artery being occluded. We can only hypothesize that information generated by the onset of occlusion may be innocuous and that the activity might elicit only some innocuous sensation. There are afferent fibers that are sensitive to mechanical deformation and pressure changes in coronary arteries (Brown and Malliani, 1971; Malliani *et al.*, 1973). We also found cells sensitive to both the onset of occlusion and myocardial ischemia (Blair *et al.*, 1984).

4. Sympathetic Afferents: Splanchnic and Gallbladder Stimulation

Angina pectoris occurs during ischemia of the myocardium, but patients may experience anginalike pain without having heart disease. These patients may have gastrointestinal disorders, particularly hiatal hernia, gastritis, gallbladder disease, splenic flexure syndrome, esophageal spasm, or peptic ulcer (Hampton *et al.*, 1959; Henderson *et al.*, 1978; Miller, 1942; Palmer, 1958; Ravdin *et al.*, 1955; Wehrmacker, 1964). No electrophysiological evidence has been provided to explain how this visceral information is integrated in the spinal cord and supraspinal structures. Our research was designed to determine the central organization of STT cells in relation to their role as a pathway for integration of anginalike pain associated with heart disease, gallbladder disease, and other abdominal pain.

Several studies have demonstrated that dorsal horn cells of the T_7 to T_{11} segments receive, in addition to somatic inputs, input during electrical stimulation of the splanchnic nerve (Fields *et al.*, 1970; Pomeranz *et al.*, 1968; Gokin *et al.*, 1977), gallbladder distention (Cervero, 1983b), or mesenteric artery injections of an algesic substance (Guilbaud *et al.*, 1977). The STT cells of the T_7–T_{11} segments receiving viscerosomatic convergence also responded to electrical stimulation of the small myelinated fibers and C fibers of the splanchnic nerve (Foreman *et al.*, 1981; Hancock *et al.*, 1975).

The first question asked was: Do STT cells in the T_1 to T_5 region receive afferent input from the abdominal region as well as the cardiopulmonary region? To answer this question, we recorded from STT cells and stimulated sympathetic afferent fibers originating from the ansa subclavia and from the splanchnic afferents (Figure 3). Splanchnic stimulation excited 63 of 85 T_1 to T_5 STT neurons in 36 monkeys (Ammons *et al.*, 1984a). All of the neurons had somatic receptive fields and were excited electrically by stimulating the cardiopulmonary sympathetic afferents. There was an increased probability of encountering the splanchnic-responding neurons when cells were recorded from more caudal spinal segments. Also, there was a tendency for a higher percentage of splanchnic responses of cells to be obtained in deeper laminae.

All 63 cells having splanchnic input exhibited early responses to both the splanchnic and cardiopulmonary sympathetic afferent stimulation (Figure 5). Average latencies for the early response to splanchnic stimulation and cardiopulmonary sympathetic afferents were 11.3 ± 2 ms and 5.4 ± 0.8 ms, respectively. In contrast to the early responses, cells with late responses to one of the visceral nerves did not always exhibit late responses to the other visceral nerve. Fifty-one percent of the cells exhibited late responses to splanchnic input, and 40% had late responses to cardiopulmonary sympathetic input. Only 17 cells had late responses to both. This activity from splanchnic afferents reached T_1 to T_5 STT neurons by propriospinal pathways and by the sympathetic chain that has afferents entering the upper thoracic spinal segments (Ammons *et al.*, 1984a). Thus, it is evident from these results that cells in the upper thoracic regions, i.e., T_1 to T_5, do receive input from splanchnic afferents.

Since splanchnic nerve stimulation is such a diffuse stimulus for activating abdominal afferents, we decided to examine the input that originated from gallbladder distention. The gallbladder has been implicated in anginalike pain; therefore, it would be a good choice to examine the effect of its distention of T_1 to T_5 STT cells. The gallbladder was exposed through a midline incision, and the cystic duct was ligated at its junction with the common hepatic duct (Figure 3; Ammons *et al.*, 1984a). A double-barrel cannula was inserted into the fundus of the gallbladder. The inner barrel was connected to a pressure

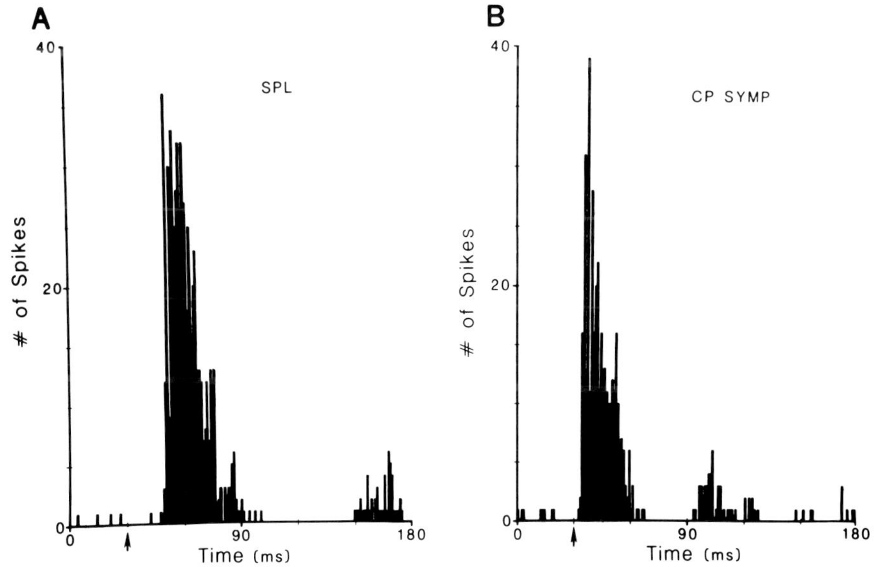

FIGURE 5. A comparison of STT cell responses to electrical stimulation of the greater splanchnic (SPL) nerve and the cardiopulmonary (CP) sympathetic fibers. Stimulus strength was intense enough to activate early and late volleys. Arrows indicate the onset of the stimulus.

transducer to measure gallbladder pressure, and saline was injected into the gallbladder by the outer barrel. Sixteen STT cells were excited during gallbladder distention. Typical responses of the cells to gallbladder distention fell into two categories. One category showed a tonic level of activity during gallbladder distention, whereas the other group showed a phasic activation of the cells during distention (Figure 6). The gallbladder pressure threshold for cell responses varied between 20 and 80 mm Hg. Maximal responses were usually obtained to 80 mm Hg. The most effective distending pressure resulted in an increase of cell activity from 13 ± 4 (control) to 24 ± 3 impulses/s (distended). These results demonstrate that increased gallbladder pressure activates upper thoracic STT neurons and may explain a number of clinical observations of chest pain resulting from gallbladder disease.

D. *Visceral Pain Mechanisms*

A common characteristic of visceral pain sensation is its referral to overlying or nearby somatic structures. In fact, referred pain is a far more common sensation than the sense that the pain is originating at a specific site in a visceral organ. The purpose of this section is to discuss neural mechanisms that have been proposed for explaining referred pain associated with visceral disease. This discussion does not include the hyperalgesia that is often associated with visceral pain.

Angina and anginalike pain are used here as the prototypical description for referred pain, since the heart and gallbladder have been studied most intensely. Angina pectoris is usually perceived in the retrosternal, precordial anterior thoracic, and anterior cervical regions of the chest; in the left and sometimes the right shoulder, arm, wrist, or hand; or in one or both jaws and may even include the teeth or posterior region of the lungs (Harrison and Reeves, 1968). Although this pain radiation is common for heart disease, it could also be associated with other, noncardiac disease such as gastrointestinal

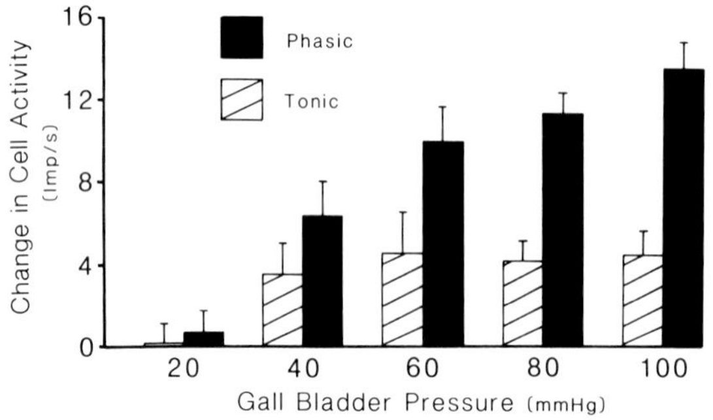

FIGURE 6. Effects of gallbladder distention on STT cell activity. Cells could be divided into phasic or tonic responders.

disorders, esophageal diseases, pulmonary disease, and musculoskeletal disorders (Christie and Conti, 1981). The locations of somatic receptive fields in STT studies correlate well with somatic locations described by patients. It should be pointed out, however, that all cell recordings have been obtained from the left gray matter, and none have been recorded from the right side.

Over the years, theories have been proposed to explain the phenomenon of referred pain. Each of the theories is described and then examined in light of our present understanding of neural mechanisms.

1. *Convergence–Facilitation Theory*

This theory was one of the earliest theories proposed to describe referred pain (MacKenzie, 1909), although Head (1893) was the first to coin the term "referred pain," and Sturge (1883) was the first to describe some type of convergence as a possible physiological mechanism underlying the referred pain associated with angina pectoris. MacKenzie (1909) was correct in suggesting that sensory impulses originating from a visceral organ are transmitted to spinal gray matter. He felt that sympathetic afferent fibers had no direct connection with somatic pain pathways but instead set up a focus of excitability in the cells near the pain pathway. Using current information to update his theory, impulses normally arriving in the spinal cord from somatic structures may cause some background discharge activity of STT cells, but after the cells are facilitated by sympathetic afferents, activity will be increased sufficiently to cause sensation of somatic pain.

Numerous studies dispute the "convergence–facilitation theory." Referred pain was not abolished when procaine was infiltrated in the area of the sternum of a patient exhibiting angina pectoris with pain referred to the sternum (Lewis, 1942). Other investigators obtained similar results in patients with various visceral diseases (Boyden and Rigler, 1934; White, 1952; Wolff and Hardy, 1947). Somatic denervation in animals also failed to abolish pain referral during coronary artery occlusion (White *et al.*, 1933) or gallbladder distention (Davis *et al.*, 1932). Although Weiss and Davis (1928) relieved referred cutaneous pain under certain conditions, S. Wolf, H. G. Wolff, and H. Goodell (unpublished data cited by Wolff and Hardy, 1947) failed to confirm these experiments.

Electrophysiological studies in the spinal gray matter also do not support the "convergence–facilitation" theory. Field potentials of similar magnitude were produced in the lumbar gray matter when somatic and visceral afferent fibers were electrically stimulated (Selzer and Spencer, 1969). The initial local activity for visceral afferent fibers, as well as for somatic afferents, was greatest in the lamina V region. If sympathetic afferent fibers produced only facilitation without causing cells to discharge, then it is unlikely that field potentials would have been generated. These results indicate that sympathetic afferent fibers can activate interneurons without requiring excitation of somatic afferent fibers. In summary, clinical and animal studies do not support the "convergence–facilitation theory" for explaining referred pain.

2. *Convergence–Projection Theory*

This theory, proposed by Ruch (1961), seems to be the most logical explanation for describing the central phenomenon of referred pain. Ruch (1961) states that "some visceral afferents converge with cutaneous pain afferents to end upon the *same* neuron at some point in the sensory pathway—spinal, thalamic or cortical—and that the system of fibers is sufficiently organized topographically to provide the dermatomal reference." Logically, the first synapse at which this convergence could occur is the STT. This theory presumes that actual monosynaptic and polysynaptic postsynaptic impulses are initiated by both somatic and visceral inputs and produce action potentials in cells of the STT. Under normal conditions, sympathetic afferent fibers may continually transmit impulses to the spinal gray matter, but during visceral pain such as angina pectoris, afferents gradually increase their discharge rate (Baker *et al.*, 1980; Malliani and Lombardi 1982). These afferent impulses increase the discharge rate of STT cells. The STT cells send signals to the ventral posterior lateral nucleus of the thalamus and from there to areas of the brain involved with conscious perception of pain.

In general, up to the third to fifth decade of a normal person's life, the STT transmits nociceptive information from somatic structures, since somatic receptors interact with a hostile external environment. In those individuals who develop angina pectoris, the increased frequency of impulses originating from the heart (Malliani, 1982) or increased number of cardiac afferents recruited (Uchida and Murao, 1974a,b) increases the discharge rate of STT cells that also receive somatic inputs. When the information activates areas of the brain involved with pain perception, it may be interpreted as coming from somatic structures because the brain may have "learned" the somatic location from previous experiences. The theory of a "learned" experience to explain how the central nervous system can interpret the somatic and visceral information seems plausible, but no experimental data support it (Mountcastle, 1980). On the other hand, there seems to be no experimental evidence to refute that supposition. This seems to be a fruitful area for further research.

Deep, dull, and poorly localized perception of pain in the area of referral is another characteristic of visceral pain. The sensation is similar to that produced by pain arising from muscles, periosteum, and joints (Lewis, 1942). This type of referred pain could be sensed if sympathetic afferent fibers synapse on STT cells that receive their primary input from muscles and deep structures. In our studies on STT cells, many cells received muscle input in addition to cutaneous input. Thus, there seems to be some relationship between the types of cells excited by both somatic and visceral input and the characteristics of somatic receptive fields.

Anginalike pain associated with gallbladder disease presents another interesting type of referred pain. Convergence onto STT cells of sympathetic input arising from two different visceral organs provides one explanation for the sensation of this type of referred pain. The interaction is more complicated, because visceral pain can often be referred to somatic structures closer to the gallbladder. No neurophysiological experiments have been done to explain why pain sometimes is referred to overlying structures and other times is referred to somatic fields that are usually the target for another visceral organ.

3. *Psychological Theory*

Another theory called the "psychological theory" needs to be discussed briefly. Theobald (1949) suggested that viscerosomatic convergence occurred only at suprasegmental levels. He felt that the "convergence–facilitation" theory was inadequate to explain referred pain; therefore, he emphasized the interactions that occur in the cerebral cortex. Only passing reference was made to convergence that might occur in the spinal cord. No doubt the cortex processes this convergent information, but the actual viscerosomatic convergence occurs predominately in cells located in the spinal cord. McLeod (1958) shows that thalamic cells respond to visceral and somatic inputs, but most likely this information is transmitted in the same STT cell. The issue suprasegmentally is how the cerebral cortex or central areas that perceive pain process information that has converged at the spinal cord level. The question of convergence occurring at the cortical level may not be as important for understanding referred pain.

So far, the emphasis for the basis of viscerosomatic convergence has centered around central interactions. Although this seems to provide a sound basis for referred pain, one cannot rule out peripheral mechanisms such as branching of dendrites. In this situation, one branch of a spinal neuron innervates a somatic structure, and one branch innervates a visceral organ (Bahr *et al.*, 1981; Sinclair *et al.*, 1948). Branching might play a minor role, but it is unlikely that a majority of sympathetic afferent fibers are branches of a spinal neuron also projecting to a somatic structure. It is more likely that the branched neurons might play a more significant role in hyperalgesia associated with visceral pain (Sinclair *et al.*, 1948).

Indirect evidence from our studies led us to the suggestion that sympathetic afferent fibers have very few branches that contribute to the phenomenon of referred pain. A population of STT cells exhibited tachyphylaxis to repeated injections of bradykinin into the heart, yet somatic manipulation elicited a response in STT cells similar to the response observed following the first bradykinin injection (Blair *et al.*, 1982b). Desensitization of cardiac receptors was not the cause of tachyphylaxis because in the same experiment, subsequent cells responded vigorously to repeated intracardiac injections. Thus, there may be central mechanisms that produce tachyphylaxis in a certain population of STT cells. If this population of cells received input from branched neurons, then one would expect tachyphylaxis for somatic input as well because the branched dendrites would converge somatic and visceral information onto the same sensory axons to affect a common pool of spinal neurons. Since somatic input was unchanged in STT cells that were tachyphylactic to visceral input, we speculate that somatic afferent input may activate cells by affecting a different pool of interneurons or by synapsing on a different region of the cell. These differential responses may require separate spinal neurons for somatic and for visceral inputs. Thus, branching may be of minor importance for explaining referred pain.

E. Contribution of Vagal Afferents

The possible influence of the cardiopulmonary vagal afferent fibers on STT cell responses needed to be considered because bradykinin and coronary artery occlusion also activate receptors of vagal afferents. Our first concern was that these vagal afferent fibers were carrying information that contributed to the excitation of STT cells observed when cardiac receptors were stimulated.

1. Vagal Afferent Fibers

Myelinated fibers arise primarily from the atria and the venal–atrial junctions (J. C. G. Coleridge *et al.*, 1957; Paintel, 1973; Thorén *et al.*, 1976). In contrast to the more localized contribution of the myelinated fibers, vagal afferent C fibers have their sensory endings distributed to all chambers of the heart (Baker *et al.*, 1979; Coleridge *et al.*, 1978; Muers and Sleight, 1972; Sleight and Widdicombe, 1965; Thorén, 1979).

Vagal afferent unmyelinated fibers can be roughly classified into two categories. One category is considered mechanosensitive and is located primarily in the atria (Thames *et al.*, 1977; Thorén *et al.*, 1976) and ventricles (Oberg and Thorén, 1973; Sleight and Widdicombe, 1965; Thorén, 1977). Unmyelinated afferent fibers of the second category have chemosensitive endings and are found in the veins, atria, and arteries (Coleridge *et al.*, 1973) as well as the ventricles (Coleridge *et al.*, 1978; Sleight and Widdicombe, 1965). These chemosensitive receptors are stimulated with a variety of endogenous chemicals and also respond to naturally occurring substances such as bradykinin (Kaufman *et al.*, 1980). Vagal afferent fibers are also excited during coronary artery occlusion (Thorén, 1976).

Vasomotor regions of the central nervous system are tonically inhibited by vagal afferent fibers from the cardiopulmonary region (Thorén *et al.*, 1976). Another demonstration of vagal interaction with sympathetic efferent fibers was that by Schwartz *et al.* (1973), who showed that excitation of vagal afferent fibers inhibited the single-unit activity of cardiac sympathetic efferent fibers. Thus, numerous studies show that a considerable amount of interaction occurs within the central nervous system when vagal afferent fibers are activated. Furthermore, these areas also mediate pain responses.

2. *Effects of Vagal Afferents on STT Activity*

Since vagal afferent fibers influence areas in the central nervous system that also function in pain, it was important to demonstrate how STT cell activity was affected during coronary artery occlusion or following injections of bradykinin into the heart. Injections of bradykinin before and after transection of the vagus produced similar STT cell responses; therefore, vagal afferents do not contribute to the overall excitation of STT cells during noxious stimulation. However, while we were recording from a cell, activity sometimes changed when vagi were in the process of being transected. This led us to consider whether vagal afferents could influence STT cells in another way, so we investigated vagal nerve stimulation as a possible means for activating vagal afferents.

The left thoracic vagus nerve was exposed, and a bipolar electrode was placed just superior to the aortic arch (Figure 3, electrode pair B). An additional electrode was placed on the cardiac branch of the vagus nerve (Figure 3, electrode pair C), and in several experiments electrodes were also placed on the vagus nerve between the heart and the abdomen (Figure 3, electrode pair D). Ligatures were placed around both vagi in the neck so that a bilateral vagotomy could be performed while recording from a cell. Stimuli were usually delivered with a 2-ms duration at a frequency at 20 Hz for 5 to 10 s. Stimulus intensity ranged from 2 to 35 V. Intensity of the stimulus was often chosen to obtain a near maximal response without appearance of the vagal stimulus artifact in the window of the discriminator. For 71 STT cells tested, 61% were inhibited by left thoracic vagal stimulation, 13% were excited, 4% were initally excited then inhibited, and 22% did not change their activity (Ammons *et al.*, 1983a). The degree of inhibition caused by left thoracic vagal stimulation was less when cell activity was greater (Ammons *et al.*, 1983).

Since vagal afferent fibers inhibited the spontaneous activity of STT cells, we wondered whether a noxious stimulus applied to the skin or skin and muscle would be modified. Left thoracic vagal stimulation inhibited 100% of the cells responding to noxious somatic stimulation (Ammons, 1983a). In addition, vagal stimulation could inhibit innocuous stimuli such as hair movement. Stimulation of the cardiac vagal branch could produce responses similar to left thoracic vagal stimulation, but stimulation of vagal fibers below the heart was unable to produce inhibition. Effects of vagal stimulation completely disappeared after the vagi were transected in the cervical region. These results indicated that activation of descending pathways initiated by cardiac or cardiopulmonary vagal afferents was powerful enough to depress cell activity even when the cell received noxious input. Thus, the input, at least on some cells, is potent.

Vagal stimulation could modulate somatic input, but does it have the ability to change the activity of a cell when sympathetic afferent fibers are stimulated? Effects of vagal stimulation on sympathetic input were evaluated in two ways. One method was to apply the conditioning–test (CT) technique. A conditioning stimulus was applied to vagal afferent fibers, and the test stimulus was applied to sympathetic afferent fibers at different intervals following the conditioning stimulus (Ammons *et al.*, 1983b). The averaged CT curve for 15 STT cells showed a triphasic curve for the vagal effects on responses to A-δ sympathetic fiber activation. Following maximal inhibition near a CT interval of 50 ms, the response began to recover at an interval of 80 ms. A secondary prolonged inhibitory trend followed for at least 200 ms. The CT curve for C-fiber input occurred with a maximal inhibition slightly earlier, and inhibition appeared to be more prolonged. These CT curves suggest that inhibition is effective for both the A-δ and C-fiber sympathetic afferents. The effects are often long lasting and seem complex in nature. The long-lasting nature of the inhibition is consistent with, although not proof of, the presence of a presynaptic inhibitory mechanism (Foreman *et al.*, 1976; Schmidt, 1971).

The second method used to determine the effects of vagal stimulation on sympathetic afferent fiber input was to inject bradykinin into the left atrium and observe the influence of vagal stimulation (Ammons *et al.*, 1983b). Figure 7 shows the average responses to intracardiac injection of bradykinin and the effects of left thoracic vagal stimulation on these responses. Bradykinin caused cells to increase their discharge rates from an average of 9.1 ± 2.1 spikes/s to 29.2 ± 3.7 spikes/s just before vagal stimulation. Vagal stimulation reduced activity by 18 spikes/s to an average of 11.7 ± 4 ($P < 0.001$). After vagal stimulation was stopped, cell activity returned to the bradykinin-stimulated level. If this same paradigm was tested after the cervical vagi were transected,

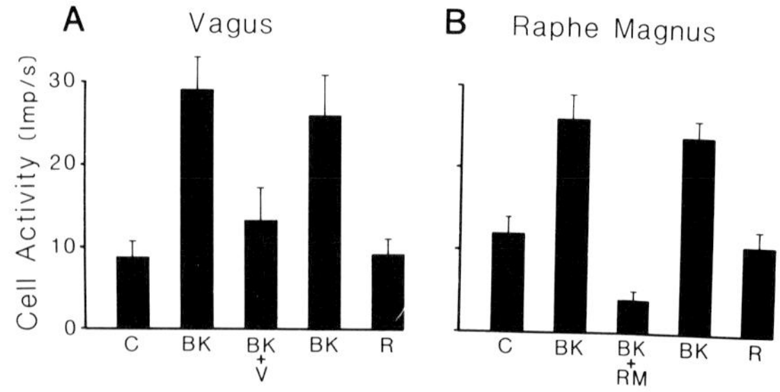

FIGURE 7. Inhibition of discharges in STT cells during their responses to injections of bradykinin into the left atrium. Inhibition was produced by electrically stimulating the vagus nerve (A) or the nucleus raphe magnus (B). Letters at the bottom of the graphs indicate the following: C, control (background activity); BK, peak response to bradykinin (BK) injection; BK + V, effect of stimulating the vagus during peak BK response; BK + RM, effect of stimulating the nucleus raphe magnus during peak BK response; R, recovery after cell had returned to control levels of activity.

no inhibition was observed. Activity of the STT cells by both electrical and natural stimulation can be modified by activation of vagal fibers.

F. Descending Inhibitory Pathways

Vagal afferent fibers elicit inhibitory effects on cells of origin of the STT. The next question to be raised is: Over what pathways is this information being transmitted? It is probable that these pathways include brainstem networks and descending bulbospinal pathways. Pain and noxious information can be modified by activating descending spinal pathways that modulate the discharge rate of dorsal horn neurons including STT cells (see comments by Hammond, Chapter 15, and Gebhart, Chapter 16). Possible pathways that could be activated during vagal afferent activation include the hypothalamus (Carstens, 1982), midbrain periaqueductal gray (Carstens *et al.*, 1979, 1981), nucleus reticularis gigantocellularis (Haber *et al.*, 1978, 1980), and nucleus raphe magnus (NRM) (Fields *et al.*, 1977; Gerhart *et al.*, 1981). Thus, it is reasonable to assume that vagal inhibition of STT neurons may be mediated by activation of descending systems that are part of the system for pain modulation.

In support of this concept is the recent evidence indicating that coronary artery occlusion altered catecholamine and serotonin levels in areas of the rat brain related to systems involved in analgesia including the NRM (Sole *et al.*, 1983). After vagal afferent fibers were interrupted, these changes were not observed. The extent to which overlap occurs between brain circuits controlling blood pressure and those modulating sensory information is not established, but interesting studies show that analgesic drugs may cause changes in blood pressure (Eckenhoff and Oech, 1960) and that rats made hypertensive are less sensitive to pain (Zamir and Segal, 1979). Furthermore, individual cells of the reticular formation receive information from somatic and visceral modalities (Blair, 1985; Langhorst *et al.*, 1983). Thus, there may be interaction between these two systems.

We have demonstrated in a recent series of studies that the NRM can inhibit input originating from the cardiopulmonary region (Ammons *et al.*, 1984b). In that study, a stimulating electrode was placed in the NRM of the monkey. Stimulation parameters for activation of the NRM were pulses of 200 μs duration, 100 Hz frequency, and mean intensity of approximately 300 μA. Stimulation of the NRM inhibited all 17 cells that responded with an increased discharge to the intracardiac injection of bradykinin (Figure 7). Bradykinin increased the discharge rate of the STT cells from an average 12 ± 2 impulses/s to 26 ± 3 impulses/s. At the peak of the response, the NRM was stimulated. This reduced the activity of the cells to an average 4 ± 1 impulses/s. After the stimulation was stopped, activity returned to 24 ± 2 spikes/s and eventually recovered to a mean of 11 ± 2 spikes/s. Thus, results of this study showed that NRM stimulation powerfully inhibited STT cell responses to noxious cardiac stimuli. In addition, NRM stimulation inhibited background activity and noxious and innocuous somatic inputs. Thus, the raphe–spinal pathway appears to be capable of exerting powerful influences on the transmission of noxious visceral information. The effectiveness of NRM stimulation on the lumbar STT response to somatic stimuli was found in other studies (Beall *et al.*, 1976; Gerhart *et al.*, 1981; McCreery *et al.*, 1979; Willis *et al.*, 1977). Our studies combined with work of these investigators clearly demonstrate that NRM is involved in the modulation of both visceral and somatic information.

Hypothetical connections can be used to explain how vagal afferent fibers can modulate STT cells by activating the descending pathway originating from NRM (Figure 8). Vagal afferent fibers in the primate terminate in or near the nucleus of the tractus solitarius (NTS) (Beckstead and Norgren, 1979). Connections between NTS and NRM are not defined anatomically or electrophysiologically, but at least in the cat and rat, efferent fibers from NTS do project to the medial reticular formation and the hypothalamus (Figure 8, dashed line) (Loewy and Burton, 1978; Ricardo and Koh, 1978). Based on our results to date, we speculate that this inhibitory effect of vagal activation may utilize the raphe–spinal system. Although this possibility seems plausible, other descending pathways including those originating from the hypothalamus, periaqueductal gray, and nucleus reticularis gigantocellularis must also be investigated.

The role of vagal afferents originating from the cardiopulmonary region and producing inhibition of STT cell activity is unknown. We can only speculate that this type of interaction could explain the silent infarct observed in patients who have severe myocardial ischemia but perceive no pain (Margolis *et al.*, 1973; Master and Geller, 1969; Uretsky *et al.*, 1977). During the right conditions, myocardial ischemia could occur without pain sensation because vagal input into the brainstem powerfully activates descending inhibitory path-

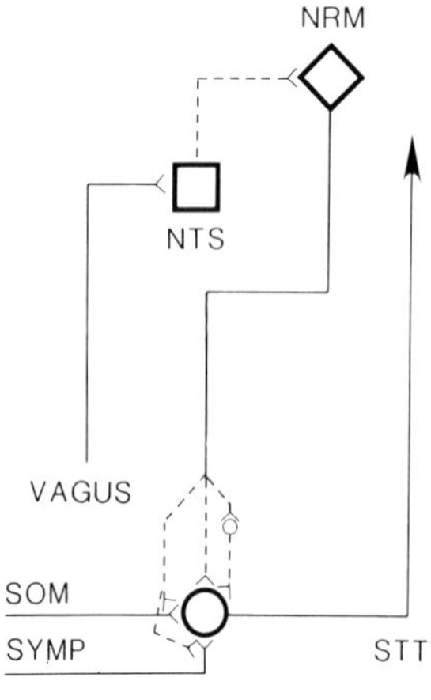

FIGURE 8. A schematic diagram showing a hypothetical pathway to explain inhibition produced during vagal stimulation and nucleus raphe magnus stimulation. Solid lines represent known pathways. Broken lines represent hypothetical connections. The descending pathway could produce inhibition via presynaptic mechanisms, direct postsynaptic inhibition, and indirect postsynaptic inhibition by way of interneurons. Abbreviations are: NTS, nucleus tractus solitarius; NRM, nucleus raphe magnus; SOM, input from somatic receptic field; SYMP, input from sympathetic afferent fibers; STT, spinothalamic tract cells.

ways. This activation could reduce the responsiveness of STT cells to the excitatory effects of sympathetic afferent fibers. This speculation represents a working hypothesis to provide the basis for further investigations to discover physiological mechanisms to explain the role of vagal afferents.

ACKNOWLEDGMENTS. The scientific experiments were supported by NIH grants HL22732, HL27260, and Research Career Development Award HL00557 from the National Heart, Lung and Blood Institute. The author wishes to thank W. Steve Ammons and Robert W. Blair for participating in these experiments. They were postdoctoral fellows supported by NIH postdoctoral fellowships HL06318 (R.W.B.) and NS071134 (W.S.A.). A special thanks to Diana Holston and Mary Martindale for technical assistance, and to Tammi Williams for preparing the figures.

References

AMMONS, W. S., BLAIR, R. W., AND FOREMAN, R. D. Vagal afferent inhibition of primate T_1–T_5 spinothalamic neurons. *J. Neurophysiol.* 50:926–940, 1983a.

AMMONS, W. S., BLAIR, R. W., AND FOREMAN, R. D. Vagal afferent inhibition of spinothalamic cell responses to sympathetic afferents and bradykinin in the monkey. *Circ. Res.* 53:603–612, 1983b.

AMMONS, W. S., BLAIR, R. W., AND FOREMAN, R. D. Greater splanchnic excitation of primate T_1–T_5 spinothalamic neurons. *J. Neurophysiol.* 51:592–603, 1984a.

AMMONS, W. S., BLAIR, R. W., AND FOREMAN, R. D. Raphe magnus inhibition of primate T_1–T_4 spinothalamic cells with cardiopulmonary visceral input. *Pain* 20:247–260, 1984b.

BAHR, R., BLUMBERG, H., AND JANIG, W. Do dichotomizing afferent fibers exist which supply visceral organs as well as somatic structures? A contribution to the problem of referred pain. *Neurosci. Lett.* 24:25–28, 1981.

BAKER, D. G., COLERIDGE, H. M., AND COLERIDGE, J. C. G. Vagal afferent C fibres from the ventricle, in: *Cardiac Receptors* (R. HAINSWORTH, C. KIDD, AND R. J. LINDEN, eds.) Cambridge University Press, Cambridge, 1979, pp. 117–137.

BAKER, D. G., COLERIDGE, H. M., COLERIDGE, J. C. G., AND NERDRUM, T. Search for a cardiac nociceptor: Stimulation by bradykinin of sympathetic afferent nerve endings in the heart of the cat. *J. Physiol. (Lond.)* 306:519–536, 1980.

BEALL, J. E., MARTIN, R. F., APPLEBAUM, A. E., AND WILLIS, W. D. Inhibition of primate spinothalamic tract neurons by stimulation in the region of the nucleus raphe magnus. *Brain Res.* 114:328–333, 1976.

BECKSTEAD, R. M., AND NORGREN, R. An autoradiographic examination of the central distribution of the trigeminal facial, glossopharyngeal and vagus nerves in the monkey. *J. Comp. Neurol.* 184:455–472, 1979.

BLAIR, R. W. Noxious cardiac input onto neurons in medullary reticular formation. *Brain Res.* 326:335–346, 1985.

BLAIR, R. W., WEBER, R. N., AND FOREMAN, R. D. Characteristics of primate spinothalmic tract neurons receiving viscerosomatic convergent inputs in T_3–T_5 segments. *J. Neurophysiol.* 46:797–811, 1981a.

BLAIR, R. W., WEBER, R. N., AND FOREMAN, R. D. Response of spinal cord neurons to electrically-induced arrhythmias. *Fed. Proc.* 40:321, 1981b.

BLAIR, R. W., HOLMES, H. R., AND FOREMAN, R. D. Excitation of feline thoracic spinal neurons by cardiac arrhythmias. *Physiologist* 25:322, 1982a.

BLAIR, R. W., WEBER, R. N., AND FOREMAN, R. D. Responses of thoracic spinothalamic neurons to intracardiac injection of bradykinin the the monkey. *Circ. Res.* 51:83–94, 1982b.

BLAIR, R. W., AMMONS, W. S., AND FOREMAN, R. D. Responses of thoracic spinothalamic and spinoreticular cells to coronary artery occlusion. *J. Neurophysiol.* 51:636–648, 1984.

BOYDEN, E. A., AND RIGLER, L. G. Localization of pain accompanying faradic excitation of stomach and duodenum in healthy individuals. *J. Clin. Invest.* 13:833–851, 1934.

BROWN, A. M. Excitation of afferent cardiac sympathetic nerve fibres during myocardial ischaemia. *J. Physiol. (Lond.)* 190:35–53, 1967.

BROWN, A. M. Cardiac reflexes, in: *Handbook of Physiology,* Vol. 1, *The Cardiovascular System, The Heart* (R. M. BERNE, ed.), American Physiological Society, Bethesda, 1979, pp. 677–689.

BROWN, A. M., AND MALLIANI, A. Spinal sympathetic reflexes initiated by coronary receptors. *J. Physiol. (Lond.)* 212:685–705, 1971.

CARSTENS, E. Inhibition of spinal dorsal horn neuronal responses to noxious skin heating by medial hypothalamic stimulation in the cat. *J. Neurophysiol.* 48:808 –822, 1982.

CARSTENS, E., YOKOTA, T., AND ZIMMERMANN, M. Inhibition of spinal neuronal responses to noxious skin heating by stimulation of mesencephalic periaqueductal gray in the cat. *J. Neurophysiol.* 42:558–568, 1979.

CARSTENS, E., FRAUNHOFFER, M., AND ZIMMERMANN, M. Serotonergic mediation of descending inhibition from midbrain periaqueductal gray, but not reticular formation, of spinal nociceptive transmission in the cat. *Pain* 10:149–167, 1981.

CASATI, R., LOMBARDI, F., AND MALLIANI, A. Afferent sympathetic unmyelinated fibres with left ventricular endings in cats. *J. Physiol. (Lond.)* 292:135–148, 1979.

CERVERO, F. Mechanisms of visceral pain, in: *Persistent Pain,* Vol. 4, (S. LIPTON AND J. MILES, eds.), Grune & Stratton, London, 1983a, pp. 1–19.

CERVERO, F. Somatic and visceral inputs in to the thoracic spinal cord of the cat: Effects of noxious stimulation of the biliary system. *J. Physiol. (Lond.)* 337:51–67, 1983b.

CHRISTIE, L. G., AND CONTI, C. R. Systematic approach to evaluation of angina-like chest pain: Pathophysiology and clinical testing with emphasis on objective documentation of myocardial ischemia. *Am. Heart J.* 102:897–912, 1981.

COLERIDGE, H. M., COLERIDGE, J. C. G., DANGEL, A., KIDD, C., LUCK, J. C., AND SLEIGHT, P. Impulses in slowly conducting vagal fibers from afferent endings in the veins atria, and arteries of dogs and cats. *Circ. Res.* 33:87–97, 1973.

COLERIDGE, H. M., COLERIDGE, J. C. G., AND KIDD, C. Afferent innervation of the heart and great vessels: A comparison of the vagal and sympathetic components. *Acta Physiol. Pol.* 29(Suppl.):55–79, 1978.

COLERIDGE, J. C. G., HEMINGWAY, A., HOLMES, R. L., AND LINDEN, R. J. The location of artial receptors in the dog: A physiological and histological study. *J. Physiol. (Lond.)* 136:174–197, 1957.

DAVIS, L., POLLACK, L. J., AND STONE, T. T. Visceral pain. *Surg. Gynaecol. Obstet.* 55:418–427, 1932.

DUBNER, R., PRICE, D. D., BEITEL, R. E., AND HU, J. W. Peripheral neural correlates of behavior in monkey and human related to sensory-discriminative aspects of pain, in: *Pain in the Trigeminal Region,* (D. J. ANDERSON AND B. MATTHEWS, eds.), Elsevier/North Holland, Amsterdam, 1977, pp. 57–66.

ECKENHOFF, J. E., AND OECH, S. R. Effects of narcotics and antagonists upon respiration and circulation in man. *Clin. Pharmacol. Ther.* 1:483–524, 1960.

FIELDS, H. L., MEYER, G. A., AND PARTRIDGE, L. D., JR. Convergence of visceral and somatic inputs onto spinal neurons. *Exp. Neurol.* 26:36–52, 1970.

FIELDS, H. L., BASBAUM, A. I., CLANTON, C. H., AND ANDERSON, S. D. Nucleus raphe magnus inhibition of spinal cord dorsal horn neurons. *Brain Res.* 126:441–453, 1977.

FOREMAN, R. D., AND OHATA, C. A. Effects of coronary artery occlusion of thoracic spinal neurons receiving viscerosomatic inputs. *Am. J. Physiol.* 238:H667–H679, 1980.

FOREMAN, R. D., APPLEBAUM, A. E., BEALL, J. E., TREVINO, D. L., AND WILLIS, W. D. Responses of primate spinothalamic tract neurons to electrical stimulation of hindlimb peripheral nerves. *J. Neurophysiol.* 38:132–145, 1975.

Foreman, R. D., Beall, J. E., Applebaum, A. E., Coulter, J. D., and Willis, W. D. Effects of dorsal column stimulation on primate spinothalamic tract neurons. *J. Neurophysiol.* 39:534–546, 1976.

Foreman, R. D., Hancock, M. B., and Willis, W. D. Responses of spinothalamic tract cells in the thoracic spinal cord of the monkey to cutaneous and visceral inputs. *Pain* 11:149–162, 1981.

Gerhart, K. D., Wilcox, T. K., Chung, J. M., and Willis, W. D. Inhibition of nociceptive and non-nociceptive responses of primate spinothalamic cells by stimulation in medial brain stem. *J. Neurophysiol.* 45:121–136, 1981.

Gokin, A. P., Kostyuk, P. G., and Preobrazhensky, N. N. Neuronal mechanisms of interactions of high-threshold visceral and somatic afferent influences in spinal cord and medulla. *J. Physiol. (Paris)* 73:319–333, 1977.

Guilbaud, G., Benelli, G., and Besson, J. M. Response of thoracic dorsal horn interneurones to cutaneous stimulation and to the administration of algogenic substances into the mesenteric artery in the spinal cat. *Brain Res.* 124:437–448, 1977.

Guzman, F., Braun, C., and Lim, R. K. S. Visceral pain and the pseudaffective response to intra-arterial injection of bradykinin and other algesic agents. *Arch. Int. Pharmacodyn. Ther.* 136:353–383, 1962.

Gybels, J., Handwerker, H. O., and Van Hees, J. A comparison between the discharges of human nociceptive nerve fibres and the subject's ratings of his sensations. *J. Physiol. (Lond.)* 292:193–206, 1979.

Haber, L. H., Martin, R. F., Chatt, A. B., and Willis, W. D. Effects of stimulation in nucleus reticularis gigantocellularis on the activity of spinothalamic tract neurons in the monkey. *Brain Res.* 153:163–168, 1978.

Haber, L. H., Martin, R. F., Chung, J. M., and Willis, W. D. Inhibition and excitation of primate spinothalamic tract neurons by stimulation in region of nucleus reticularis gigantocellularis. *J. Neurophysiol.* 43:1578–1593, 1980.

Hampton, A. G., Beckwith, J. R., and Wood, J. E., Jr. The relationship between heart disease and gall bladder disease. *Ann. Intern. Med.* 50:1135–1148, 1959.

Hancock, M. B., Foreman, R. D., and Willis, W. D. Convergence of visceral and cutaneous input onto spinothalamic tract cells in the thoracic spinal cord of the cat. *Exp. Neurol.* 47:240–248, 1975.

Harrison, T. R., and Reeves, R. J. *Principles and Problems of Ischemic Heart Disease,* Year Book Medical Publishers, Chicago, 1968, pp. 197–204.

Hashimoto, K., Hirose, M., Furukawa, S., Haykawa, H., and Kimura, E. Changes in hemodynamics and bradykinin concentration in coronary sinus blood in experimental coronary artery occlusion. *Jpn. Heart J.* 18:679–689, 1977.

Head, H. On disturbances of sensation with special reference to the pain of visceral disease. *Brain* 16:1–133, 1893.

Henderson, R. D., Wigle, E. D., Sample, K., and Manyat, G. Atypical chest pain of cardiac and esophageal origin. *Chest* 73:24–41, 1978.

Hoffman, D. S., Dubnar, R., Hayes, R. L., and Medlin, T. P. Neuronal activity in medullary dorsal horn of awake monkeys trained in the thermal discrimination task. I. Responses to innocuous and noxious thermal stimuli. *J. Neurophysiol.* 46:409–427, 1981.

Holmes, H. R., Armour, J. A., Chapman, C. D., Foreman, R. D., and Blair, R. W. Receptor mechanics of cardiovascular afferents. *Physiologist.* 25:236, 1982.

Holmes, H. R., Chapman, C. D., Armour, J. A., and Foreman, R. D. Receptive field mechanics of left ventricular sympathetic afferent fibers. *Fed. Proc.* 42:1119, 1983.

Kaufman, M. P., Baker, D. G., Coleridge, H. M., and Coleridge, J. C. G. Stimulation by bradykinin of afferent vagal C-fibers with chemosensitive endings in the heart and aorta of the dog. *Circ. Res.* 46:476–484, 1980.

KIMURA, E., HASHIMOTO, K., FURUKAWA, S., AND HAYAKAWA, H. Changes in bradykinin level in coronary sinus blood after the experimental occlusion of coronary artery. *Am. Heart J.* 85:635–647, 1973.

KOSTREVA, D. R., ZUPERKU, E. J., HESS, R. L., COON, R. L., AND KAMPINE, J. P. Pulmonary afferent activity recorded from sympathetic nerves. *J. Appl. Physiol.* 39:37–40, 1975.

LAMOTTE, R. H., AND CAMPBELL, J. N. Comparison of responses of warm and nociceptive C-fiber afferents in monkey with human judgments of thermal pain. *J. Neurophysiol.* 41:509–528, 1978.

LANGHORST, P., SCHULZ, B., SCHULZ, G., AND LAMBERTZ, M. Reticular formation of the lower brainstem. A common system for cardio-respiratory and somatomotor functions: Discharge patterns of neighboring neurons influenced by cardiovascular and respiratory afferents. *J. Autonom. Nerv. Syst.* 9:411–432, 1983.

LANGLEY, J. N. The autonomic nervous system. *Brain* 26:1–26, 1903.

LEWIS, T. *Pain,* Macmillan, London, 1942, p. 192.

LOEWY, A. D., AND BURTON, H. Nuclei of the solitary tract: Efferent projections to the lower brain stem and spinal cord of the cat. *J. Comp. Neurol.* 181:421–450, 1978.

LOMBARDI, F., MALLIANI, A., AND PAGANI, M. Nervous activity of afferent sympathetic fibers innervating the pulmonary veins. *Brain Res.* 113:197–200, 1976.

LOMBARDI, F., DELLA BELLA. P., CASATI, R., AND MALLIANI, A. Effects of intracoronary administration of bradykinin on the impulse activity of afferent sympathetic unmyelinated fibers with left ventricular endings in the cat. *Circ. Res.* 48:69–75, 1981.

MACKENZIE, J. *Symptoms and Their Interpretation,* Shaw & Sons, London, 1909.

MALLIANI, A. Cardiovascular sympathetic afferent fibers. *Rev. Physiol. Biochem. Pharmacol.* 94:11–74, 1982.

MALLIANI, A., AND LOMBARDI, F. Consideration of the fundamental mechanisms eliciting cardiac pain. *Am. Heart J.* 103:575–578, 1982.

MALLIANI, A., AND PAGANI, M. Afferent sympathetic nerve fibres with aortic endings. *J. Physiol. (Lond.)* 263:157–169, 1976.

MALLIANI, A., PETERSON, D. F., BISHOP, V. S., AND BROWN, A. M. Spinal sympathetic cardiocardiac reflexes. *Circ. Res.* 30:158–166, 1972.

MALLIANI, A., RECORDATI, G., AND SCHWARTZ, P. J. Nervous activity of afferent cardiac sympathetic fibres with atrial and ventricular endings. *J. Physiol. (Lond.)* 229:457–469, 1973.

MALLIANI, A., LOMBARDI, F., PAGANI, M., RECORDATI, G., AND SCHWARTZ, P. J. Spinal cardiovascular reflexes. *Brain Res.* 87:239–246, 1975.

MARGOLIS, J. R., KANNEL, W. S., FEINLEIB, M., DAWBER, T. R., AND MCNAMARA, P. W. Clinical features of unrecognized myocardial infarction—silent and symptomatic: Eighteen year followup: The Framingham Study. *Am. J. Cardiol.* 32:1–7, 1973.

MASTER, A. M., AND GELLER, A. J. The extent of completely asymptomatic coronary artery disease. *Am. J. Cardiol.* 23:173–179, 1969.

MCCREERY, D. B., BLOEDEL, J. R., AND HARNES, E. G. Effects of stimulating in raphe nuclei and in reticular formation on response of spinothalamic neurons to mechanical stimuli. *J. Neurophysiol.* 42:166–182, 1979.

MCLEOD, J. G. The representation of splanchnic afferent pathways in the thalamus of the cat. *J. Physiol. (Lond.)* 140:462–478, 1958.

MILLER, H. R. The interrelationship of disease of coronary arteries and gall bladder. *Am. Heart J.* 24:579–587, 1942.

MILNE, R. J., FOREMAN, R. D., GIESLER, G. J., JR., AND WILLIS, W. D. Convergence of cutaneous and pelvic viseral nociceptive inputs onto primate spinothalamic neurons. *Pain* 11:163–183, 1981.

MOUNTCASTLE, V. B. Pain and temperature sensibilities, in: *Medical Physiology,* ed. 14 (V. B. MOUNTCASTLE, ed.). C. V. Mosby, St. Louis, 1980, pp. 391–427.

MUERS, M. F., AND SLEIGHT, O. Action potentials from ventricular mechanoreceptors stimulated by occlusion of the coronary sinus in the dog. *J. Physiol. (Lond.)* 221:283–309, 1972.

NISHI, K., SAKANASHI, M., AND TAKENAKA, F. Afferent fibres from pulmonary arterial baroreceptors in the left cardiac sympathetic nerve of the cat. *J. Physiol. (Lond.)* 240:53–66, 1974.

NISHI, K., SAKANASHI, M., AND TAKENAKA, F. Activation of afferent cardiac sympathetic nerve fibres of the cat by pain producing substances and by noxious heat. *Pfluegers Arch.* 372:53–61, 1977.

OBERG, B., AND THORÉN, P. Circulatory responses to stimulation of medullated and non-medullated afferents in the cardiac nerve in the cat. *Acta Physiol. Scand.* 87:121–132, 1973.

PAINTAL, A. S. Vagal sensory receptors and their reflex effects. *Physiol. Rev.* 53:159–227, 1973.

PALMER, E. D. Chest pain of colon origin. *Gastroenterologia* 90:15–21, 1958.

POMERANZ, B., WALL, P. D., AND WEBER, W. V. Cord cells responding to fine myelinated afferents from viscera, muscle and skin. *J. Physiol. (Lond.)* 199:511–532, 1968.

RAVDIN, I. S., FITZ-HUGH, T., JR., WOLFERTH, C. C., BARBIERI, E. A., AND RAVDIN, R. G. Relation of gallstone disease to angina pectoris. *Arch. Surg.* 70:333–342, 1955.

RICARDO, J. A., AND KOH, E. T. Anatomical evidence of direct projections from the nucleus of the solitary tract to the hypothalamus, amygdala and other forebrain structures in the rat. *Brain Res.* 153:1–26, 1978.

RUCH, T. C. Pathophysiology of pain, in: *Neurophysiology* (T. C. RUCH, H. D. PATTON, J. W. WOODBURY, AND A. L. TOWE, eds). W. B. Saunders, Philadelphia, 1961, pp.350–368.

SCHERF, D., AND BOYD, L. J. *Cardiovascular Diseaes.* Grune & Stratton, New York, 1958, pp. 637–638.

SCMIDT, R. F. Presynaptic inhibition in the vertebrate central nervous system. *Ergeb. Physiol.* 63:20–101, 1971.

SCHWARTZ, P. J., PAGANI, M., LOMBARDI, F., MALLIANI, A., AND BROWN, A. M. A cardiocardiac sympathovagal reflex in the cat. *Circ. Res.* 32:215–220, 1973.

SEAGARD, J. L., PEDERSON, H. J., KOSTREVA, D. R., VAN HORN, D. L., CUSIK, J. F., AND KAMPINE, J. P. Ultrastructural identification of afferent fibers of cardiac origin in thoracic sympathetic nerves in the dog. *Am. J. Anat.* 153:217–232, 1978.

SELZER, M., AND SPENCER, W. A. Convergence of visceral and cutaneous afferent pathways in the lumbar spinal cord. *Brain Res.* 14:331–348, 1969.

SINCLAIR, D. C., WEDDELL, G., AND FEINDEL, W. H. Referred pain and associated phenomena. *Brain* 71:184–212, 1948.

SLEIGHT, P., AND WIDDICOMBE, J. G. Action potentials of the dog's left ventricle. *J. Physiol. (Lond.)* 181:235–258, 1965.

SOLE, M. J., VERSTEEG, D. H. G., DEKLOET, E. R., HUSSAIN, N., AND LIXFELD, W. The identification of specific serotonergic nuclei inhibited by cardiac vagal afferents during acute myocardial ischemia in the rat. *Brain Res.* 265:55–61, 1983.

STURGE, W. A. The phenomena of angina pectoris and their bearing upon the theory of counter-irritation. *Brain* 5:492–510, 1883.

THAMES, M. D., DONALD, D. E., AND SHEPHERD, J. T. Behavior of cardiac receptors with non-myelinated vagal afferents during spontaneous respiration in cats. *Circ. Res.* 41:694–701, 1977.

THEOBALD, G. W. The role of the cerebral cortex in the apperception of pain. *Lancet* 2:41–47, 94–97, 1949.

THORÉN, P. N. Activation of left ventricular receptors with nonmedullated vagal afferent fibers during occlusion of a coronary artery in the cat. *Am. J. Cardiol.* 37:1046–1051, 1976.

THORÉN, P. N. Characteristics of left ventricular receptors with nonmedullated vagal afferents in cats. *Circ. Res.* 40:415–421, 1977.

THORÉN, P. N. Role of cardiac vagal C-fibers in cardiovascular control. *Rev. Physiol. Biochem. Pharmacol.* 86:1–94, 1979.

THORÉN, P. N., DONALD, D. E., AND SHEPHERD, J. T. Role of heart and lung receptors with nonmedullated vagal afferents in circulatory control. *Circ. Res.* 38:(Suppl. II)II-2–II-9, 1976.

TOREBJÖRK, H. E., AND HALLIN, R. G. Identification of afferent C units in intact human skin nerves. *Brain Res.* 67:387–403, 1974.

UCHIDA, Y. Afferent sympathetic nerve fibers with mechanoreceptors in the right heart. *Am. J. Physiol.* 228:223–230, 1975a.

UCHIDA, Y. Afferent aortic nerve fibers with their pathways in cardiac sympathetic nerves. *Am. J. Phsyiol.* 228:990–995, 1975b.

UCHIDA, Y., AND MURAO, S. Excitation of afferent cardiac sympathetic nerve fibers during coronary occlusion. *Am. J. Physiol.* 226:1094–1099, 1974a.

UCHIDA, Y., AND MURAO, S. Bradykinin induced excitation of afferent cardiac sympathetic nerve fibers. *Jpn. Heart J.* 15:84–91, 1974b.

UEDA, H., UCHIDA, Y., AND KAMISAKA, K. Distribution and responses of the cardiac sympathetic receptors to mechanically induced circulatory changes. *Jpn. Heart J.* 10:70–81, 1969.

URETSKY, B. F., FARQUBAR, D. S., BEREZIN, A. F., AND HOOD, W. G., JR. Symptomatic myocardial infarction without chest pain: Prevelance and clincial course. *Am. J. Cardiol.* 40:498–503, 1977.

VAN HEES, J., AND GYBELS, J. M. C nociceptor activity in human nerve during painful and nonpainful skin stimulation. *J. Neurol. Neurosurg. Psychiatry* 44:600–607, 1981.

WEHRMACHER, E. H. *Pain in the Chest,* Charles C. Thomas, Springfield, IL, 1964, pp. 342–361.

WEISS, S., AND DAVIS, D. The significance of the afferent impulses from the skin in the mechanism of visceral pain. Skin infiltration as useful therapeutic measure. *Am. J. Med. Sci.* 176:517–536, 1928.

WHITE, J. C. Conduction of visceral pain. *N. Engl. J. Med.* 246:686–691, 1952.

WHITE, J. C., GARREY, W. E., AND ATKINS, J. A. Cardiac innervation: Experimental and clinical studies. *Arch. Surg.* 26:765–786, 1933.

WILLIS, W. D., AND COGGESHALL, R. E. *Sensory Mechanisms of the Spinal Cord,* Plenum Press, New York, 1978, p. 485.

WILLIS, W. D., TREVINO, D. L., COULTER, J. D., AND MAUNZ, R. D. Responses of primate spinothalamic tract neurons to natural stimulation of hindlimb. *J. Neurophysiol.* 37:358–372, 1974.

WILLIS, W. D., HABER, L. H., AND MARTIN, R. F. Inhibition of spinothalamic tract cells and interneurons by brainstem stimulation in the monkey. *J. Neurophysiol.* 40:968–981, 1977.

WOLFF, H. G., AND HARDY, J. D. On the nature of pain. *Physiol. Rev.* 27:167–199, 1947.

ZAMIR, N. AND SEGAL, M. Hypertension-induced analgesia: Changes in pain sensitivity in experimental hypertensive rats. *Brain Res.* 160:170–173, 1979.

11 Ascending Somatosensory Systems

WILLIAM D. WILLIS, JR.

A. *Introduction*

The ascending somatosensory pathways signal to the brain information concerning stimuli that are applied to the body or head. This chapter considers only those pathways that convey sensory information from the body. The term "somatosensory" is somewhat misleading, since the somatosensory pathways are used for the perception of signals originating from the viscera (see Foreman, Chapter 10) in addition to those coming from sensory receptors located in such somatic structures as the skin, muscles, and joints. Thus, the pathways to be discussed mediate both somatic and visceral sensation.

The principal ascending somatosensory pathways that connect the spinal cord with the brain in mammals include the dorsal column path, the postsynaptic dorsal column path, the spinocervical tract, and the spinomedullary tract in the dorsal half of the cord and the spinothalamic, spinoreticular, and spinomesencephalic tracts in the ventral half of the cord (Willis and Coggeshall, 1978). Since the cerebellum can be removed without any change in somatic sensation, the ascending pathways that distribute directly to the cerebellum or indirectly by way of such precerebellar nuclei as the inferior olive, the lateral reticular nucleus, and the pontine nuclei (Brodal, 1981) are not considered parts of the ascending somatosensory system but rather afferent limbs of motor system pathways, except when a somatosensory path is collateral to a spinocerebellar path (e.g., as appears to be the case for the spinomedullary tract).

There have been several recent reviews that deal extensively with various

WILLIAM D. WILLIS, JR. • Marine Biomedical Institute and Departments of Physiology and Biophysics and Anatomy, University of Texas Medical Branch, Galveston, Texas 77550.

aspects of the ascending somatosensory pathways (Besson *et al.*, 1982; Brown, 1981; Mountcastle, 1984; Perl, 1984; Willis and Coggeshall, 1978).

B. Ascending Somatosensory Pathways in the Dorsal Spinal Cord

1. Dorsal Column Path: Primary Afferent Collaterals

The dorsal column path at the spinal cord level consists of the ascending branches of large myelinated primary afferent fibers that traverse either the fasciculus gracilis or the fasciculus cuneatus to terminate synaptically in the nucleus gracilis or nucleus cuneatus in the caudal part of the medulla oblongata (Figure 1; Ferraro and Barrera, 1935a,b; Walker and Weaver, 1942). The axons of the fasciculus gracilis enter the spinal cord over ipsilateral dorsal

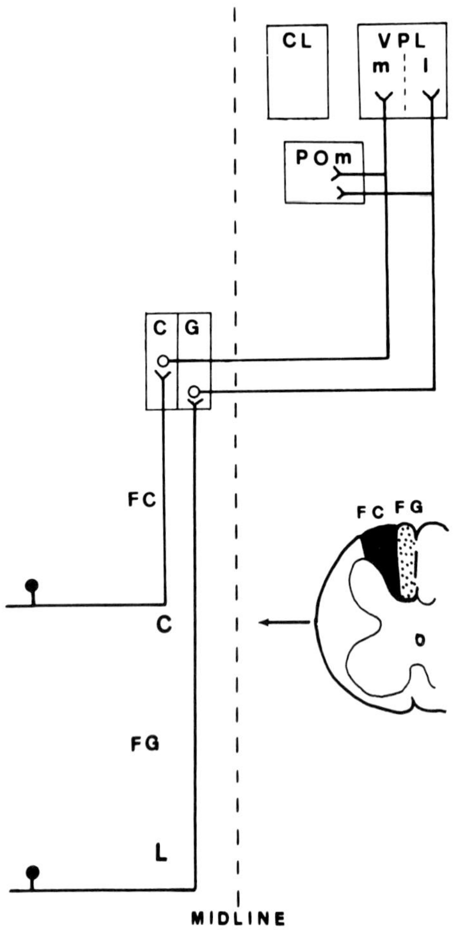

FIGURE 1. The dorsal column pathway. Axons of primary afferents are shown entering the cord over cervical (C) and lumbar (L) dorsal roots and turning rostrally to ascend in the fasciculus cuneatus (FC) or fasciculus gracilis (FG) to end in the nucleus cuneatus (C) or nucleus gracilis (G). The second-order neurons in the dorsal column nuclei then project contralaterally through the medial lemniscus to end in the medial part of the posterior complex (PO_m) and in the ventral posterior lateral nucleus (VPL). The nucleus cuneatus projects to the medial and the nucleus gracilis to the lateral portions (m,l) of VPL. The drawing of a cross section of the cord indicates the locations of the FC and FG. (From Willis and Coggeshall, 1978).

roots from midthoracic segmental levels caudally, whereas those in the fasciculus cuneatus enter through the dorsal roots from midthoracic levels and more rostrally (Carpenter *et al.*, 1968; Shriver *et al.*, 1968; Walker and Weaver, 1942). Thus, the part of the dorsal column path that is in the fasciculus gracilis is concerned largely with signals derived from sensory receptors on the ipsilateral hindlimb and lower trunk, whereas the fasciculus cuneatus conveys information originating chiefly from the forelimb and upper trunk.

If the dorsal column is examined at a given level of the spinal cord, only a fraction of the axons can be shown to belong to the dorsal column pathway proper (i.e., they project all the way to the medulla). Glees and Soler (1951) found that only 22% of the primary afferent axons entering the lumbosacral enlargement reach the nucleus gracilis. The remainder terminate within the spinal cord, either at the segmental level or at a more rostral or caudal level (Horch *et al.*, 1976). For instance, many of the large afferent fibers from the stretch receptors of muscle and from slowly adapting joint receptors that enter the lumbar cord ascend through the fasciculus gracilis only to the level of Clarke's column, where they terminate (Clark, 1972; Lloyd and McIntyre, 1950). In addition to the axons of primary afferent fibers, the dorsal column contains many axons that belong to neurons intrinsic to the spinal cord, including propriospinal neurons (Nathan and Smith, 1959) and the cells of origin of the postsynaptic dorsal column pathway (Angaut-Petit, 1975a; Rustioni, 1973, 1974; Uddenberg, 1968b). There are also axons in the dorsal column that descend from neurons in the brain. Examples of such projections include a descending pathway from neurons within the dorsal column nuclei (Bromberg *et al.*, 1981; Burton and Loewy, 1977) and, in some animals such as rodents, the corticospinal tract (Valverde, 1966). Although most of the axons in the dorsal column are myelinated, some are unmyelinated (Langford and Coggeshall, 1981). The origin of the unmyelinated component of the dorsal column is as yet unclear.

The primary afferent axons that form the dorsal column path proper undergo a spatial rearrangement as they ascend the spinal cord. At the level of entry of a given dorsal root, the ascending branches of the axons of that dorsal root form a relatively compact bundle. If activity is sampled using microelectrode recordings from axons in the bundle that supply cutaneous receptors, adjacent axons in the bundle will be found to innervate receptive fields within the same dermatome (the area of skin supplied by a particular dorsal root). However, two adjacent axons in the bundle could supply receptive fields on quite separate parts of the dermatome (Whitsel *et al.*, 1970). For example, one axon in the fasciculus gracilis could innervate the skin on one finger and another axon nearby the skin on another finger (Figure 2; B. H. Pubols *et al.*, 1965). However, near the medulla, recordings from the fasciculus gracilis show that the axons of a given dorsal root have become rearranged and are intermingled with axons from other dorsal roots. A microelectrode that samples the activity of adjacent axons will no longer demonstrate that the receptive fields are on different parts of the same dermatome. Instead,

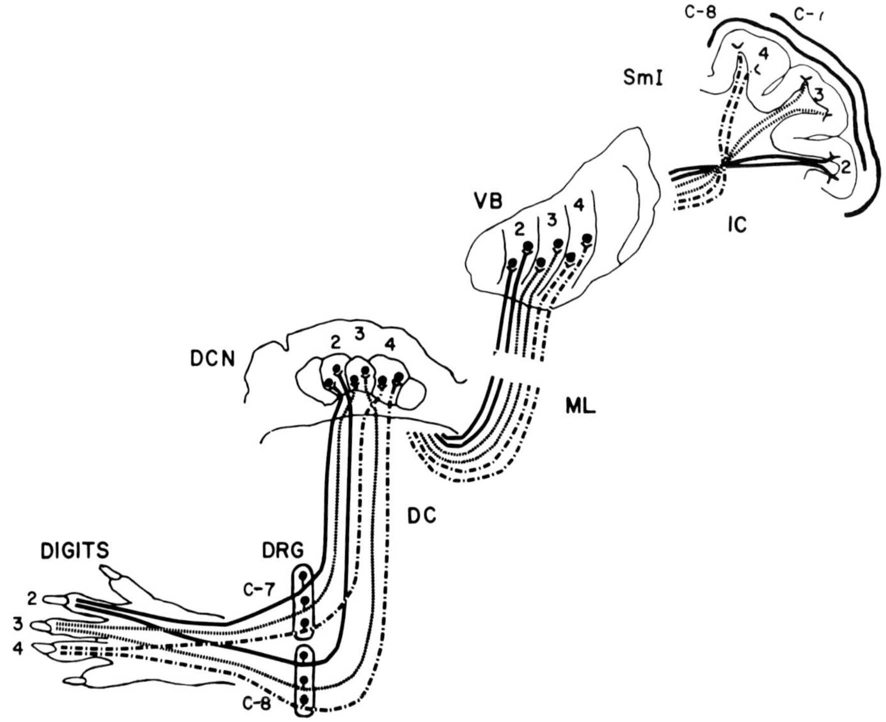

FIGURE 2. Diagram showing how fiber resorting accounts for a change from a dermatomal to a somatotopic organization in the dorsal column pathway. Abbreviations: DRG, dorsal root ganglion; DC, dorsal column; DCN, dorsal column nuclei; ML, medial lemniscus; VB, ventrobasal complex of thalamus; IC, internal capsule; SmI, sensorimotor area I. (From B. H. Pubols *et al.*, 1965.)

adjacent axons now innervate the same or closely adjacent parts of the body surface (Whitsel *et al.*, 1970). The axons of the rostral fasciculus gracilis have a somatotopic rather than a dermatomal organization. Resorting in the fasciculus cuneatus appears to be incomplete between the lower and upper cervical levels; presumably the resorting is completed as the ascending fibers enter the nucleus cuneatus (Pubols and Pubols, 1973).

Not all types of somatosensory receptors project in the dorsal column path. Recordings from primary afferent axons in the fasciculus gracilis show that the vast majority come from rapidly adapting cutaneous mechanoreceptors, such as hair follicle receptors, the RA (for rapidly adapting) receptors of glabrous skin, and Pacinian corpuscles (Brown, 1968; Horch *et al.*, 1976; Petit and Burgess, 1968). Only a small percentage of the axons in the fasciculus gracilis comes from muscle stretch receptors or slowly adapting joint receptors (Burgess and Clark, 1969; Whitsel *et al.*, 1969). However, it should be stressed that the fasciculus cuneatus does contain the axons of many slowly adapting receptors, including the ascending branches of muscle stretch receptors (Bromberg and Whitehorn, 1974; Pubols and Pubols, 1973; Uddenberg, 1968a; Whitsel *et al.*, 1969). Thus, the fasciculi gracilis and cuneatus are not exact equivalents.

The primary afferent fibers in the dorsal column path synapse on neurons in the dorsal column nuclei (Hand, 1966; Rustioni and Macchi, 1968; Rustioni and Sotelo, 1974; Walberg, 1965). The synaptic termination zone is chiefly in the middle portion of the dorsal column nuclei on neurons of the "cell cluster region" (Biedenbach, 1972; Cajal, 1909; Kuypers and Tuerk, 1964). A somatotopic organization is characteristic of the cell cluster region, presumably because of the somatotopic arrangement of the afferent projections in the dorsal column and their orderly pattern of termination in the dorsal column nuclei. The somatotopic arrangement is demonstrated in microelectrode recordings from the cell cluster region by a progressive shift in the receptive fields of neurons along both the mediolateral and the dorsoventral axes of the dorsal column nuclei but not along the rostrocaudal axis (Johnson *et al.*, 1968; Kruger *et al.*, 1961; Millar and Basbaum, 1975). Medially placed neurons have caudally situated receptive fields, and laterally placed neurons have rostral fields (Figure 3). Dorsally located neurons have fields on the distal parts of the extremities, and ventral neurons have proximal fields.

The neurons of the dorsal column nuclei that receive their input from the dorsal column path tend to have small, ipsilateral receptive fields (Gordon

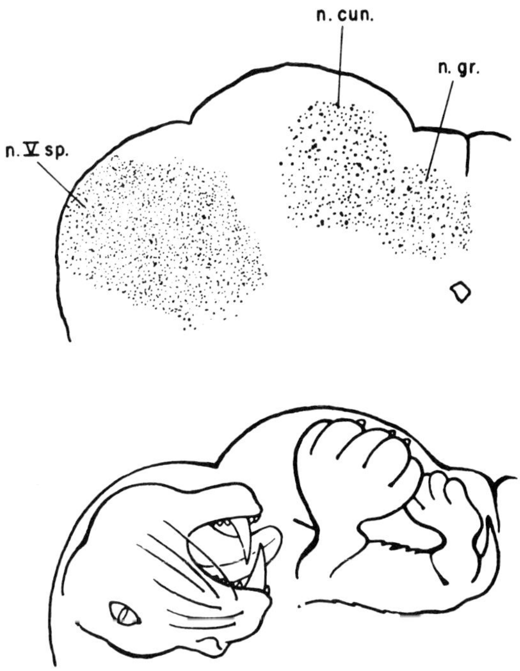

FIGURE 3. The dorsal column nuclei of the cat (n. cun., nucleus cuneatus; n. gr., nucleus gracilis) and the spinal nucleus of the trigeminal, pars caudalis (n. V sp.). Bottom: A "feliculus," showing the somatotopic organization of the somatosensory nuclei of the caudal medulla. (From Kruger *et al.*, 1961.)

and Jukes, 1964; Kruger *et al.*, 1961; McComas, 1963; Perl *et al.*, 1962), although large receptive fields have been reported for cells in the rostral part of the nucleus gracilis (Gordon and Jukes, 1964) and for cells with slowly adapting responses to tactile stimuli (Perl *et al.*, 1962). Furthermore, it is common for a given neuron to receive its sole, or at least dominant, input from a particular class of sensory receptor (Douglas *et al.*, 1978; Dykes *et al.*, 1982; Gordon and Jukes, 1964; Kruger *et al.*, 1961; Perl *et al.*, 1962). Thus, many neurons of the dorsal column nuclei are said to be modality specific (Mountcastle, 1984), since such cells relay information concerning a particular aspect of a stimulus and presumably participate in the mediation of a particular sensory quality.

A major difference between the cells of the dorsal column nuclei and the primary afferent fibers of the dorsal column is that many of the cells in the dorsal column nuclei are subject to inhibitory as well as excitatory actions following peripheral stimulation (Gordon and Jukes, 1964; Jänig *et al.*, 1977). The receptive fields of such neurons can be arranged in a center-surround fashion, with an excitatory receptive field surrounded by an inhibitory one (Figure 4A). However, this arrangement actually arises from overlapping excitatory and inhibitory receptive fields that have different gradients of effectiveness (Figure 4B; Jänig *et al.*, 1977). The responses of a particular neuron in a dorsal column nucleus are excitatory when a stimulus is applied near the center of the combined fields because the excitatory input is more powerful than the inhibitory input. However, the potency of the excitatory field decreases spatially more rapidly than does that of the inhibitory field, and so stimuli applied more peripherally cause predominantly an inhibitory action.

Cells of the dorsal column nuclei that relay information to higher levels of the somatosensory system for further processing project to the thalamus or midbrain. Neurons in the cell cluster region, for example, send their axons across the midline to ascend in the medial lemniscus to the thalamus (Berkley, 1980; Boivie, 1971a, 1978; Ellis and Rustioni, 1981; Hand and Van Winkle, 1977; Jones and Burton, 1974; Rasmussen and Peyton, 1948). The most prominent terminations of the medial lemniscus are in the ventral posterior lateral (VPL) nucleus of the ventrobasal complex. Another termination zone that may be important for somatic sensation is in the medial part of the posterior complex (PO_m nucleus; Berkley, 1980; Boivie, 1971a, 1978). In addition, connections are made from the dorsal column nuclei to a number of other brainstem regions, including several nuclei of the midbrain (Björkland, 1984; Blomqvist *et al.*, 1978; Hand and Van Winkle, 1977). Very few neurons of the dorsal column nuclei send collateral projections to both the thalamus and midbrain, and so these projections are distinct (Berkley *et al.*, 1980).

Neurons of the VPL nucleus often have small contralateral excitatory cutaneous receptive fields, sometimes with surround inhibition (Iwamura and Inubushi, 1974; Jänig *et al.*, 1979; Loe *et al.*, 1977; Poggio and Mountcastle, 1960, 1963; Pubols, 1968). The receptive field organization presumably re-

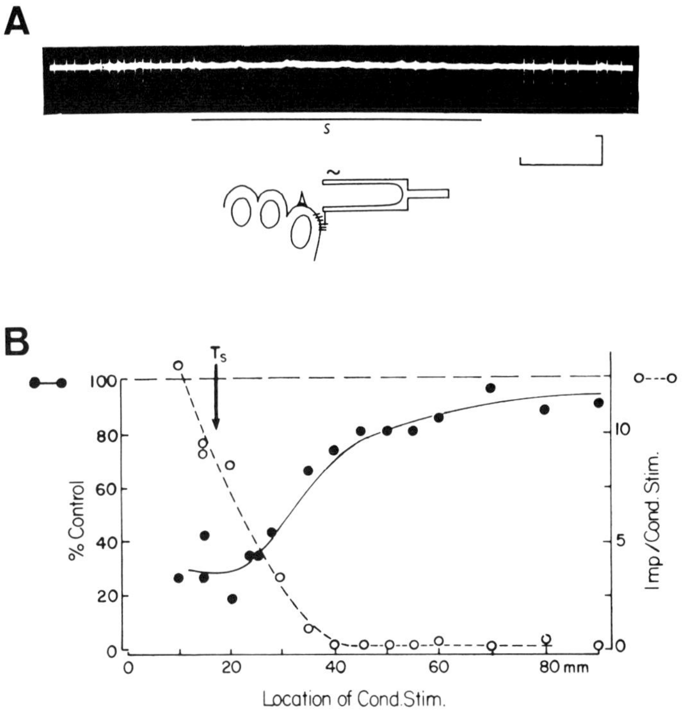

FIGURE 4. A: Inhibition of a neuron in the nucleus gracilis of the cat. The excitatory receptive field was at the base of the claw (black region in inset), and the background discharge of the cell could be inhibited by a vibratory stimulus applied to a wide region of the ipsilateral body surface, including the location indicated in the inset (100 Hz vibration). (From Gordon and Jukes, 1964.) B: The spatial distribution of the excitatory and inhibitory receptive fields of a neuron in the cuneate nucleus of the cat. The cell projected to the thalamus, and it was excited by hair movement over the region shown by the open circles in the graph. When the test stimulus was placed at a fixed position (Ts), it was found that a conditioning stimulus applied at the points shown by the filled circles produced an inhibition over a broad region as measured from the tip of the toes, which served as the reference point for plotting stimulus location. Both the test and conditioning stimuli were calibrated air puffs. Inhibition is expressed as percentage of unconditioned response (left ordinate). Excitation by conditioning stimulus is plotted as impulses per stimulus (right ordinate). (From Jänig *et al.*, 1977.)

flects that of the dorsal column nuclei. However, it should be noted that some contribution could be made by other ascending somatosensory pathways, since several of these also terminate in the VPL nucleus (Berkley, 1980; Boivie, 1970, 1979, 1980). The more rostral a neuron is in the somatosensory system, the more difficult it becomes to define the source(s) of its input. Surround inhibition is based on a similar organization of overlapping excitatory and inhibitory receptive fields, with a broader extension of the inhibitory than of the excitatory field, as in the dorsal column nuclei (Iwamura and Inubushi, 1974; Jänig *et al.*, 1979).

The neurons of the VPL nucleus have a somatotopic organization that is essentially an inverted version of that already described for the dorsal column nuclei (Figures 2 and 5; Jones and Friedman, 1982; Jones *et al.*, 1979; Mountcastle and Henneman, 1952; Nelson and Kaas, 1981; Kaas *et al.*, 1984; Poggio and Mountcastle, 1963). The contralateral hindlimb is represented laterally and the forelimb medially; the trunk is represented dorsally, and distal areas ventrally. The face area is in the ventral posterior medial (VPM) nucleus.

The VPL nucleus projects to the several different cytoarchitectural areas of the first (SI) somatosensory area of the cerebral cortex (Figure 6) and also to the SII region (Friedman and Jones, 1981; Jones and Friedman, 1982; Jones and Powell, 1970; Jones *et al.*, 1979; Nelson and Kaas, 1981; Whitsel *et al.*, 1978). In primates, the SI cortex includes cytoarchitectural areas 3a, 3b, 1, and 2 of the postcentral gyrus (Powell and Mountcastle, 1959a), and the SII cortex is in the cortex overlying the lateral fissure (Woolsey, 1958).

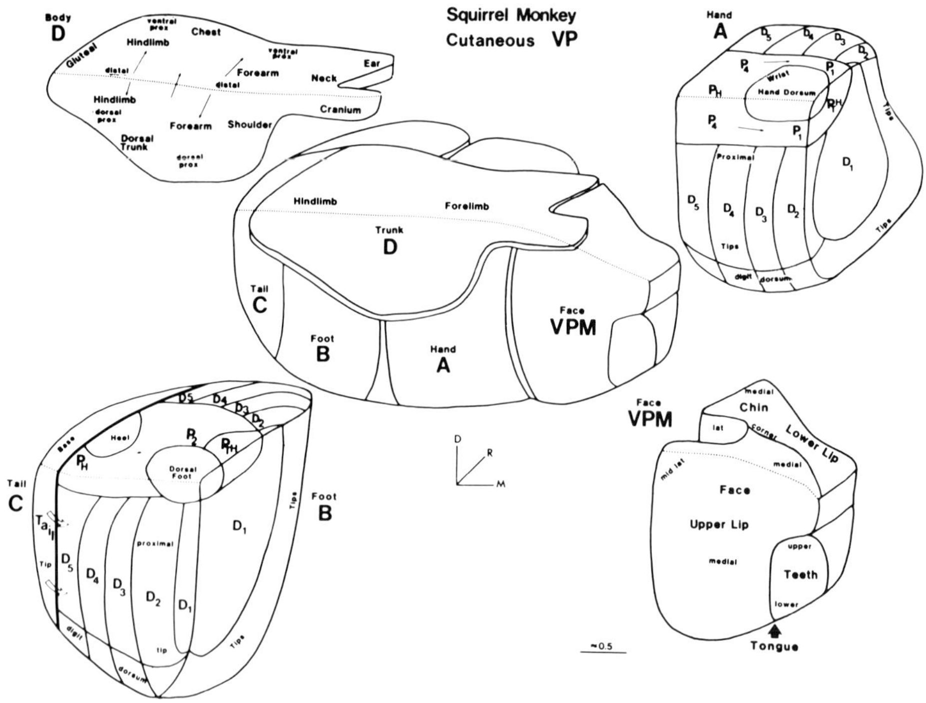

FIGURE 5. Somatotopic organization of the ventrobasal complex (on left side of brain). The ventral posterior lateral (VPL) nucleus is subdivided into subnuclei labeled A–D. The hand is represented in A, the foot in B, the tail in C, and the trunk in D. The ventral posterior medial (VPM) nucleus contains the face representation. D_{1-5} are the digits, P_{1-4} the pads of the hand and foot, P_H the hypothenar pad, and P_{TH} the thenar pad. Directions on indicator are dorsal, D; rostral, R; and medial, M. (From Kaas *et al.*, 1984.)

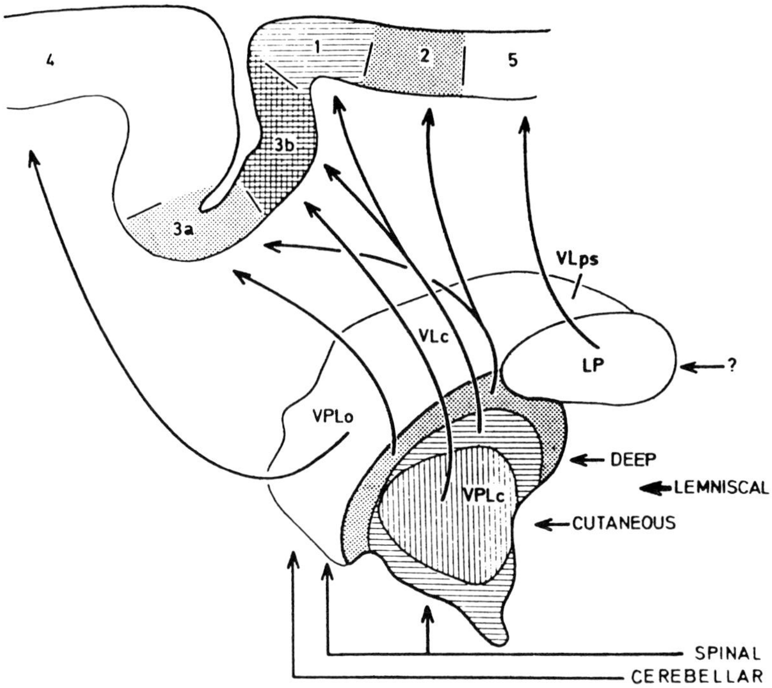

FIGURE 6. Cortical projections of the ventrobasal complex and adjacent thalamic nuclei. Different concentric zones of the ventral posterior lateral (VPL_c) nucleus are shown by dots and horizontal and vertical hatching. The thalamus and SI somatosensory cortex are shown in sagittal section. (From Jones and Friedman, 1982.)

Some of the neurons of the VPL nucleus project to both the SI and the SII cortex, whereas most neurons appear to project to just one or the other (Fisher *et al.,* 1983; Spreafico *et al.,* 1981). There is controversy as to whether or not separate neurons project to the different cytoarchitectural zones within the SI cortex (Jones *et al.,* 1979; Landry and Deschenes, 1981; Lin *et al.,* 1979).

Neurons in the SI cortex tend to respond to different kinds of sensory receptors depending on the cytoarchitectural area in which the neurons are located. For example, neurons in areas 3a and 2 are more likely to have receptive fields in deep tissues, such as muscle, than in skin, whereas neurons in areas 3b and 1 are more likely to have cutaneous receptive fields (Dreyer *et al.,* 1974, 1975; Phillips *et al.,* 1971; Powell and Mountcastle, 1959b; Tanji and Wise, 1981). Zones containing neurons with cutaneous receptive fields may be devoted to inputs either from slowly adapting or from rapidly adapting receptors (Paul *et al.,* 1972; Sretavan and Dykes, 1983; Sur *et al.,* 1981).

The receptive fields of neurons in the SI cortex tend to be small and contralateral, just as in the dorsal column nuclei and in the VPL nucleus of the thalamus (Merzenich *et al.,* 1978; Mountcastle and Powell, 1959; Sur *et al.*, 1980), although exceptions have been reported (e.g., Mountcastle and Powell, 1959). There may be surround inhibition of cortical neurons (Mountcastle and Powell, 1959; Sur, 1980), as in the nuclei at lower levels of the pathway. Thus, in many ways the responses of neurons in the SI cortex can be accounted for rather well on the basis of the response properties of neurons of the dorsal column nuclei and the VPL nucleus, especially neurons in area 3b. However, some of the neurons in the SI cortex have more elaborate response characteristics that are quite different from those of neurons in the dorsal column nuclei or the VPL nucleus. These neurons appear to function in feature extraction. For example, some neurons in the SI cortex may respond better to a stimulus moved in one direction across the receptive field than to a stimulus moved in the opposite direction (Costanzo and Gardner, 1980). Presumably these more elaborate responses depend on intracortical processing of information along lines similar to those that have been studied extensively in the visual system (Hubel and Wiesel, 1977).

The neurons encountered by a microelectrode inserted normally to the surface of the SI cortex will all (except those in the most superficial layers, according to McKenna *et al.*, 1984) have very similar receptive field properties, whereas those encountered by an electrode passing parallel to the surface of the cortex will show sudden shifts in receptive field properties every 0.5 mm or so (Mountcastle, 1957). These observations are taken to indicate that the SI cortex has a "columnar" organization (Mountcastle, 1984). Again, similar findings have been reported for the visual cortex (Hubel and Wiesel, 1977).

The SI cortex has a somatotopic organization. In primates and man, the hindlimb is represented medially on the postcentral gyrus, and the forelimb laterally (Penfield and Jasper, 1954; Whitsel *et al.*, 1971). Actually, there is now evidence that there is a separate somatotopic map for each of the four cytoarchitectural areas of the SI cortex (Figure 7; Kaas, 1983; Kaas *et al.*, 1979; Merzenich *et al.*, 1978; Nelson *et al.*, 1980), although this is disputed (Duncan *et al.*, 1982; McKenna *et al.*, 1982).

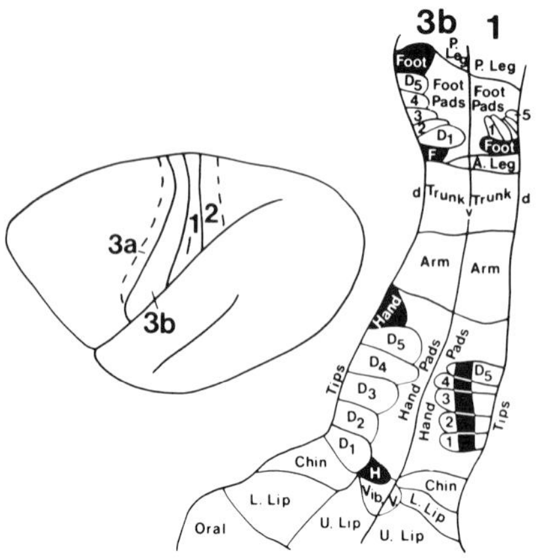

FIGURE 7. The multiple representation of the body surface in different cytoarchitectural fields of the SI cortex of the owl monkey. The drawing at the left shows the orientation of areas 3a, 3b, 1, and 2 of the SI cortex. The maps at the right show the representation patterns for areas 3b and 1. Shaded areas are for the hairy surfaces of the hand and foot. D_{1-5} are digit representations. (From Kaas, 1983.)

The SI cortex receives an input not only from the VPL nucleus but also from the intralaminar complex of the thalamus, in particular from the central lateral (CL) nucleus (Jones and Leavitt, 1974). However, the synaptic terminals of the VPL projection are concentrated in cortical layers 3 and 4, whereas the terminals of the CL projection are chiefly in layers 1 and 6, suggesting a different function (Jones, 1984).

The SI and SII areas of the cerebral cortex are interconnected; they project back on the thalamic nuclei from which they receive an input; and they make corticocortical associational and commissural connections with a number of other cortical areas (reviewed in Mountcastle, 1984). Thus, the higher processing of somatosensory information depends on activity not only in the SI and SII regions but also in many other cortical and subcortical regions with which these connect.

2. *Dorsal Column Path: Postsynaptic Elements*

As already mentioned, the dorsal column contains not only the axons of primary afferent fibers that project to the dorsal column nuclei but also axons belonging to several other systems. Among these is the postsynaptic dorsal column pathway (Uddenberg, 1968b).

The cells of origin of the postsynaptic dorsal column pathway have been found to lie mostly in laminae III and IV of the dorsal horn (Figure 8; Bennett *et al.*, 1983; Giesler *et al.*, 1984; Rustioni *et al.*, 1979; Rustioni and Kaufman, 1977). Cells in the lumbosacral enlargement project to the nucleus gracilis, and those in the cervical enlargement to the nucleus cuneatus (Rustioni, 1973, 1974). Two exceptions to this organization should be noted. Some of the axons of dorsal horn neurons ascending in the dorsal column terminate outside the dorsal column nuclei, specifically in nucleus Z (Rustioni, 1973). Furthermore, some of the axons that project to the dorsal column nuclei do so by way of the dorsal lateral funiculus (DLF) rather than by way of the dorsal column (Nijensohn and Kerr, 1975; Rustioni *et al.*, 1979). This arrangement makes the name "postsynaptic dorsal column pathway" a misnomer. An alternative nomenclature would be to include the axons in the DLF with the spinomedullary pathway (Mountcastle, 1984). The spinomedullary tract has generally been regarded as a pathway that receives an input from proprioceptive afferents and that projects to nucleus Z (see below). However, "spinomedullary" is a general term that could include these pathways and also the postsynaptic dorsal column path proper (with axons in the dorsal columns) and elements of the spinoreticular tract that project to the medullary reticular formation. If such a general meaning is assigned to the "spinomedullary pathways," then it would be best to specify which particular component is meant.

The response properties of the cells belonging to the postsynaptic dorsal column pathway are different from those characteristic of the neurons in the

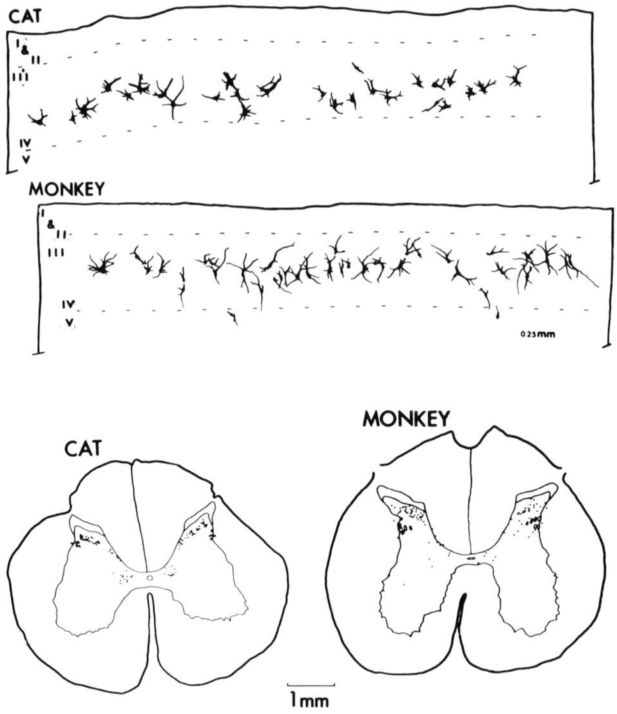

FIGURE 8. Cells of origin of the postsynaptic dorsal column pathway. The neurons giving rise to the postsynaptic dorsal column pathway in the cat and monkey were labeled by retrogradely transported horseradish peroxidase that had been injected into the dorsal column nuclei. The labeled cells are shown in sagittal section at the top, and the locations of the cells are plotted on drawings of transverse sections of the spinal cord below. (From Bennett *et al.*, 1983.)

cell cluster region of the dorsal column nuclei. Although some neurons of the postsynaptic dorsal column pathway appear to receive an input from a homogeneous population of cutaneous mechanoreceptors, most are activated by convergent inputs from both mechanoreceptors and nociceptors (Angaut-Petit, 1975b; Bennett *et al.*, 1983; Brown and Fyffe, 1981; Lu *et al.*, 1983; Uddenberg, 1968b). A few of the neurons in this pathway have been reported to receive a purely nociceptive input (Angaut-Petit, 1975b), although this has not been confirmed in recent experiments (Lu *et al.*, 1983). Cells with a convergent input from both mechanoreceptors and nociceptors have been termed "wide-dynamic-range" (WDR) neurons (Mendell, 1966) because they can be excited by a wide range of intensities of mechanical stimuli applied to the skin. However, it has recently been suggested that the term "multiconvergent" might be preferable (Brown and Réthelyi, 1981).

The postsynaptic dorsal column pathway does not end on neurons in the cell cluster region of the dorsal column nuclei (Rustioni, 1973, 1974). Instead, it ends in the more rostral and ventral parts of these nuclei. Some neurons in the rostral dorsal column nuclei do project to the thalamus (Berkley, 1975; Gordon and Jukes, 1964), and neurons in the rostral dorsal column nuclei have been found with response characteristics similar to those of the cells of the postsynaptic dorsal column pathway (Angaut-Petit, 1975b). However, it has not been conclusively shown that cells in the dorsal column nuclei are activated by the postsynaptic dorsal column pathway, nor that these cells do in fact project to the thalamus. Nor is it clear where in the thalamus such neurons would terminate. Lacking this information, it is impossible at the moment to evaluate possible actions of the postsynaptic dorsal column pathway at a thalamic or cortical level.

3. Spinocervical Tract

The spinocervical tract derives its name from the fact that this projection relays in the cervical spinal cord in a nucleus called the lateral cervical nucleus, which is located in the first two cervical segments (Figure 9; Brodal and Rexed, 1953). The functional properties of the pathway were first described by Morin (1955), and it has been thoroughly investigated by Brown and his associates (reviewed in Brown, 1981).

The spinocervical tract, like the postsynaptic dorsal column pathway (see above), originates from neurons located in laminae III and IV of the dorsal horn (Figure 10). Several types of response have been recorded either from the cells of origin of the path or from axons that ascend in the DLF. Some spinocervical tract (SCT) cells can be activated only by a homogeneous set of mechanoreceptors, whereas other SCT neurons are excited by convergent inputs from both sensitive mechanoreceptors and nociceptors (Brown, 1981; Brown and Franz, 1969; Cervero *et al.*, 1977; Hong *et al.*, 1979). Several classes of mechanoreceptive inputs to cat spinocervical tract cells have been described, but these can be altered through the action of inhibitory control systems originating in the brainstem (Brown, 1971; Brown and Franz, 1969). The dominant input is from the various types of hair follicle receptors. Responses of SCT cells to noxious stimuli are also under the influence of descending inhibitory controls and can be substantially enhanced following elimination of the descending controls by application of a cold block to the spinal cord (Brown, 1971; Cervero *et al.*, 1977; Hong *et al.*, 1979).

The lateral cervical nucleus (LCN) has been examined anatomically and electrophysiologically by several laboratories (Craig, 1978; Craig and Burton, 1979; Craig and Tapper, 1978; Giesler *et al.*, 1979b; Horrobin, 1966; Kitai *et al.*, 1965; Oswaldo-Cruz and Kidd, 1964). In the cat and dog, most of the neurons in the LCN appear to be excited only by sensitive mechanoreceptors. However, some nociceptive responses have been recorded from LCN neurons (Horrobin, 1966; Oswaldo-Cruz and Kidd, 1964). Nociceptive cells in the

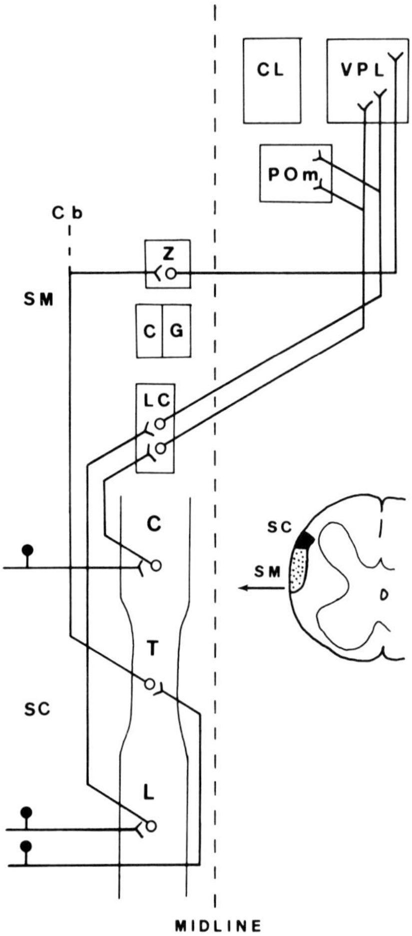

FIGURE 9. Sensory pathways of the dorsal lateral fasciculus. The organization of the spinocervical and spinomedullothalamic pathways is shown. Primary afferent fibers end on cells of the dorsal horn in the cervical (C) and lumbar (L) enlargements. The second-order neurons project through the spinocervical tract (SC) to the lateral cervical nucleus (LC). The axons of third-order cells decussate and project through the medial lemniscus to the medial part of the posterior nuclear complex (PO_m) and the ventral posterior lateral (VPL) nucleus of the thalamus. Other primary afferent fibers ascend in the dorsal column to the thoracic cord (T), where they synapse on cells in Clarke's column (and also on cells caudal to Clarke's column), which in turn project in the spinomedullary tract (SM) to nucleus Z. Some of these axons also project to the cerebellum (Cb). Nucleus Z projects contralaterally to the VPL and adjacent parts of the ventral lateral nucleus. The transverse section of the spinal cord indicates the locations of the spinocervical and spinomedullary pathways. (From Willis and Coggeshall, 1978.)

medial part of the nucleus did not appear to project to the thalamus (Craig and Tapper, 1978). In the rat, many of the cells of the LCN show nociceptive responsiveness (Giesler *et al.*, 1979b).

The lateral cervical nucleus has a somatotopic organization (Craig and Burton, 1979). Neurons of the LCN project contralaterally by way of the spinal cord ventral white commissure, and the ascending axons enter the brainstem and eventually join the medial lemniscus en route to the thalamus (Ha, 1971). There is a substantial synaptic termination of the cervicothalamic axons in the VPL nucleus (Berkley, 1980; Boivie, 1979, 1980; Ha, 1971), and there are also other termination zones in the medial part of the posterior complex (PO_m; Berkley, 1980; Boivie, 1980) and in several nuclei of the midbrain (Björkland, 1984). The termination zone of the cervicothalamic projection in the VPL nucleus overlaps that of the dorsal column nuclei,

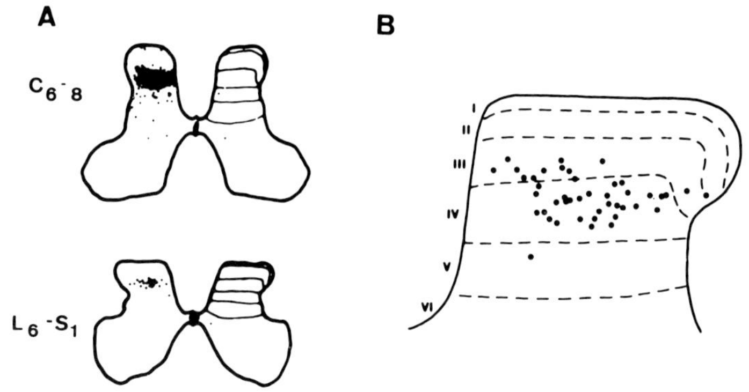

FIGURE 10. Locations of the cells of origin of the spinocervical tract. The distribution of neurons labeled retrogradely by horseradish peroxidase after injection into the region of the lateral cervical nucleus are shown in A. The distribution of intracellularly injected spinocervical tract cells identified by antidromic activation are shown in B. (A is from Craig, 1976; B is from Brown, 1981.)

although there is a tendency for the heaviest concentration of endings for these different pathways to be on separate populations of VPL neurons (Berkley, 1980). However, some VPL neurons appear to receive a convergent input from both the dorsal column and the spinocervicothalamic pathways (Landgren *et al.*, 1965).

Selective lesions have been made in some studies to eliminate transmission of activity to the brain over the dorsal column (Andersson *et al.*, 1972; Dreyer *et al.*, 1974; Levitt and Levitt, 1968). Such investigations show that the SCT influences neurons at higher levels of the somatosensory pathways, but the special significance of the spinocervicothalamic pathway is still unclear.

4. *Spinomedullary Path to Nucleus Z*

The spinomedullothalamic pathway by way of nucleus Z appears to be the proprioceptive system for the hindlimb (Figure 9; see reviews by Mountcastle, 1984; Willis and Coggeshall, 1978). The afferent input to this pathway is from stretch receptors of muscle, including group Ia and II afferents from muscle spindles (Landgren and Silfvenius, 1971; Magherini *et al.*, 1975) and afferents from joint receptors (Clark *et al.*, 1973). The ascending tract appears to originate at least in part from Clarke's column as collaterals of the dorsal spinocerebellar tract (Johansson and Silfvenius, 1977). There is a medullary relay in nucleus Z, a small group of neurons just rostral to the nucleus gracilis (Nijensohn and Kerr, 1975; Pompeiano and Brodal, 1957). This cell group projects to the contralateral thalamus by way of the medial lemniscus, terminating in the rostral part of the VPL nucleus and in the ventral lateral nucleus (Grant *et al.*, 1973). It is presumed that activity recorded in the somatosensory cerebral cortex in response to stimulation of group I fibers in hindlimb muscle nerves is transmitted by this pathway (Landgren and Silfvenius, 1969).

The proprioceptive system for the forelimb appears to involve the dorsal column path proper rather than a spinomedullothalamic system. Proprioceptive afferent fibers ascend through the fasciculus cuneatus and end in the main cuneate nucleus (as well as in the external cuneate nucleus; Rosen, 1969; Rosen and Sjolund, 1973). The proprioceptive neurons of the main cuneate nucleus are largely in the ventral part of the nucleus. Information from these neurons is forwarded to the VPL thalamus and somatosensory cortex by way of the medial lemniscus (Rosen, 1969). In the cat, the external cuneate nucleus projects just to the cerebellum and so should not be considered part of the somatosensory projection system. However, in the monkey, this nucleus projects to both the cerebellum and the thalamus (Boivie and Bowman, 1981; Boivie *et al.*, 1975). It is not clear what difference there may be in the functions of the projections to the thalamus from the main and external cuneate nuclei.

C. Ascending Somatosensory Pathways in the Ventral Spinal Cord

1. Spinothalamic Tract

The spinothalamic tract is largely a crossed ascending path (Figure 11). It originates from neurons located not only in the dorsal horn but also in the intermediate region and ventral horn (Figure 12), as shown by several anatomic techniques, including retrograde chromatolysis (Foerster and Gagel, 1932; Kerr, 1975a; Kuru, 1949) and retrograde transport of horseradish peroxidase (Carstens and Trevino, 1978; Giesler *et al.*, 1979a; Willis *et al.*, 1979) and by electrophysiological mapping of antidromically activated neurons by a stimulating electrode placed in the thalamus (Albe-Fessard *et al.*, 1974; Dilly *et al.*, 1968; Trevino *et al.*, 1972, 1973).

The axons of the spinothalamic tract decussate within a few segments of the cell body (or even immediately, within a single 50-μm section; Willis *et al.*, 1979), crossing in the ventral white commissure to enter the contralateral ventrolateral white matter. As the axons ascend towards the brain, they shift from a medial to a more lateral position. Axons crossing to more rostral levels of the spinal cord assume a position medial to that of axons crossing at more caudal levels, giving the tract a somatotopic organization (Applebaum *et al.*, 1975; Weaver and Walker, 1941), with the lower extremity represented ventromedially and the upper extremity dorsolaterally in the cervical spinal cord.

The spinothalamic tract ascends through the medulla in a position just dorsolateral to the inferior olivary nucleus; in the pons and midbrain, it occupies a position just dorsolateral to the medial lemniscus (Kerr, 1975b; Kerr and Lippman, 1974; Mehler, 1962; Mehler *et al.*, 1960; Rasmussen and Peyton, 1948). The tract terminates in the thalamus in several different thalamic nuclei, including the VPL nucleus (in primates and rodents but not in

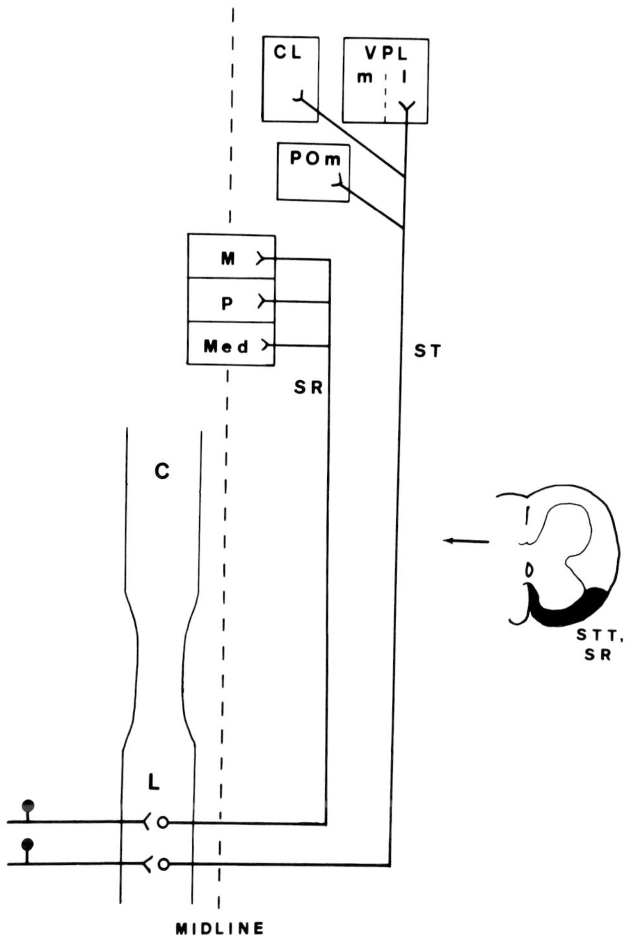

FIGURE 11. The spinothalamic, spinoreticular, and spinomesencephalic tracts. For simplicity, the pathways through the cervical (C) enlargement are not shown. Primary afferents enter the lumbar (L) cord and synapse on tract cells. Second-order projections in the spinothalamic tract (ST) decussate and ascend to end in the medial part of the posterior complex (PO_m), the central lateral (CL) intralaminar nucleus, and the ventral posterior lateral (VPL) nucleus (lateral part, l). The spinoreticular tract (SR) is shown decussating also, but it is a bilateral pathway. It terminates in a variety of nuclei of the reticular formation of the brainstem (Med, medulla; P, pons; M, midbrain). The portion of the pathway that ends in the midbrain can be considered the spinomesencephalic tract. The transverse section of the spinal cord shows the location of the spinothalamic tract (STT) and the spinoreticular tract (SR) in the ventral quadrant. (From Willis and Coggeshall, 1978.)

the cat), the medial part of the posterior complex, the intralaminar nuclei (particularly in the central lateral nucleus), the nucleus submedius, and several others (Berkley, 1980; Boivie, 1971b, 1979; Bowsher, 1957, 1961; Burton and Craig, 1983; Craig and Burton, 1981; Jones and Burton, 1974; Kerr, 1975b; Kerr and Lippman, 1974; Lund and Webster, 1967; Mantyh, 1983;

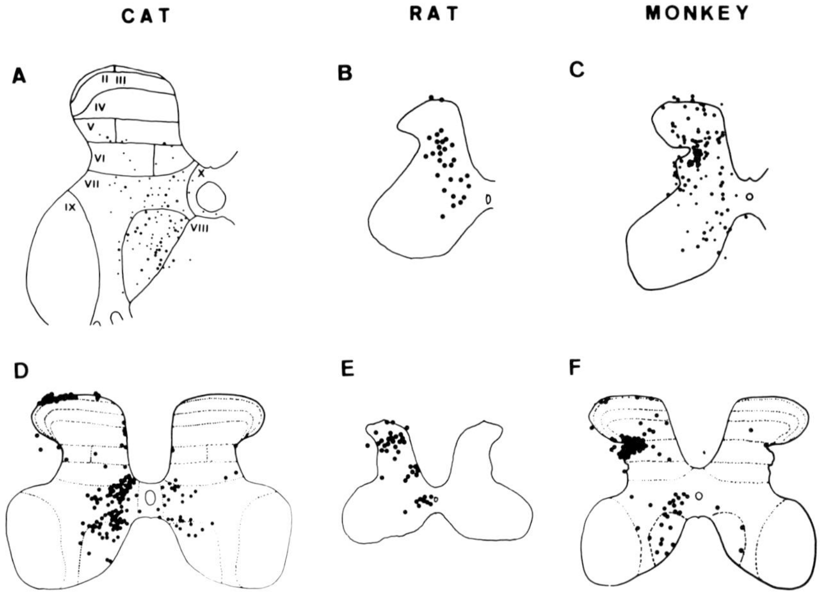

FIGURE 12. A–C: Recording sites from which antidromic action potentials could be recorded from spinothalamic tract cells in the lumbosacral enlargement of the cat, rat and monkey following stimulation in the contralateral thalamus. (A is from Trevino *et al.*, 1973; B from Giesler *et al.*, 1976; C from Trevino *et al.*, 1973). D–F: Location of spinothalamic tract cells labeled retrogradely following injection of horseradish peroxidase into the thalamus in cat, rat, and monkey. (D and F from Trevino and Carstens, 1975; E from Giesler *et al.*, 1979a.)

Mehler, 1962; Mehler *et al.*, 1960; Peschanski *et al.*, 1983). In cats, the spinothalamic tract has few endings in the VPL nucleus but instead terminates in a "shell" region surrounding this nucleus (Berkley, 1980; Boivie, 1971b; Burton and Craig, 1983; Jones and Burton, 1974; Mantyh, 1983). The terminations in the VPL nucleus of the primate and rodent are somatotopic (Boivie, 1979; Lund and Webster, 1967; Mehler *et al.*, 1960; Peschanski *et al.*, 1983).

The input to spinothalamic tract cells has been investigated using both electrically evoked volleys in peripheral nerves and natural forms of stimulation of the skin, muscle, and viscera. Many spinothalamic tract (STT) cells are activated by A-α,β, A-δ, and C fibers in cutaneous nerves (Beall *et al.*, 1977; Chung *et al.*, 1979; Foreman *et al.*, 1975). However, in some cases the input may be restricted to the smaller afferent fiber groups (Foreman *et al.*, 1975). The responses to natural forms of stimulation of the skin and deep structures have led to the following classification of STT cells: low threshold (activated by innocuous but not by noxious cutaneous stimuli); wide dynamic range (activated by innocuous stimuli, but better by noxious stimuli applied to the skin); high threshold (activated only by noxious stimulation of the skin); and deep (activated only or best by subcutaneous receptors) (Chung *et al.*,

1979; Giesler *et al.*, 1976; Price *et al.*, 1978). Most STT cells appear to be of the wide-dynamic-range ("multireceptive") or the high-threshold classes. In addition to their responses to mechanical stimuli, many STT cells can be activated by the application of noxious heat stimuli to the skin (Kenshalo *et al.*, 1979). Only a few STT cells have been shown to respond to input from specific thermoreceptors (Craig and Kniffki, 1982). Many STT cells respond not only to cutaneous stimulation but also to the activation of receptors in muscle or viscera (Foreman *et al.*, 1979; Foreman and Weber, 1980; Milne *et al.*, 1981).

The excitatory receptive fields of most STT cells that project to the VPL nucleus have a restricted size, and they are located contralaterally to the thalamic projection zone (Applebaum *et al.*, 1975; Giesler *et al.*, 1981). However, there are some STT cells that appear to project just to medial parts of the thalamus, such as the central lateral nucleus, and that have excitatory receptive fields over the entire surface of the body and face (Giesler *et al.*, 1981). It seems likely that STT cells with restricted contralateral receptive fields are able to signal stimulus location, whereas STT cells with very large bilateral receptive fields may be involved in tasks other than sensory discrimination.

The STT cells also have inhibitory receptive fields. These may be organized in a surround fashion, in which case the effective afferents seem to include those supplying sensitive mechanoreceptors (Milne *et al.*, 1981), or they may be distributed over much of the body surface, in which case the inhibition depends on the activation of nociceptors (Gerhart *et al.*, 1981). Inhibition of a long-lasting type (duration about half an hour) can be produced by prolonged repetitive stimulation of a peripheral nerve (Chung *et al.*, 1984a,b). This type of inhibition has several features that call to mind the characteristics of the analgesia produced by transcutaneous nerve stimulation.

Nociceptive responses have been recorded from neurons of the thalamus that are in nuclei that receive terminations of the spinothalamic tract. These include the VPL nucleus in the primate and the rat and the "shell" region around VPL in the cat (Casey and Morrow, 1983; Gaze and Gordon, 1954; Guilbaud *et al.*, 1980; Honda *et al.*, 1983; Kenshalo *et al.*, 1980; Kniffki and Mizumura, 1983; Mitchell and Hellon, 1977; Perl and Whitlock, 1961; Peschanski *et al.*, 1980; Pollin and Albe-Fessard, 1979) as well as the PO_m nucleus (Guilbaud *et al.*, 1977; Poggio and Mountcastle, 1960) and the intralaminar complex (Albe-Fessard and Kruger, 1962; Dong *et al.*, 1978; Peschanski *et al.*, 1981). In some experiments, it has been possible to show that these nociceptive responses depend on activity conveyed by axons ascending in the ventrolateral white matter of the spinal cord, possibly in the spinothalamic tract (Dong *et al.*, 1978; Kenshalo *et al.*, 1980; Perl and Whitlock, 1961; Pollin and Albe-Fessard, 1979). Nociceptive responses have also been recorded from neurons in the SI region of the cerebral cortex (Kenshalo and Isensee, 1983; Lamour *et al.*, 1983a,b). Evidently, it is possible that the sensory processing of information related to pain depends on a mechanism that parallels that of the dorsal column pathway for tactile sensation. However, in addition, other thalamic connections presumably mediate such aspects of the pain reaction as the motivational–affective component.

2. *Spinoreticular Tract*

Although the spinoreticular tract is depicted in Figure 11 as a crossed tract, it actually includes both crossed and uncrossed components (Kerr and Lippman, 1974). In the monkey, counts of spinoreticular neurons labeled retrogradely following unilateral injections of horseradish peroxidase into the medullary reticular formation show that many of the cells in the cervical enlargement project ipsilaterally; most of the spinoreticular cells of the lumbosacral enlargement, however, project contralaterally (Kevetter *et al.*, 1982).

The cells of origin of the spinoreticular tract are concentrated in Rexed's laminae VII and VIII, although some are also found in the dorsal horn, including a few in lamina I (Figure 13; Abols and Basbaum, 1981; Andrezik *et al.*, 1981; Chaouch *et al.*, 1983; Kevetter *et al.*, 1982; Kevetter and Willis, 1983). Some spinoreticular neurons project to both the reticular formation and the thalamus (Kevetter and Willis, 1982, 1983).

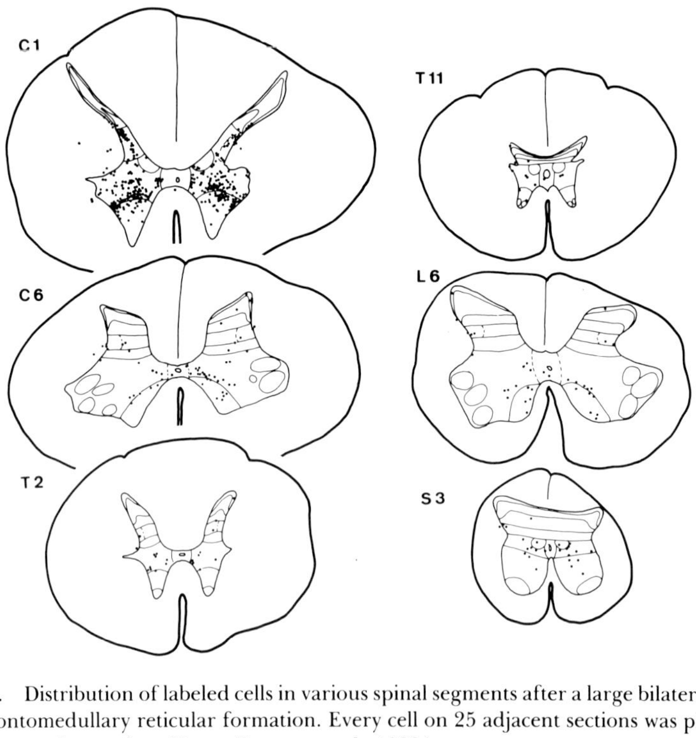

FIGURE 13. Distribution of labeled cells in various spinal segments after a large bilateral injection into the pontomedullary reticular formation. Every cell on 25 adjacent sections was plotted onto each representative section. (From Kevetter *et al.*, 1982.)

The spinoreticular tract projects to a number of nuclei in the pontomedullary reticular formation (Kerr, 1975b; Mehler *et al.*, 1960). The target nuclei include the retroambiguus nucleus, the nucleus supraspinalis, the dorsal and ventral parts of the nucleus medullae oblongatae centralis, the lateral reticular nucleus, the nucleus gigantocellularis, the nucleus interfascicularis hypoglossi, the nucleus of Roller, the inferior olivary nucleus, the nuclei paragigantocellularis lateralis and dorsalis, the nuclei pontis centrali caudalis and oralis, and the subcoeruleus complex (Mehler *et al.*, 1960). Some of these nuclei form parts of the motor system, but others, such as the nucleus gigantocellularis, are likely to play an important role in sensory processing.

Recordings have been made from spinoreticular neurons (Fields *et al.*, 1975, 1977; Haber *et al.*, 1982; Maunz *et al.*, 1978). Many of the cells have complicated receptive fields, but they often receive a nociceptive input and thus may play a role in nociception. However, it seems unlikely that the reticular formation would be concerned with sensoridiscriminative functions; rather, it is more likely to contribute to such activities as alerting, selective attention, and motivational–affective behavior.

3. Spinomesencephalic Tract

The spinomesencephalic tract is a largely crossed pathway (Figure 11). The cells of origin of the spinomesencephalic pathway have been demonstrated by retrograde labeling with horseradish peroxidase (Liu, 1983; Menetrey *et al.*, 1982; Trevino, 1976; Willis *et al.*, 1979). They are concentrated in laminae I and V of the dorsal horn in the same regions as spinothalamic tract cells that project to the VPL nucleus (Figure 14). In fact, several neurons in the study by Price *et al.* (1978) could be activated antidromically from both

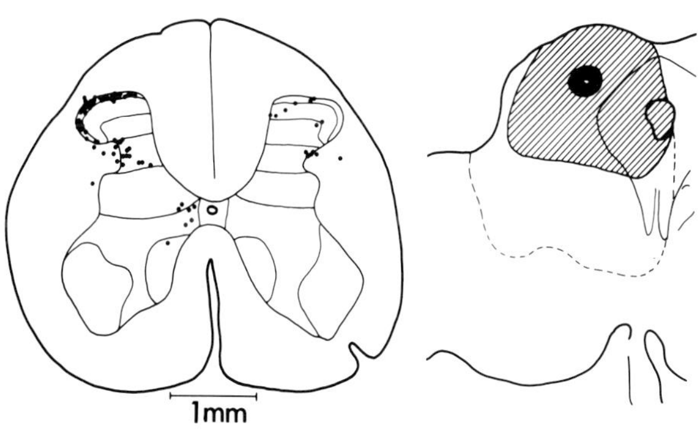

FIGURE 14. Cells of origin of the spinomesencephalic tract in monkey. Left: Composite plot of all of the labeled cells found in 15 alternate serial sections in the lumbosacral enlargement. Right: Drawing of the injection site, showing three intensities of staining for HRP. (From Willis *et al.*, 1979.)

the midbrain and the thalamus, indicating that the same neurons can project to both targets.

Recordings have been made from spinomesencephalic tract cells of the rat and cat (Menetrey *et al.*, 1980; Yezierski and Schwartz, 1984). Many of the cells have a nociceptive input and so could participate in nociception. However, it is not clear if these cells have primarily a sensory role or a feedback function in regulating sensory transmission.

D. Sensory Functions of the Ascending Somatosensory Pathways

The ascending somatosensory pathways of the spinal cord are responsible for signaling information that is used for a variety of sensory modalities (see review by Willis and Coggeshall, 1978). These modalities include touch–pressure, flutter–vibration, pain, temperature sense, position sense, and visceral sense.

Systematic studies in man and animal, as discussed by Vierck and colleagues (Chapter 12), have indeed demonstrated that certain pathways exist whereby these stimuli affect the brainstem. Yet, from the evidence that is at hand, it appears that several different funicular and projection pathways are likely to contribute to many of these sensory modalities. Thus, touch–pressure may well be subserved not only by the dorsal column pathway but also by the postsynaptic dorsal column path, the spinocervical tract, and the spinothalamic tract. Flutter probably uses the same set of pathways, although vibration may be the exclusive domain of the dorsal column pathway. Pain may depend not only on the spinothalamic tract (especially for its sensoridiscriminative aspects) but also on the spinoreticular and spinomesencephalic tracts (perhaps for motivational–affective aspects and also for regulation). It is also possible that pain can be signaled by the postsynaptic dorsal column pathway and/or the spinocervical tract under certain circumstances. Such multiple pathways may in part explain the recovery of sensory function observed following partial spinal lesions. Temperature sense seems to be dependent on the spinothalamic tract, although the evidence is surprisingly weak. Mediation of position sense is complicated. For the hindlimb, the spinomedullary pathway through nucleus Z appears to be responsible, whereas for the forelimb the main pathway involved seems to be the dorsal column path. Visceral sense is not generally of much consequence unless there is visceral pain, and this may then be overwhelming. Visceral pain appears to be mediated largely by the spinothalamic tract and the accompanying pathways of the anterolateral quadrant, including the spinoreticular tract (see comments by Foreman, Chapter 10).

An important question is, however, what role these multiple pathways play. Though they may appear redundant, it appears likely that the multiplicity reflects the subtlety of the role these several systems may play in coding the sensory message. As discussed by others, it is clear that the coding of sensory information is exceedingly complex, even at the level of the dorsal horn, when only a limited population of spinal neurons is considered (see discussion by Le Bars *et al.*, Chapter 19, and Price, Chapter 18). The "meaning" of the sensory message being sent concurrently over any one of the given lines discussed above may be interpretable only in the context of the activity of information concurrently arriving over the several lines. When one considers that the arriving message may activate spinofugal inhibitory and excitatory influences on spinal projection neurons, the true complexity of the organization of the ascending sensory system may be appreciated.

E. Closing Remarks

It was a pleasure for me to receive an invitation to contribute a chapter on the topic of the ascending somatosensory pathways to a volume dedicated to the memory of Dr. F. W. L. Kerr. Fred Kerr devoted much of his research effort to the somatosensory system, being concerned especially with pain mechanisms. His work on the somatosensory system involved chiefly anatomic techniques for the study of the organization of the pain transmission system. Fred brought to his work not only his rich basic science experience but also his clinical experience, which gave a unique perspective to his approach. His influence will persist through his writings and through the memories of his friends and colleagues.

ACKNOWLEDGMENTS. The author thanks his colleagues for the experiments mentioned here that were done in his laboratory and also Helen Willcockson and Griselda Gonzales for their expert technical assistance. He also thanks Phyllis Waldrop for typing the manuscript. The experiments in the author's laboratory were supported by NIH grants NS 09743 and NS 11255.

References

ABOLS, I. A., AND BASBAUM, A. I. Afferent connections of the rostral medulla of the cat: A neural substrate for midbrain-medullary interactions in the modulation of pain. *J. Comp. Neurol.* 201:285–297, 1981.

ALBE-FESSARD, D., AND KRUGER, L. Duality of unit discharges from cat centrum medianum in response to natural and electrical stimulation. *J. Neurophysiol.* 25:3–20, 1962.

ALBE-FESSARD, D., LEVANTE, A., AND LAMOUR, Y. Origin of spinothalamic tract in monkeys. *Brain Res.* 65:503–509, 1974.

ANDERSSON, S. A., NORRSELL, K., AND NORRSELL, U. Spinal pathways projecting to the cerebral first somatosensory area in the monkey. *J. Physiol. (Lond.)* 225:589–597, 1972.

ANDREZIK, J. A., CHAN-PALAY, V., AND PALAY, S. L. The nucleus paragigantocellularis lateralis in the rat. Demonstration of afferents by the retrograde transport of horseradish peroxidase. *Anat. Embryol.* 161:373–390, 1981.

ANGAUT-PETIT, D. The dorsal column system: I. Existence of long ascending postsynaptic fibres in the cat's fasciculus gracilis. *Exp. Brain Res.* 22:457–470, 1975a.

ANGAUT-PETIT, D. The dorsal column system: II. Functional properties and bulbar relay of the cat's fasciculus gracilis. *Exp. Brain Res.* 22:471–493, 1975b.

APPLEBAUM, A. E., BEALL, J. E., FOREMAN, R. D., AND WILLIS, W. D. Organization and receptive fields of primate spinothalamic tract neurons. *J. Neurophysiol.,* 38:572–586, 1975.

BEALL, J. E., APPLEBAUM, A. E., FOREMAN, R. D., AND WILLIS, W. D. Spinal cord potentials evoked by cutaneous afferents in the monkey. *J. Neurophysiol.,* 40:199–211, 1977.

BENNETT, G. J., SELTZER, Z., LU, G. W., NISHIKAWA, N., AND DUBNER, R. The cells of origin of the dorsal column projection in the lumbosacral enlargements of cats and monkeys. *Somatosens. Res.* 1:131–149, 1983.

BERKLEY, K. J. Different targets of different neurons in nucleus gracilis of the cat. *J. Comp. Neurol.* 163:285–304, 1975.

BERKLEY, K. J. Spatial relationships between the terminations of somatic sensory and motor pathways in the rostral brainstem of cats and monkeys. I. Ascending somatic sensory inputs to lateral diencephalon. *J. Comp. Neurol.* 193:283–317, 1980.

BERKLEY, K. J., BLOMQVIST, A., PELT, A., AND FLINK, R. Differences in the collateralization of neuronal projections from the dorsal column nuclei and lateral cervical nucleus to the thalamus and tectum in the cat: An anatomical study using two different double-labeling techniques. *Brain Res.* 202:273–290, 1980.

BESSON, J. M., GUILBAUD, G., ABDELMOUMENE, H., AND CHAOUCH, A. Physiologie de la nociception. *J. Physiol. (Paris)* 78:7–107, 1982.

BIEDENBACH, M. A. Cell density and regional distribution of cell types in the cuneate nucleus of the rhesus monkey. *Brain Res.* 45:1–14, 1972.

BJÖRKLAND, M. *Anatomical Studies on the Somatosensory Projections to the Midbrain from the Spinal Cord and Dorsal Column Nuclei in the Cat,* Dissertation, Karolinska Institutet, Stockholm, 1984.

BLOMQVIST, A., FLINK, R., BOWSHER, D., GRIPH, S., AND WESTMAN, J. Tectal and thalamic projections of dorsal column and lateral cervical nuclei: A quantitative study in the cat. *Brain Res.* 141:335–341, 1978.

BOIVIE, J. The termination of the cervicothalamic tract in the cat. An experimental study with silver impregnation methods. *Brain Res.* 19:333–360, 1970.

BOIVIE, J. The termination in the thalamus and the zona incerta of fibres from the dorsal column nuclei (DCN) in the cat. An experimental study with silver impregnation methods. *Brain Res.* 28:459–490, 1971a.

BOIVIE, J. The termination of the spinothalamic tract in the cat. An experimental study with silver impregnation methods. *Exp. Brain Res.* 12:331–353, 1971b.

BOIVIE, J. Anatomical observations on the dorsal column nuclei, their thalamic projection and the cytoarchitecture of some somatosensory thalamic nuclei in the monkey. *J. Comp. Neurol.* 178:17–48, 1978.

BOIVIE, J. An anatomical reinvestigation of the termination of the spinothalamic tract in the monkey. *J. Comp. Neurol.* 186:343–370, 1979.

BOIVIE, J. Thalamic projections from lateral cervical nucleus in the monkey. A degeneration study. *Brain Res.* 198:13–26, 1980.

BOIVIE, J., AND BOMAN, K. Termination of a separate (proprioceptive?) cuneothalamic tract from external cuneate nucleus in monkey. *Brain Res.* 224:235–246, 1981.

BOIVIE, J., GRANT, G., ALBE-FESSARD, D., AND LEVANTE, A. Evidence for a projection to the thalamus from the external cuneate nucleus in the monkey. *Neurosci. Lett.* 1:3–8, 1975.

BOWSHER, D. Termination of the central pain pathway in man: The conscious appreciation of pain. *Brain* 80:606–622, 1957.

BOWSHER, D. The termination of secondary somatosensory neurons within the thalamus of *Macaca mulatta:* An experimental degeneration study. *J. Comp. Neurol.* 117:213–227, 1961.

BRODAL, A. *Neurological Anatomy in Relation to Clinical Medicine,* Oxford University Press, New York, 1981.

BRODAL, A., AND REXED, B. Spinal afferents to the lateral cervical nucleus in the cat. An experimental study. *J. Comp. Neurol.* 98:179–211, 1953.

BROMBERG, M. B., AND WHITEHORN, D. Myelinated fiber types in the superficial radial nerve of the cat and their central projections. *Brain Res.* 78:157–163, 1974.

BROMBERG, M. B., BURNHAM, J. A., AND TOWE, A. L. Doubly projecting neurons of the dorsal column nuclei. *Neurosci. Lett.* 25:215–220, 1981.

BROWN, A. G. Cutaneous afferent fibre collaterals in the dorsal columns of the cat. *Exp. Brain Res.* 5:293–305, 1968.

BROWN, A. G. Effects of descending impulses on transmission through the spinocervical tract. *J. Physiol. (Lond.)* 219:103–125, 1971.

BROWN, A. G. *Organization in the Spinal Cord.* Springer-Verlag, New York, 1981.

BROWN, A. G., AND FRANZ, D. N. Responses of spinocervical tract neurones to natural stimulation of identified cutaneous receptors. *Exp. Brain Res.* 7:231–249, 1969.

BROWN, A. G., AND FYFFE, R. E. W. Form and function of dorsal horn neurones with axons ascending the dorsal columns in the cat. *J. Physiol. (Lond.)* 321:31–47, 1981.

BROWN, A. G., AND RÉTHELYI, M. (eds.) *Spinal Cord Sensation: Sensory Processing in the Dorsal Horn,* Scottish Academic Press, Edinburgh, 1981, p. 332.

BURGESS, P. R., AND CLARK, F. J. Dorsal column projection of fibres from the cat knee joint. *J. Physiol. (Lond.)* 203:301–315, 1969.

BURTON, H., AND CRAIG, A. D. Spinothalamic projections in cat, raccoon and monkey: A study based on anterograde transport of horseradish peroxidase, in: *Somatosensory Integration in the Thalamus* (G. MACCHI, A. RUSTIONI, AND R. SPREAFICO, eds.), Elsevier, Amsterdam, 1983, pp. 17–41.

BURTON, H., AND LOEWY, A. D. Projections to the spinal cord from medullary somatosensory relay nuclei. *J. Comp. Neurol.* 173:773–793, 1977.

CAJAL, S. R. Y *Histologie du Système Nerveux de l'Homme et des Vertébrés,* Vol. I, Institute, Cajal, Madrid, 1909, reprinted 1952.

CARPENTER, M. B., STEIN, B. M., AND SHRIVER, J. E. Central projections of spinal dorsal roots in the monkey. II. Lower thoracic, lumbosacral and coccygeal dorsal roots. *Am. J. Anat.* 123:75–118, 1968.

CARSTENS, E., AND TREVINO, D. L. Laminar origins of spinothalamic projections in the cat as determined by the retrograde transport of horseradish peroxidase. *J. Comp. Neurol.* 182:151–166, 1978.

CASEY, K. L., AND MORROW, T. J. Ventral posterior thalamic neurons differentially responsive to noxious stimulation of the awake monkey. *Science* 221:675–677, 1983.

CERVERO, F., IGGO, A., AND MOLONY, V. Responses of spinocervical tract neurones to noxious stimulation of the skin. *J. Physiol. (Lond.)* 267:537–558, 1977.

CHAOUCH, A., MENETREY, D., BINDER, D., AND BESSON, J. M. Neurons at the origin of the medial component of the bulbopontine spinoreticular tract in the rat: An anatomical study using horseradish peroxidase retrograde transport. *J. Comp. Neurol.* 214:309–320, 1983.

CHUNG, J. M., KENSHALO, D. R., JR., GERHART, K. D., AND WILLIS, W. D. Excitation of primate spinothalamic neurons by cutaneous C-fiber volleys. *J. Neurophysiol.* 42:1354–1369, 1979.

CHUNG, J. M., FANG, Z. R., HORI, Y., LEE, K. H., AND WILLIS, W. D. Prolonged inhibition of primate spinothalamic tract cells by peripheral nerve stimulation. *Pain* 19:259–274, 1984a.

CHUNG, J. M., LEE, K. H., HORI, Y., ENDO, K., AND WILLIS, W. D. Factors influencing peripheral nerve stimulation produced inhibition of primate spinothalamic tract cells. *Pain* 19:277–293, 1984b.

CLARK, F. J. Central projections of sensory fibers from the cat knee joint. *J. Neurobiol.* 3:101–110, 1972.

CLARK, F. J., LANDGREN, S., AND SILFVENIUS, H. Projections to the cat's cerebral cortex from low threshold joint afferents. *Acta Physiol. Scand.* 89:503–521, 1973.

COSTANZO, R. M. AND GARDNER, E. P. A quantitative analysis of responses of direction-sensitive neurons in somatosensory cortex of awake monkeys. *J. Neurophysiol.* 43:1319–1341, 1980.

CRAIG, A. D. Spinocervical tract cells in cat and dog, labeled by the retrograde transport of horseradish peroxidase. *Neurosci. Lett.* 3:173–177, 1976.

CRAIG, A. D. Spinal and medullary input to the lateral cervical nucleus. *J. Comp. Neurol.* 181:729–744, 1978.

CRAIG, A. D., AND BURTON, H. The lateral cervical nucleus in the cat: Anatomic organization of cervicothalamic neurons. *J. Comp. Neurol.* 185:329–346, 1979.

CRAIG, A. D., AND BURTON, H. Spinal and medullary lamina I projection to nucleus submedius in medial thalamus: A possible pain center. *J. Neurophysiol.* 45:443–466, 1981.

CRAIG, A. D., AND KNIFFKI, K. D. Lumbosacral lamina I cells projecting to medial and/or lateral thalamus in the cat. *Soc. Neurosci. Abstr.* 8:95, 1982.

CRAIG, A. D., AND TAPPER, D. N. Lateral cervical nucleus in the cat: Functional organization and characteristics. *J. Neurophysiol.* 41:1511–1534, 1978.

DILLY, P. N., WALL, P. D., AND WEBSTER, K. E. Cells of origin of the spinothalamic tract in the cat and rat. *Exp. Neurol.* 21:550–562, 1968.

DONG, W. K., RYU, H., AND, WAGMAN, I. H. Nociceptive responses of neurons in medial thalamus and their relationship to spinothalamic pathways. *J. Neurophysiol.* 41:1592–1613, 1978.

DOUGLAS, P. R., FERRINGTON, D. G., AND ROWE, M. R. Coding of information about tactile stimuli by neurones of the cuneate nucleus. *J. Physiol. (Lond.)* 285:493–513, 1978.

DREYER, D. A., SCHNEIDER, R. J., METZ, C. B., AND WHITSEL, B. L. Differential contributions of spinal pathways to body representation in postcentral gyrus of *Macaca Mulatta*. *J. Neurophysiol.* 37:119–145, 1974.

DREYER, D. A. LOE, P. R., METZ, C. B., AND WHITSEL, B. L. Representation of head and face in postcentral gyrus of the macaque. *J. Neurophysiol.* 38:714–733, 1975.

DUNCAN, G. H., DREYER, D. A., MCKENNA, T. M., AND WHITSEL, B. L. Dose- and time-dependent effects of ketamine on SI neurons with cutaneous receptive fields. *J. Neurophysiol.* 47:677–699, 1982.

DYKES, R. W., RASMUSSEN, D. D., SRETAVAN, D., AND REHMAN, N. B. Submodality segregation and receptive-field sequences in the cuneate, gracile, and external cuneate nuclei of the cat. *J. Neurophysiol.* 47:389–416, 1982.

ELLIS, L. C., AND RUSTIONI, A. A correlative HRP, Golgi, and EM study of the intrinsic organization of the feline dorsal column nuclei. *J. Comp. Neurol.* 197:341–367, 1981.

FERRARO, A., AND BARRERA, S. E. The nuclei of the posterior funiculi in *Macacus rhesus*. *Arch. Neurol. Psychiatry* 33:262–275, 1935a.

FERRARO, A., AND BARRERA, S. E. Posterior column fibers and their termination in *Macacus rhesus*. *J. Comp. Neurol.* 62:507–530, 1935b.

FIELDS, H. L., WAGNER, G. M., AND ANDERSON, S. D. Some properties of spinal neurons projecting to the medial brain-stem reticular formation. *Exp. Neurol.* 47:118–134, 1975.

FIELDS, H. L., CLANTON, C. H., AND ANDERSON, S. D. Somatosensory properties of spinoreticular neurons in the cat. *Brain Res.* 120:49–66, 1977.

FISHER, G. R., FREEMAN, B., AND ROWE, M. J. Organization of parallel projections from Pacinian afferent fibers to somatosensory cortical areas I and II in the cat. *J. Neurophysiol.* 49:75–97, 1983.

FOERSTER, O., AND GAGEL, O. Die Vorderseitenstrangdurschneidung beim Menschen. Eine klinisch-patho-physiologisch-anatomische Studie. *Z. Ges. Neurol. Psychiatrie* 138:1–92, 1932.

FOREMAN, R. D., AND WEBBER, R. N. Responses from neurons of the primate spinothalamic tract to electrical stimulation of afferents from the cardiopulmonary region and somatic structures. *Brain Res.* 186:463–468, 1980.

FOREMAN, R. D., APPLEBAUM, A. E., BEALL, J. E., TREVINO, D. L., AND WILLIS, W. D. Responses of primate spinothalamic tract neurons to electrical stimulation of hindlimb peripheral nerves. *J. Neurophysiol.* 38:132–145, 1975.

FOREMAN, R. D., SCHMIDT, R. F., AND WILLIS, W. D. Effects of mechanical and chemical stimulation of fine muscle afferents upon primate spinothalamic tract cells. *J. Physiol. (Lond.)* 286:215–231, 1979.

FRIEDMAN, D. P., AND JONES, E. G. Thalamic input to areas 3a and 2 in monkeys. *J. Neurophysiol.* 45:59–85, 1981.

GAZE, R. M., AND GORDON, G. The representation of cutaneous sense in the thalamus of the cat and monkey. *Q. J. Exp. Physiol.* 39:279–304, 1954.

GERHART, K. D., YEZIERSKI, R. P., GIESLER, G. J., AND WILLIS, W. D. Inhibitory receptive fields of primate spinothalamic tract cells. *J. Neurophysiol.* 46:1309–1325, 1981.

GIESLER, G. J., MENETREY, D., GUILBAUD, G., AND BESSON, J. M. Lumbar cord neurons at the origin of the spinothalamic tract in the rat. *Brain Res.* 118:320–324, 1976.

GIESLER, G. J., MENETREY, D., AND BASBAUM, A. I. Differential origins of spinothalamic tract projections to medial and lateral thalamus in the rat. *J. Comp. Neurol.* 184:107–126, 1979a.

GIESLER, G. J., URCA, G., CANNON, J. T., AND LIEBESKIND, J. C. Response properties of neurons of the lateral cervical nucleus in the rat. *J. Comp. Neurol.* 186:65–78, 1979b.

GIESLER, G. J., YEZIERSKI, R. P., GERHART, K. D., AND WILLIS, W. D. Spinothalamic tract neurons that project to medial and/or lateral thalamic nuclei: Evidence for a physiologically novel population of spinal cord neurons. *J. Neurophysiol.* 46:1285–1308, 1981.

GIESLER, G. J., NAHIN, R. L., AND MADSEN, A. M. Postsynaptic dorsal column pathway of the rat. I. Anatomical studies. *J. Neurophysiol.* 51:260–275, 1984.

GLEES, P., AND SOLER, J. Fibre content of the posterior column and synaptic connections of nucleus gracilis. *Z. Zellforsch.* 36:381–400, 1951.

GORDON, G., AND JUKES, M. G. M. Dual organization of the exteroceptive components of the cat's gracile nucleus, *J. Physiol. (Lond.)* 173:263–290, 1964.

GRANT, G., BOIVIE, J., AND SILFVENIUS, H. Course and termination of fibres from the nucleus Z of the medulla oblongata. An experimental light microscopical study in the cat. *Brain Res.* 55:55–70, 1973.

GUILBAUD, G., CAILLE, D., BESSON, J. M., AND BENELLI, G. Single unit activities in ventral posterior and posterior group thalamic nuclei during nociceptive and non-nociceptive stimulations in the cat. *Arch. Ital. Biol.* 115:38–56, 1977.

GUILBAUD, G., PESCHANSKI, M., GAUTRON, M., AND BINDER, D. Neurones responding to noxious stimulation of VB complex and caudal adjacent regions in the thalamus of the rat. *Pain* 8:303–318, 1980.

HA, H. Cervicothalamic tract in the rhesus monkey. *Exp. Neurol.* 33:205–212, 1971.

HABER, L. H., MOORE, B. D., AND WILLIS, W. D. Electrophysiological response properties of spinoreticular neurons in the monkey. *J. Comp. Neurol.* 207:75–84, 1982.

HAND, P. J. Lumbosacral dorsal root terminations in the nucleus gracilis of the cat. *J. Comp. Neurol.* 126:137–156, 1966.

HAND, *P. J.*, AND VAN WINKLE, T. The afferent connections of the feline nucleus cuneatus. *J. Comp. Neurol.* 171:83–110, 1977.

HONDA, C. N., MENSE, S., AND PERL, E. R. Neurons in ventrobasal region of the cat thalamus selectively responsive to noxious mechanical stimulation. *J. Neurophysiol.* 49:662–673, 1983.

HONG, S. K., KNIFFKI, K. D., MENSE, S., SCHMIDT, R. F., AND WENDISCH, M. Descending influences on the responses of spinocervical tract neurones to chemical stimulation of fine muscle afferents. *J. Physiol. (Lond.)* 290:129–140, 1979.

HORCH, K. W., BURGESS, P. R., AND WHITEHORN, D. Ascending collaterals of cutaneous neurons in the fasciculus gracilis of the cat. *Brain Res.* 117:1–17, 1976.

HORROBIN, D. F. The lateral cervical nucleus of the cat; an electrophysiological study. *Q. J. Exp. Physiol.* 51:351–371, 1966.

HUBEL, D. H., AND WIESEL, T. N. Functional architecture of macaque monkey visual cortex, *Proc. R. Soc. Lond. [Biol.]* 198:1–59, 1977.

IWAMURA, Y., AND INUBUSHI, S. Regional diversity in excitatory and inhibitory receptive-field organization of cat thalamic ventrobasal neurons. *J. Neurophysiol.* 37:910–919, 1974.

JÄNIG, W., SCHOULTZ, T., AND SPENCER, W. A. Temporal and spatial parameters of excitation and afferent inhibition in cuneothalamic relay neurons. *J. Neurophysiol.* 40:822–835, 1977.

JÄNIG, W., SPENCER, W. A., AND YOUNKIN, S. G. Spatial and temporal features of afferent inhibition of thalamocortical relay cells. *J. Neurophysiol.* 42:1450–1460, 1979.

JOHANSSON, H., AND SILFVENIUS, H. Axon-collateral activation by dorsal spinocerebellar tract fibers of group I relay cells of nucleus Z in the cat medulla oblongata. *J. Physiol. (Lond.)* 265:341–369, 1977.

JOHNSON, J. I., WALKER, W. I., AND PUBOLS, B. H. Somatotopic organization of raccoon dorsal column nuclei. *J. Comp. Neurol.* 132:1–44, 1968.

JONES, E. G. Organization of the thalamocortical complex and its relation to sensory processes, in: *Handbook of Physiology, The Nervous System III,* (I. DARION-SMITH, ed.) American Physiological Society, Bethesda, 1984, pp. 149–212.

JONES, E. G., AND BURTON, H. Cytoarchitecture and somatic sensory connectivity of thalamic nuclei other than the ventrobasal complex. *J. Comp. Neurol.* 154:395–432, 1974.

JONES, E. G., AND FRIEDMAN, D. P. Projection pattern of functional components of thalamic ventrobasal complex on monkey somatosensory cortex. *J. Neurophysiol.* 48:521–544, 1982.

JONES, E. G., AND LEAVITT, R. Y. Retrograde axonal transport and the demonstration of non-specific projections to the central cortex and striatum from thalamic intralaminar nuclei in the rat, cat, and monkey. *J. Comp. Neurol.* 154:349–378, 1974.

JONES, E. G., AND POWELL, T. P. S. Connexions of the somatic sensory cortex of the rhesus monkey. III. Thalamic connexions. *Brain* 93:37–56, 1970.

JONES, E. G., WISE. S. P., AND COULTER, J. D. Differential thalamic relationships of sensory-motor and parietal cortical fields in monkeys. *J. Comp. Neurol.* 183:833–882, 1979.

KAAS, J. H. What, if anything, is SI? Organization of first somatosensory area of cortex. *Physiol. Rev.* 63:206–231, 1983.

KAAS, J. H., NELSON, R. J., SUR, M., LIN, C. S., AND MERZENICH, M. M. Multiple representations of the body within the primary somatosensory complex of primates. *Science* 204:521–523, 1979.

KAAS, J. H., NELSON, R. J., SUR, M., DYKES, R. W., AND MERZENICH, M. M. The somatotoptic organization of the ventroposterior thalamus of the squirrel monkey, *Saimiri sciureus*. *J. Comp. Neurol.* 226:111–140, 1984.

KENSHALO, D. R., JR., LEONARD, R. B., CHUNG, J. M., AND WILLIS, W. D. Responses of primate spinothalamic neurons to graded and to repeated noxious heat stimuli. *J. Neurophysiol.* 42:1370–1389, 1979.

KENSHALO, D. R., JR., AND ISENSEE, O. Responses of primate SI cortical neurons to noxious stimuli. *J. Neurophysiol.* 50:1479–1496, 1983.

KENSHALO, D. R., JR., GIESLER, G. J., LEONARD, R. B., AND WILLIS, W. D. Responses of neurons in primate ventral posterior lateral nucleus to noxious stimuli. *J. Neurophysiol.* 43:1594–1614, 1980.

KERR, F. W. L. Neuroanatomical substrates of nociception in the spinal cord. *Pain* 1:325–356, 1975a.

KERR, F. W. L. The ventral spinothalamic tract and other ascending systems of the ventral funiculus of the spinal cord. *J. Comp. Neurol.* 159:335–356, 1975b.

KERR, F. W. L., AND LIPPMAN, H. H. The primate spinothalamic tract as demonstrated by anterolateral cordotomy and commissural myelotomy. *Adv. Neurol.* 4:147–156, 1974.

KEVETTER, G. A., AND WILLIS, W. D. Spinothalamic cells in the rat lumbar cord with collaterals to the medullary reticular formation. *Brain Res.* 238:181–185, 1982.

KEVETTER, G. A., AND WILLIS, W. D. Collaterals of spinothalamic cells in the rat. *J. Comp. Neurol.* 215:453–464, 1983.

KEVETTER, G. A., HABER, L. H., YEZIERSKI, R. P., CHUNG, J. M., MARTIN, R. F., AND WILLIS, W. D. Cells of origin of the spinoreticular tract in the monkey. *J. Comp. Neurol.* 207:61–74, 1982.

KITAI, S. T., HA, H., AND MORIN, F. Lateral cervical nucleus of the dog: Anatomical and microelectrode studies. *Am. J. Physiol.* 209:307–311, 1965.

KNIFFKI, K. D., AND MIZUMURA, K. Responses of neurons in VPL and VPL-VL region of the cat to algesic stimulation of muscle and tendon. *J. Neurophysiol.* 49:649–661, 1983.

KRUGER, L., SIMINOFF, R., AND WITKOVSKY, P. Single neuron analysis of dorsal column nuclei and spinal nucleus of trigeminal in cat. *J. Neurophysiol.* 24:333–349, 1961.

KURU, M. *Sensory Paths in the Spinal Cord and Brain Stem of Man*, Sogensya, Tokyo, 1949.

KUYPERS, H. G. J. M., AND TUERK, J. D. The distribution of the cortical fibres within the nuclei cuneatus and gracilis in the cat. *J. Anat.* 98:143–162, 1964.

LAMOUR, Y., GUILBAUD, G., AND WILLER, J. C. Rat somatosensory (SmI) cortex. II. Laminar and columnar organization of noxious and non-noxious inputs. *Exp. Brain Res.* 49:46–54, 1983a.

LAMOUR, Y., WILLER, J. C., AND GUILBAUD, G. Rat somatosensory (SmI) cortex. I. Characteristics of neuronal responses to noxious stimulation and comparison with responses to non-noxious stimulation. *Exp. Brain Res.* 49:35–45, 1983b.

LANDGREN, S., AND SILFVENIUS, H. Projection to cerebral cortex of group I muscle afferents from the cat's hind limb. *J. Physiol. (Lond.)* 200:353–372, 1969.

LANDGREN, S., AND SILFVENIUS, H. Nucleus Z, the medullary relay in the projection path to the cerebral cortex of group I muscle afferents from the cat's hind limb. *J. Physiol. (Lond.)* 218:551–571, 1971.

LANDGREN, S. A., NORDWALL, A., AND WENGSTRÖM, C. The location of the thalamic relay in the spino–cervical–lemniscal path. *Acta Physiol. Scand.* 65:164–175, 1965.

LANDRY, P., AND DESCHENES, M. Intracortical arborizations and receptive fields of identified ventrobasal thalamocortical afferents to the primary somatic sensory cortex in the cat. *J. Comp. Neurol.* 199:345–371, 1981.

LANGFORD, L. A., AND COGGESHALL, R. E. Unmyelinated axons in the posterior funiculi. *Science* 211:176–177, 1981.

LEVITT, M., AND LEVITT, J. Sensory hind limb representation in the SmI cortex of the cat after spinal tractotomies. *Exp. Neurol.* 22:276–302, 1968.

LIN, C. S., MERZENICH, M. M., SUR, M., AND KAAS, J. H. Connections of areas 3b and 1 of the parietal somatosensory strip with the ventroposterior nucleus in the owl monkey *(Aotus trivirgatus). J. Comp. Neurol.* 185:355–372, 1979.

LIU, R. P. C. Laminar origins of spinal projection neurons to periaqueductal gray of the rat. *Brain Res.* 264:118–122, 1983.

LLOYD, D. P. C., AND MCINTYRE, A. K. Dorsal column conduction of group I muscle afferent impulses and their relay through Clarke's column. *J. Neurophysiol.* 13:39–54, 1950.

LOE, P. R., WHITSEL, B. L., DREYER, D. A., AND METZ, C. B. Body representation in ventrobasal thalamus of macaque: A single-unit analysis. *J. Neurophysiol.* 40:1339–1355, 1977.

LU, G. W., BENNETT, G. J., NISHIKAWA, N., HOFFERT, M. J., AND DUBNER, R. Extra- and intracellular recordings from dorsal column postsynaptic spinomedullary neurons in the cat. *Exp. Neurol.* 82:456–477, 1983.

LUND, R. D., AND WEBSTER, K. E. Thalamic afferents from the spinal cord and trigeminal nuclei. An experimental anatomical study in the rat. *J. Comp. Neurol.* 130:313–328, 1967.

MAGHERINI, P. C., POMPEIANO, O., AND SEGUIN, J. J. Responses of nucleus Z neurons to vibration of hindlimb extensor muscles in the decerebrate cat. *Arch. Ital. Biol.* 113:150–187, 1975.

MANTYH, P. W. The terminations of the spinothalamic tract in the cat. *Neurosci. Lett.* 38:119–124, 1983.

MAUNZ, R. A., PITTS, N. G., AND PETERSON, B. W. Cat spinoreticular neurons: Locations, responses and changes in responses during repetitive stimulation. *Brain Res.* 148:365–379, 1978.

MCCOMAS, A. J. Responses of the rat dorsal column system to mechanical stimulation of the hind paw. *J. Physiol. (Lond.)* 166:435–448, 1963.

MCKENNA, T. M., WHITSEL, B. L., AND DREYER, D. A. Anterior parietal cortical topographic organization in macaque monkey: A reevaluation. *J. Neurophysiol* 48:289–317, 1982.

MCKENNA, T. M., LIGHT, A. R., AND WHITSEL, B. L. Neurons with unusual response and receptive-field properties in upper laminae of cat SI cortex. *J. Neurophysiol.* 51:1055–1076, 1984.

MEHLER, W. R. The anatomy of the so-called "pain tract" in man: An analysis of the course and distribution of the ascending fibers of the fasciculus anterolateralis, in: *Basic Research in Paraplegia* (J. D. FRENCH AND R. W. PORTER, eds.), Charles C. Thomas, Springfield, IL, 1962, pp. 26–55.

MEHLER, W. R., FEFERMAN, M. E., AND NAUTA, W. J. H. Ascending axon degeneration following anterolateral cordotomy. An experimental study in the monkey. *Brain* 83:718–751, 1960.

MENDELL, L. M. Physiological properties of unmyelinated fiber projection to the spinal cord. *Exp. Neurol.* 16:316–332, 1966.

MENETREY, D., CHAOUCH, A., AND BESSON, J. M. Location and properties of dorsal horn neurons at origin of spinoreticular tract in lumbar enlargement of the rat. *J. Neurophysiol.* 44:862–877, 1980.

MENETREY, D., CHAOUCH, A., BINDER, D., AND BESSON, J. M. The origin of the spinomesencephalic tract in the rat: An anatomical study using the retrograde transport of horseradish peroxidase. *J. Comp. Neurol.* 206:193–207, 1982.

MERZENICH, M. M., KAAS, J. H., SUR, M., AND LIN, C. S. Double representation of the body surface within cytoarchitectonic areas 3b and 1 in 'SI' in the owl monkey *(Aotus trivirgatus). J. Comp. Neurol.* 181:41–73, 1978.

MILLAR, J., AND BASBAUM, A. I. Topography of the projection of the body surface of the cat to cuneate and gracile nuclei. *Exp. Neurol.* 49:281–290, 1975.

MILNE, R. J., FOREMAN, R. D., GIESLER, G. J., AND WILLIS, W. D. Convergence of cutaneous and pelvic visceral nociceptive inputs onto primate spinothalamic neurons. *Pain* 11:163–183, 1981.

MITCHELL, D., AND HELLON, R. F. Neuronal and behavioural responses in rats during noxious stimulation of the tail. *Proc. R. Soc. Lond. [Biol.]* 197:169–194, 1977.

MORIN, F. A new spinal pathway for cutaneous impulses. *Am. J. Physiol.* 183:245–252, 1955.

MOUNTCASTLE, V. B. Modality and topographic properties of single neurons of cat's somatic sensory cortex. *J. Neurophysiol.* 20:408–434, 1957.

MOUNTCASTLE, V. B. Central nervous mechanisms in mechanoreceptive sensibility, in: *Handbook of Physiology, The Nervous System III,* (I. DARIAN-SMITH, ed.), American Physiological Society, Bethesda, 1984, pp. 789–878.

MOUNTCASTLE, V. B., AND HENNEMAN, E. The representation of tactile sensibility in the thalamus of the monkey. *J. Comp. Neurol.* 97:409–440, 1952.

MOUNTCASTLE, V. B., AND POWELL, T. P. S. Neural mechanisms subserving cutaneous sensibility, with special reference to the role of afferent inhibition in sensory perception and discrimination. *Bull. Johns Hopkins Hosp.* 105:201–232, 1959.

NATHAN, P. W., AND SMITH, M. C. Fasciculi proprii of the spinal cord in man: Review of present knowledge. *Brain* 82:610–668, 1959.

NELSON, R. J., AND KAAS, J. H. Connections of the ventroposterior nucleus of the thalamus with the body surface representations in cortical areas 3b and 1 of the cynomolgus macaque, *(Macaca fascicularis). J. Comp. Neurol.* 199:29–64, 1981.

NELSON, R. J., SUR, M., FELLEMAN, D. J., AND KAAS, J. H. Representations of the body surface in postcentral parietal cortex of *Macaca fascicularis. J. Comp. Neurol.* 192:611–643, 1980.

NIJENSOHN, D. E., AND KERR, F. W. L. The ascending projections of the dorsolateral funiculus of the spinal cord in the primate. *J. Comp. Neurol.* 161:459–470, 1975.

OSWALDO-CRUZ, E., AND KIDD, C. Functional properties of neurons in the lateral cervical nucleus of the cat. *J. Neurophysiol.* 27:1–14, 1964.

PAUL, R. L., MERZENICH, M., AND GOODMAN, H. Representation of slowly and rapidly adapting cutaneous mechanoreceptors of the hand in Brodmann's areas 3 and 1 of *Macaca mulatta. Brain Res.* 36:229–249, 1972.

PENFIELD, W., AND JASPER, H. *Epilepsy and the Functional Anatomy of the Human Brain,* Little, Brown, Boston, 1954.

PERL, E. R. Pain and nociception, in: *Handbook of Physiology,* Section 1, Vol. III, *Sensory Processes,* Part 2 (I. DARIAN-SMITH, ed.), American Physiological Society, Bethesda, 1984, pp. 915–975.

PERL, E. R., AND WHITLOCK, D. G. Somatic stimuli exciting spinothalamic projections to thalamic neurons in cat and monkey. *Exp. Neurol.* 3:256–296, 1961.

PERL, E. R., WHITLOCK, D. G., AND GENTRY, J. R. Cutaneous projection to second-order neurons of the dorsal column system. *J. Neurophysiol.* 25:337–358, 1962.

PESCHANSKI, M., GUILBAUD, G., GAUTRON, M., AND BESSON, J. M. Encoding of noxious heat messages in neurons of the ventrobasal thalamic complex of the rat. *Brain Res.* 197:401–413, 1980.

PESCHANSKI, M., GUILBAUD, D., AND GAUTRON, M. Posterior intralaminar region in rat: Neuronal responses to noxious and nonnoxious cutaneous stimuli. *Exp. Neurol.* 72:226–238, 1981.

PESCHANSKI, M., MANTYH, P. W., AND BESSON, J. M. Spinal afferents to the ventrobasal thalamic complex in the rat: An anatomical study using wheatgerm agglutinin conjugated to horseradish peroxidase. *Brain Res.* 278:240–244, 1983.

PETIT, D., AND BURGESS, P. R. Dorsal column projection of receptors in cat hairy skin supplied by myelinated fibers. *J. Neurophysiol.* 31:849–855, 1968.

PHILLIPS, C. G., POWELL, T. P. S., AND WIESENDANGER, M. Projection from low-threshold muscle afferents of hand and forearm to area 3a of baboon's cortex. *J. Physiol. (Lond.)* 21:419–446, 1971.

POGGIO, G. F., AND MOUNTCASTLE, V. B. A study of the functional contributions of the lemniscal and spinothalamic systems to somatic sensibility. *Bull. Johns Hopkins Hosp.* 106:266–316, 1960.

POGGIO, G. F., AND MOUNTCASTLE, V. B. The functional properties of ventrobasal thalamic neurons studied in unanesthetized monkeys. *J. Neurophysiol.* 26:775–806, 1963.

POLLIN, B., AND ALBE-FESSARD, D. Organization of somatic thalamus in monkeys with and without section of dorsal spinal tracts. *Brain Res.* 173:431–449, 1979.

POMPEIANO, O., AND BRODAL, A. Spino-vestibular fibers in the cat; an experimental study. *J. Comp. Neurol.* 108:353–382, 1957.

POWELL, T. P. S., AND MOUNTCASTLE, V. B. The cytoarchitecture of the postcentral gyrus of the monkey *Macaca mulatta*. *Bull. Johns Hopkins Hosp.* 105:108–131, 1959a.

POWELL, T. P. S., AND MOUNTCASTLE, V. B. Some aspects of the functional organization of the cortex of the postcentral gyrus of the monkey: A correlation of findings obtained in a single unit analysis with cytoarchitecture. *Bull. Johns Hopkins Hosp.* 105:133–162, 1959b.

PRICE, D. D., HAYES, R. L., RUDA, M. A., AND DUBNER, R. Spatial and temporal transformation of input to spinothalamic tract neurons and their relation to somatic sensations. *J. Neurophysiol.* 41:933–947, 1978.

PUBOLS, B. H., WELKER, W. I., AND JOHNSON, J. I. Somatic sensory representation of forelimb in dorsal root fibers of raccoon, coatimundi, and cat. *J. Neurophysiol.* 28:312–341, 1965.

PUBOLS, L. M. Somatic sensory representation in the thalamic ventrobasal complex of the spider monkey *(Ateles)*. *Brain Behav. Evol.* 1:305–323, 1968.

PUBOLS, L. M., AND PUBOLS, B. H. Modality composition and functional characteristics of dorsal column mechanoreceptive afferent fibers innervating the raccoon's forepaw. *J. Neurophysiol.* 36:1023–1037, 1973.

RASMUSSEN, A. T., AND PEYTON, W. T. The course and termination of the medial lemniscus in man. *J. Comp. Neurol.* 88:411–424, 1948.

ROSEN, I. Afferent connexions to group I activated cells in the main cuneate nucleus of the cat. *J. Physiol. (Lond.)* 205:209–236, 1969.

ROSEN, I., AND SJOLUND, B. Organization of group I activated cells in the main and external cuneate nuclei of the cat: Identification of muscle receptors. *Exp. Brain Res.* 16:221–237, 1973.

RUSTIONI, A. Non-primary afferents to the nucleus gracilis from the lumbar cord of the cat. *Brain Res.* 51:81–85, 1973.

RUSTIONI, A. Non-primary afferents to the cuneate nucleus in the brachial dorsal funiculus of the cat. *Brain Res.* 75:247–259, 1974.

RUSTIONI, A., AND KAUFMAN, A. B. Identification of cells of origin of nonprimary afferents to the dorsal column nuclei of the cat. *Exp. Brain Res.* 27:1–14, 1977.

RUSTIONI, A., AND MACCHI, G. Distribution of dorsal root fibers in the medulla oblongata of the cat. *J. Comp. Neurol.* 134:113–126, 1968.

RUSTIONI, A., AND SOTELO, C. Synaptic organization of the nucleus gracilis of the cat. Experimental identification of dorsal root fibers and cortical afferents. *J. Comp. Neurol.* 155:441–468, 1974.

RUSTIONI, A., HAYES, N. L., AND O'NEILL, S. Dorsal column nuclei and ascending spinal afferents in macaques. *Brain* 102:95–125, 1979.

SHRIVER, J. E., STEIN, B. M., AND CARPENTER, M. B. Central projections of spinal dorsal roots in the monkey. I. Cervical and upper thoracic dorsal roots. *Am. J. Anat.* 123:27–74, 1968.

SPREAFICO, R., HAYES, N. L., AND RUSTIONI, A. Thalamic projections to the primary and secondary somatosensory cortices in cat: Single and double retrograde tracer studies. *J. Comp. Neurol.* 203:67–90, 1981.

SRETAVAN, D., AND DYKES, R. W. The organization of two cutaneous submodalities in the forearm region of area 3b of cat somatosensory cortex. *J. Comp. Neurol.* 213:381–398, 1983.

SUR, M. Receptive fields of neurons in areas 3b and 1 of somatosensory cortex in monkeys. *Brain Res.* 198:465–471, 1980.

SUR, M., MERZENICH, M. M., AND KAAS, J. H. Magnification, receptive-field area, and "hypercolumn" size in areas 3b and 1 of somatosensory cortex in owl monkeys. *J. Neurophysiol.* 44:295–311, 1980.

SUR, M., WALL, J. T., AND KAAS, J. H. Modular segregation of functional cell classes within the postcentral somatosensory cortex of monkeys. *Science* 212:1059–1061, 1981.

TANJI, J., AND WISE, S. P. Submodality distribution in sensorimotor cortex of the unanesthetized monkey. *J. Neurophysiol.* 45:467–481, 1981.

TREVINO, D. L. The origin and projections of a spinal nociceptive and thermoreceptive pathway, in: *Sensory Functions of the Skin in Primates, with Special Reference to Man* (Y. Zotterman, ed.), Pergamon Press, New York, 1976, pp. 367–376.

TREVINO, D. L., AND CARSTENS E. Confirmation of the location of spinothalamic neurons in the cat and monkey by the retrograde transport of horseradish peroxidase. *Brain Res.* 98:177–182, 1975.

TREVINO, D. L., MAUNZ, R. A., BRYAN, R. N., AND WILLIS, W. D. Location of cells of origin of the spinothalamic tract in the lumbar enlargement of cat. *Exp. Neurol.* 34:64–77, 1972.

TREVINO, D. L., COULTER, J. D., AND WILLIS, W. D. Location of cells of origin of spinothalamic tract in lumbar enlargement of the monkey. *J. Neurophysiol.* 36:750–761, 1973.

UDDENBERG, N. Differential localization in dorsal funiculus of fibres originating from different receptors. *Exp. Brain Res.* 4:367–376, 1968a.

UDDENBERG, N. Functional organization of long, second-order afferents in the dorsal funiculus. *Exp. Brain Res.* 4:377–382, 1968b.

VALVERDE, F. The pyramidal tract in rodents. A study of its relations with the posterior column nuclei, dorsolateral reticular formation of the medulla oblongata and cervical spinal cord (Golgi and electron microscopic observations). *Z. Zellforsch.* 71:297–363, 1966.

WALBERG, F. Axoaxonic contacts in the cuneate nucleus, probable basis for presynaptic depolarization. *Exp. Neurol.* 13:218–231, 1965.

WALKER, A. E., AND WEAVER, T. A. The topical organization and termination of the fibers of the posterior columns in *Macaca mulatta. J. Comp. Neurol.* 76:145–158, 1942.

WEAVER, T. A., AND WALKER, A. E. Topical arrangement within the spinothalamic tract of the monkey. *Arch. Neurol. Psychiatry* 46:877–883, 1941.

WHITSEL, B. L., PETRUCELLI, L. M., AND SAPIRO, G. Modality representation in the lumbar and cervical fasciculus gracilis of squirrel monkeys. *Brain Res.* 15:67–78, 1969.

WHITSEL, B. L., PETRUCELLI, L. M., SAPIRO, G., AND HA, H. Fiber sorting in the fasciculus gracilis of squirrel monkeys. *Exp. Neurol.* 29:227–242, 1970.

WHITSEL, B. L., DREYER, D. A., AND ROPPOLO, J. R. Determinants of body representation in postcentral gyrus of macaques. *J. Neurophysiol.* 34:1018–1034, 1971.

WHITSEL, B. L., RUSTIONI, A., DREYER, D. A., LOE, P. R., ALLEN, E. E., AND METZ, C. B. Thalamic projections to S-I in macaque monkey. *J. Comp. Neurol.* 178:385–410, 1978.

WILLIS, W. D., AND COGGESHALL, R. E. *Sensory Mechanisms of the Spinal Cord,* New York, Plenum Press, 1978.

WILLIS, W. D., KENSHALO, D. R., AND LEONARD, R. B. The cells of origin of the primate spinothalamic tract. *J. Comp. Neurol.* 188:543–574, 1979.

WOOLSEY, C. N. Organization of somatic sensory and motor areas of the cerebral cortex, in: *Biological and Biochemical Bases of Behavior* (H. F. HARLOW AND C. N. WOOLSEY, eds.), University of Wisconsin Press, Madison, 1958, pp. 63–81.

YEZIERSKI, R. P., AND SCHWARTZ, R. H. Receptive field properties of spinomesencephalic tract (SMT) cells. *Pain [Suppl.]* 2:184, 1984.

12 The Spinal Pathways Contributing to the Ascending Conduction and the Descending Modulation of Pain Sensations and Reactions

CHARLES J. VIERCK, JR., JOEL D. GREENSPAN, LOUIS A. RITZ, AND DAVID C. YEOMANS

A. *Introduction*

Recent advances in pain research have strongly implicated a variety of transmitters within the dorsal horn of the spinal cord as modulators of conduction from peripheral nociceptors to ascending pathways (see Hammond, Chapter 15; Ruda, Chapter 7; Yaksh, Chapter 8; and several recent reviews including: Basbaum and Fields, 1984; La Motte and de Lanerolle, 1983; Light *et al.*, 1983; Schmauss and Yaksh, 1984; Westlund *et al.*, 1984). These findings have supplemented and refined a wealth of anatomic and physiological information on synaptic interactions within the dorsal horn that are relevant to pain coding (see Willis, Chapter 11; Cervero, Chapter 9). The weakest link in this intense effort to understand the totality of influences on pain transmission within the spinal cord (Kerr, 1975b) has been the behavioral analysis of pain sensitivity in human patients and laboratory animals (primarily rats, cats, and monkeys).

CHARLES J. VIERCK, JR., AND DAVID C. YEOMANS • Department of Neuroscience and Center for Neurobiological Sciences, University of Florida College of Medicine, Gainesville, Florida 32610. JOEL D. GREENSPAN • Department of Physiology, University of North Carolina School of Medicine, Chapel Hill, North Carolina 27514. LOUIS A. RITZ • Departments of Neurological Surgery and Neuroscience, University of Florida College of Medicine, Gainesville, Florida 32610.

At this time, we are presented with a multitude of presumptive circuits for pain transmission (Kerr, 1975c) to which different "responsibilities" for discriminable pain experiences have been attributed (Berkley, 1985). For example, chronic pain changes in character after recovery from mesencephalic spinothalamic tractotomy (Bowsher, 1983; Drake and McKenzie, 1953; Walker, 1943), which leaves intact a spinoreticulothalamic system of projection (Nauta and Kuypers, 1958). It is these systems that have received most attention as pain pathways, and for a behavioral analysis of their functions, we are aided by a clinical literature that describes the consequences of surgically controlled lesions involving different combinations of spinothalamic and spinoreticular components.

A lesion of one anterolateral column of the spinal cord interrupts spinothalamic and spinoreticulospinal tracts of contralateral origin and ipsilateral spinoreticular and reticulospinal tracts. The effects of this lesion, termed spinothalamic tractotomy or anterolateral chordotomy, have been described in considerable detail by intuitively skilled clinician–scientists. Their written account often is frustrating for a lack of psychophysical data and specification of test stimuli, and the locations of the lesions often have not been verified histologically. But the clinical literature on the pain pathways is rich with interesting and valid comparisons of sensory effects that result from lesions of different pathways that have been attributed a role in pain coding. For example, a number of observers have compared the effects of selective lesions on pain from different sources (e.g., cutaneous versus deep, somatic versus visceral, acute versus chronic, fast versus slow, and thermal versus mechanical versus chemical) and also on nonnociceptive sensations.

Once the human capability of verbal expression is applied to effect a complete description of the deficits produced by lesions of pathways for pain conduction and control, it is possible to identify hallmark signs that can be tested in animal models, which, in turn, (1) permit a more complete analysis of the neural mechanisms for unfortunate consequences of damage to the pain pathways (e.g., hyperpathia or recovery from analgesia) and (2) provide the opportunity to search for lesions that optimize the desirable effects of ameliorative surgery. Because the pain pathways have evolved to a unique organization in primates (Mehler, 1969), this review concentrates on evidence from humans and nonhuman primates concerning the sensory functions of presumed pathways for pain.

Traumatic lateral hemisection of the spinal cord in human patients (the Brown-Sequard syndrome) is accompanied by contralateral decreases of pain intensity (Brown-Sequard, 1868; Head and Thompson, 1906; Turner, 1891), and intentional interruption of the lateral spinothalamic tract by anterolateral chordotomy produces significant diminution of chronic pain (e.g., Spiller and Martin, 1912). The importance of the anterolateral column has been demonstrated especially by a few clinicians who have observed the effects of chordotomies on pain and have evaluated histological sections of the spinal cords of these patients to specify the critical lesion configuration (Amromin and

Crue, 1975; Gardner and Cuneo, 1945; Hyndman and Van Epps, 1939; Moffie, 1975; Lahuerta *et al.*, 1984; Nathan and Smith, 1966, 1979; White *et al.*, 1956; White and Sweet, 1969). For human patients and in corroborating investigations of monkeys (King, 1957; Vierck *et al.*, 1983c; White and Sweet, 1969), contralateral spinal lesions produce pervasive reductions in pain, with apparent analgesia for some forms and hypalgesia for others.

Many patients recover pain sensitivity to a considerable degree after spinal lesions that appear to transect the white matter containing the crossed spinothalamic tract (Graf, 1960; Foerster and Gagel, 1932; White, 1968). Thus, some of the rostral connections of the contralateral lateral column are necessary for perception of some forms of pain, but remaining pathways (to similar rostral sites?) can eventually compensate for an anterolateral spinal lesion. As a beginning to an understanding of these processes, the course and rostral terminations of axons in the ventral spinal quadrant of primates have been identified.

B. Anatomy of the Anterolateral and Ventral Spinal Columns

Figure 1 presents examples of diagrams published by investigators who have plotted the location of ascending axonal degeneration or have correlated sensory levels with the locations of anterolateral chordotomies (Smith, 1957; Taren *et al.*, 1969; Walker, 1940). Also, Figure 2 summarizes the distribution of spinothalamic fibers in the white matter of monkeys as determined by recording from axons that are backfired from the ipsilateral somatosensory thalamus (Applebaum *et al.*, 1975) or by plotting degeneration resulting from commissural myelotomy (Kerr and Lippman, 1974). Although the crossed spinothalamic tract (cSTT) occupies slightly different regions at different rostrocaudal levels (Smith, 1957) and in different individuals (French and Peyton, 1948; Papo, 1979b; Voris, 1951; Walker, 1940), spinothalamic axons are most highly concentrated near the periphery of the anterolateral column, with caudal segments dorsal and cervical segments ventral (Figures 1 and 2). Axonal degeneration from a caudal lesion shifts peripherally with progression to rostral spinal levels (Gardner and Cuneo, 1945; Poirier and Bertrand, 1955; Weaver and Walker, 1941), indicating that superficial lesions of the anterolateral column would be especially effective for reduction of pain from segments well below the lesion.

Anatomic studies of degeneration following anterolateral chordotomy have shown that axons are interrupted for many pathways in primates that may have importance for coding of pain sensations (see Table I for details).

The lateral spinothalmic tract (STT) projects to a variety of thalamic nuclei that have been categorized simplistically by most authors as lateral neospinothalamic terminations (e.g., in nucleus ventralis posterolateralis) and medial paleospinothalamic terminations (e.g., in nucleus centralis lateralis, one of a dozen medial nuclei receiving spinothalamic afferents).

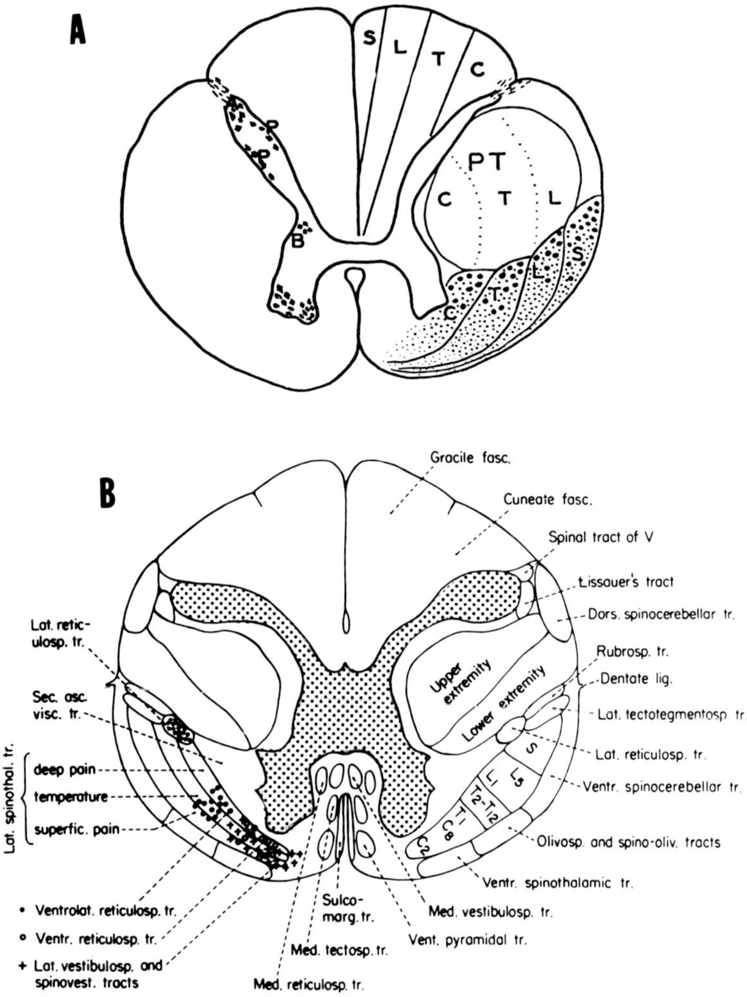

FIGURE 1. Distributions of spinothalamic axons in spinal cords of human patients based on correlations of sensory losses with the locations of lesions and degeneration as determined histologically. (A) Walker's (1940) diagram portrays drop-shaped distributions for axons representing sacral (S), lumbar (L), thoracic (T), and cervical (C) dermatomes, implying somatotopic organization in the anterolateral column but considerable overlap in the ventromedial portion of the STT. Somatotopic organization also is given for the dorsal columns and the pyramidal tract (PT). For the spinothalamic tract, the large dots represent locations of axons mediating thermoreception, the medium dots indicate localization for pain, and the fine dots represent touch and pressure sensitivities. (B) A diagram from Taren *et al.* (1969) showing dermatomal order (right side: S–C2) and submodality segregation (left side) for the STT. Other long pathways in the vicinity of the STT are indicated. (C) Smith's (1957) diagrams of shifts in location of spinothalamic and other pathways at different cervical levels of the spinal cord.

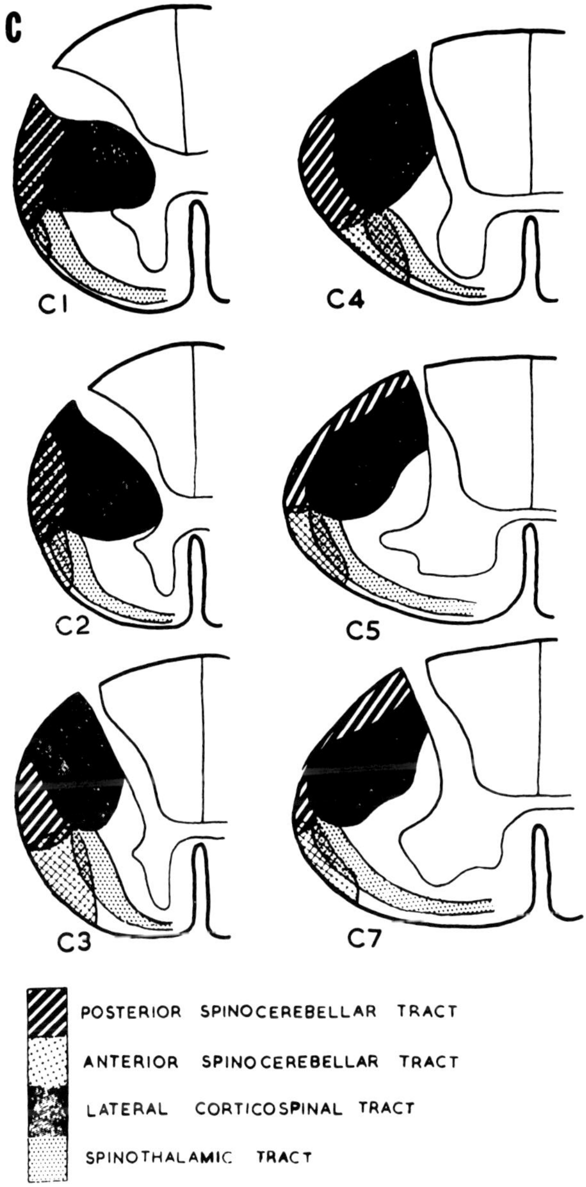

FIGURE 1. (*Continued*)

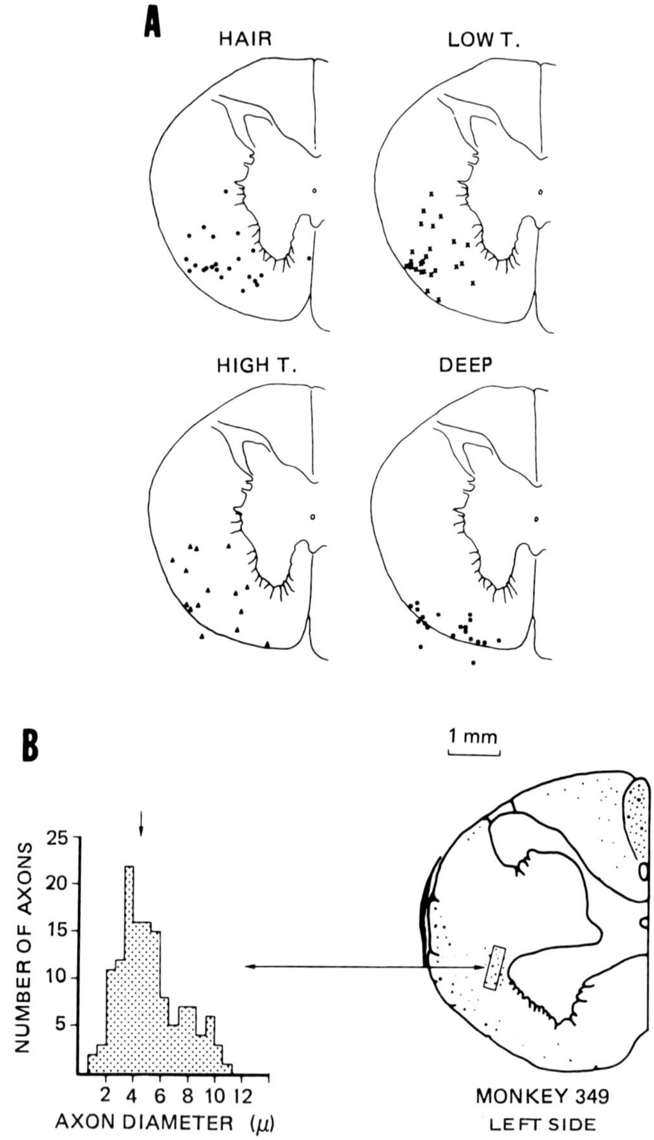

FIGURE 2. (A) A diagram from Applebaum *et al.* (1975) showing the location of axons in the upper lumbar cord that were backfired from the thalamus. Different functional categories of STT axons are presented separately. The deep category does not imply deep pain but could be proprioceptive. Low T refers to low-threshold sensitivity to touch of the skin. (B) Kerr and Lippman (1974) presented a histogram of the diameters of degenerating axons following midline myelotomy. The axons were measured within the rectangle within the cervical section shown on the right. A surprising paucity of unmyelinated axons was noted (Lippman and Kerr, 1972).

Table I
Ascending Projections of the Anterolateral and Ventral Columns[a]

Regions of termination	Myelotomy	Lateral chordotomy or hemisection		Ventral chordotomy
	monkey	Man	Monkey	Monkey
Spinal cord				
Ventral horn			x	
Medulla				
Central N., medulla oblongata	x	x	x	
Paragigantocellular N., dorsal	x	x	x	
Lateral reticular N.	x	x		
Ventral accessory olive	x			
Gigantocellular N.		x	x	x
N. raphe pallidus		x	xx	
Parvocellular N.		x	x	
Paragigantocellular N.		x	xx	
N. retroambigualis			x	
N. supraspinalis			x	
Interfascicular hypoglossal N.			x	
Lateral N., medulla oblongata			x	
Inferior olivary complex			x	
Dorsal accessory olivary lamina			x	
Pons				
Pontine gigantocellular N.	x	x	x	x
Pontine griseum centrale			x	x
Pedunculopontine tegmental N.			x	x
N. subcoeruleus			x	x
N. pontis oralis and caudalis			x	x
Midbrain				
Periaqueductal gray	x	x	x	x
N. Darkschewitz	x			
Superior colliculus			x	
Intercollicular N.			x	
Paralemniscal N.		x		
Interstitial N. Cajal		x		
N. cuneiformis				x
Diencephalon				
Posterior hypothalamus	x		x	
Posterior N., thalamus	x	x	x	x
N. ventralis posterolateralis	x	x	x	x
N. ventralis lateralis	x	x	x	
N. centralis lateralis	x	x	x	
Parafascicular N.	x	x	x	
Dorsomedial thalamic N.	x	x	x	
Paralaminar N.			x	
Thalamic reticular N.	x			
N. limitans		*		
Medial dorsal–lateral habenular N.		*		
Paracentral N.		*		
Central medial N.		*		
N. submedius		*		
N. reuniens		*		
Periventricular N.		*		

[a] X denotes Nauta or Fink–Heimer degeneration as noted by Boivie (1979), Bowsher (1957), Kerr (1975a), Kerr and Lippman (1974), or Mehler *et al.* (1960). XX notes regions receiving substantial contralateral projections. Asterisk denotes terminations in the thalamus that have been observed only following anterograde transport of wheat-germ agglutinin conjugated to horseradish peroxidase following spinal injection in the region of a lateral hemisection (Mantyh, 1983).

Spinoreticular tracts (SRT) terminate in as many as ten medullary, five pontine, and seven mesencephalic nuclei. Some of these brainstem nuclei contribute ascending projections (e.g., to the hypothalamus and the medial group of thalamic nuclei).

Some of the brainstem nuclei listed in Table I also provide descending projections that have been strongly implicated in inhibition of pain (e.g., the periaqueductal gray, the raphe nuclei, and the gigantocellular reticular nuclei; see Hammond, Chapter 15). A noradrenergic tract that originates in part in the nucleus subcoeruleus, which receives spinoreticular input, is interrupted by anterolateral chordotomy (see Crutcher and Bingham, 1978; Westlund *et al.*, 1984).

When a chordotomy includes the ventral column, ventral spinothalamic and spinoreticular connections are interrupted to some of the nuclei receiving input from anterolateral axons.

Table I allows comparison of nuclei in the brainstem and diencephalon of primates that receive projections from different components of the homolateral lateral and ventral columns, as determined in degeneration or transport studies following spinal hemisection, anterolateral chordotomy, ventral chordotomy, or commissurotomy. Important elements in this comparison were provided by Fred Kerr, permitting evaluation of spinoreticular and spinothalamic connections that arise from contralateral cell bodies (interrupted by commissural myelotomy) or from ipsilateral cell bodies (by subtraction of the commissurotomy results from the chordotomy results). Interpretation of the contralateral sensory deficits that result from chordotomy should give special consideration to the subset of nuclei receiving input from the contralateral gray matter, but many of these (e.g., the ventral accessory olive, lateral reticular nucleus, and nucleus Darkschewitz) are likely involved with sensorimotor functions rather than coding of pain sensations.

C. Sensory Effects of Anterolateral Chordotomy

Anterolateral chordotomy has been utilized primarily for chronic pain from distortion of tissue by carcinomas, and dramatic relief can occur (e.g., Papo, 1979a). Many qualities of pain are produced by cancer, and they vary according to the composition of the nerve(s) involved. Direct infiltration of the afferents in a peripheral nerve can produce pain, or inflammation and excitation of mechanical nociceptors can result from tumor growth (Wall, 1984). Often the pain is of visceral origin, where mechanoreceptivity and chemoreceptivity have been demonstrated for nociceptors (e.g., Uchida *et al.*, 1971, 1974).

Numerous accounts of the effects of anterolateral chordotomy on pain in humans have been published, but it is difficult to glean from these reports the magnitude of reductions for different sources of pain input. Many authors speak of analgesia, implying an absence of all varieties of pain, but evidence of careful semantic distinctions or psychophysical evaluations usually is not given. Other reports specify that clinical pain and pain elicited by the examiner often are attenuated but not eliminated by section of the spinothalamic tract (Head and Thompson, 1906; King, 1957; Ray and Wolff, 1945; White and Sweet, 1969). Finally, there are reports that some forms of pain are absent and others are spared. For example, muscular cramps or testicular compression can be perceived as painful following chordotomies that are otherwise effective (White, 1968). Sparing of pain sensitivity from superficial stimulation seems to be especially noticeable following interruption of crossing spinothalamic axons by midline myelotomy (Cook *et al.*, 1984; Papo and Luongo, 1976).

1. *Superficial Sensations*

In the following sections we deal with the effects of chordotomy on the sensations generated by classes of stimuli affecting superficial afferent terminals (see Winklemann, Chapter 2; Dyck, Chapter 14).

a. Pain Evoked by Electrocutaneous Stimulation

Testing of patients for their sensitivities to phasic cutaneous pain after spinothalamic chordotomy has revealed elevations of threshold for pain elicited by electrical stimulation (King, 1957). Similarly, thresholds for elicitation of escape reactions with electrocutaneous stimulation of cats or monkeys are elevated following complete spinothalamic chordotomy (Figure 3) or mesencephalic tractotomy (Kelly and Glusman, 1968), but escape reactions to strong stimulation are not eliminated. When escape reactions have been compared before and after complete section of the contralateral ventral spinal quadrant (Figure 3), the functions relating stimulus intensity to the speed and vigor of the pain reactions indicate a depression throughout the normal pain sensitivity range without a change in slope. Thus, spinothalamic chordotomy elevates thresholds for electrocutaneous pain and reduces the intensity of phasically elicited pain sensations (human subjects) and pain reactions (monkeys).

Electrocutaneous stimulation activates large myelinated afferents (subserving sensations of touch) and small myelinated afferents sensitive to touch or to mechanical and thermal stimuli within the painful range of intensities. Although electrocutaneous stimulation can activate unmyelinated nociceptors (e.g., above 1 mA/mm^2 with focal stimulation; Vierck and Cooper, 1984), the resulting pain sensation occurs late (beyond 1.5 s with stimulation of the legs) in response only to strong stimulation, and the second pains are less intense than preceding first pains. Therefore, psychophysical evaluations of electrocutaneous pain are determined primarily by input from myelinated afferents, and the escape responses of laboratory animals generally occur before onset

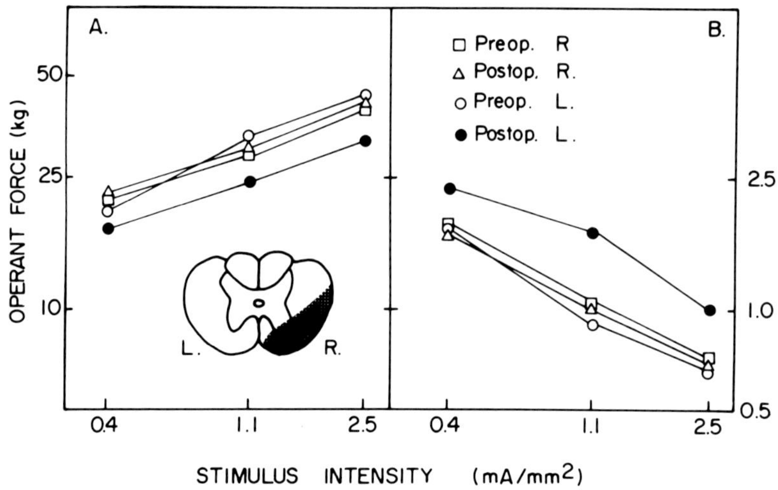

FIGURE 3. The force and latency of operant responses to escape focal electrical stimulation are plotted as functions of normally painful stimulus intensities. Nine monkeys produced nearly identical functions relating escape vigor to stimulus intensities applied to either leg preoperatively and to the left leg (ipsilateral to a chordotomy) in the postoperative period. Contralateral pain reactivity was clearly and consistently attenuated contralateral to chordotomy, reducing response vigor (A) and increasing response latency (B).

of second pain attributable to excitation of unmyelinated afferents (Vierck *et al.*, 1983b). Thus, reactions to electrocutaneous pain ordinarily provide a model for acute pain from myelinated nociceptors.

Spinothalamic projection cells with axons in the anterolateral column receive input from myelinated nociceptors (Albe-Fessard *et al.*, 1974; Foreman *et al.*, 1975) and are considered the principal projection system for rapidly conducted, well-localized pain (Price and Dubner, 1977; Willis and Coggeshall, 1978), suggesting that models of first-pain intensity are appropriate for assessing the effects of chordotomy. Collins *et al.*, (1960) have demonstrated this point conclusively by stimulating peripheral nerves at intensities sufficient to excite A-δ afferents and produce pain before, but not after, anterolateral chordotomy. On the other hand, pain elicited by high levels of electrocutaneous stimulation can be perceived following chordotomy (King, 1957; Figure 3). Similarly, Collins *et al.*, (1960) report that chordotomy blunted but did not eliminate pain resulting from stimulus levels sufficient to activate C afferents. Thus, it is important to attend to different sources of natural stimulation that serve as adequate stimuli for classes of myelinated and unmyelinated nociceptors to determine whether certain sources of pain are transmitted preferentially by the cSTT. Also, because spinothalamic projection neurons receive input from receptors subserving painless somatosensory qualities, it is of interest to determine whether chordotomy produces defects in nonnociceptive sensations.

b. Pain Evoked by Thermal Stimulation

Variation of temperatures applied to the skin can selectively activate different combinations of small peripheral afferents: (1) unmyelinated nonnociceptors (warm stimuli up to 44°C), (2) myelinated and unmyelinated nonnociceptors (cold stimuli), and (3) myelinated and unmyelinated nociceptors (hot stimuli above 45°C). Unfortunately, most clinical studies of chordotomy have reported on thermal sensitivity without specification of the temperatures delivered or the methods of stimulation. Commonly, thermosensitivity is not tested, or it is simply stated that pain and temperature sensations are lost or diminished contralateral to a spinothalamic chordotomy (Gardner and Cuneo, 1945; Moffie, 1975; Nathan and Smith, 1966; Ray and Wolff, 1945; Taren and Kahn, 1966; Turnbull, 1940; Walker, 1940). Occasionally, it is made clear that neither ice water nor noxious heat (above 45°C) is perceived as painful by the patients when stimulated in the distribution of the severed spinothalamic tract (Hyndman, 1942; Hyndman and Wolkin, 1943). In other studies, sensations of "warm and cold" are reported as lost following chordotomy (Hyndman and Wolkin, 1943; Nathan and Smith, 1966; White and Sweet, 1969), implying that nonnoxious thermal sensations are not elicited. A most interesting observation of Hyndman and Wolkin (1943) was that patients placed in a heating cabinet or refrigerator did not feel warmth or cold in the analgesic zone produced by chordotomy. Because of the spatial summation characteristic of thermal sensitivity (Marks and Stevens, 1973; Price *et al.*, 1978), focal stimulation could have been a misleading representation of thermal sensitivity to stimuli normally encountered in the environment.

Input to the spinal cord from both myelinated and unmyelinated thermosensitive afferents often is not effective in eliciting painful or innocuous thermal sensations in the early period following chordotomy. Thus, behavioral evidence from human patients focuses attention on the STT as the most important of the different ascending spinal pathways that receive input from thermoreceptors (e.g., the postsynaptic dorsal column pathway, the spinocervicothalamic tract, Lissauer's tract, and ipsilateral spinoreticular axons; Willis and Coggeshall, 1978). Spinothalamic projection cells responsive to thermal stimuli can receive convergent inputs from superficial mechanical, deep somatic, and visceral nociceptors (Foreman *et al.*, 1977; Hancock *et al.*, 1975; Price and Mayer, 1975; Willis *et al.*, 1974), and some STT cells respond selectively to input from thermoreceptive afferents (Kumazawa *et al.*, 1975; Willis *et al.*, 1974). The axons of these nociceptor-specific cells appear to be intermingled with the other categories of STT axons (Applebaum *et al.*, 1975), and, therefore, a chordotomy should impair all qualities of nociception represented by spinothalamic cells. This has generally been the result when it has been put to the test by appropriate sensory testing (Hyndman and Wolkin, 1943; White and Sweet, 1969). However, there also are examples of dissociation between the early effects of chordotomy on thermal sensitivity versus clinical pain or pin-prick sensitivity.

Occasionally, innocuous and painful thermal sensations are intact in the distribution of hypalgesia or analgesia for mechanical stimulation of the skin with a pin following chordotomy (Head and Thompson, 1906; Sherman and Arief, 1948; Stookey, 1929; Walker, 1940). This has been explained on the basis of a slightly more central location of thermoreceptive STT axons (Schneider, 1982; Walker, 1940; Figure 1). Presumably, a high percentage of the mechanical nociceptive cells are transected by superficial lesions of the STT. Radiofrequency lesions that progress outward from a central locus have been shown to decrease thermal pain before superficial pain from mechanical stimulation (Taren *et al.*, 1969).

When both mechanical and thermal pain are diminished following chordotomy, the decrease in thermal sensitivity can be more enduring than the effects on superficial mechanical and deep clinical pain, which often recover with time (White and Sweet, 1969). Perhaps the thermoreceptive spinothalamic axons are more focally located within the anterolateral column, as suggested by reports that levels of thermoanesthesia frequently are closer to the level of chordotomy than are levels for pinprick or deep, clinical pain (see below). That is, thermoreceptive spinothalamic axons representing a given dermatone may be minimally distributed in the anteroposterior dimension, diminishing the likelihood of sparing after subtotal anterolateral lesions. Alternatively, thermoreception could be represented more exclusively in the spinothalamic tract than are other submodalities of nociception.

c. Pain Evoked by Mechanical Stimulation

A number of clinicians have asserted that pin-prick sensitivity is profoundly affected by chordotomy, reporting analgesia for cutaneous stimulation with a pin (e.g., Amromin and Crue, 1975; Hyndman and Wolkin, 1943; Moffie, 1975; Nathan and Smith, 1979; Ray and Wolff, 1945; White and Sweet, 1969). But the term analgesia should not be applied to the effect of chordotomy on the mild pain sensations elicited by pin-prick testing. More intense sensations from mechanical stimulation of the skin may not be eliminated by chordotomy. For example, temporal summation by repeated pin pricks in dermatomes below a chordotomy can elicit pain when insensitivity to single pricks or scratches has been observed (Lalonde and Poirier, 1959; Nathan and Smith, 1979; Walker, 1943).

Some investigators have shown that the sensation of sharpness is lost following chordotomy, irrespective of whether the sharp quality is regarded as painful. For example, White and Sweet (1969) tested patients by pressing the skin lightly with a fingertip on some trials and the finger plus a sharp point on other trials. Chordotomy eliminated discrimination of the presence of the punctate stimulus, but the light pressure sensation was perceived. Loss or diminution of sensations of sharpness can be understood as a reflection of projections from high-threshold mechanoreceptors onto STT projection neurons (Foreman *et al.*, 1975). High-threshold mechanoreceptors can be expected to be selectively sensitive to the high forces produced at the tip of a pin even when the extent of the stimulus or of the tissue disruption (with release of natural algesic substances) is insufficient to produce substantial levels of pain.

Ordinarily, evaluation of the effects of chordotomy involves reports on clinical pain (often "deep pain") and determination of the dermatomes over which pin-prick sensations are diminished or absent. Based on a high correlation of clinical with pin-prick pain, the use of punctate cutaneous stimulation has been successful as a diagnostic tool. The examiner can learn to deliver a range of forces that consistently elicit mild pain in normal subjects, and the effects of chordotomy on the sensations of sharpness and focal pain are quite clear and are observed reliably by scratching or punching the skin. The usual result is that clinical pain is relieved effectively when the upper level of pin-prick loss is higher than the most rostral dermatome involved by the chronic pain.

A partial involvement by clinical pain of dermatomes above the "pin-prick level" portends a poor result. Clinical pain can be perceived as severe in cases in which the rostral level of pin-prick hypalgesia is less than three segments above the upper level of clinical pain (Nathan and Smith, 1979), and regression of pin-prick levels over time is often accompanied by return of clinical pain (Horrax, 1929; Hyndman and Van Epps, 1939). Small patches of normal sensations of sharpness below the sensory level also appear to correlate strongly with retention or recovery of clinical pain (Graf, 1960; Kahn and Rand, 1952). Repeat chordotomies following spared islands or low levels of pin-prick sensation have often been successful in reducing or eliminating clinical pain that was spared by an initial chordotomy (Kahn and Rand, 1952; White 1963; see below).

d. Itch and Tickle

In recent experiments, human subjects have reported on the sensations elicited by direct electrical stimulation of single peripheral afferents and by natural stimulation that drives these units. Itch can be produced by application of pruritic substances (e.g., histamine) that induce discharge in small peripheral afferents (Bickford, 1938; Tuckett, 1980), and intraneural microstimulation of a subpopulation of C-polymodal nociceptors produces itch sensations rather than the dull pain elicited by stimulation of other polymodal nociceptors (Ochoa, 1984). Thus, itch appears to result from activity in a subpopulation of afferents rather than from a unique firing pattern in all C-polymodal nociceptors. Consistent with observations that unmyelinated peripheral afferents contact spinothalamic neurons for rostral conduction (Chung *et al.*, 1979), itch sensations are lost within dermatomes caudal and contralateral to an anterolateral chordotomy (Graf, 1960; Hyndman and Wolkin, 1943; Arthur and Shelley, 1959; Taren and Kahn, 1966; White and Sweet, 1969).

Sensations of tickle are produced by light tactile stroking that does not irritate the skin but excites cutaneous touch receptors that are highly sensitive to movement across the skin surface. Slowly conducting tactile afferents have been implicated in the coding of tickle by nerve-blocking procedures (Bickford, 1938), and C mechanoreceptors have been described in the hairy skin of cats that respond at low threshold to movement across the skin surface (Iggo, 1974). The nonnociceptive C mechanoreceptors require very slow rates of movement over the skin, and the optimum rate of stimulus movement for elicitation of tickle is comparable. The C mechanoreceptors appear to be suited for elicitation of a unique sensation of tickle, but these afferents have not been reported to supply the glabrous skin of humans, where tickle can be elicited readily. Thus, without identification of a specific receptor population mediating tickle sensations, they may be presumed to result from unique spatiotemporal patterns of activity in central projection cells responding to certain combinations of input from low-threshold cutaneous mechanoreceptors. Evaluation of tickle sensations following section of the spinothalamic tract has revealed preservation contralaterally and caudal to the lesion (Hyndman and Wolkin, 1943; White and Sweet, 1969), but deficits also have been reported (Foerster and Gagel, 1932; Schwartz and O'Leary, 1942; Walker, 1943).

e. Touch

The methods ordinarily utilized to test patients for light touch have been to stroke the skin with cotton wool or to determine thresholds with von Frey hairs. The sensations elicited by stroking with a "wisp" of cotton vary greatly, depending on the region of skin stimulated (e.g., hairy or hairless), the size of the wisp, and the pressure exerted by the examiner. Stimulation with von Frey hairs appears to be more reliable, but a large data base is required to determine thresholds accurately, and the attention and biases of the subjects must be taken into account. Extensive testing of symmetric sites preoperatively and then ipsilateral and contralateral to a unilateral chordotomy is required, and the subjects must be alert and experienced. These factors are important because threshold sensations of touch are ephemeral.

In early reports (Brown-Sequard, 1868; Head and Thompson, 1906; May, 1906; Petren, 1902), sensations of light touch were attributed to conduction over the contralateral spinal cord, and textbooks have repeatedly identified a ventral spinothalamic pathway as necessary for sensations of light touch. However, patients with selective section of the ventral columns have not been tested for tactile thresholds. The effects of chordotomy on light tactile sensitivity are subtle if present. Walker (1940) reported that the number of touch spots was reduced contralateral to STT section. White and Sweet (1969) have reported that touch thresholds on glabrous skin were increased by chordotomies received by "the majority" of their patients, but touch sensitivity on hairy skin "remains remarkably acute." The patients of White and Sweet were instructed that they would "be able to detect a mosquito when he alights [on hairy skin], although they will not be able to feel him bite nor be annoyed by the subsequent itch." Preservation of light tactile sensitivity on hairy skin is consistent with the substantial rostral projection of inputs from hair receptors by the lemniscal spinal pathways (Bryan *et al.*, 1974; Whitsel *et al.*, 1969).

The conclusion that thresholds for light touch are affected only slightly by chordotomy has been confirmed in an investigation of monkeys trained to detect minimal electrical stimulation of the lateral calf (Figure 4). A psychophysical evaluation of four monkeys showing substantial losses of pain reactivity contralateral to ventral quadrant lesions (of the anterolateral and ventral columns) has demonstrated slightly higher contralateral thresholds for detection of electrical stimulation. However, the postoperative differences in thresholds from the hindlimbs resulted from consistent increases contralaterally and decreases ipsilaterally, comparing each limb to preoperative performance on the discrimination task. Thus, the slight differences in light tactile sensitivity that have been observed after chordotomy may result in part from an ipsilateral hypersensitivity. Clearly, it can be said that section of the lateral and ventral spinothalamic tracts does not result in substantial elevations of absolute thresholds for light cutaneous stimulation.

Light tactile input onto spinothalamic cells has been demonstrated (Price *et al.*, 1978; Willis *et al.*, 1974), and the interdigitation of spinothalamic with lemniscal projections to the diencephalon (Berkley, 1980) makes understandable a slight deficit of touch detection from chordotomy on the basis of a partial reduction in driving of cells in the thalamic nucleus ventralis posterolateralis. Thus, light touch cannot be regarded as a function that is critically dependent on spinothalamic conduction. However, light tactile sensitivity is also spared following interruption of the ipsilateral lemniscal pathways (Vierck,

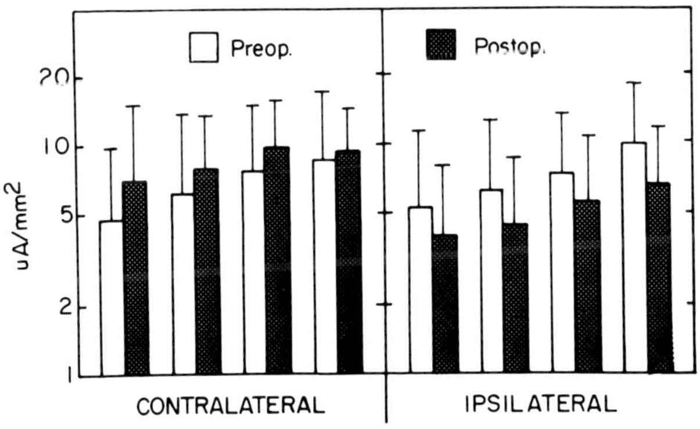

FIGURE 4. Thresholds for detection of electrocutaneous stimulation are shown for four monkeys sustaining anterolateral spinal lesions that attenuated contralateral pain reactivity. On the left side, contralateral to the chordotomies, detection thresholds were elevated relative to preoperative values from the same leg. On the right, ipsilateral to the chordotomies, postoperative thresholds were decreased. These effects were small but present in each animal.

1977; Wall and Norodenbos, 1977). These findings of bilateral sparing of touch sensitivity following unilateral hemisection demonstrate that simple recognition of touch is redundantly mediated by ipsilateral and contralateral pathways. The early reports of substantial light touch deficits contralateral to spinal lesions did not include histological confirmation that the interruption of white matter was strictly unilateral, and because these lesions were accidental, the probability of bilateral damage was high.

Most investigators of patients with spinothalamic chordotomy have focused their attention of pain sensations and reactions and have not carefully tested capacities for spatial, temporal, or spatiotemporal resolution of somatosensory stimuli. However, based on questioning of patients and routine clinical testing for "epicritic" capacities, Head and Thompson (1906) and others have reported normal spatiotactile resolution (e.g., two-point tactile sensitivity) and proprioception contralateral to spinal lesions that produce contralateral losses of pain and temperature sensations. Similarly, STT lesions do not produce impairments of spatiotactile or limb position thresholds in monkeys (Levitt and Schwartzman, 1966; Vierck, 1984). However, slight deficits in two-point discrimination by chordotomy patients have been reported by Kruger and Mosso (1974). Also, cSTT interruption can reinstate impairments of spatiotactile resolution that have recovered following ipsilateral lesion of the dorsal columns (Vierck *et al.*, 1983a). Thus, the STT appears not to be necessary for spatial resolution, but it supplies some information that can support spatial resolution (in collaboration with ipsilateral lemniscal pathways).

One way to evaluate the discriminative capacities of the crossed spinal pathways is to isolate them by ipsilateral lesions of the lemniscal pathways in the dorsal and dorsolateral columns. When this has been accomplished, many forms of spatial resolution were impaired (e.g., sensitivity for the direction of movement across the skin, point localization, two-point discrimination, and tactile size discrimination; Levitt and Schwartzman, 1966; Vierck, 1973, 1974, 1984; Vierck *et al.*, 1983a). However, capacities for absolute localization of cutaneous stimuli have not been tested following STT isolation, and simple localization is not affected by lesions of the dorsal column component of the ipsilateral lemniscal system (Vierck and Rand, 1979). Furthermore, nociceptor-specific STT cells could provide unique spatial codes (Yezierski *et al.*, 1983) that would be revealed by the use of strong levels of stimulation. For example, previous studies testing spatial resolution for radiant thermal stimulation in the warm range have shown very poor facility (Cain, 1973) or thresholds slightly higher than for light tactile stimulation (Nathan and Rice, 1966), but there are indications that painful thermal stimulation may be localized accurately (Nathan and Rice, 1966; Bekesy, 1962).

f. Other Superficial Sensations

Many STT cells are multireceptive, receiving input from low- and high-threshold afferent categories (Price and Mayer, 1975; Willis *et al.*, 1974; see

Willis, Chapter 11), and some qualitatively distinct somatosensations other than pain can be expected to depend critically on certain patterns of activity in these neurons. That is, if diminished pain sensitivity by chordotomy depends in part on axotomy of multireceptive neurons (Mayer *et al.*, 1975), then nonnociceptive sensations coded by low rates of discharge among these cells should be impaired as well. Multireceptive neurons with similar physiological properties project rostrally via the STT and ipsilateral dorsal and dorsolateral pathways (see Willis and Coggeshall, 1978), and it is important to define specificities of the multireceptive projection pathways for different somesthetic sensations.

Several sensory experiences consequent to light tactile stimulation may be lost following anterolateral chordotomy. For example, sensations of wetness have been reported to be eliminated contralaterally (Hyndman and Wolkin, 1943). Ordinarily, sensations of wetness include the presence of mechanical and thermal stimuli, but the necessary conditions have not been delineated, and the methods of testing patients have not been detailed appropriately.

Another unique sensation that has been reported to be lost after bilateral chordotomy is the voluptuous sensation elicited by genital stimulation (Hyndman and Wolkin, 1943; Kahn and Barney, 1937; Taren and Kahn, 1966). Again, the stimulus conditions are complex, and in this case psychophysical investigations are unlikely. The prolonged sensations elicited by genital stimulation are interesting in relation to the tendency of multireceptive cells to afterdischarge (Mendell and Wall, 1965; Price *et al.*, 1978). However, Hyndman and Wolkin (1943) implicate a parasympathetic pathway on the basis of midlateral spinal lesions that produce loss of the voluptuous sensation but do not eliminate pain sensitivity for the genitalia.

2. *Deep Somatic Sensations*

In a few investigations of the effects of chordotomy, deep somatic pain has been assessed by application of weights to compress tissue over bones (White and Sweet, 1969) or by squeezing of the Achilles tendon (Lalonde and Poirer, 1959; Yoss, 1953). There appears to be uniform agreement that deep somatic pain is substantially reduced by anterolateral chordotomy. In fact, Nathan and Smith (1979) state that deep pain, as assessed with a pressure algesiometer, correlates best with the clinical results of chordotomy. For example, they cite cases in which the upper levels for loss of pain from cancer and from application of pressure are three or four dermatomes lower than the levels determined with pin-prick testing. This finding could result from larger peripheral receptive fields for deep nociceptors or from a longer rostrocaudal spread of the dorsal horn map for deep nociception. Another suggestion for a wider dispersal of deep pain than of superficial pain has been offered by cases in which there was selective referral of pain to the side ipsilateral to chordotomy when the contralateral stimulation involved deep somatic receptors (Ray and Wolff, 1945).

Spinothalamic axons transmitting deep somatic pain may be located dorsolaterally relative to axons supplying superficial sites within the same dermatomes, as suggested by effects that depend on extension of chordotomies above the dentate ligament (Kahn and Rand, 1952; Lalonde and Poirier, 1959; see Foreman, Chapter 10 and Willis, Chapter 11 for further discussion). However, cases with syringomyelia and reports during stereotactic chordotomies have suggested a medial location of STT axons subserving deep pain (Schneider, 1982; Taren *et al.*, 1969). Isolated cases of chordotomy producing deep pain losses but preservation of pin-prick sensations (e.g., Amromin and Crue, 1975) reinforce the possibility that the spinothalamic somatotopies differ for deep and superficial pain or that deep pain is mediated by the cSTT and a different, more medial pathway (see below).

Proprioceptive senses of limb movement and position are represented by muscle and joint afferent input onto a small percentage of spinothalamic tract cells (see Figure 2A; Applebaum *et al.*, 1975), and some residual capacity for discriminating limb position sense is preserved after ipsilateral hemisection in monkeys (Vierck, 1984). Thresholds for discrimination of hindlimb positions were doubled by isolation of contralateral spinal pathways. However, isolation of the contralateral anterolateral column in a human patient has been reported not to spare sensations of joint movement (Wall and Noordenbos, 1977). Possibly, the ipsilateral lemniscal pathways are more critical for phasic sensations of limb movement then for static sensations of position. In either case, the cSTT contributes little information in support of proprioceptive sensations. Interruption of the cSTT produces no proprioceptive deficit that has been discerned in monkeys or human subjects (Vierck, 1984; White and Sweet, 1969).

3. Visceral Pain

Visceral sensation has been tested objectively in a few investigations involving distension of the ureter or of intestinal loops (Drakes and McKenzie, 1953; White and Sweet, 1969), and substantially elevated thresholds following STT section substantiate numerous cases reports demonstrating relief of clinical pains of visceral origin by chordotomy or midline myelotomy (e.g., Hyndman and Wolkin, 1943; Nathan, 1956; Papo and Luongo, 1976; Taren and Kahn, 1966; White, 1968). Visceral inputs have been shown to converge with somatic afferents onto spinothalamic neurons (Foreman *et al.*, 1981), providing an anatomic substrate for referred visceral pain and for the effectiveness of chordotomy for both visceral and somatic pain. Different levels of entry to the spinal cord of visceral and somatic nerves may well account for variance in the distributions of visceral and superficial pain losses following chordotomy (White, 1943). According to some surgeons, chordotomies for control of visceral pain should extend medially to the gray matter (consistent with observations for deep somatic pain) and should be bilateral (Cook *et al.*, 1984;

Taren *et al.*, 1969; Hyndman and Wolkin, 1943). The need for bilateral lesions could reflect bilateral innervation of many visceral structures (White and Sweet, 1969).

4. *Sources of Pain Not Relieved by Chordotomy*

In the early period following anterolateral chordotomy, nearly all categories of acute and chronic pain are attenuated (or lost) if the lesion involves enough of the cSTT to produce an adequate level of effect. However, pain of an upper extremity has been reported to be retained more often following chordotomy than is pain in the legs (e.g., Grant and Wood, 1958). High cervical chordotomies can involve a respiratory pathway (near the ventral horn; Lipton, 1979; Nathan, 1963), eliminating bilateral chordotomies from consideration. Unilateral high cervical chordotomies have been performed, generally producing appropriate levels of hypalgesia when extended ventrally to interrupt cervical STT axons (French *et al.*, 1966; Horrax and Price, 1954; Ogle *et al.*, 1956; Roulhac, 1953; Schwartz, 1962; White and Sweet, 1969). Also, medullary lesions of the STT are equally effective for pain in the upper and lower extremities (Birkenfeld and Fisher, 1963; Schwartz and O'Leary, 1942), indicating that STT inputs from cervical and lower levels do not differ qualitatively. These findings also suggest that the more substantial ipsilateral spinoreticular projections from the forelimbs (Kerr and Lippman, 1974; Kevetter *et al.*, 1982) subserve functions other than coding of pain sensations and reactions.

Some sources or varieties of pain may be especially insensitive to attenuation by chordotomy. For example, White (1943) contends that testicular compression or muscular cramps will elicit pain contralateral to chordotomies that are otherwise successful. Other observers reiterate the relative sparing of muscular pain or of pain in caudal segments after STT section (e.g., the cervix, testicles, or rectum; Cook and Kamakawi 1977; Drake and McKenzie, 1953; Head and Thompson, 1906; Papo and Luongo, 1976). Statements such as these may indicate a projection outside the STT of pain from deep stimulation, but they also can reflect the degree of bilateral innervation of the structure stimulated or the location of the chordotomy. Also, comparisons of relative sparing require precise estimates of the magnitudes of the different pain stimuli. When cutaneous stimuli have been utilized to evaluate sensitivity following interruption of the STT, strong, repetitive stimulation has produced pain in otherwise analgesic areas (King, 1957; Lalonde and Poirier, 1959; Nathan and Smith, 1979; Walker, 1943; White and Sweet, 1969).

Chronic pain produced by invasion of peripheral nerves by carcinomas is relieved effectively by chordotomy under most conditions, but good results are less reliably produced for pain of long standing (Taren and Kahn, 1966; White and Sweet, 1969). In addition, different forms of invasion or degeneration within the spinal cord can produce chronic pain that survives chordotomy. This is especially found for cases in which there is direct involvement of sensory axons within the spinal cord (Melzack and Loeser, 1978; White and Sweet, 1969) and applies to avulsion of the brachial plexus, arachnoiditis, herpes zoster, tabes dorsalis, or transection of peripheral nerves (Browder and Gallagher, 1948; Cook and Kawakami, 1977; Falconer, 1966; King, 1977; Papo and Luongo, 1976; Taren and Kahn, 1966). The effectiveness of chordotomy for these conditions is controversial (White and Sweet, 1969), but an apparently high incidence of failures may be related to establishment of unusual rates and/or durations of activity in cells with axons outside the contralateral anterolateral column. For example, deafferentation of spinal neurons can result in development of high levels of spontaneous activity (Loeser and Ward, 1967).

5. *Levels of Pain Relief Following Chordotomy*

A cursory reading of clinical reports in which the upper levels of hypalgesia or analgesia have been determined following chordotomy suggests that the results are extremely variable, ranging from one or two segments to seven or eight segments below the chordotomy. Clearly, the distribution of effects is subject to individual differences in organization of the pain pathways, but the few studies that have presented histological confirmation of the location and extent of chordotomies reinforce a statement by Kahn and Rand (1952) that ". . . chordotomy is a precision operation. The procedure should not be condemned if a poor result follows faulty technique." That is, most of the variation in the levels of pain attenuation can be described to lesions that involve the anterolateral columns to different degrees.

When a surgeon completely interrupts the white matter of one anterolateral column (extending from above the dentate ligament through the exit zone of the ventral roots), pain sensitivity is attenuated within two or three levels below the chordotomy (e.g., Hyndman and Van Epps, 1939; Kahn and Rand, 1952; Moffie, 1975; Nathan, 1956; Nathan and Smith, 1966, 1979; Ray and Wolff, 1945), and exact correspondence of sensory and lesion levels has been claimed (e.g., Cook *et al.*, 1984). Exceptions can occur as a result of slight shifts within the lateral column of the STT axons supplying a given area (Smith, 1957; Figure 1). For example, sacral sparing would be seen with cervical lesions that miss dorsally shifted axons from caudal dermatones. Also, anterolateral axons supplying near caudal segments are relatively diffusely scattered medially and ventrally (Poirier and Bertrand, 1955; White *et al.*, 1956), and thus a chordotomy must extend into or near the ventral column to produce a sensory level near that of the lesion. Because surgeons are reluctant to cut near the ventral spinal artery, many chordotomies have produced upper levels of cutaneous "analgesia" that are more than three segments below the chordotomy. Therefore, the most valid evaluations of the results of chordotomy are those involving histological confirmation of lesions well above the most rostral dermatome involved by the source of pain.

Following complete interruption of the STT, the upper level of maximal pain reduction might be expected to be many segments below the level of section, because small primary afferents extend as many as five segments rostral to their entry point (Carpenter *et al.*, 1968; Culberson and Brown, 1984; Nadelhaft *et al.*, 1983). To the extent that contributions to Lissauer's tract from the substantia gelatinose distribute nociceptive input to rostral spinal cells for conduction of pain (Szentagothai, 1964), the upper levels of analgesia could be displaced even further. However, the limiting factor in generation of sensations localized to a given region is the distribution of spinal neurons with corresponding receptive fields.

Somatotopic maps of feline spinal cords have revealed that cells responsive to a given locus extend three segments rostral and caudal to the central root (Brown and Fuchs, 1975), but maps for primate cells driven by nociceptive stimuli are needed. The distribution of "analgesia" following anterolateral chordotomy indicates that the functional "map" for cutaneous nociception extends two to six segments above a dermatome, depending on the stimuli utilized to test the sensory level. Explicit comparisons of the upper levels of hypalgesia for different sources of pain have indicated that the rostral level of thermoanesthesia can be slightly higher than the level for pin-prick analgesia (Taren and Kahn, 1966; White and Sweet, 1969). Also, the level for experimentally induced or clinical deep pain can be three or four segments below the level for light stimulation with a pin (Nathan and Smith, 1979). These observations indicate that dorsal horn cells responding to deep pain from a given myotome extend further rostrally than the corresponding dermatomal map of the skin.

Demonstrations of the importance of the dorsal root entry zone (including Lissauer's tract) for dispersion of nociceptive inputs over several segments have been provided by procedures in which ipsilateral lesions at the tip of the dorsal horn have been combined with contralateral chordotomy (Hyndman, 1942). In the few cases reported, levels of hypalgesia were reported to correspond to the segment of the lesions. Several of these patients received bilateral lesions of the STT but only unilateral interruption of Lissauer's tract, and the correspondence of the sensory level with the lesion occurred only ipsilateral to the dorsal lesion.

If Lissauer's tract modulates the excitability of neurons that code pain from segments rostral to a given input level, then a source of chronic pain within dermatomes below a chordotomy would be expected to modify sensitivity to stimulation above the level of the lesion. When chordotomies effectively eliminate pain from caudal segments, freeing attention to more subtle sensations, rostral effects do become apparent to the patients. Evidence of rostral excitatory influences on pain by Lissauer's tract is presented by referral of pain from an analgesic zone (caudal to a chordotomy) to levels rostral to the lesion. Repetitive, vigorous stimulation with a hot object or a pin can be perceived as touch within the analgesic area, and a slowly incrementing, long-lasting, burning pain can be perceived above the analgesic level (Nathan, 1956; Nathan and Smith, 1979). The probability of rostral referral and the effective distance (between the stimulus or "trigger point" and the analgesic level) are related to stimulus intensity. Thus, rostral conduction of pain by the dorsal propriospinal system can occur with particularly intense, prolonged stimulation, but rostral referral is not common or is observed only locally (near the lesion) for most forms of pain.

D. Sensory Functions of the Ventral Columns

Early conjecture concerning the presence of ventral spinothalamic axons and their role(s) in sensory coding has not led to definitive physiological and behavioral experiments that would distinguish functions for the anterolateral and ventral columns. This issue was of special interest to Fred Kerr, who performed a unique experiment involving selective unilateral interruption of the ventral columns in monkeys. He found that rostral projections of the ventral columns overlap to some extent with anterolateral STT projections in thalamic nucleus ventralis posterolateralis, gigantocellularis nuclei of the medulla and pons, the periaqueductal gray, nucleus cuneiformis, and paralaminar and posterior thalamic nuclei (Kerr, 1975a; Table 1).

Given the similarities in anatomic projections of the ventral and anterolateral columns, it is expected that ventral quadrant lesions would produce more substantial decreases in pain sensitivity than anterolateral lesions. Furthermore, chordotomies that extend to the ventral columns typically involve axons in and near the gray matter to a greater extent than pure anterolateral lesions. Although patients with confirmed lesions of the ventral columns have been infrequent, making valid comparisons with anterolateral chordotomy difficult, the results of several series indicate that involvment of the ventral column does not increase the effects of chordotomy on pain (Lahuerta *et al.*, 1984; Nathan and Smith, 1966).

Another way to evaluate the importance of the ventral columns for pain transmission is potentially available by isolating (sparing) the ventral columns and transecting all other white matter. Such a preparation has been produced rarely but was approximated fortuitously in several rats that received spaced lateral hemisections to evaluate the functions of the propriospinal system of bilateral spinal projections (Basbaum, 1973). The animals with ventral column sparing differed from rats sustaining complete lesions in that the rats with incomplete lesions vocalized in response to strong stimulation. Thresholds for escape of electrical stimulation were not significantly lower for the ventral column isolates than for animals with complete hemisections, suggesting that pain sensitivity was not increased by ventral column sparing in these animals. The release of vocalizations may result from a projection of the ventral columns to the periaqueductal gray (Kerr, 1975a), where vocalizations can be elicited by direct stimulation (Jurgens and Pratt, 1979; Larson and Kistler, 1984).

Pain-elicited vocalizations have been utilized as measures of pain sensitivity in a variety of animals (particularly rodents), but a potentially reflexive connection from the spinal cord to the periaqueductal gray and then to the nucleus ambigous questions whether loss of vocalizations would necessarily indicate loss of pain. For example, vocalizations are inhibited in primates with dosages of systemic morphine that do not produce analgesia (Vierck *et al.*, 1983b,c), suggesting a direct effect on vocalization via neurons in the periaqueductal gray with morphine receptors. Thus, contralateral axons of nociceptive cells projecting to the periaqueductal gray may elicit vocalizations without contributing directly to pain sensations.

Denny-Brown (1979) has observed behavioral reactions of monkeys following lesions of one anterolateral column, following lateral hemisection, and after hemisection with interruption of both ventral columns. Untrained reactions of the animals to thermal and pin-prick stimulation were observed. Depending on the lesion, the animals either responded normally by briefly scratching the area previously stimulated (i.e., with local sign), ipsilateral to interruption of the lateral and dorsal columns, and attention frequently was not directed to a limb stimulated contralateral to lateral and dorsal lesions (Figure 5, top), or exaggerated reactions were observed contralateral to interruption of either ventral column (Figure 5, middle and bottom).

Because the stimuli utilized in Denny-Brown's study have been used extensively to document the effects of chordotomy in humans, it is of interest to search the chordotomy literature for the consequences of including the ventral column(s) with interruption of an anterolateral column. Denny-Brown's

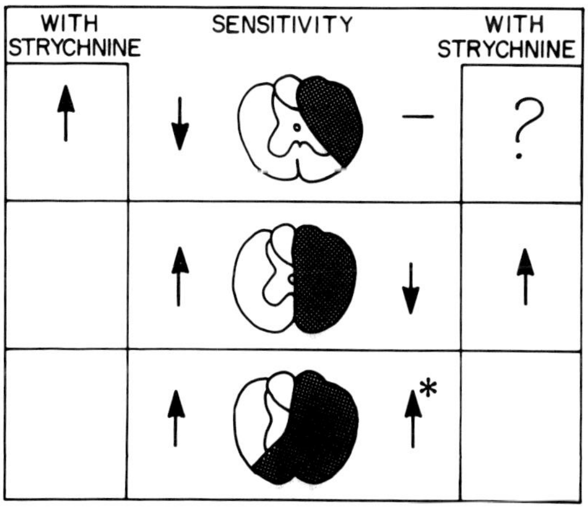

FIGURE 5. A diagrammatic representation of Denny-Brown's (1979) effects of spinal cord lesions on scratch reflexes with local sign. Sensitivity was decreased (fewer scratch responses were observed) contralateral to interruption of the dorsal and lateral columns. More extensive lesions produced frequent and exaggerated reactions contralateral to section of either ventral column. Asterisk indicates that the hypersensitivity developed gradually. When sensitivity was decreased (contralateral to the upper lesion but ipsilateral to the middle lesion), it could be restored by injections of strychnine.

result suggests that a lesion of the contralateral ventral quadrant would produce hyperalgesia or would diminish the hypalgesia commonly observed with restricted section of the anterolateral column. Although cases with confirmed interruption of the ventral quadrant have been reported (Amromin and Crue, 1975; Hyndman and Van Epps, 1939; Moffie, 1975; Nathan and Smith, 1966; White *et al.*, 1956), hypalgesia (or "analgesia") was observed, and contralateral hypersensitivity does not appear to have occurred preferentially in these patients. In the absence of further documentation of a release of nociceptive sensations contralateral to ventral quadrant lesions, an explanation for Denny-Brown's result is that monkey's local sign reactions were reflexive in nature and were modulated by influences not acting on rostrally conducting neurons important for sensation.

E. Sensory Functions of Other Spinofugal Systems

1. The Propriospinal Systems

Anatomic investigations of the spinal cord have revealed a number of specific pathways in the propriospinal system of projections within the spinal gray matter and on its periphery (Molenaar and Kuypers, 1978; Nathan and Smith, 1959). These subsystems take origin from different sets of neurons, contribute axons to distinct locations, and terminate reliably in different patterns. Propriospinal projections ascend and descend to terminate back in the spinal cord, and targets within the brainstem have been discerned but are poorly described. In addition to classical descriptions of normal material (e.g., Ramon y Cajal, 1909; Rexed, 1952), investigators have cut the spinal white matter, allowed long-tract degeneration to clear (e.g., for 70 weeks), and then introduced a second lesion of propriospinal axons that survived the first lesion (Barilari and Kuypers, 1969; Szentagothai, 1964; Tower *et al.*, 1941; Figure 6A). The terminations of propriospinal axons were observed to be similarly distributed for ascending and descending projections. The long, large intraspinal axons that are visualized most readily with silver stains after lateral hemisection terminate predominantly in the intermediate gray and ventral horn (laminae V through VIII), where the cell bodies or dendrites of some spinothalamic and many spinoreticular cells are located. Many of the propriospinal axons are small, and a recent estimate of 97% has been offered for the proportion of propriospinal axons to the total of all axons in the spinal cord (Chung *et al.*, 1984). The extensive system of small, short intraspinal axons interconnects neurons with similar laminar locations, and all parts of the gray matter receive and send spinal–spinal connections (Nathan and Smith, 1959).

The possibility that propriospinal systems relay information to the CNS that is interpreted as aversive has been supported by experiments involving lateral hemisections that are spaced more than several segments apart (Bas-

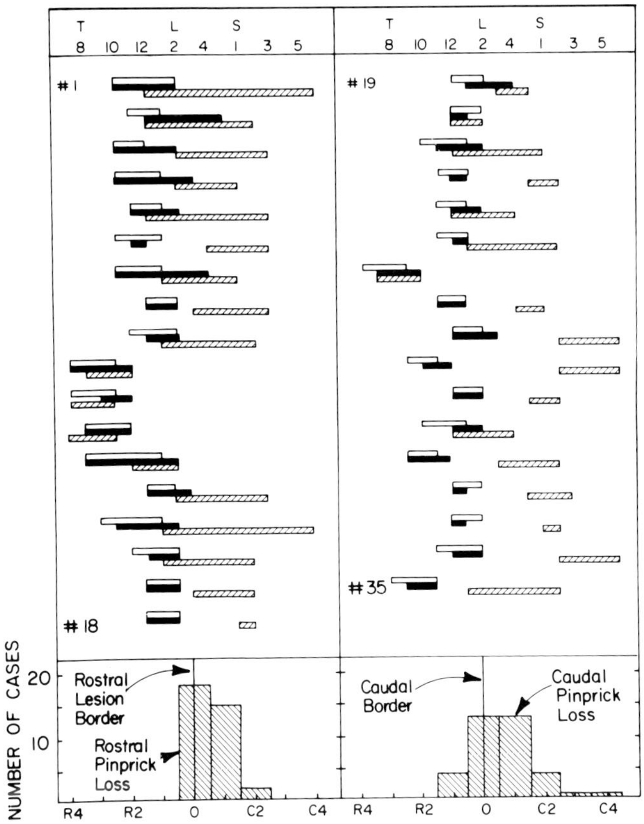

FIGURE 6. A graphical representation of Sourek's (1977) description of the spinal levels (on the abscissa) in which the dorsal and ventral midline spinal commisures were sectioned (open rectangles) or the dermatomes (T8 through S5) over which pin-prick sensitivity was diminished (black rectangles) or deep clinical pain was attenuated (hatched rectangles). The rostral and caudal borders of the clinical pain depend on the locus of pathology and do not imply that pain from other dermatomes was unaffected. The histograms display the variability in rostral and caudal pin-prick levels relative to the rostral and caudal borders of the myelotomies. The sensory levels occurred most frequently at the lesion borders (0) but could be as many as four levels caudal to the lesion border (C4).

baum, 1973; Breazile and Kitchell, 1968; Karplus and Kreidl, 1925). As expected, thresholds for aversive reactions were elevated, but carnivores and rodents escaped (terminated) normally suprathreshold painful stimuli after receiving hemisections of both the left and right halves of the spinal cord, leaving rostral conduction to the system of short-axoned interneurons that communicate up, down, and across the spinal cord. These experiments appear to discourage efforts to produce analgesia by lesions of the spinal cord, except that Karplus and Kriedl (1925) report no pain sensitivity in monkeys with spaced lateral hemisections. If replicated, this important finding indicates that (1) crossing and recrossing is not a significant factor for conduction of pain by propriospinal systems of primates or that (2) the propriospinal connections in primates do not contribute to the rostral conduction of nociception.

Interruption of axons bordering the ventral horn involves a portion of the propriospinal system termed the lateral ground bundle (Nathan and Smith, 1959). This region receives collaterals from the anterolateral column (Figure 6D), but the functions of the ventral propriospinal system are likely to be motoric. Accordingly, involvement of propriospinal axons bordering the ventral columns does not produce greater losses of pain than more superficial chordotomies (Lahuerta *et al.*, 1984; Nathan and Smith, 1979; see also Figure 9A,B). This suggests that the ventral portion of the lateral ground bundle contributes to reflexive activities rather than to the rostral transmission of pain. However, dorsal propriospinal pathways terminate extensively within the superficial laminae of the dorsal horn and are expected to contribute to nociception.

Only a few long propriospinal axons have been observed in the dorsal propriospinal system, but dense projections of short and small intraspinal axons are apparent within Lissauer's tract and at the base of the dorsal columns, in the cornu commissural tract (Figure 6A,C). These spinal–spinal connections are primarily ipsilateral but also contralateral (Barilari and Kuypers, 1969). Hence, if interruption of these systems were to impair pain sensitivity, deficits should be primarily ipsilateral with unilateral lesions, and the most severe deficits should occur with bilateral lesions. Note that Figures 6A and 6C show only the locations of propriospinal axons in the white matter; axons within the gray matter may contribute critically to nociception.

2. *The Dorsal Columns and Dorsal Propriospinal Pathways*

Interruption of the ipsilateral dorsal column produces a significant decrease in pain reactivity when added to contralateral chordotomy (Figure 7A; Vierck *et al.*, 1971; Vierck and Luck, 1979). Also, primary interruption of the dorsal column in monkeys produces a slight but enduring decrease in pain reactivity (Vierck *et al.*, 1971). This effect could result from interruption of the postsynaptic dorsal column pathway or of a propriospinal system such as Lissauer's tract or the cornu commissural tract. The postsynaptic pathway of the dorsal columns is made up largely of multireceptive neurons from laminae IV–VI of the dorsal horn (Rustioni and Kaufman, 1977), and this pathway is likely to be damaged by midline myelotomies that produce remote hypalgesia. However, few axons of nocimultireceptive neurons in the postsynaptic dorsal column pathway (PSDC) should be interrupted by a midline lesion. Axons of the PSDC tract could provide nociceptive input to dorsal column cells that project back to the dorsal horn (Burton and Loewy, 1977) or to regions supplied by the STT (e.g., thalamic nucleus ventralis posterolateralis), but lemniscal influences on pain have generally been regarded as inhibitory rather than facilitatory (Sheally *et al.*, 1970; Willis, 1982).

Lissauer's tract can be considered a portion of the propriospinal system

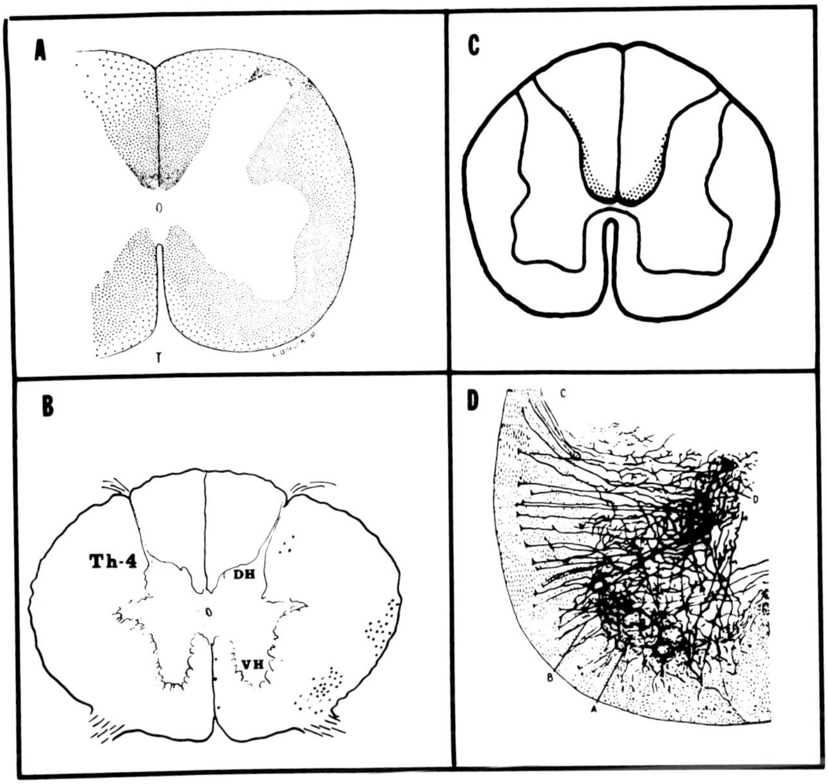

FIGURE 7. (A) A schematic plotting of the relative number of propriospinal axons in different portions of the spinal white matter of monkeys (Tower *et al.* 1941). (B) A diagram from Crutcher and Bingham (1978) illustrating the location of fluorescent rings on the right side, indicating the distribution of descending monoaminergic axons in spinal cords of monkeys. The dots on the left plot the distribution of catecholamine vericosities at T4. (C) A diagram indicating the pre-sumed location of the cornu commissural tract in the white matter of primates (from Nathan and Smith, 1959). (D) A drawing from Golgi sections by Ramon y Cajal (1909) showing collaterals into the ventral horn from anterolateral spinal axons.

given over especially to distribution of activity from small peripheral afferents (Ranson, 1914; Kerr, 1975c; Kumazawa and Perl, 1978), and local effects of lesions at the tip of the dorsal horn have been demonstrated (Hyndman, 1942). Also, a nociceptive pressor reflex in cats is affected by bilateral lesions in Lissauer's tract and the dorsal portion of the lateral ground bundle (Ranson and Von Hess, 1915). However, the available evidence does not support the possibility that this lesion produces remote caudal deficits of pain sensitivity. For example, monkeys have received bilateral interruption of Lissauer's tract after recovery of pain sensitivity following a unilateral chordotomy (Vierck and Luck, 1979), and the dorsal lesions did not produce detectable deficits in pain reactivity (Figure 7B). Similarly, Hyndman (1942) did not report remote caudal deficits following section of Lissauer's tract in humans.

The pain deficit that occurs caudal to midline myelotomy (sparing Lissauer's tract) is likely to result from interruption of propriospinal axons at the base of the dorsal columns (e.g., the cornu commissural tract). This conclusion is supported by cases who have received electrical stimulation in the core region of the spinal cord, eliciting reports of bilateral burning sensations (Schvarcz, 1976). Also, Davis *et al.*, (1929) have claimed that visceral pain in dogs is dependent on conduction in the core region. For humans, the remote caudal effect of midline myelotomy on deep pain is more enduring and extensive than is the influence on superficial cutaneous sensations of pain (Cook *et al.*, 1984; King, 1977; Sourek, 1977). The hypalgesia for cutaneous pain in the segments of the myelotomy can recede and disappear, in contrast with prolonged and remote relief of deep pain. Thus, if the cutaneous hypalgesia from dorsal column lesions results from damage to the core region, the effect is expected to be mild relative to bilateral lesions and deep pain sensations. The decrease in reactivity to cutaneous pain is subtle but enduring (Vierck *et al.*, 1971).

Rostrally directed axons along or near the base of the dorsal columns originate deeply within the dorsal horn, the substantia gelatinosa (Van Gehuchten, 1906), lamina I (Rexed, 1952), and possibly lamina X (Matsushita *et al.*, 1979; Molenaar and Kuypers, 1978). These regions receive nociceptive afferents (Light and Perl, 1979a). The ascending pathway(s) for lamina X neurons is not known but is of particular interest because of a prominent input from deep nociceptors and from midline structures that are most resistant to analgesia from anterolateral chordotomy (Honda, 1984; Nahin *et al.*, 1983). Nociceptor-specific and nocimultireceptive neurons have been described recently in lamina X of cats and rats (Honda, 1984; Honda and Perl, 1984; Nahin *et al.*, 1983), and rostral targets of lamina X include regions of the brainstem reticular formation that respond to nociceptive stimuli (Nahin *et al.*, 1983). Comparable studies in primates are needed.

3. *The Dorsolateral Columns*

Nociceptive afferents approach the dorsal horn via the lateral division of the dorsal roots (Ranson, 1914; Light and Perl, 1979b), and propriospinal axons along the lateral border of the dorsal horn (the dorsal portion of the lateral ground bundle; Nathan and Smith, 1959) might convey nociceptive information (Szentagothai, 1964). Also, behavioral and physiological investigations of nociceptive responses in cats have called attention to the possibility that dorsolateral spinal axons might be important for pain reactivity. Cells of the dorsal horn that project superficially in the ipsilateral dorsolateral column (e.g., via the spinocervicothalamic tract of cats or primates; Brown, 1981; Nijensohn and Kerr, 1975) or the contralateral dorsolateral column (in rodents; McMahon and Wall, 1983) receive input from nociceptors. And dorsal hemisection attenuates pain reactivity or thermosensitivity in cats (Kennard,

1954; Casey *et al.*, 1981). However, dorsolateral pathways in carnivores are prominent relative to primates and the STT (Andersson *et al.*, 1972; Berkley, 1985), and dorsal hemisection involves all of the dorsal propriospinal system in addition to the dorsolateral tracts.

For primates, ipsilateral lesions involving the dorsolateral column have produced hyperalgesia (Pool, 1946; Turner, 1891; Vierck *et al.*, 1971), and contralateral pain sensitivity is not decreased (Nathan and Smith, 1966; Vierck *et al.*, 1971). Thus, interruption of descending inhibitory pathways (Basbaum *et al.*, 1978) produces a disinhibition of pain, but it appears that dorsolateral pathways contribute little to the rostral conduction of pain sensations. These ascending pathways include (1) axons of dorsal horn cells that terminate in the dorsal column nuclei or the lateral cervical nucleus, (2) spinocerebellar axons, (3) the dorsal part of the lateral ground bundle, and (4) Lissauer's tract.

4. The Spinoreticular Pathways

Spinoreticular cells course in the anterolateral and ventral columns (Kerr, 1975a; Mehler *et al.*, 1960) and project bilaterally from the cervical enlargement (Kerr and Lippman, 1974; Kevetter *et al.*, 1982) or originate primarily from contralateral cells in the lumbosacral enlargement (Kevetter *et al.*, 1982). Spinoreticular terminations in the brainstem (see Table 1) are in regions that have been implicated in the rostral conduction of pain (e.g., to the intralaminar thalamic nuclei), in regions that project back to the spinal cord to exert excitatory or inhibitory influences in the dorsal, intermediate, or ventral horn (e.g., from the periaqueductal gray and from the subcoeruleus, raphe, and gigantocellularis nuclei), and in regions concerned with motor control (e.g., the lateral reticular nucleus). The issue of motor versus sensory coding is unresolved for spinoreticular or reticulothalamic connections (Jones, 1983; Maunz *et al.*, 1978; Mehler, 1966) and for the reticulospinal projections to the dorsal, intermediate, and ventral horns because it is difficult to distinguish sensory from motor effects in laboratory animals. Therefore, reports of chordotomy patients with interruption of the contralateral STT and SRT provide opportunities to evaluate sensory capacities for the iSRT.

Spinoreticular cells reveal both small receptive fields and large, often bilateral, receptive fields (Fields *et al.*, 1977; Giesler *et al.*, 1981; Maunz *et al.*, 1978). Because of a preponderance of large fields and bilateral projections to a bilateral reticulothalamic system, it is expected that any residual pain following contralateral chordotomy will be poorly localized. However, the question of whether "discriminative" pain sensations remain after interruption of the cSTT and cSRT has not been resolved. When pain sensations have been elicited by stimulation within regions supplied by the iSRT but deprived of representation by contralateral pathways, clinical reports have not made a special point of poor localization. However, the patients should be tested with stimuli that do not provide localizing cues via the ipsilateral lemniscal pathways.

Another aspect of relative discriminability for the spinothalamic and spinoreticular systems of projection pertains to the growth of sensation intensity with increases in stimulus strength. When the slopes of stimulus–response functions have been compared for the contralateral and ipsilateral limbs of monkeys receiving unilateral chordotomy (Figure 3), significant differences have not been obtained. This result may reflect the similar patterns of multireceptive convergence onto spinothalamic and spinoreticular projection cells (Fields *et al.*, 1977; Giesler *et al.*, 1981), but similar data from human patients are needed to determine the extent to which discriminations of pain intensity are eliminated by contralateral lesions of the STT. For example, because of the high proportion of large receptive fields among SRT cells, it is of interest to determine whether chordotomized patients would confuse increases in intensity with increases in extent of the sensation.

The literature concerning neural mechanisms of pain is replete with comments to the effect that spinal pathways to the brainstem reticular formation and medial thalamic nuclei support motivational–emotional reactions to pain that are distinct from sensory-discriminative functions attributed to the STT (e.g., Bowsher, 1983; Fields *et al.*, 1977; Giesler *et al.*, 1981; Melzack and Casey, 1968). Accordingly, contralateral chordotomies or midline myelotomies that interrupt the spinothalamic tract but spare significant ipsilateral projections to the brainstem reticular formation might produce a situation in which strong stimulation produces arousal without pain. However, chordotomy and myelotomy appear to eliminate pain sensations, arousal, and emotional reactions to strong stimulation or all these reactions are produced with very strong stimulation (or after recovery). Similarly, brainstem lesions that interrupt the cSTT but preserve the spinoreticulothalamic system can produce disturbing paresthesias (Drake and McKenzie, 1953), but emotional reactions are accompanied by eliciting sensations. The relationship between aversion and stimulus intensity can be altered in the direction of hyperesthesia or hyperpathia, implying a release from inhibition (Bowsher, 1983) rather than a dissociation of sensory and emotional responses. The emotional reactions appear to be secondary to perceptions of pain regardless of the spinal pathway(s) of conduction.

Spinothalamic tractotomy within the midbrain can produce hyperreactivity to pain and/or spontaneous paresthesias (Drake and McKenzie, 1953; Nashold *et al.*, 1974), but medullary tractotomy appears to be more effective in producing hypalgesia without the development of disturbing sensations (Birkenfeld and Fisher, 1963; White and Sweet, 1969). An explanation offered for the effects of mesencephalic lesions is that spinoreticular connections are uniquely spared by the high tractotomy (see Bowsher, 1983; White and Sweet, 1969). Each lesion interrupts input from the STT directly to the medial and lateral thalamus (Table 1), but medullary and spinal tractotomies interrupt spinoreticular connections to pontomedullary regions that project to the medial thalamus and to the spinal cord. The reticulothalamic projection involves medially located axons that are spared by the mesencephalic lesion (Nauta and Kuypers, 1958; Schiebel and Scheibel, 1966).

The "unpleasant dysesthesias" (Cassinari and Pagni, 1969) that appear following mesencephalic tractotomy are accompanied by suffering that can exceed reactions to the chronic pain sensations present before the surgery (Drake and McKenzie, 1953; White and Sweet, 1969). But several large series of mesencephalic tractotomies have revealed that disturbing dysesthesias occur in fewer than 15% of the patients (Cassinari and Pagni, 1969; Mazars *et al.*, 1960; Walker, 1950; Wycis and Spiegel, 1962). A small number of cases reporting dysesthesia after mesencephalic tractotomy have established a reputation for this procedure for producing a particularly severe, burning paresthesia (Drake and McKenzie, 1953). However, the dysesthesias are not always described as severe (Mikula *et al.*, 1959; Wycis and Spiegel, 1962). It is difficult to conclude from the literature that spinothalamic tractotomy in the midbrain produces more frequent or severe dysesthesias than do lesions of the spinal cord. For example, as Cassinari and Pagni (1969) point out, mesencephalic tractotomies often involve the medial lemniscus with the STT, and combined dorsal column and STT section by midline myelotomy reliably produces paresthesias (Broager, 1974; Cook and Kawakami, 1977; Papo and Luongo, 1976).

A variety of lesion configurations are included among mesencephalic tractotomies, involving the medial lemniscus and reticular formation to different extents. Therefore, we cannot define the lesion size and location necessary to produce a variety of abnormalities: a sensation of "pins and needles" (paresthesias; Mikula *et al.*, 1959) or "burning dysesthesias" (Drake and McKenzie, 1953) or hyperpathia with elevated nociceptive thresholds but increased sensitivity to strong thermal and mechanical stimuli (Torvik, 1959). Reports of cases exhibiting one or more of these abnormalities following lesions that involve large portions of the reticular formation (Wycis and Spiegel, 1962) create difficulties for the notion that reticulothalamic sparing is necessary for development of abnormalities of pain. Possibly the dysesthesias are a consequence of direct neural damage to the pain pathway(s), as seen with spinal involvement (including cord transection; Melzack and Loeser, 1978).

F. Bilateral Conduction of Pain

1. Conduction Pathways

Following unilateral chordotomy, a variety of sensory experiences of patients indicate that ipsilateral conduction of pain can occur. Infrequently, ipsilateral or bilateral hypalgesia has been observed following a unilateral anterolateral lesion (French and Peyton, 1948; Voris, 1951; Walker, 1940; White and Sweet, 1969), suggesting individual differences in the degree to which pain is lateralized within the ascending spinal pathways. Also, electrical stimulation within one anterolateral column can elicit sensations of tingling, warmth, cold, or pain that are localized ipsilaterally (Lipton, 1979; Tasker and Organ, 1973). And repetitive nociceptive stimuli can evoke potentials in the rostral spinal cord or brainstem after myelotomy and block of A-fiber conduction (Sheally *et al.*, 1966). A small number of STT cells in primates can be backfired, labeled, or made chromatolytic from manipulations of ipsilateral spinothalamic axons (Berkley, 1985; Foerster and Gagel, 1932; Kerr, 1975c; Kuru, 1949; Trevino and Carstens, 1975; Trevino *et al.*, 1973), and some spinoreticular axons originate from ipsilateral cell bodies (the iSRT; Kerr and Lippman, 1974; Kevetter *et al.*, 1982). Bilateral receptive fields have been demonstrated for some spinothalamic and many spinoreticular projection cells (Fields *et al.*, 1977; Giesler *et al.*, 1981). And axonal terminals of nociceptive afferents are not always confined to the ipsilateral dorsal horn but can cross at some cord levels (e.g., with fused dorsal horns) to terminate in deeper layers that give rise to spinoreticular and some of the spinothalamic axons (Light and Perl, 1979a; Matshushita and Tanami, 1983; Nadelhaft *et al.*, 1983; Willis *et al.*, 1979). Thus, in principle, rostral conduction of pain from a unilateral source can occur via three major pathways: contralateral axons of ipsilateral cells (the cSTT and cSRT tracts) or ipsilateral axons of ipsilateral cells (the iSRT) and two components that are presumed to be minor or inconsequential, contralateral or ipsilateral conduction from cells in the contralateral dorsal horn (see Willis, Chapter 11, for further discussion).

Occasionally, when patients report that chronic pain is strictly unilateral before surgery, discomfort is perceived ipsilateral to a chordotomy (Taren *et al.*, 1969; White and Sweet, 1969). In these cases, it is possible that the pain ipsilateral to the chordotomy resulted from peripheral sources on that side but was masked preoperatively by more severe contralateral pain (White and Sweet, 1969). Nathan (1956) discounts this explanation on the basis of careful observations of patients with well-lateralized pain; he prefers to implicate ipsilateral referral of pain from the contralateral source. Referral of pain to the normal side (ipsilateral to a chordotomy) has also been observed to occur with natural stimulation within the contralateral, hypalgesic zone (French *et al.*, 1966; Nathan, 1956; Ray and Wolff, 1945). Light contralateral stimulation was correctly perceived and localized, but intense stimulation (e.g., 60°C but not 50°C) could evoke pain referred ipsilateral to the lesion, particularly if it was applied repetitively. The qualities of the referred sensations have not been described by many authors, but Nathan (1956) refers to pains that "seem to come from within," are usually localized homotypically, could occur at short latency or spread gradually, and are prolonged (minutes). Thus, pain of ipsilateral origin can arise from contralateral neurons with dominant contralateral receptive fields. But referral does not occur reliably (18% of Nathan's chordotomy patients), indicating that special conditions must be present.

2. *Effects of Spinal Commissurotomy*

One lesion of importance for evaluating ipsilateral conduction of pain is spinal commissurotomy, deafferenting the cSTT and cSRT from lesioned segments and preserving the iSRT (and other ipsilateral pathways). If pain sensations depend entirely on contralateral spinal pathways, the effects of spinal commissurotomy on somatosensations should be as follows:

1. Deficits should occur bilaterally within the dermatomes corresponding to spinal levels with the commissure severed.
2. The sensory deficits observed following chordotomy should result from commissural myelotomy as well. Cutaneous pain from mechanical or thermal stimulation, sensations of sharpness and itch, deep somatic pain, and visceral nociception are regarded as spinothalamic, and these sensations should be affected by both lesions.
3. Given a myelotomy extent of at least five levels (to sever the axons of all STT cells gathering input from a single dermatomal area), the deficits from myelotomy should be comparable in magnitude to those observed after chordotomy.

In general, the correspondence of effects from chordotomy and commissural myelotomy is good, but some important surprises result from the comparison.

Studies involving comprehensive sensory testing of patients following midline myelotomy of the spinal cord have reported that pin-prick and thermal nociception are usually attenuated within some of the dermatomes lesioned, and both visceral and deep somatic, clinical pain are decreased reliably (Cook and Kawakami, 1977; Cook *et al.*, 1984; King, 1977; Papo and Luongo, 1976; Putnam, 1934; Sourek, 1969). As expected, interruption of the crossing fibers is especially effective for control of midline pain or nociception from bilaterally innervated structures (Lippert *et al.*, 1974; Papo, 1979a). Compared with chordotomy, some apparent differences in the effects of myelotomy are:

1. An increased incidence of paresthesias, probably from involvement of medial fibers of the dorsal columns (Broager, 1974; Cook and Kawakami, 1977; King, 1977; Lippert *et al.*, 1974; Papo and Luongo, 1976; Sourek, 1969).
2. No decrease in the magnitude of elicited cutaneous pain and/or more frequent and obvious recovery of superficial pain (Cook *et al.*, 1984; Hitchcock, 1974; Papo, 1979a; Putnam, 1934; Schvarcz, 1976).
3. Preserved sharp–dull discrimination (Hitchcock, 1974; Schvarcz, 1976).
4. Pronounced losses of deep pain that are relatively enduring (Lippert *et al.*, 1974; Sourek, 1969, 1977).

When clinical pain has returned, it has been described as less sharp and more tolerable than preoperative pain, but a burning quality often is present (Putnam, 1934; Sourek, 1969).

Because of rostral and caudal afferent collateralization in Lissauer's tract, sensory deficits resulting from commissurotomy should be distributed over fewer segments than the extent of the myelotomy. However, when Sourek (1969) and King (1977) documented the effects of commissural myelotomy at cervical and thoracic levels, the regions in which hypalgesia could be demonstrated were larger than expected. Rostral borders of pin-prick hypalgesia occurred most often in the segment of the rostral limit of the myelotomy but could be two segments caudal to the rostral lesion border (Sourek, 1977; Figure 8). The caudal extent of pin-prick hypalgesia was as many as four segments below the caudal limit of the myelotomy in Sourek's cases, and King described even longer caudal extents for pin-prick hypalgesia (up to ten segments below myelotomies of three segments). The most limited of these areas of cutaneous hypalgesia seem large (covering the most rostral and/or caudal dermatomes lesioned), considering the partial involvement of STT neurons supplying the border segments. However, the rapid recovery of superficial pain following myelotomies of limited extent suggests that operative trauma is a factor in early deficits. Recovery is expected because of the rostral–caudal extent of spinal projection cells representing each dermatome.

The reported distributions of clinical pain relief following myelotomy are especially impressive in size. Clinical pain involving lumbar and sacral der-

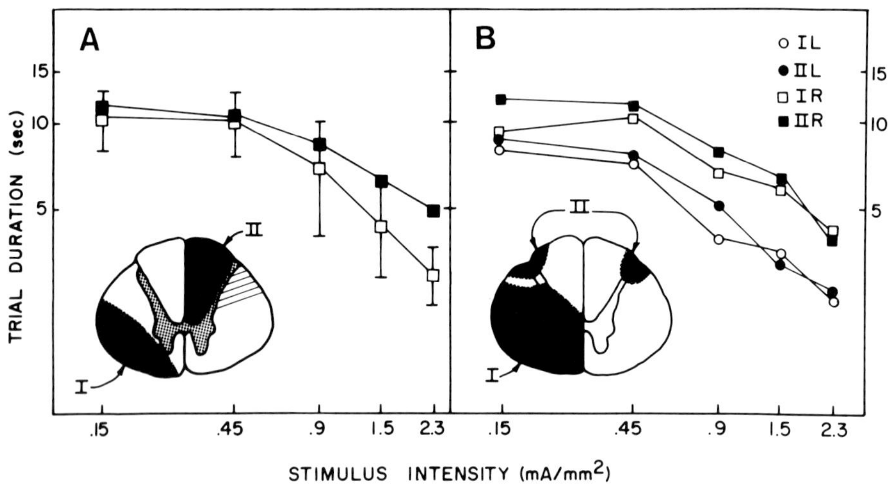

FIGURE 8. On the left, average trial durations for four monkeys are plotted as functions of electrocutaneous stimulation intensities delivered months following contralateral chordotomy (open squares) or after secondary lesions to the ipsilateral dorsal column (closed squares). For two animals, the dorsal lesion included the dorsolateral column (hatched area). For each monkey, pain reactivity was significantly reduced by addition of the dorsal lesion to the chordotomy. On the right, results are presented from testing a monkey months after receiving a large chordotomy on the left (open symbols) followed by bilateral section of Lissauer's tract (solid symbols). Pain reactivity was not significantly elevated for either hind limb after the dorsal lesions.

matomes can be attenuated or lost following thoracic or cervical myelotomies involving only a few segments (Hitchcock, 1970; King, 1977; Sourek, 1977) and producing limited or no hypalgesia for cutaneous stimulation (Cook *et al.*, 1984; Lippert *et al.*, 1974; Papo and Luongo, 1976; Putnam, 1934). If these results occurred only following upper cervical myelotomies, it would be tempting to suspect that interruption of crossing spinocervical tract axons produces remote caudal effects, but the success of thoracic myelotomies in providing hypalgesia in remote segments indicates that the effect applies to most or all levels of the spinal cord. Thus, myelotomy appears to interrupt an ascending pain pathway (in addition to crossing STT axons) that is critical to the full sensory impact of chronic, deep pain.

Nonsurgical myelotomy can occur in cases of syringomyelia, involving a focused cavitation in the central canal region, gradually increasing in size (rostrally, caudally, and radially). Detailed correlations of the sizes and locations of syringomyeli with sensory deficits have not been presented, but "typically," deep pain is lost first; then thermal nociception and then superficial mechanical nociception are lost over the segments involved by the tumor and then caudally (Netsky, 1953; Schneider, 1982). Head and Thompson (1906) described progressive blunting of thermal sensitivity as follows: 50°C could be felt as warm but not painful, and 40°C was not perceived; then warmth could not be elicited by even intense thermal stimulation. As the disease progresses, local wasting of muscles becomes apparent from involvement of the ventral horn, and lemniscal signs usually appear late (i.e., deficits of spatiotactile and limb position sensitivity). The point to be emphasized is that deep sensitivity was lost first and is presumed, therefore, to be conducted via centrally located axons. This observation reinforces the extensive and powerful effects of midline myelotomy on deep clinical pain. The effects of myelotomy and syringomyelia implicate centrally located propriospinal axons in the rostral conduction of deep pain (Broager, 1974; Brown-Sequard, 1868; Hitchcock, 1974; Nathan, 1956; Noordenbos, 1959; Schvarcz, 1976).

G. *Recovery of Pain Sensitivity Following Spinal Lesions*

Perhaps one of the more intriguing aspects of the effects produced by selective spinal lesions is the recovery of sensation following the lesion. Whether this occurs as a result of anatomic changes (e.g., sprouting of new connections; see discussion by Micevych and colleagues, Chapter 17) or by a functional reorganization of pathways not previously relevant to the coding of that sensory modality is not clear. As discussed above, it appears likely that pain may be transmitted by ipsilateral or contralateral systems, though the acute efficacy of a unilateral chordotomy is a striking phenomenon. Moreover, as discussed previously (see above and further discussion by Willis, Chapter 11), the likelihood of multiple pathways relevant to particular sensations appears very great. In the following sections, we review some of the characteristics of recovery from chordotomy.

1. Unilateral Chordotomy: Recovery of Contralateral Hypalgesia

White and Sweet (1969) report that 53% of patients with appropriate early levels of pain relief experience a return, within 2 years, of clinical pain contralateral to unilateral chordotomy. The percentages of recovered patients vary considerably among investigators as expected from the limited samples and difficulties in conducting thorough examinations at regular intervals, but many agree that pain can return following complete anterolateral lesions (Bumke and Foerster, 1936; White, 1963; White and Sweet, 1969). The time course of pain return varies considerably and includes patients with onsets of recovery beyond 2 years (Graf, 1960). These important observations have limited the use of chordotomy to patients with short life expectancies. However, there are a number of difficulties inherent to the clinical data base.

Early relief of pain can occur because of operative trauma that produces temporary loss of conduction by STT axons not transected by the lesion. For example, when levels of pin-prick hypalgesia regress early in the postoperative period, the lesion is likely to have traumatized but spared ventral axons in the STT (Hyndman and Van Epps, 1939). These cases should not be categorized as recovered from complete contralateral chordotomy, particularly when histological confirmation of the lesion is not available. However, cases have been reported in which very late contraction of an "analagesic" zone left long rostral and/or caudal borders of hypalgesia (Nathan, 1963).

Some patients appear to have recovered pain sensitivity throughout the original zone of "analgesia," but clinical pain ordinarily is not static; it can spread to involve tissues supplied by spared spinothalamic cells. Similarly, the source of pain can progressively increase the intensity of its excitation of peripheral nociceptors. In this case, an increase in pain sensations could be misinterpreted as a recovery of function within the pain pathways. That is, increases of clinical pain do not necessarily imply a change in the excitability of spared central projection cells or an increase in the number of cells capable of conveying nociception.

Establishment of a nonhuman primate model of pain reactivity that reflects the effectiveness of chordotomy in producing hypalgesia could permit a valid analysis of recovery over time. Accordingly, in experiments with *Cebus albifrons* or *Macaca nemestrina* monkeys (Greenspan *et al.*, 1982; Ritz *et al.*, 1981; Vierck and Luck, 1979), electrical stimulation has been utilized to evoke reactions to pain elicited by stimulation at levels well below complete lesions of the contralateral spinothalamic tract. Electrical stimulation of the skin of either lateral calf was chosen for a variety of reasons:

1. Pain elicited by electrocutaneous stimulation is reliably reduced in humans by chordotomy (King, 1957), and cutaneous hypalgesia generally accompanies effective relief of chronic pain by chordotomy (e.g., Hyndman and Wolkin, 1943; White and Sweet, 1969).
2. With appropriate temporal and intensive structuring, electrocuta-

neous stimulation produces focal, brief, and discriminative sensations that can be rated objectively and reliably by human observers. The pain is real but tolerable (humane), and many levels of intensity can be discriminated within the pain sensitivity range (from pain detection to pain tolerance thresholds; Vierck *et al.,* 1983b).

3. Electrocutaneous stimulation can be nontraumatic to the skin, producing consistent sensation levels from day to day with application of the electrodes to identical stimulus sites on awake subjects. Electrocutaneous pain intensities are relatively uninfluenced by movements of the subject, and the onset of pain is "immediate," preventing the subjects from avoiding pain by responding to nonnociceptive cues (e.g., as provided by the gradual warming of a thermode and the skin).
4. Behavioral reactions of humans and nonhuman primates that terminate painful electrical stimuli are graded similarly in magnitude and speed as functions of stimulus intensity (in milliamperes per square millimeter), and thresholds for escape of shock by the monkeys correspond to pain thresholds of humans (Vierck *et al.,* 1983b).
5. Of most importance, substantial reductions of reactivity to normally painful stimuli are reliably observed following anterolateral chordotomy in the monkeys (Vierck and Luck, 1979; Figure 9).

When hypalgesia is demonstrated contralateral to chordotomy in monkeys, it is possible to assess whether changes in pain sensitivity occur for stimuli that remain constant, and the long-term effectiveness of lesions differing in location or size can be compared. Preliminary results of this analysis are presented in Figure 9. Clearly, recovery to normal or near-normal levels of pain sensitivity can occur for primates following lesions that completely interrupt the contralateral ventral quadrant (Figure 9A), confirming experiences with chronic pain in humans. In both cases, the time course of recovery was long, spanning months (White and Sweet, 1969; Figure 9). For the monkeys, the earliest increase in contralateral sensitivity ordinarily reached a peak within 20 postoperative weeks, and then contralateral reactivity waxed and waned at or below preoperative or ipsilateral values over subsequent weeks (up to 65 weeks of testing in some animals). Thus, return of pain reactivity depends on a delayed and gradual process of central reorganization that is not dependent on shifts or increases in the peripheral source of pain, and the pathway(s) subserving recovery is (are) located outside the classical distribution of the cSTT and cSRT in the anterolateral and ventral columns.

As is the case with chordotomy in humans, some monkeys with apparently complete section of the STT revealed considerable contralateral recovery, and others did not (e.g., Figure 9A–C). A large number of cases with long-term testing and histological confirmation of the lesions will be required to identify the lesion configurations that consistently produce prolonged hypalgesia or recovery, but several conclusions are suggested by the data available. For example, superficial lesions of the anterolateral column can produce enduring hypalgesia (Figure 9B). This observation is supported by Nathan and Smith (1979), who strongly advocate chordotomy as an effective long-term treatment for chronic pain; the cases they present to support this position received restricted and superficial lesions of one anterolateral column (Figure 10).

Deep lesions of a ventral spinal quadrant can produce a pronounced contralateral hypalgesia that recovers to normal sensitivity (Figure 9A), confirming results from patients with ventral quadrant lesions (Nathan and Smith, 1966; White *et al.*, 1956). That is, involvement of medial or ventral axons may permit recovery that would not have been seen with a smaller anterolateral lesion. Involvement of the ventral columns could produce a caudal disinhi-

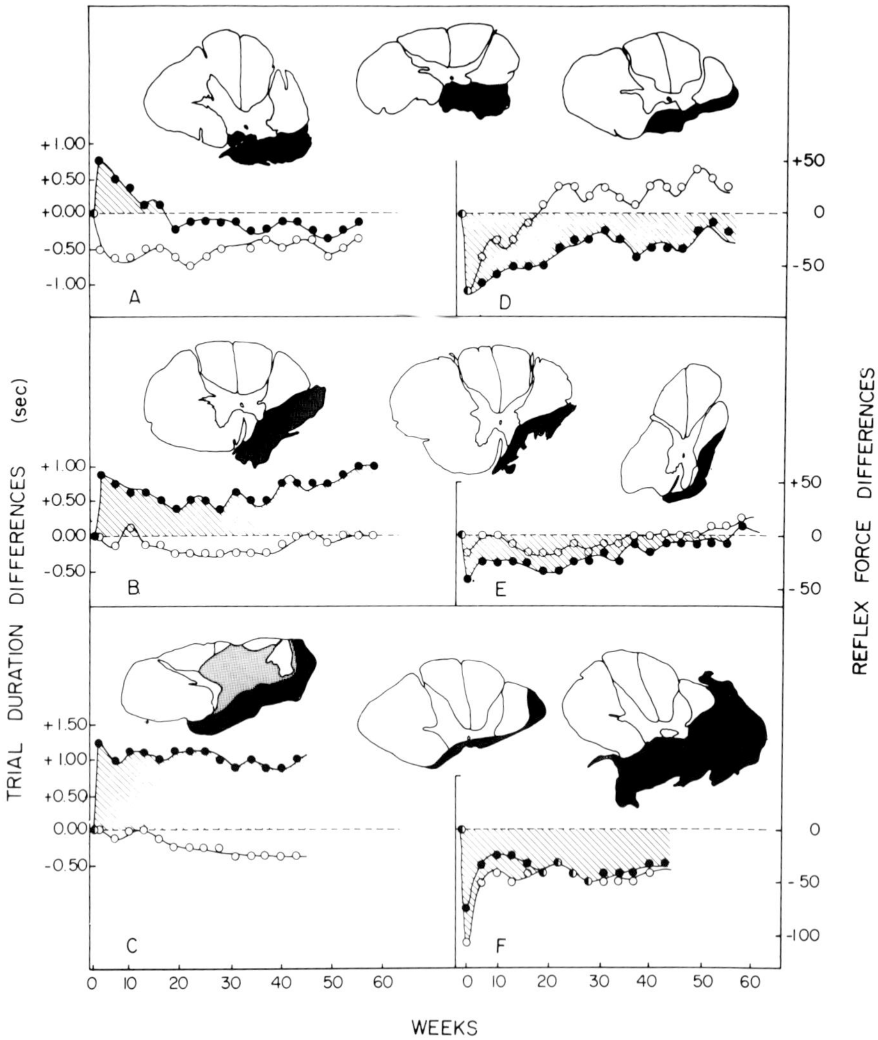

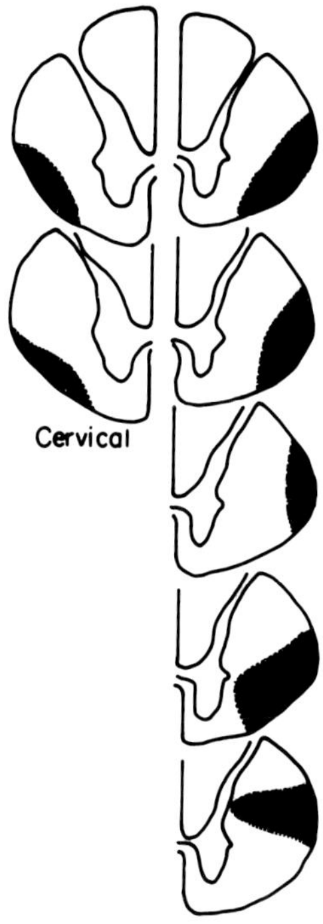

FIGURE 10. Superficial lesions of the cervical spinal cord (left column) and at thoracic levels (right column) that produced enduring contralateral attenuation of pain in humans. (Adapted from Nathan and Smith, 1979.)

←

FIGURE 9. Differences between preoperative and postoperative reactivity to electrocutaneous stimulation are presented for monkeys that are grouped according to lesion configuration and behavioral effects. Operant pain reactivity is presented in the left column (A–C), where the average duration of shock tolerated preoperatively is subtracted from the duration received contralateral to a chordotomy (solid circles; left leg) and ipsilateral to the lesion (open circles; right leg) over successive weeks of postoperative testing. For the left column, decreased operant pain reactivity is indicated by points above the dashed line representing no difference from preoperative performance. The duration and magnitude of contralateral hyporeactivity are indicated by shading. The magnitude of reflexive flexion of the stimulated leg is shown in the right column (D–F), where the average force of preoperative responses is subtracted from postoperative values for the left (contralateral) and right legs. Hyporeflexia is indicated by points below the dashed lines, and contralateral hyporeactivity is indicated by shading. Three monkeys with large lesions recovered to normal levels of contralateral pain reactivity (A). In contrast, more superficial lesions (middle row) produced little or no contralateral recovery (B), and three monkeys with extensive involvement of the ventral and central gray matter did not recover pain reactivity contralaterally (C). Contralateral reflexes were strongly depressed by the larger lesions and did not recover to normal levels (D and F), but reflexes were slightly affected after superficial chordotomies, recovering to normal levels (E). The monkeys that recovered operant pain reactivity were distinguished by development of an ipsilateral hyperreflexia (D), but large lesions that prevented recovery of pain reactivity produced an enduring, bilateral depression of flexion reflexes (F).

bition, as suggested by the apparently reflexive effects demonstrated by Denny-Brown (1979; see above). Similarly, to the extent that descending inhibitory systems are located medial to the STT axons, the larger lesions may contribute to the return of pain sensitivity or to the presence of postoperative paresthesias by reducing inhibitory influences on the remaining projection neurons. Also, extensive involvement of the lateral ground bundle, including long propriospinal axons, could lead to partial deafferentation of cells in the deep laminae (e.g., V–VII) of the dorsal horn caudal to the lesion (Molenaar and Kuypers, 1978), changing the responsivities over time of intact projection cells.

Paresthesias, dysesthesias, or hyperpathias resulting from a caudal disinhibition of other causes of hypersensitivity of spared projection cells are seen in a minor percentage of chordotomy patients (e.g., 11%; White, 1968). These disorders of sensation tend to occur within segments near the lesion level, where pain can be referred (Nathan, 1956), or where special conditions of reaction to trauma can lead to abnormal discharge in spared cells (Loeser and Ward, 1967). Therefore, it is important to specify the spatial distribution of disordered sensations and distinguish border pain from a distribution throughout segments caudal to the lesion. On the basis of the available information, it is not justifiable to conclude that the spinocerebral systems spared by chordotomy become hypersensitive or hyperactive as a generalized reaction to STT section. That is, when pain sensitivity recovers from chordotomy, there ordinarily is a gradual return to levels near those experienced preoperatively, without development of exaggerated pain that is out of proportion to the stimulus intensity (e.g., Figure 9B).

A most puzzling difference in the longevity of hypalgesia is presented by monkeys with large ventral quadrant lesions that permitted recovery (Figure 9A) or produced enduring hypalgesia (Figure 9C). Apparently, slight differences in lesion configuration can differentially include critical axons or trigger a recovery process. For example, small differences in the bilateral dorsomedial extent of a dorsal quadrant lesion could determine a critical involvement of the core system of ascending projections. The lesions of animals in group C (demonstrating no recovery of hypalgesia) interrupt the ventral horns and core region to a greater extent than the ventral lesions of group A that permitted recovery.

2. *Unilateral Chordotomy: Ipsilateral Hyperalgesia*

A noradrenergic projection from the pons and midbrain is located in the anterolateral columns (Crutcher and Bingham, 1978) and terminates bilaterally in the spinal dorsal horn (primarily ipsilaterally; Hodge *et al.*, 1981; Westlund *et al.*, 1984), and iontophoretic application of norepinephrine inhibits activity of STT cells in the spinal cord (Willcockson *et al.*, 1984). Unilateral chordotomy provides an interesting test of the tonic influences of descending anterolateral pathways because descending projections are reduced bilaterally to projection cells with intact axons. Also, with repeated testing following chordotomy, it is possible to evaluate whether interruption of descending inputs to dorsal horn cells leads to an ipsilateral hypersensitivity that could parallel recovery of contralateral pain sensitivity. For example, if compensatory processes important for recovery occur on both sides after a unilateral lesion, then ipsilateral hyperalgesia could develop as contralateral hypalgesia recovers.

Some of the many clinicians who have examined chordotomy patients postoperatively have noted the appearance of new chronic pain or unusual sensations caudal and ipsilateral to the lesion level (Nathan, 1956; Taren *et al.*, 1969; White and Sweet, 1969). However, these effects may be consequences of referral from contralateral sources of pain, and ipsilateral pathology cannot be ruled out for these patients. Reports of hypersensitivity to stimulation throughout the segments caudal and ipsilateral to chordotomy have not been found, but evaluations of chordotomy patients have concentrated on contralateral effects and have not included tests for subtle changes in ipsilateral sensitivity.

Direct comparisons of preoperative and postoperative ipsilateral sensitivity of monkeys are available with stimulation over months with the same stimulus intensities (Figure 9A–F). For each of three groups of three animals, operant pain reactivity ipsilateral to chordotomy was greater for much of the postoperative testing period, in comparison to preoperative performance with stimulation of the same leg. Overall, the effect was slight, as expected for a partial deafferentation from supraspinal inputs, and for most animals the ipsilateral hyperreactivity appeared after months of postoperative testing. It is, of course, possible that the animals would have become more sensitive over time in the absence of a spinal lesion, but reactivity is expected to decrease with habituation over months of testing. Of particular interest are differences in the time course and magnitude of ipsilateral sensitivity changes that occurred over time for the three groups of monkeys (Figure 9) that (1) recovered from contralateral hypalgesia after unilateral interruption of the anterolateral column and bilateral involvement of the ventral columns, (2) showed little or no contralateral recovery after lesions restricted to one anterolateral column, or (3) did not recover from hypalgesia following large lesions of one anterolateral column, both ventral columns, and the ventral gray matter. The earliest, most pronounced, and most enduring ipsilateral hyperalgesia (relative to preoperative values) occurred for the animals that recovered contralateral operant reactivity (Figure 9A). This result suggests that a generalized caudal disinhibition can occur following chordotomy, leading to eventual return of contralateral pain sensitivity.

Another opportunity to evaluate the effects of unilateral chordotomy on caudal spinal neurons is provided by measurements of the magnitude of reflexive responses to electrical stimulation of either leg (Figure 9D–F). Flexor reflex responses were elicited reliably by 50-ms trains of electrical stimulation to the lateral calf. The stimulated limb responded within 38 ms of stimulus onset, and the amplitude of the leg flexion increased with stimulus intensity through approximately 1 mA/mm^2. Thus, the response was elicited by non-nociceptive stimulus intensities, but it was maximal at weak to moderate levels of pain (Vierck and Cooper, 1984). Following unilateral chordotomy, reflex force was sharply diminished bilaterally (Figure 9D–F), and some recovery was observed with stimulation of either limb. Confirming the ipsilateral effects of chordotomy on operant reactions, the clearest hyperreflexia was observed for the ipsilateral limbs of monkeys that recovered from contralateral hypalgesia (Figure 9A, D). Also, the largest and most enduring hyporeflexia occurred following large lesions that produced an enduring hypalgesia (Figure 9C, F). Again, the groups with large ventral lesions differed with respect to evidence for ipsilateral hyperreactivity; contralateral recovery was accompanied by ipsilateral hypersensitivity.

3. Bilateral Chordotomy

A prime candidate for the location of pathways of pain conduction after chordotomy is the ipsilateral ventral quadrant, with spinoreticular and possibly spinothalamic projections (Kerr and Lippman, 1974; Kevetter *et al.,* 1982). Unfortunately, studies of chronic pain patients have not revealed greater or more enduring deficits of pain sensitivity following bilateral anterolateral lesions (White and Sweet, 1969). Sequential lesions can produce a temporary decrease in pain sensitivity ipsilateral to the second procedure (French *et al.,* 1966; Nathan and Smith, 1966; Vierck and Luck, 1979), but the long-term effects of bilateral chordotomy appear not to be noticeably different from the effects of unilateral interruption of the anterolateral column (White and Sweet, 1969).

The lack of permanent analgesia following bilateral chodotomy indicates that the iSRT is not an important channel for sensations of pain. This finding in turn forces the question of whether interruption of the cSRT contributes substantially to the hypalgesia produced by anterolateral chordotomy. Some cSRT neurons appear to code stimulus intensity within the pain range (Fields *et al.,* 1977), but others are inhibited by strong stimulation (Maunz *et al.,* 1978). Repetition of nociceptive stimuli enhances pain sensitivity contralateral to a chordotomy (Nathan, 1956; White and Sweet, 1969), but many SRT neurons habituate to repetitive stimulation (Maunz *et al.,* 1978). Finally, many of the targets of SRT projection are to areas that inhibit pain or contribute to the programming of motor processes (Basbaum and Fields, 1984; Jones, 1983; Willis, 1982; Table 1).

If spinocerebral conduction of pain sensations is spared following bilateral lesions of the lateral STT, it is likely that the ventral columns or the propriospinal system (or both) is the relevant channel. In regard to the ventral columns, some interesting comparisons are available. When contralateral or bilateral interruption of the ventral column(s) has been added to contralateral chordotomy, hypalgesia (not analgesia) has resulted (e.g., Figure 9A, C; Lahuerta *et al.*, 1984). Thus, addition of both ventral columns or of the ipsilateral anterolateral column (iALC) appears to add little to the hypalgesia produced by a contralateral cordotomy (see Nathan and Smith, 1966).

4. Ventral Hemisection

When the ventral spinal artery becomes occluded or severed, the ventral two-thirds of the spinal cord becomes infarcted. Although there are few reports of careful testing for pain sensitivity in human cases of confirmed ventral hemisection, Nathan and Smith (1979) report a patient for whom intense stimulation within dermatomes below the infarct produced sensations of touch on the stimulated spot and burning pain that was referred above the level of the lesion. With respect to sensations localized within the affected dermatomes, the patient was analgesic. Similarly, a monkey has been tested with electrocutaneous stimulation for 305 days following ventral hemisection, and virtual analgesia was observed throughout that period (Vierck and Luck, 1979). Escape responses occurred on occasion, but spontaneous rates of pulling the manipulandum could account for the low rate of responding to the strong stimulus intensities. Hence, although ventral hemisection cannot, in strict terms, be said to produce analgesia because of referred pain, ventral hemisection may eliminate transmission of pain by spinocerebral systems that represent the affected area spatially.

A patient with traumatic isolation of one anterolateral column has been tested over a long period of time and continues to reveal loss of thermal sensations and discriminations of sharpness on the side of the spared axons (Wall and Noordenbos, 1977). This result and reports that bilateral chordotomy does not eliminate pain suggest that analgesia from ventral hemisection results from involvement of the STT and axons within or around the gray matter. For example, central axons in the depths of the dorsal columns or in the central spinal gray can be involved by ventral hemisection but are spared by bilateral chordotomies. The existence of an important pathway for pain in the spinal core region has been suggested frequently (Broager, 1974; Brown-Sequard, 1868; Foerster and Gagel, 1932; Noordenbos, 1959; Sourek, 1977; Tower *et al.*, 1941; Vierck *et al.*, 1971). In contrast, Nathan and Smith (1979) argue against any importance for pain conduction of axons surrounding the ventral horns, and it is likely that this is a system of motor control.

The discovery that neurons in the central zone of the spinal gray matter (lamina X) receive nociceptive inputs from superficial and deep locations (Honda, 1985; Honda and Perl, 1985; Light and Perl, 1979; Nahin *et al.*, 1983) and also receive modulatory influences from peptides and monoamines present in the superficial dorsal horn (LaMotte *et al.*, 1982; Light, 1983; see LaMotte, Chapter 5, and Seybold, Chapter 6, for further discussion) demands attention to this system as an important source of pain conduction. The remote caudal effects of midline myelotomy on clinical pain (Hitchcock, 1974; King, 1977; Sourek, 1969) especially implicate the central core of the spinal cord in rostral conduction of pain, but it is important to define the location, length, and termination sites for axons emanating from this region. Thus, the effectiveness of ventral hemisections in producing analgesia may depend on involvement of the central core region in addition to interruption of contralateral spinothalamic (and spinoreticular) pathways.

H. Summary

Anterolateral chordotomy has been utilized successfully to control "intractable" pain since 1912, after Spiller noticed vacuoles in the anterolateral columns of a tuberculosis patient with hypalgesia. Chordotomy produces a comprehensive and substantial reduction of pain sensitivity contralaterally, and isolation of the anterolateral columns leaves simian and human primates with pain and temperature sensitivity intact (Vierck and Luck, 1979; Wall and Noordenbos, 1977; White and Sweet, 1969). Painful sensations produced by superficial mechanical, thermal, and electrical stimulation are attenuated by chordotomy, as are deep somatic and visceral pain. The deficits are not restricted to painful sensations but include itch, sharpness, warmth and cold, wetness, and sensations that accompany orgasm. Thresholds for touch can be elevated contralaterally to a slight degree, and touch thresholds are insignificantly elevated following isolation of the cALC (Vierck, 1977; Wall and Noordenbos, 1977). Discriminative cutaneous sensations (e.g., spatial resolution for touch) and proprioception are generally reported as fully intact following chordotomy, but isolation of the cALC severely deteriorates spatiotactile and proprioceptive capacities (Vierck, 1984; Wall and Noordenbos, 1977).

Somatotopic organization of the STT projection in the anterolateral columns has been demonstrated conclusively by correlating regions of hypalgesia with the extent of histologically confirmed lesions. When the STT is sectioned completely on one side of the cord, upper levels of pain relief extend to within several segments of the lesion, and additional interruption of Lissauer's tract (ipsilaterally, at the level of the chordotomy) can bring the sensory level to the surgical level. Chordotomy has been claimed to produce analgesia over caudal, contralateral segments, but careful evaluations have generally described a hypalgesia (King, 1957). Thresholds for pain are elevated, and suprathreshold stimuli elicit pain according to a shifted growth function that is similar in slope to preoperative stimulus–response relationships (Figure 3). Pain sensitivity can recover substantially with time after chordotomy, even when the lesion extends throughout the contralateral ventral quadrant of the cord (Figure 9).

Stimulation within the hypalgesic zone produced by chordotomy can lead to referral of sensation rostrally (to segments near the level of the lesion) or contralaterally (to homotopic regions) when high-intensity stimulation is delivered. Paresthesias or dysesthesias can develop following chordotomy, but they ordinarily are present within segments near the lesion. This and other evidence indicate that the propriospinal and ipsilateral spinoreticular pathways effectively transmit nociceptive inputs only to limited sets of projection neurons in the early postoperative period. After recovery, when pain is evoked by stimulation within the region of early hypalgesia, it can be localized contralateral to and below the lesion, but the accuracy of localization and qualitative features of the pain have not been well described. In order to characterize the varieties of pain that can be coded and transmitted by extraspinothalamic pathways, careful testing of chordotomized patients is indicated. Theoretical formulations of the capacities of pain pathways other than the neospinothalamic tract have suggested that residual pain following chordotomy should be diffuse and should elicit exaggerated emotional reactions, but these predictions have not been supported strongly.

Laboratory animal models of nocifensive reactivity by primates have replicated the major effects of chordotomy in humans: contralateral hypalgesia with delayed and slow recovery in some subjects. This provides opportunities to clearly define the pathways contributing to and necessary for pain conduction, but an important gap in the anatomic and physiological literature makes this task difficult. Studies of ascending and descending projections contributing to pain sensitivity have concentrated on origins and terminations and generally have not charted the course of the axons in the white matter. Hence, it is difficult to know the proportions of spinothalamic, spinoreticular, and propriospinal pathways interrupted by lesions involving different portions of the spinal white and gray matter. Furthermore, the anatomic information must be obtained from primates, because carnivores and rodents have revealed substantial differences in organization of their pain pathways. Cats have a poorly developed STT but prominent spinocervicothalamic and spinoreticular tracts, and pain conduction is not affected greatly by anterolateral spinal lesions (Casey *et al.*, 1981; Kennard, 1954; Ranson and Von Hess, 1915). In rats, the lateral and medial thalamic projection systems appear to be separated into the anterolateral and ventral columns (Giesler *et al.*, 1979). Furthermore, SRT projections from lamina I of rodents via the contralateral dorsolateral column are distinct from more ventral axons of multireceptive neurons (McMahon and Wall, 1983). Both rodents and carnivores may depend on bilateral spinal conduction of pain to a greater extent than primates (Karplus and Kriedl, 1925).

Potential pathways of pain conduction in the ventral columns, the ipsilateral anterolateral column, Lissauer's tract, and the ipsilateral dorsolateral column appear to contribute little to the rostral conduction of appropriately localized pain sensations in primates. However, midline myelotomy has revealed a remote, caudal hypalgesia for deep pain (e.g., Cook *et al.*, 1984; King, 1977; Sourek, 1977) that focuses attention on axons in the region of the central spinal core (e.g., the cornu commissural tract). When unilateral lesions of the dorsal columns interrupt the predominant ipsilateral component of this bilateral propriospinal system, pain reactivity is diminished, and the effects of contralateral chordotomy are accentuated (Vierck *et al.*, 1971; Vierck and Luck, 1979; Figure 8). Also, the analgesias produced by dorsal hemisections in cats (Kennard, 1954) and ventral hemisections in primates (Nathan, 1956;

Vierck and Luck, 1979) may depend on combined section of pathways in the lateral columns and the core of the spinal cord.

The preceding discussion leads to a proposal for the minimal lesion that will lead to an enduring loss of lateralized chronic pain. Superficial section of one anterolateral column (extending into the dorsolateral and ventral funiculi) produces enduring hypalgesia for contralateral nociceptive stimulation (Figure 9) and for clinical pain (Figure 10). For cutaneous pain, a superficial lesion produces early effects comparable to those of a deeper section that includes the ventral horns, and greater recovery of pain sensitivity can occur with the more extensive lesion (Figure 9A, B). Lesions approaching complete section of a ventral quadrant should be avoided because interruption of medial projection systems in the ventral quadrant increases the incidence of undesirable deficits (e.g., orthostatic hypotension, motoric weakness, disturbances of bowel and bladder functions, and respiratory depression if the lesion is at upper cervical levels; Nathan 1963; Nathan and Smith, 1958). The large lesions can produce an ipsilateral hyperalgesia and hyperreflexia (Figure 9A, D). These and other effects are ascribed to interruption of projection systems that include axons near the ventral horn.

At the level of a superficial section of the cALC, a lesion of the central core of the spinal cord could be made by inserting an electrode in the dorsomedial septum, minimizing damage to the dorsal columns. Radio-frequency or electrolytic lesions can be regulated in size and have been utilized for midline myelotomy and chordotomy (Hitchcock, 1974; Mullen *et al.,* 1965). The central core lesion is expected to add considerably to the effects of anterolateral chordotomy on pain (especially deep and midline pain; Honda, 1985; Sourek, 1977). Few side effects are produced by superficial chordotomy or midline myelotomy (involving the core region), but paresthesias can occur after each lesion. In the case of myelotomy involving both the STT and the core regions, paresthesias are common but brief, lasting several weeks. Avoiding extensive damage to primary axons in the dorsal columns may prevent appearance of the mild paresthesias that are produced by myelotomy, and cutting the cSTT superficially (Figure 11) could prevent a disinhibition that may contribute to the development of paresthesias (Figure 9).

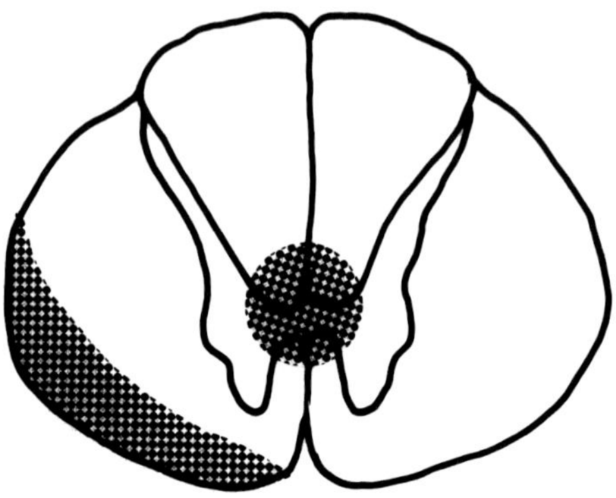

FIGURE 11. A diagram of lesions that are proposed to be effective in producing enduring loss of pain contralateral to the chordotomy with minimal involvement of pathways other than the STT and the central core. Addition of the core lesion to chordotomy should be particularly effective for deep pain and for pain that includes midline regions.

ACKNOWLEDGMENTS. Research presented in this chapter has been supported by grants NS 07261, NS 14899, NS 06347, NS 06835, and NS 07166 from the National Institute of Neurological and Communicative Disorders and Stroke.

References

ALBE-FESSARD, D., LEVANTE, A., AND LAMOUR, Y. Origin of spino-thalamic tract in monkeys. *Brain Res.* 65:503–509, 1974.

AMROMIN, G. D., AND CRUE, B. L., JR. Pathological specimens from cases undergoing posterior approach percutaneous stereotactic radiofrequency cervical cordotomy, in: *Pain Research and Treatment* (B. L. CRUE, JR., ed.), Academic Press, New York, 1975, pp. 213–225.

ANDERSSON, S. A., NORRSELL, K., AND NORSELL, U. Spinal pathways projecting to the cerebral first somatosensory area in the monkey. *J. Physiol. (Lond.)* 225:589–597, 1972.

APPLEBAUM, A. E., BEALL, J. E., FOREMAN, R. D., AND WILLIS, W. D. Organization and receptive fields of primate spinothalamic tract neurons. *J. Neurophysiol.* 38:572–586, 1975.

ARTHUR, R. P., AND SHELLEY, W. B. The peripheral mechanisms of itch in man, in: *Pain and Itch* (G. E. W. WOLSTENHOLME AND M. O'CONNOR eds.), American Physiological Society, Washington, 1959, pp. 84–97.

BARILARI, M. G., AND KUYPERS, H. G. J. M. Propriospinal fibers interconnecting the spinal enlargements in the cat. *Brain Res.* 14:321–330, 1969.

BASBAUM, A. I. Conduction of the effects of nocious stimulation by short-fiber multisynaptic systems of the spinal cord in the rat. *Exp. Neurol.* 40:699–716, 1973.

BASBAUM, A. I., AND FIELDS, H. L. Endogenous pain control systems: Brainstem spinal pathways and endorphin circuitry. *Annu. Rev. Neurosci.* 7:309–338, 1984.

BASBAUM, A. I., CLANTON, C. H., AND FIELDS, H. L. Three bulbospinal pathways from the rostral medulla of the cat: An autoradiographic study of pain modulating systems. *J. Comp. Neurol.* 178:2109–224, 1978.

BEKESY, G. VON. Lateral inhibition of heat sensations on the skin. *J. Appl. Physiol.* 17:1003–1008, 1962.

BERKLEY, K. J. Spatial relationships between the terminations of somatic sensory and motor pathways in the rostral brainstem of cats and monkeys. I. Ascending somatic sensory inputs to lateral diencephalon. *J. Comp. Neurol.* 193:283–317, 1980.

BERKLEY, K. J. Projections to the diencephalon arising from limbs, trunk and viscera, in: *Diencephalic Mechanisms of Pain Sensations* (D. ALBE-FESSARD, K. J. BERKLEY, L. KRUGER, K. J. RALSTON, III, AND W. D. WILLIS, eds.), *Brain Res. Rev.*, vol. 9. pp. 217–296, 1985.

BICKFORD, R. G. Experiments relating to the itch sensation, its peripheral mechanism, and central pathways. *Clin. Sci.* 3:377–386, 1938.

BIRKINFELD, R., AND FISHER, R. G. Successful treatment of causalgia of upper extremity with medullary spinothalamic tractotomy. Case report and review of the literature. *J. Neurosurg.* 20:303–311, 1963.

BOIVIE, J. An anatomical reinvestigation of the termination of the spinothalamic tract in the monkeys. *J. Comp. Neurol.* 186:343–369, 1979.

BOWSHER, D. Termination of the central pain pathway in man: The conscious appreciation of pain. *Brain* 80:606–622, 1957.

BOWSHER, D. Pain pathways and mechanisms, in: *Relief of Intractable Pain* (M. SWERDLOW, ed.), Elsevier, Amsterdam, 1983, pp. 1–23.

BREAZILE, J. E., AND KITCHELL, R. L. A study of fiber systems within the spinal cord of the domestic pig that subserve pain. *J. Comp. Neurol.* 133:373–382, 1968.

BROAGER, B. Commissural myelotomy. *Surg. Neurol.* 2:71–74, 1974.

BROWDER, J. AND GALLAGHER, J. P. Dorsal cordotomy for painful phantom limb. *Ann. Surg.* 128:456–469, 1948.

BROWN, A. G. *Organization in the Spinal Cord*, Springer-Verlag, New York, 1981.

BROWN, P. B. AND FUCHS, J. L. Somatotopic representation of hindlimb skin in cat dorsal horn. *J. Neurophysiol.* 38:1–9, 1975.

BROWN-SEQUARD, E. Lectures on the physiology and pathology of the nervous system. *Lancet* 2:593–596, 755–757, 821–823, 1868.

BRYAN, R. N., COULTER, J. D., AND WILLIS, W. D. Cells of origin of the spinocervical tract in the monkey. *Exp. Neurol.* 42:574–586, 1974.

BUMKE, O., AND FOERSTER, O. *Handbuch der Neurologie,* Springer-Verlag, Berlin, 1936.

BURGESS, P. R., AND PERL, E. R. Cutaneous mechanoreceptors and nociceptors, in: *Handbook of Sensory Physiology, Somatosensory System,* Vol. II (A. IGGO, ed.), Springer-Verlag, Berlin, 1973, pp. 29–79.

BURTON, H., AND LOEWY, A. D. Projections to the spinal cord from medullary somatosensory relay nuclei. *J. Comp. Neurol.* 173:773–792, 1977.

CAIN, W. S. Spatial discrimination of cutaneous warmth. *Am. J. Psychol.* 86:169–181, 1973.

CARPENTER, M. G., STEIN, B. M., AND SHRIVER, J. E. Central projections of spinal dorsal roots in the monkey II. Lower Thoracic, lumbosacral and coccygeal dorsal roots. *Am. J. Anat.* 123:75–118, 1968.

CASEY, K. L., AND MORROW, T. J. Supraspinal pain mechanisms in the cat, in: *Animal Pain Perception and Alleviation* (R. L. KITCHELL AND H. H. ERICKSON, eds.), American Physiological Society, Bethesda, 1983, pp. 63–82.

CASEY, K. L, HALL, B. R, AND MORROW, T. J. Effect of Spinal cord lesions on responses of cats to thermal pulses. *Pain* (Suppl. 1):S130, 1981.

CASSINARI, V., AND PAGNI, C. A. *Central Pain: A Neurosurgical Survey,* Harvard University Press, Cambridge, 1969.

CHUNG, J. M., KENSHALO, D. R., GERHART, K. D., AND WILLIS, W. D. Excitation of primate spinothalamic neurons by cutaneous C-fiber volleys. *J. Neurophysiol.* 42:1354–1369, 1979.

CHUNG, J. M., KEVETTER, G. A., WILLIS, W. D., AND COGGESHALL, R. E. An estimate of the ratio of propriospinal to long tract neurons in the sacral spinal cord of the rat. *Neurosci. Lett.* 44:173–177, 1984.

COLLINS, W. F., NULSEN, F. E., AND RANDT, C. T. Relation of peripheral nerve fibre size and sensation in man. *Arch. Neurol.* 3:381–385, 1960.

COOK, A. W., AND KAWAKAMI, Y. Commissural myelotomy. *J. Neurosurg.* 47:1–6, 1977.

COOK, A. W., NATHAN, P. W., AND SMITH, M. C. Sensory consequences of commissural myelotomy. *Brain* 107:547–568, 1984.

CRUTCHER, K. A., AND BINGHAM, W. G. Descending monoaminergic pathways in the primate spinal cord. *Am. J. Anat.* 153:159–164, 1978.

CULBERSON, J. L., AND BROWN, P. B. Projections of hindlimb dorsal roots to lumbosacral spinal cord of cat. *J. Neurophysiol.* 51:516–528, 1984.

DAVIS, L. E., HART, J. T., AND CRAIN, R. C. The pathway for visceral afferent impulses within the spinal cord. II. Experimental dilatation of the biliary ducts. *Surg. Gynecol. Obstet.* 48:647–651, 1929.

DENNY-BROWN, D. The enigma of crossed sensory loss with cord hemisection. *Adv. Pain Res. Ther.* 3:889–895, 1979.

DRAKE, C. G., AND MCKKENZIE, K. G. Mesencephalic tractotomy for pain. Experience with six cases. *J. Neurosurg.* 10:457–462, 1953.

FALCONER, M. A. Relief of phantom pain by cordotomy, in: *Pain* (R. S. KNIGHTON AND P. R. DUMKE, eds.), Little, Brown, Boston; 1966, p. 273–278.

FIELDS, H. L., CLANTON, C. H., AND ANDERSDON, S. D. Somatosensory properties of spinoreticular neurons in the cat. *Brain Res.* 120:49–66, 1977.

FOERSTER, O., AND GAGEL, O. Die Vordersetienstrangdurchschneidung beim Menshen. *Z. Ges. Neurol. Psychiatrie* 138:1–92, 1932.

FOREMAN, R. D., APPLEBAUM, A. E., BEALL, J. E., TREVINO, D. L., AND WILLIS, W. D. Responses of primate spinothalamic tract neurons to electrical stimulation of hindlimb peripheral nerves. *J. Neurophysiol.* 38:132–145, 1975.

FOREMAN, R. D., SCHMIDT, R. F., AND WILLIS, W. D. Convergence of muscle and cutaneous input onto primate spinothalamic tract neurons. *Brain Res.* 124:555–560, 1977.

FOREMAN, R. D., HANCOCK, M. B., AND WILLIS, W. D. Responses of spinothalamic tract cells in the thoracic spinal cord of the monkey to cutaneous and visceral inputs. *Pain* 11:149–162, 1981.

FRENCH, L. A., AND PEYTON, W. T. Ipsilateral sensory loss following cordotomy. *J. Neurosurg.* 5:403–404, 1948.

FRENCH, L. A., CHOU, S. N., AND STORY, J. L. Cervical tractotomy: Technique and clinical usefulness, in: *Pain* (R. S. KNIGHTON AND P. R. DUMKE, eds.), Little, Brown, Boston, 1966, pp. 311–320.

GARDNER, E., AND CUNEO, H. M. Lateral spinothalamic tract and associated tracts in man. *Arch. Neurol. Psychiatry* 53:423–430, 1945.

GIESLER, G. J., JR., MENETREY, D., AND BASBAUM, A. I. Differential origins of spinothalamic tract projections to medial and lateral thalamus in the rat. *J. Comp. Neurol.* 184:107–126, 1979.

GIESLER, G. J., YEZIERSKI, R. P., GERHART, K. D., AND WILLIS, W. D. Spinothalamic tract neurons that project to medial and/or lateral thalamic nuclei: Evidence for a physiologically novel population of spinal cord neurons. *J. Neurophysiol.* 46:1285–1308, 1981.

GRAF, C. J. Consideration in loss of sensory level after bilateral cervical cordotomy. *Arch. Neurol.* 3:410–415, 1960.

GRANT, F. C., AND WOOD, F. A. Experience with chordotomy. *Clin. Neurosurg.* 5:38–64, 1958.

GREENSPAN, J. D., RITZ, L. A., AND VIERCK, C. J., JR. Relationship between locus of chordotomy and time-course of hyporeactivity to noxious stimulation in monkeys. *Soc. Neurosci. Abstr.* 8:264, 1982.

HANCOCK, M. B., FOREMAN, R. D., AND WILLIS, W. D. Viscerosomatic interactions in lumbar spinal cord of the cat. *J. Neurophysiol.* 47:240–248, 1975.

HEAD, H., AND THOMPSON, T. The grouping of afferent impulses within the spinal cord. *Brain* 29: 537–741, 1906.

HITCHCOCK, E. Stereotactic cervical myelotomy. *J. Neurol. Neurosurg. Psychiatry* 33:224–230, 1970.

HITCHCOCK, E. Stereotactic myelotomy. *Proc. R. Soc. Med.* 67:771–772, 1974.

HODGE, C. J., APKARIAN, A. V., STEVENS, R., VOGILSANG, G., AND WISNICKI, H. J. Locus coeruleus modulation of dorsal horn unit responses to cutaneous stimulation. *Brain Res.* 204:415–420, 1981.

HONDA, C. Convergence of visceral and somatic afferent covergence onto neurons near the central canal in the sacral spinal cord of the cat. *J. Neurophysiol.* 53:1059–1078, 1985.

HONDA, C., AND PERL, E. R. Functional and morphological features of neurons in the midline region of the caudal spinal cord of the cat. *Brain Res.* (in press), 1985.

HORRAX, G. Experiences with chordotomy. *Arch. Surg.* 18:1140–1164, 1929.

HORRAX, G., AND PRICE, W. T., JR. High cervical chordotomy for relief of intractable pain in the arm, shoulder and upper chest. *Ann. Surg.* 139:567–585, 1954.

HYNDMAN, O. R. Lissauer's tract section; a contribution to chordotomy for the relief of pain. *J. Int. Coll. Surg.* 5:394–400, 1942.

HYNDMAN, O. R., AND VAN EPPS, C. Possibility of differential section of the spinothalamic tract. *Arch. Surg.* 38:1036–1053, 1939.

HYNDMAN, O. R., AND WOLKIN, J. Anterior chordotomy. *Arch. Neurol. Psychiatry* 50:129–148, 1943.

IGGO, A. Cutaneous receptors, in: *The Peripheral Nervous System,* Vol. 4 (J. I. HUBBARD, ed.), Plenum Press, New York, 1974, pp. 347–404.

JONES, E. G. The thalamus, in: *Chemical Neuroanatomy* (P. C. EMSON, ed.), Raven Press, New York, 1983, pp. 257–293.

JURGENS, U., AND PRATT, R. J. Role of the periaqueductal grey in vocal expression of emotion. *Brain Res.* 167:367–378, 1979.

KAHN, E. A., AND BARNEY, B. F. Anterolateral chordotomy for intractable pain of tabes dorsalis. *Arch. Neurol. Psychiatry* 38:467–472, 1937.

KAHN, E. A., AND RAND, R. W. On the anatomy of anterolateral cordotomy. *J. Neurosurg.* 9:611–619, 1952.

KARPLUS, J. P., AND KREIDEL, A. Ein Beitrag zur Kenntnis der Schmerzleitung im Ruckenmark. II. Mitteilung. *Pflugers Arch. Ges. Physiol.* 2107:134–139, 1925.

KELLY, D. D., AND GLUSMAN, M. Aversive thresholds following midbrain lesions. *J. Comp. Physiol. Psychol.* 66:25–34, 1968.

KENNARD, M. A. The course of ascending fibers in the spinal cord of the cat essential to the recognition of painful stimuli. *J. Comp. Neurol.* 100:511–524, 1954.

KERR, F. W. L. The ventral spinothalamic tract and other ascending systems of the ventral funiculus of the spinal cord. *J. Comp. Neurol.* 159:335–357, 1975a.

KERR, F. W. L. Pain, a new central inhibitory balance theory. *Mayo Clin. Proc.* 50:685–690, 1975b.

KERR, F. W. L. Neuroanatomical substrates of nociception in the spinal cord. *Pain* 1:325–356, 1975c.

KERR, F. W. L., AND LIPPMAN, H. H. The primate spinothalamic tract as demonstrated by anterolateral cordotomy and commissural myelotomy. *Adv. Neurol.* 4:147–156, 1974.

KEVETTER, G. A., HABER, L. H., YEZIERSKI, R. P. CHUNG, J. M., MARTIN, R. F., AND WILLIS, W. W. Cells of origin of the spinoreticular tract in the monkey. *J. Comp. Neurol.* 207:61–74, 1982.

KING, R. B. Postchordotomy studies of pain threshold. *Neurology (Minneap.)* 7:610–614, 1957.

KING, R. B. Anterior commissurotomy for intractable pain. *J. Neurosurg.* 47:7–11, 1977.

KRUGER, L., AND MOSSO, J. A. An evaluation of duality in the trigeminal afferent system. *Adv. Neurol.* 4:73–82, 1974.

KUMAZAWA, T., AND PERL, E. R. Excitation of marginal and substantia gelatinosa neurons in the primate spinal cord: Indications of their place in dorsal horn functional organization. *J. Comp. Neurol.* 177:417–434, 1978.

KUMAZAMA, T., PERL, E. R., BURGESS, P. R., AND WHITEHORN, D. Ascending projections from marginal zone (lamina I) neurons of the spinal dorsal horn. *J. Comp. Neurol.* 162:1–11, 1975.

KURU, M. *Sensory Paths in the Spinal Cord and Brain Stem of Man,* Sogensya, Tokyo, 1949.

LAHUERTA, J., LIPTON, S. AND BOWSHER, D. Anatomical correlations in human cutaneous pinprick analgesia and pain relief following unilateral cervical cordotomy. *Pain* (Suppl.) 2:S312, 1984.

LALONDE, J.-L., AND POIRIER, L. J. Study of various modalities of pain sensation in the monkey. *J. Comp. Neurol.* 112:185–195, 1959.

LAMOTTE, C. C., AND DE LANEROLLE, N. C. Ultrastructure of chemically defined neuron systems on the dorsal horn of the monkey. III. Serotonin immunoreactivity. *Brain Res.* 274:65–77, 1983.

LAMOTTE, C. C., JOHNS, D. R., AND DE LANEROLLE, N. C. Immunohistochemical evidence of indolamine neurons in monkey spinal cord. *J. Comp. Neurol.* 206:359–370, 1982.

LARSON, C. R., AND KISTLER, M. K. Periaqueductal gray neuronal activity associated with laryngeal EMG and vocalization in the awake monkey. *Neurosci. Lett.* 46:261–266, 1984.

LEVITT, M., AND SCHWARTZMAN, R. J. Spinal sensory tracts and two-point tactile sensitivity. *Anat. Rec.* 154:377, 1966.

LIGHT, A. R. Spinal projections of physiological identified axons from the rostral medula of cats. *Adv. Pain Res. Ther.* 5:373–379, 1983.

LIGHT, A. R., AND PERL, E. R. Spinal termination of functionally identified primary afferent neurons with slowly conducting myelinated fibers. *J. Comp. Neurol.* 186:133–150, 1979a.

LIGHT, A. R., AND PERL, E. R. Reexamination of the dorsal root projection to the spinal dorsal horn including observations on the differential termination of coarse and fine fibers. *J. Comp. Neurol.* 186:117–131, 1979b.

LIGHT, A. R., KAVOOKJIAN, A. M., AND PETRUSZ, P. The ultrastructure and synaptic connections of serotonin-immunoreactive terminals in spinal laminae I and II. *Somatosen. Res.* 1:33–50, 1983.

LIPPERT, R. G., HOSOBUCHI, Y., AND NIELSEN, S. L. Spinal commissurotomy. *Surg. Neurol.* 2:373–377, 1974.

LIPPMAN, H. H., AND KERR, F. W. L. Light and electron microscopic study of crossed ascending pathways in the anterolateral funiculus in monkey. *Brain Res.* 40:496–499, 1972.

LIPTON, S. Percutaneous cervical cordotomy. *Adv. Pain Res. Ther.* 2:425–438, 1979.

LOESER, J. D., AND WARD, A. A. Some effects of deafferentation on neurons of the cat spinal cord. *Arch. Neurol.* 17:629–636, 1967.

MANTYH, P. W. The spinothalamic tract in the primate: A re-examination using wheatgerm agglutinin conjugated to horseradish peroxidase. *Neuroscience* 9:847–862, 1983.

MARKS, L. E., AND STEVENS, J. C. Spatial summation of warmth: Influence of duration and configuration of the stimulus. *Am. J. Psychol.* 86:251–267, 1973.

MATSUSHITA, M., AND TANAMI, T. Contralateral termination of primary afferent axons in the sacral and caudal segments of the cat, as studied by anterograde transport of horseradish peroxidase. *J. Comp. Neurol.* 220:206–218, 1983.

MATSUSHITA, M., HOSOYA, Y. AND IKEDA, M. Anatomical organization of the spinocerebellar system in the cat, as studied by retrograde transport of horseradish peroxidase. *J. Comp. Neurol.* 184:81–106, 1979.

MAUNZ, R. A., PITTS, M. G., AND PETERSON, B. W. Cat spinoreticular neurons: Locations, responses and changes in responses during repetitive stimulation. *Brain Res.* 148:365–379, 1978.

MAY, W. P. The afferent path. *Brain* 29:742–803, 1906.

MAYER, D. J., PRICE, D. D., BECKER, D. P., AND YOUNG, H. F. Threshold for pain from anterolateral quadrant stimulation as a predictor of success of percutaneous cordotomy for relief of pain. *J. Neurosurg.* 43:445–447, 1975.

MAZARS, G., ROSE, R., AND PANSINI, A. Stereotactic coagulation of the spinothalamic tract for intractable trigeminal pain. *J. Neurol. Neurosurg. Psychiatry* 23:352–361, 1960.

MCMAHON, S. B., AND WALL, P. D. A system of rat spinal cord lamina 1 cells projecting through the contralateral dorsolateral funiculus. *J. Comp. Neurol.* 214:217–223, 1983.

MEHLER, W. R. Some observations on secondary ascending afferent systems in the central nervous system, in: *Pain* (R. S. KNIGHTON AND P. R. DUMKE, eds.), Little, Brown, Boston, 1966, pp. 11–32.

MEHLER, W. R. Some neurological species differences—*a posteriori*. *Ann. N.Y. Acad. Sci.* 167:424–468, 1969.

MEHLER, W. R. Central pain and the spinothalamic tract. *Adv. Neurol.* 4:127–146, 1974.

MEHLER, W. R., FEFERMAN, M. E., AND NAUTA, W. J. H. Ascending axon degeneration following anterolateral cordotomy. An experimental study in the monkey. *Brain* 83:718–750, 1960.

MELZACK, R., AND CASEY, K. L. Sensory, motivational, and central control determinants of pain, in: *The Skin Senses* (D. R. KENSHALO, ed.), Charles C. Thomas, Springfield, IL, 1968, pp. 423–439.

MELZACK, R., AND LOESER, J. D. Phantom body pain in paraplegics: Evidence for a central "pattern generating mechanism" for pain. *Pain* 4:195–210, 1978.

MENDELL, L. M., AND WALL, P. D. Responses of single dorsal cord cells to peripheral cutaneous unmyelinated fibers. *Nature* 206:97–99, 1965.

MIKULA, F., SIROKY, J., AND ZAPLETAL, B. Le traitement des crises gastraligiques par la tractotomie mesencephalique bilaterale et ses complications auditives inattendues. *Rev. Otoneurooftal. (Buenos Aires)* 31:456–463, 1959.

MOFFIE, D. Spinothalamic fibres, pain conduction and cordotomy. *Clin. Neurol. Neurosurg.* 4:261–268, 1975.

MOLENAAR, I., AND KUYPERS, H. G. J. M. Cells of origin of propriospinal fibers and of fibers ascending to supraspinal levels. A HRP study in cat and rhesus monkey. *Brain Res.* 152:429–450, 1978.

MULLEN, S., HEKMATPANAH, J., DOBBEN, G., AND BECKMAN, B. A. Percutaneous, intramedullary cordotomy utilizing the unipolar anodal electrolytic lesion. *J. Neurosurg.* 22:548–553, 1965.

NADELHAFT, I., ROPPOLO, J., MORGAN, D., AND DE GROAT, W. D. Parasympathetic preganglionic neurons and visceral primary afferents in monkey sacral spinal cord revealed following application of horseradish peroxidase to pelvic nerve. *J. Comp. Neurol.* 216:36–52, 1983.

NAHIN, R. L., MADSEN, A. M., AND GEISLER, G. J., JR. Anatomical and physiological studies of the gray matter surrounding the spinal cord central canal. *J. Comp. Neurol.* 220:321–335, 1983.

NASHOLD, B. S., JR. WILSON, W. P., AND SLAUGHTER, G. The midbrain and pain. *Adv. Neurol.* 4:191–196, 1974.

NATHAN, P. W. Reference of sensation at the spinal level. *J. Neurol. Neurosurg. Psychiatry* 19:88–100, 1956.

NATHAN, P. W. Results of antero-lateral cordotomy for pain in cancer. *J. Neurol. Neurosurg. Psychiatry* 26:353–362, 1963.

NATHAN, P. W., AND RICE, R. C. The localization of warm stimuli. *Neurology (Minneap.)* 16:533–540, 1966.

NATHAN, P. W., AND SMITH, M. C. The centrifugal pathway for micturition within the spinal cord. *J. Neurol. Neurosurg. Psychiatry* 21:177–18"9, 1958.

NATHAN, P. W., AND SMITH, M. C. Fasciculi proprii of the spinal cord in man. *Brain* 82:610–668, 1959.

NATHAN, P. W., AND SMITH, M. C. Some tracts of the anterior and lateral columns of the spinal cord, in: *Pain* (R. S. KNIGHTON AND P. R. DUMKE, eds.), Little, Brown, Boston, 1966, pp. 47–57.

NATHAN, P. W., AND SMITH, M. C. Clinico–anatomical correlation in anterolateral cordotomy. *Adv. Pain Res. Ther.* 3:921–926, 1979.

NAUTA, W. J. H., AND KUYPERS, H. G. J. M. Some ascending pathways in the brain stem reticular formation, in: *Reticular Formation of the Brain* (H. H. JASPER, L. D. PROCTOR, R. S. KNIGHTON, W. C. NOSHAY AND R. T. COSTELLO, eds.), Little, Brown, Boston, 1958, pp. 3–30.

NETSKY, M. G. Syringomyelia. *Arch. Neurol. Psychiatry* 70:741–777, 1953.

NIJENSOHN, D. E., AND KERR, F. W. L. The ascending projections of the dorsolateral funiculus of the spinal cord in the primate. *J. Comp. Neurol.* 161:459–470, 1975.

NOORDENBOS, W. *Pain,* Elsevier, New York, 1959.

OCHOA, J. Peripheral unmyelinated units in man: Structure, function, disorder and role in sensation. *Adv. Pain Res. Ther.* 6:53–68, 1984.

OGLE, W. S., FRENCH, L. A., AND PEYTON, W. T. Experiences with high cervical chordotomy. *J. Neurosurg.* 13:81–87, 1956.

PAPO, I. Spinal posterior rhizotomy and commissural myelotomy in the treatment of cancer pain. *Adv. Pain Res. Ther.* 2:439–448, 1979a.

PAPO, I. Open cordotomy in the treatment of cancer pain. *Adv. Pain Res. Ther.* 2:449–452, 1979b.

PAPO, I., AND LUONGO, A. High cervical commissural myelotomy in the treatment of pain. *J. Neurol. Neurosurg. Psychiatry* 39:705–710, 1976.

PETREN, K. Ein Beitrag zur Pfage vom Verlaufe der Bahnen der Hautsinne im Ruckenmarke. *Scand. Arch. Physiol.* 13:9–98, 1902.

POIRIER, L. J., AND BERTRAND, C. Experimental and anatomical investigation of the lateral spinothalamic and spinotectal tracts. *J. Comp. Neurol.* 102:745–758, 1955.

POOL., J. L. Posterior cordotomy for relief of phantom limb pain. *Ann. Surg.* 124:386–391, 1946.

PRICE, D. D., AND DUBNER, R. Neurons that subserve the sensory discriminative aspects of pain. *Pain* 3:307–338, 1977.

PRICE, D. D., AND MAYER, D. J. Neurophysiological characterization of anterolateral quadrant neurons subserving pain in *M. mulatta. Pain* 1:59–72, 1975.

PRICE, D. D., HAYES, R. L., RUDA, M., AND DUBNER, R. Spatial and temporal transformations of input to spinothalamic tract neurons and their relation to somatic sensations. *J. Neurophysiol.* 41:993–947, 1978.

PUTNAM, T. J. Myelotomy of the commissure. *Arch. Neurol. Psychiatry* 32:1189–1193, 1934.

RAMON Y CAJAL, S. *Histologie du Systeme Nerveux de l'Homme et des Vertebres,* Vol. I, Instituto Cajal, Madrid, 1909.

RANSON, S. W. The tract of Lissauer and the substantia gelatinosa Rolandi. *Am. J. Anat.* 16:97–126, 1914.

RANSON, S. W., AND VON HESS, C. L. The conduction within the spinal cord of the afferent impulses producing pain and the vasomotor reflexes. *Am. J. Physiol.* 38:128–152, 1915.

RAY, B. S., AND WOLFF, H. G. Studies on pain. "Spread of pain"; evidence on site of spread within the neuraxis of effects of painful stimulation. *Arch. Neurol. Psychiatry* 53:257–261, 1945.

REXED, B. The cytoarchitectonic organization of the spinal cord in the cat. *J. Comp. Neurol.* 196:415–466, 1952.

RITZ, L. A., GREENSPAN, J. D. AND VIERCK, C. J. JR. Behavioral tests of the effects of anterolateral chordotomy in primates. *Pain* (Suppl.) 1: 289, 1981.

ROULHAC, C. E. High cervical chordotomy. A preliminary report. *Surgery* 34:288–295, 1953.

RUSTIONI, A. AND KAUFMAN, A. B. Identification of cells of origin of non-primary afferents to the dorsal column nuclei of the cat. *Exp. Brain Res.* 27:1–14, 1977.

SCHEIBEL, M. E., AND SCHEIBEL, A. B. Patterns of organization in specific and non-specific thalamic fields, in: *The Thalamus,* (D. P. PURPURA and M. D. YAHR, eds.), Columbia University Press, New York, 1966, pp. 13–47.

SCHMAUSS, C., AND YAKSH, T. L. *In vivo* studies on spinal opiate receptor systems mediating antinociception. II. Pharmacological profiles suggesting a differential association of *mu, delta* and *kappa* receptors with visceral chemical and cutaneous thermal stimuli in the rat. *J. Pharmacol. Exp. Ther.* 228:1–12, 1984.

SCHNEIDER, R. C. Syringomyelia, in: *Correlative Neurosurgery* (R. C. SCHNEIDER, E. A. KAHN, E. C. CROSBY, AND J. TAREN, eds.), Charles C. Thomas, Springfield, IL, 1982, pp. 1010–1049.

SCHVARCZ, J. R. Stereotactic extralemniscal myelotomy. *J. Neurol. Neurosurg. Psychiatry* 39:53–57, 1976.

SCHVARCZ, J. R. Functional exploration of the spinomedullary junction. *Acta Neurochir.* 24 (Suppl.): 179–185, 1977.

SCHWARTZ, H. G. High cervical cordotomy—technique and results. *Clin. Neurosurg.* 8:282–293, 1962.

SCHWARTZ, H. G., AND O'LEARY, J. L. Section of the spinothalamic tract at the level of the inferior olive. *Arch. Neurol. Psychiatry* 47:293–304, 1942.

SHEALLY, C. N., TYNER, C. F., AND TASLITZ, N. Physiological evidence of bilateral spinal projections of pain fibers in cats and monkeys. *J. Neurosurg.* 24:708–713, 1966.

SHEALLY, C. N., MORTIMER, J. T., AND HAGFORS, N. R. Dorsal column electroanalgesia. *J. Neurosurg.* 32:560–564, 1970.

SHERMAN, J. C., AND ARIEFF, A. J. Dissociation between pain and temperature in spinal cord lesions. *J. Nerv. Ment. Dis.* 108:285–292, 1948.

SMITH, M. C. Observations on the topography of the lateral column of the human cervical spinal cord. *Brain* 80:263–272, 1957.

SOUREK, K. Commissural myelotomy. *J. Neurosurg.* 31:524–527, 1969.

SOUREK, K. Mediolongitudinal myelotomy. *Prog. Neurol. Surg.* 8:15–34, 1977.

SPILLER, W. G., AND MARTIN, E. The treatment of persistent pain of organic origin in the lower part of the body by division of the anterolateral column of the spinal cord. *J.A.M.A.* 58:1489–1490, 1912.

STOOKEY, B. Further light on the transmission of pain and temperature within the spinal cord: Human cordotomy to abolish pain sense without destroying temperature sense. *J. Nerve. Ment. Dis.* 69:552–557, 1929.

SZENTAGOTHAI, J. Neuronal and synaptic arrangement in the substantia gelatinosa Rolandi. *J. Comp. Neurol.* 122:219–240, 1964.

TAREN, J. A., AND KAHN, E. A. Thoracic anterolateral cordotomy, in: *Pain* (R. S. KNIGHTON and P. R. DUMKE, eds.), Little, Brown, Boston, 1966, pp. 299–310.

TAREN, J. A. DAVIS, R., AND CROSBY, E. C. Target physiologic corroboration in stereotaxic cervical cordotomy. *J. Neurosurg.* 30:569–584, 1969.

TASKER, R. R., AND ORGAN, L. W. Percutaneous cordotomy. *Confin. Neurol.* 35:110–117, 1973.

TORVIK, A. Sensory motor and reflex changes in two cases of intractable pain after stereotactic mesencephalic tractotomy. *J. Neurol. Neurosurg. Psychiatry* 22:299–305, 1959.

TOWER, S., BODIAN, D., AND HOWE, H. Isolation of intrinsic and motor mechanisms of the monkey's spinal cord. *J. Neurophysiol.* 4:338–397, 1941.

TREVINO, D. L., AND CARSTENS, E. Confirmation of the location of spinothalamic neurons in the cat and monkey by the retrograde transport of horseradish peroxidase. *Brain Res.* 98:177–182, 1975.

TREVINO, D. L., COULTER, J. D., AND WILLIS, W. D. Location of cells of origin of spinothalamic tract in lumber enlargement of the monkey. *J. Neurophysiol.* 36:750–761, 1973.

TUCKETT, R. P. Response of cutaneous receptors to a pruritic stimulus. *Soc. Neurosci. Abstr.* 6:428, 1980.

TURNBULL, F. Cordotomy for thalamic pain. *Yale J. Biol. Med.* 11:411–414, 1940.

TURNER, W. A. On hemisection of the spinal cord. *Brain* 14:496–522, 1891.
UCHIDA, Y., AND MURAO, S. Bradykinin-induced excitation of afferent cardiac sympathetic nerve fibers. *Jpn. Heart J.* 15:84–91, 1974.
UCHIDA, Y., KAMISAKA, K., AND UEDA, H. Two types of renal mechanoreceptors. *Jpn. Heart J.* 12:233–241, 1971.
UCHIDA, Y., KAMISAKA, K., MURAO, S., AND UEDA, H. Mechanosensitivity of afferent cardiac sympathetic nerve fibers. *Am. J. Physiol.* 226:1088–1093, 1974.
VAN GEHUCHTEN, A., *Anatomie du Systeme Nerveux de l'Homme,* Louvain, 1906.
VIERCK, C. J., JR. Alterations of spatio-tactile discrimination after lesions of primate spinal cord. *Brain Res.* 58:69–79, 1973.
VIERCK, C. J., JR. Tactile movement detection and discrimination following dorsal column lesions in monkeys. *Exp. Brain Res.* 20:311–346, 1974.
VIERCK, C. J., JR. Absolute and differential sensitivities to touch stimuli after spinal cord lesions in monkeys. *Brain Res.* 146:279–294, 1977.
VIERCK, C. J., JR. The spinal lemniscal pathways, in: Handbook of the Spinal Cord (R. DAVIDOFF, ed.), Marcel Dekker, New York, 1984, pp. 673–750.
VIERCK, C. J., JR., AND COOPER, B. Y. Guidelines for assessing pain reactions and pain modulation in laboratory animal subjects. *Adv. Pain Res. Ther.* 6:305–322, 1984.
VIERCK, C. J., JR., AND LUCK, M. M. Loss and recovery of reactivity to noxious stimuli in monkeys with primary spinothalamic chordotomies, followed by secondary and tertiary lesions of other cord sectors. *Brain* 102:233–248, 1979.
VIERCK, C. J., JR., AND RAND, R. Localization of touch on glabrous skin following dorsal column lesion in a primate. *Soc. Neurosci. Abstr.* 5:715, 1979.
VIERCK, C. J., JR., HAMILTON, D. M., AND THORNBY, J. I. Pain reactivity of monkeys after lesions to the dorsal and lateral columns of the spinal cord. *Exp. Brain Res.* 13:140–158, 1971.
VIERCK, C. J., JR., COHEN, R. H., AND COOPER, B. Y. Effect of spinal tractotomy on spatial sequence recognition in macaques. *J. Neurosci.* 3:280–290, 1983a.
VIERCK, C. J., JR., COOPER, B. Y., AND COHEN, R. H. Human and non-human primates reactions to painful electrocutaneous stimuli and to morphine, in: *Animal Pain Perception and Alleviation* (R. L. KITCHELL AND H. H. ERICKSON, eds.), American Physiological Society, Bethesda, 1983b, pp. 117–132.
VIERCK, C. J., JR., COOPER, B. Y., FRANZEN, O., RITZ, L. A., AND GREENSPAN, J. D. Behavioral analysis of CNS pathways and transmitter systems involved in conduction and inhibition of pain sensations and reactions in primates, in: *Progress in Psychobiology and Physiological Psychology,* Vol. 10 (J. SPRAGUE AND A. EPSTEIN, eds.), Academic Press, New York, 1983c, pp. 113–165.
VORIS, H. C. Ipsilateral sensory loss following chordotomy: Report of a case. *Arch. Neurol. Psychiatry* 65:95–96, 1951.
WALKER, A. E. The spinothalamic tract in man. *Arch. Neurol. Psychiatry* 43:284–298, 1940.
WALKER, A. E. Central representation of pain. *Proc. Assoc. Res. Nerv. Ment. Dis.* 23:63–85, 1943.
WALKER, A. E. The neurosurgical treatment of intractable pain. *Lancet* 70:279–282, 1950.
WALL, P. D. Cancer pain—neurogenic mechanisms. *Pain* (Suppl.) 2: S197, 1984.
WALL, P. D., AND NOORDENBOS, W. Sensory functions which remain in man after complete transection of dorsal columns. *Brain* 100:641–653, 1977.
WEAVER, T. A., AND WALKER, A. E. Topical arrangement within the spinothalamic tract of the monkey. *Arch. Neurol. Psychiatry* 46:877–883, 1941.
WESTLUND, K. N., BOWKER, R. M., ZIEGLER, M. G., AND COULTER, J. D. Origins and terminations of descending noradrenergic projections to the spinal cord of monkey. *Brain Res.* 292:1–16, 1984.
WHITE, J. C. Sensory innervation of the viscera. Studies on visceral afferent neurones in man based on neurosurgical procedures for the relief of intractable pain. *Proc. Assoc. Res. Nerv. Ment. Dis.* 23:373–390, 1943.
WHITE, J. C. Anterolateral cordotomy—its effectiveness in relieving pain of non-malignant disease. *Neurochirurgia* 6:83–102, 1963.

WHITE, J. C. Operations for the relief of pain in the torso and extremities: Evaluation of their effectiveness over long periods, in: *Pain* (A. SOULAIRAC, J. CAHN, AND J. CHARPENTIER, eds.), Academic Press, New York, 1968, pp. 503–519.

WHITE, J. C., AND SWEET, W. H. *Pain and the Neurosurgeon: A Forty-Year Experience,* Charles C. Thomas, Springfield, IL, 1969.

WHITE, J. C., SWEET, W. H., HAWKINS, R., AND NILGES, R. G. Anterolateral cordotomy: Results, complications and causes of failure. *Brain* 73:346–367, 1950.

WHITE, J. C., RICHARDSON, E. P., JR, AND SWEET, W. H. Upper thoracic cordotomy for relief of pain. *Ann. Surg.* 144:407–420, 1956.

WHITSEL, B. L., PETRUCELLI, L. M., AND SAPIRO, G. Modality representation in the lumbar and cervical fasiculus gracilis of squirrel monkey. *Brain Res.* 15:67–78, 1969.

WILLCOCKSON, W. S., CHUNG, J. M., HORI, Y., LEE, K. H., AND WILLIS, W. D. Effects of iontophoretically released amino acids and amines on primate spinothalamic tract cells. *J. Neurosci.* 4:732–740, 1984.

WILLIS, W. D. Control of nociceptive transmission in the spinal cord, in: *Progress in Sensory Physiology,* Vol. 3 (D. OTTOSON, ed.), Springer-Verlag, New York, 1982, pp. 1–159.

WILLIS, W. D., AND COGGESHALL, R. E. *Sensory Mechanisms of the Spinal Cord,* Plenum Press, New York, 1978.

WILLIS, W. D., TREVINO, D. L., COULTER, J. D., AND MAUNZ, R. A. Responses of primate spinothalamic tract neurons to natural stimulation of hindlimb. *J. Neurophysiol.* 37:358–372, 1974.

WILLIS, W. D., KENSHALO, D. R., JR. AND LEONARD, R. B. The cells of origin of the primate spinothalamic tract. *J. Comp. Neurol.* 188:543–574, 1979.

WYCIS, H. T., AND SPIEGEL, E. A. Long-range results in the treatment of intractable pain by stereotaxic midbrain surgery. *J. Neurosurg.* 19:101–107, 1962.

YEZIERSKI, R. P. GERHART, K. D., SCHROCK, F. J., AND WILLIS, W. D. A further examination of effects of cortical stimulation on primate spinothalamic tract cells. *J. Neurophysiol.* 49:424–441, 1983.

YOSS, R. C. Studies of the spinal cord. Part 3. Pathways for deep pain within the spinal cord and brain. *Neurology (Minneap.)* 3:163–175, 1953.

13
Sensory-Discriminative Capacities of Nociceptive Pathways and Their Modulation by Behavior

RONALD DUBNER, M. CATHERINE BUSHNELL, AND GARY H. DUNCAN

A. *Introduction*

Considerable progress has been made on the characterization of neural pathways participating in the sensory component of pain sensations. The sensory component of pain refers to the quality as well as the location, intensity, and temporal aspects of noxious or tissue-damaging stimuli. Recent advances include knowledge about the coding of pain signals and how these signals can be modified by control systems originating at other brain sites.

B. *Coding of Sensory-Discriminative Information*

It often is assumed that neural pathways involved in signaling pain merely provide information about the threat of tissue-damaging stimulation and have minimal capacities for providing information about fine discriminative aspects of the stimulus. This assumption has led to the idea that sensations of pain are the result of excessive stimulation of all types of peripheral receptors (Melzack, 1973).

RONALD DUBNER, M. CATHERINE BUSHNELL, AND GARY H. DUNCAN • Neurobiology and Anesthesiology Branch, National Institute of Dental Research, National Institutes of Health, Bethesda, Maryland 20892.

Alternative theories advocate the presence of specialized neural pathways that are exclusively involved in the coding of pain (see Dubner *et al.*, 1978; Melzack, 1973; Perl, 1971). This notion has received support from the recent findings that specific nociceptors in skin, muscle, and viscera and neurons in the medullary and spinal dorsal horns provide sensory-discriminative information about the intensity and location of noxious stimuli (see Dubner and Bennett, 1983, for review). For example, only two classes of peripheral nociceptors respond to noxious heat (temperatures of 45°C or greater) as well as to other forms of intense stimulation. One class, the unmyelinated polymodal nociceptors, respond to intense thermal, mechanical, and chemical stimuli and have remarkably similar characteristics in many different species (see Burgess and Perl, 1973; Price and Dubner, 1977; Dubner and Bennett, 1983, for review). The other class, called heat nociceptors or mechanothermal nociceptors, has myelinated axons that conduct in the A-δ range. They have been found only in monkey (see Dubner and Bennett, 1983) and human (Adriaensen *et al.*, 1983). Both A-δ heat nociceptors (AHNs) and C polymodal nociceptors (CPNs) respond differentially to temperatures in the 45–49°C range (Figure 1). However, from such findings alone, one cannot conclude that there are exclusive, specialized nociceptive pathways in the brain or that the central nervous system utilizes specific information about stimulus quality and intensity coded by nociceptive neurons. The alternative interpretation, that pain sensations are coded by the combined activity of all afferent fibers activated by the stimulus and that nociceptive pathways merely provide information about the presence of noxious stimuli, cannot be ruled out.

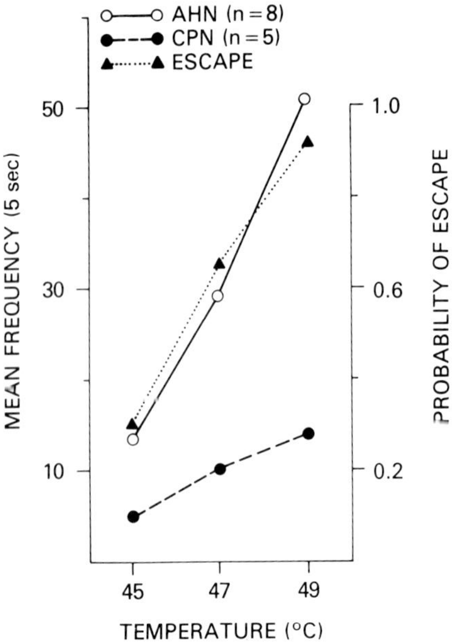

FIGURE 1. Range of maximum thermal sensitivity of AHNs and CPNs compared with the temperature range over which monkeys escape noxious (>45°C) thermal stimuli. Magnitude of the neuronal response, expressed as the mean frequency of impulses in the 5-s period after stimulus onset, is plotted against final temperatures. The probability of escape to 45°, 47°, and 49°C in two monkeys is plotted on the same graph.

The importance of specialized neural pathways in the perception of pain can be more firmly established when neural studies are combined with behavioral data related to the sensory-discriminative aspects of pain. One strategy is to examine the response range of nociceptive neurons and to determine which class or classes of such neurons can provide the minimal amount of information necessary to account for a particular behavior related to pain. For example, if an animal can be trained to discriminate different intensities of noxious heat stimulation and only one class of nociceptive neurons exhibits similar or greater thermal sensitivity, then these neurons most likely are essential for that discriminative behavior. Furthermore, evidence that animals can make fine discriminations in the noxious range would establish that the specificity observed in peripheral nociceptive pathways is preserved centrally as precisely as it is in nonnociceptive pathways (Burgess and Perl, 1973; Dubner *et al.,* 1978).

C. *Specialized Peripheral Nociceptive Pathways Essential for Pain Discrimination*

We have trained monkeys to discriminate and escape noxious thermal stimuli applied to the face (Dubner *et al.,* 1976, 1977). In this task, the monkey presses a panel to initiate a trial, and at the same time the temperature at the skin–thermode junction changes from 35°C to final temperatures varying from 37° to 51°C. To receive a grape juice reward, the monkey must continue to press the panel button until the temperature returns to the 35°C baseline, a random time period of 2 to 8 s. If the temperature shift is aversive to the animal, he can release the button and escape the stimulus but receives no reward. Figure 1 shows that the temperature range over which monkeys escape noxious thermal stimuli (>45°C) corresponds closely to the range of maximum sensitivity of AHNs and CPNs.

Escape probabilities ranged from approximately 0.3 at 45°C to 0.9 at 49°C. A further examination of the escape latency distribution revealed that twice as many escapes occurred within 3.0 s of stimulus onset on 51°C trials as on 49°C trials. Comparing this latency distribution to the latency of discharge of AHNs and CPNs revealed that these fast escapes were dependent on the discharge of AHNs. Within 2.5 s of stimulus onset, the cumulative discharge of AHNs on 51°C trials was significantly different from the discharge on 49°C trials ($P < 0.025$, paired *t*-test). This difference occurred early enough to account for the higher proportion of fast escapes to 51°C than to 49°C. We conclude from these findings that AHNs are the only nociceptors that can provide the minimal information necessary for the monkeys' fast escapes. They provide unique and specific information about noxious thermal input that is essential in the performance of this learned behavior.

This behavioral escape task, however, does not provide information on the monkeys' ability to make fine thermal discriminations within the noxious heat range. Evidence for such discriminative capacity would clearly establish that nociceptive pathways code stimulus intensity and that such capabilities are dependent on the activity of specific nociceptors.

We addressed this question by having humans and one monkey perform two-choice discriminations between simultaneous noxious heat stimuli applied to both sides of the face (Bushnell *et al.*, 1983b; Dubner *et al.*, 1983). Subjects positioned two contact thermodes above their upper lip while seated in front of a panel with three response buttons. When the lower button was pressed, the temperature at the thermode–skin interface changed from 35°C to some predetermined temperature, with one thermode reaching a higher final temperature than the other. Subjects released the lower button and pressed the right upper button if the right probe was hotter and the left upper button if the left probe was hotter. A beep sounded after correct responses. A male rhesus monkey was trained to perform the task in the same experimental situation with water used as a reinforcer.

All subjects were presented stimulus pairs in the innocuous and noxious ranges. The humans received three standard stimuli, 39°, 43°, and 47°C, and the monkey received two standard stimuli, 39° and 47°C. Each standard stimulus was paired with six comparison stimuli presented on the other side of the face. The comparison stimuli ranged from 0.0°C to 1.0°C less than the standard for the humans and from 0.0°C to 4.0°C less than the standard for the monkey. Mean percent correct was calculated for the 100 trials of each temperature pair presented. The minimum stimulus difference required to produce a sensation difference 50% of the time, known as the difference threshold, was determined. Since this was a two-choice paradigm, 75% correct implied that the subject was discriminating the temperature difference 50% of the time.

Figure 2 shows that humans and the monkey produced more accurate discriminations at 47°C than at 39°C for every temperature difference greater than zero. The mean percent correct for all humans studied was significantly greater at 47°C than at 39°C (paired *t*-test, $P < 0.05$). Figure 2 also shows that the monkey's performance was virtually indistinguishable from that of the humans at 47°C. At 39°C, the monkey never performed as well as the humans, although he was given extensive training in the innocuous warming range. Note that the monkey performed more accurately at 47°C than at 39°C despite the extensive training received at 39°C.

Every human subject and the monkey produced smaller difference thresholds at 47°C than at 39°C. The mean difference threshold for humans of 0.31°C at 47°C was significantly different from the mean difference threshold for humans of 0.52°C at 39°C (paired *t*-test, $P < 0.05$). The 47°C difference threshold of the monkey was 0.27°C, a value comparable to that of the human subjects. At 39°C, the monkey showed a difference threshold of 1.50°C, a value larger than any of the human 39°C difference thresholds.

These findings demonstrate that human and monkey can discriminate small differences between noxious thermal stimuli applied to the face and that the discriminative capabilities of the two species are quite similar within

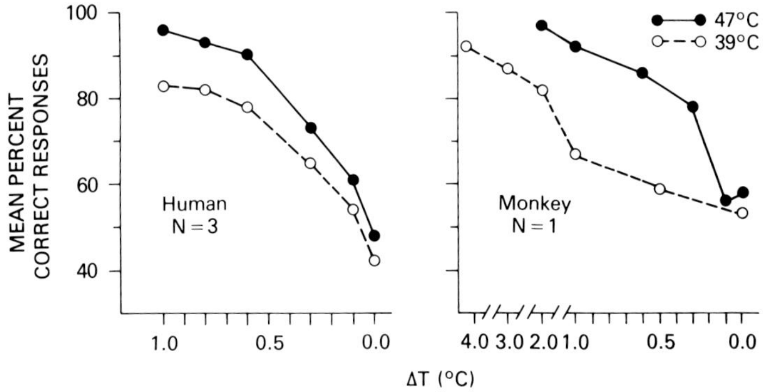

FIGURE 2. Percentage of correct responses averaged for three human subjects and for a monkey at all temperature differences (ΔT) when the standard stimulus was 47°C (solid lines) and 39°C (dashed lines). Each point is the average of 100 trials. Data from the fourth subject was similar but has been omitted because standard stimuli were slightly different. The performance of the human subjects at 43°C has been omitted for ease of visual comparison to the monkey data but was intermediate to that of 39°C and 47°C. (Adapted from Bushnell *et al.*, 1983b.)

the noxious range. Other studies have reported detection thresholds on human palmar skin of 0.1°C at 47°C (Robinson *et al.*, 1983) and on human digital pads of 0.3° at 40°C (Handwerker *et al.*, 1982), comparable to our results. It appears that thermal sensitivity in the noxious range is not peculiar to facial cutaneous zones but rather is a general characteristic of thermal nociceptive pathways in primates.

The comparable discriminative ability of human and monkey in the noxious heat range suggests that heat sensitivity likely is coded by similar nociceptive afferents in these species. The AHNs and CPNs innervating the monkey facial skin are the only two afferent populations capable of providing this information (Beitel and Dubner, 1976; Dubner and Hu, 1977; Dubner *et al.*, 1977). Warm fibers that exhibit maximum responses to warming of the skin (Sumino *et al.*, 1973) are not sensitive to changes in stimulus intensity in this range and cannot provide such discriminative information (LaMotte and Campbell, 1978; Sumino *et al.*, 1973).

Using another approach, recent studies have correlated human pain report with the discharge of monkey nociceptors. There is evidence that AHNs alone are sufficient to account for the highly localized, heat-induced, first pain sensation in humans (Price *et al.*, 1977). It also has been shown that activity in monkey and human CPNs increases in a parallel fashion with human judgments of pain magnitude, supporting a role for unmyelinated nociceptors in coding pain sensations (LaMotte and Campbell, 1978).

These results indicate that peripheral nociceptors can code unique and specific information that is essential for the fine discrimination of noxious heat. The findings provide definitive evidence that activity in specific peripheral nociceptive pathways is essential for fine discriminations of stimulus intensity in the noxious range.

D. *Specialized Central Nociceptive Pathways Essential for Pain Discrimination*

Two general classes of projection neurons and interneurons in the medullary and spinal dorsal horns receive input from peripheral nociceptors (Dubner and Bennett, 1983; Price and Dubner, 1977; Willis and Coggeshall, 1978. See Cervero, Chapter 9; Price, Chapter 18; and Le Bars *et al.*, Chapter 19). One class, referred to as nociceptive-specific (NS) neurons, responds only to intense mechanical stimuli or mechanical and thermal stimuli and receives input exclusively from different types of nociceptors. The second class, called wide-dynamic-range (WDR) neurons, is activated by hair movement and other weak mechanical stimuli but responds maximally to intense and potentially tissue-damaging mechanical stimulation. Many WDR neurons respond to noxious heat. Wide-dynamic-range neurons receive input from myelinated, low-threshold mechanoreceptors as well as from nociceptors.

We addressed the question of whether these neurons could code sensory discriminative information required for the carrying out of the behavioral tasks. We examined the response properties of NS and WDR neurons while rhesus monkeys performed a modification of the behavioral escape task described earlier (Hoffman *et al.*, 1981; Bushnell *et al.*, 1984). In this paradigm, reward was delivered for correct detection of the termination of temperature shifts in the 37–43°C range. Detection of temperature shifts in the noxious range of 45–49°C was not rewarded, but the monkey could terminate and escape the stimulus by releasing the panel button. Therefore, monkeys learned to discriminate temperatures in the 37–43°C range from those in the 45–49°C range; the correct responses on innocuous temperature trials compared with panel button releases on noxious temperature trials provided measures of such discrimination. The monkeys released the panel button earlier on noxious heat trials to terminate unreinforced trials and presumably also to escape the stimulus.

Consistent with findings in our previous behavioral task, discrimination or escape latencies decreased with increases in stimulus intensity. The activity of medullary dorsal horn thermal nociceptive neurons was correlated with the monkeys' behavior. For 11 of 12 WDR neurons and two of three NS neurons, there was an inverse relationship between neuronal response magnitude and behavioral discrimination latency. Figure 3 shows this relationship for 13 trigeminothalamic neurons. Generally, 49°C stimuli produced larger neuronal responses and shorter-latency behavioral responses than 47°C stimuli. On a few occasions, however, behavioral discrimination latency correlated better with the neuronal response than with the stimulus intensity (see neurons marked B in Figure 3). Thus, the monkeys' ability to discriminate noxious thermal stimuli is closely related to the neuronal discharge frequency of both WDR and NS projection neurons.

In other studies, humans and monkeys have been trained to detect small increases in temperature in the noxious heat range (Bushnell *et al.*, 1983a; Maixner *et al.*, 1984). Detection thresholds of the order of 0.2°C were found

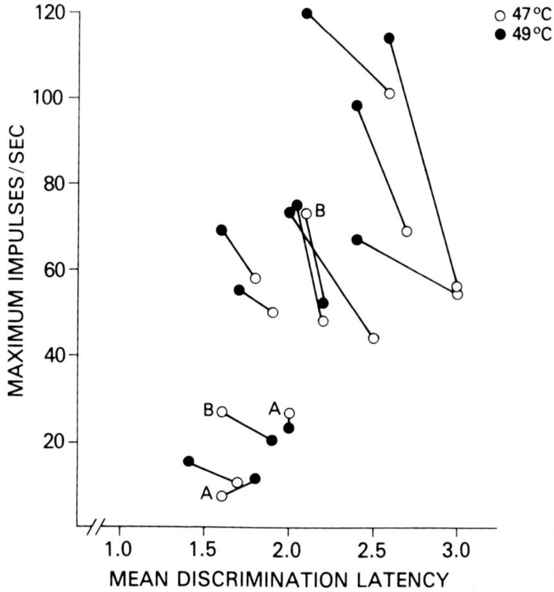

FIGURE 3. Graphic representation of the correlation between average neuronal activity (presented as maximum impulses per second) and average behavioral discrimination latency on 47° and 49°C trials for 13 cells. Each point represents the average of one to four trials. Open circles represent 47°C, and filled circles represent 49°C. The 47° and 49° points for each cell are connected by a line. All lines with negative slopes depict instances in which higher neural discharge rates are associated with shorter behavioral discrimination latencies. Note that this relationship holds for all cells except the two marked A. The two cells marked B show instances in which the neural discharge was greater at 47°C than at 49°C; correspondingly, the behavioral latency was shorter at 47°C. Latencies varied from neuron to neuron depending on the thermode location on the face. (From Bushnell *et al.*, 1984.)

from baseline temperatures of 46°C, consistent with detection thresholds reported on human palmar skin (Robinson *et al.*, 1983). Combined behavioral and neuronal studies in monkeys using this task (Maixner *et al.*, 1984) revealed that medullary dorsal horn WDR and NS neurons were responsive to these small temperature shifts and that the magnitude of the response was inversely related to detection latencies. These findings provide evidence that both NS and WDR neurons are critical for the detection of small temperature changes in the noxious heat range and that central nociceptive pathways code stimulus intensity as precisely as nonnociceptive pathways involved in tactile and innocuous thermal discriminations (Dubner *et al.*, 1978).

We conclude from the above correlative behavioral and neuronal studies that thermal nociceptive neurons in the medullary dorsal horn code stimulus intensity in the noxious heat range. The findings support the concept that pain is signaled by specialized central neural pathways carrying information about stimulus quality, intensity, and location.

E. Behavioral Modulation in Central Neural Pathways Coding Pain Sensations

Behavioral factors are known to modify pain experience. For example, how humans respond to pain depends on the situation in which the pain occurs, previous pain experience, cultural background, or the belief that an analgesic treatment will be effective (Melzack, 1973; Dubner *et al.*, 1978). Recent studies provide evidence these pain signals can be modified at the first central synapse in the spinal cord or the brainstem. Dorsal horn output pathways are not immutable and are subject to descending control from more rostral brainstem sites (see Basbaum and Fields, 1978; Dubner and Bennett, 1983; Willis, 1982, for review). Electrical stimulation or administration of opiate or morphinelike drugs activates these descending pathways and produces a profound behavioral analgesia. Naloxone, a specific opiate antagonist, reverses these effects. A number of recent reviews have provided evidence in support of these opioid-mediated systems (Mayer and Price, 1976; Sherman and Liebeskind, 1980; Yaksh and Rudy, 1978). Other findings indicate that neuropeptides such as the enkephalins and the endorphins represent the naturally occurring opioid compounds that act at some of these receptor sites (Kosterlitz, 1983). Activation of these pathways by stressful procedures (Dubner and Bennett, 1983, for review) also can produce analgesia. In addition, non-opioid-related descending pathways have been identified and involve the release of neurotransmitters such as norepinephine and serotonin in the medullary and spinal dorsal horns (Dubner and Bennett, 1983).

In our correlative behavioral and neural studies, we examined whether behavioral variables such as stimulus relevance and attentional factors modulate the thermal responses of dorsal horn nociceptive neurons (Hayes *et al.*, 1981; Dubner *et al.*, 1983; Bushnell *et al.*, 1984). The responses to noxious heat during the task were first compared with responses to similar stimuli presented between trials and not related to the animals' behavior in the task. Figure 4 shows the responses of a WDR trigeminothalamic neuron to a 49°C stimulus presented during these two conditions. When the monkey was using the stimulus as a discriminative cue during the task, the magnitude of the neuronal discharge was greater and the response latency was shorter than when the stimulus was unrelated to the monkey's behavior. The stimulus response function in Figure 4 illustrates the response of the same cell to temperatures in the 43° to 49°C range. There was a greater response at every temperature above threshold when the monkey was using the stimulus for discriminative information than when he was not.

The difference in neuronal responsivity in and out of the thermal task could be related to differences in arousal, attention, and motivation. In order to control for general arousal and motivational effects, we compared responses to thermal stimuli in the thermal task to responses to behaviorally irrelevant thermal stimuli presented during another task, called the visual task. In the visual task, the monkey pressed the panel for a variable time period and was rewarded for releasing the panel when a second light cue appeared. Thermal stimuli sometimes were presented before the onset of the second light cue but provided no information about its time of occurrence. Thus, in this task, thermal stimuli were not relevant to the monkeys' successful completion of the task. Monkeys readily learned to switch from one task to the other during the experimental session.

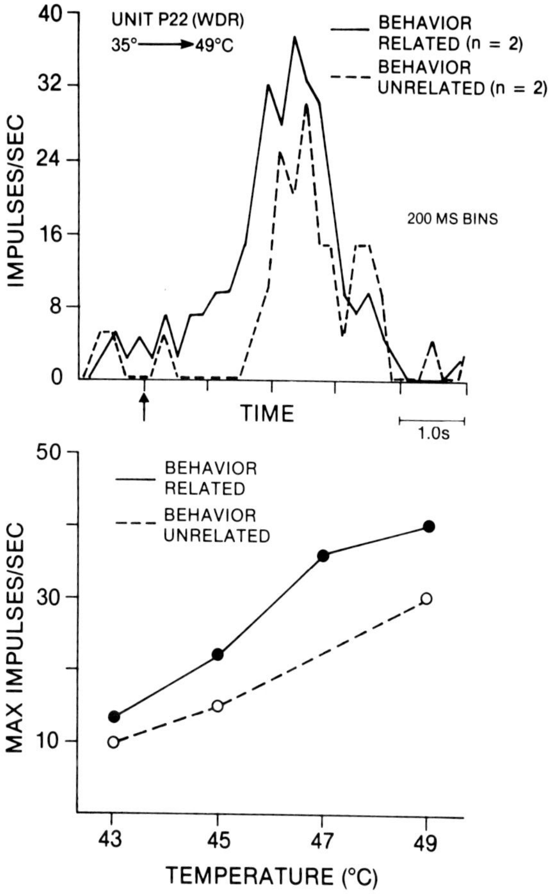

FIGURE 4. Responses of a WDR thalamic projection neuron to thermal stimuli presented during the thermal task (behavior related) and presented during the intertrial interval (behavior unrelated). The top graph compares peristimulus histograms of responses to identical 49°C stimuli. The arrow under the abscissa shows time of stimulus onset. The bottom graph shows stimulus–response functions for the same cell during each condition. Each point represents one to five trials. The abscissa shows final stimulus temperature on each trial. No 47°C behaviorally unrelated temperatures were presented. The ordinate indicates the average peak discharge rate, using 200-ms bins. Higher response rates occurred in the behavior-related condition than in the behavior-unrelated condition for every temperature tested. (From Bushnell *et al.*, 1984.)

Figure 5 compares the neuronal responses of a WDR thalamic projection neuron under the two conditions: in the thermal task, when thermal stimulation was the relevant cue, and in the visual task, when the light stimulus was the relevant cue. The neuronal response was enhanced in the thermal task relative to the visual task in two ways. First, the thermal threshold was lower in the thermal task (43°C) than in the visual task (41°C). Second, the magnitude of the response was greater in the thermal task than in the visual task at all temperatures above threshold.

These findings suggest that behavioral factors such as attentional differences may be significant in the enhancement of the response of medullary dorsal horn projection and nonprojection neurons during these behavioral tasks. Psychophysical studies show that attention to a noxious thermal stimulus improves a subject's ability to detect small changes in that stimulus (Bushnell *et al.*, 1983a). Thus, this enhancement of dorsal horn neuronal activity may be the neural substrate of improved performance in the task. Such behavioral

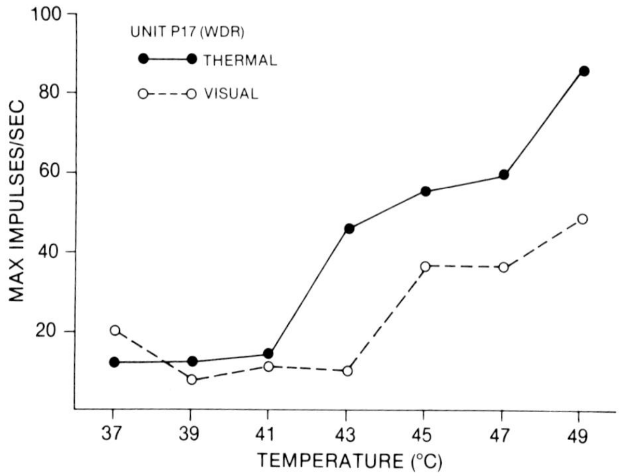

FIGURE 5. Stimulus–response functions for a WDR thalamic projection neuron during the thermal and visual tasks. The solid line represents responses to behaviorally relevant stimuli presented during the thermal task, and the dashed line represents responses to behaviorally irrelevant stimuli presented during the visual task. Each point represents two to seven trials. The ordinate indicates the average peak discharge rate, using 200-ms bins, and the abscissa represents final temperature of the stimulus. Higher response rates occurred in the thermal task than in the visual task for every temperature above threshold. Response rates were the same below threshold. (From Bushnell *et al.*, 1984.)

modulation may be related to descending pathways originating from more rostral brain sites such as the cerebral cortex and midline brainstem raphe nuclei (Hayes *et al.*, 1981).

F. Activation of Specialized Nociceptive Pathways by Behaviorally Relevant Stimuli Unrelated to Pain Discrimination

Some medullary dorsal horn nociceptive neurons activated by noxious thermal stimuli exhibit additional responses during behavior that are unrelated to pain discrimination and independent of stimulus parameters or stimulus modality (Dubner *et al.*, 1981; Bushnell *et al.*, 1984). These task-related responses sometimes occur at trial initiation and sometimes after the signal to release the response button, irrespective of whether that sensory cue was thermal or visual. Similar stimuli that do not have any behavioral relevance outside of the task do not produce these responses. Task-related responses are associated with sensory cues that are components of the sequence of behavioral events leading to reception of the reward. These responses occur in mechanoreceptive as well as in nociceptive neurons and therefore are not necessarily related to the discrimination of noxious stimuli.

Figure 6 shows an example of a task-related response of one cell while the monkey performed the thermal and visual tasks. When characterized outside the behavioral task, this neuron was classified as WDR with a large receptive field encompassing half the face. In addition, the cell had no thermal response to any temperature tested. Nevertheless, it produced a response during the trial and a response burst after the signal to release the key for reward. Similar task-related responses occurred in the thermal (Figure 6A)

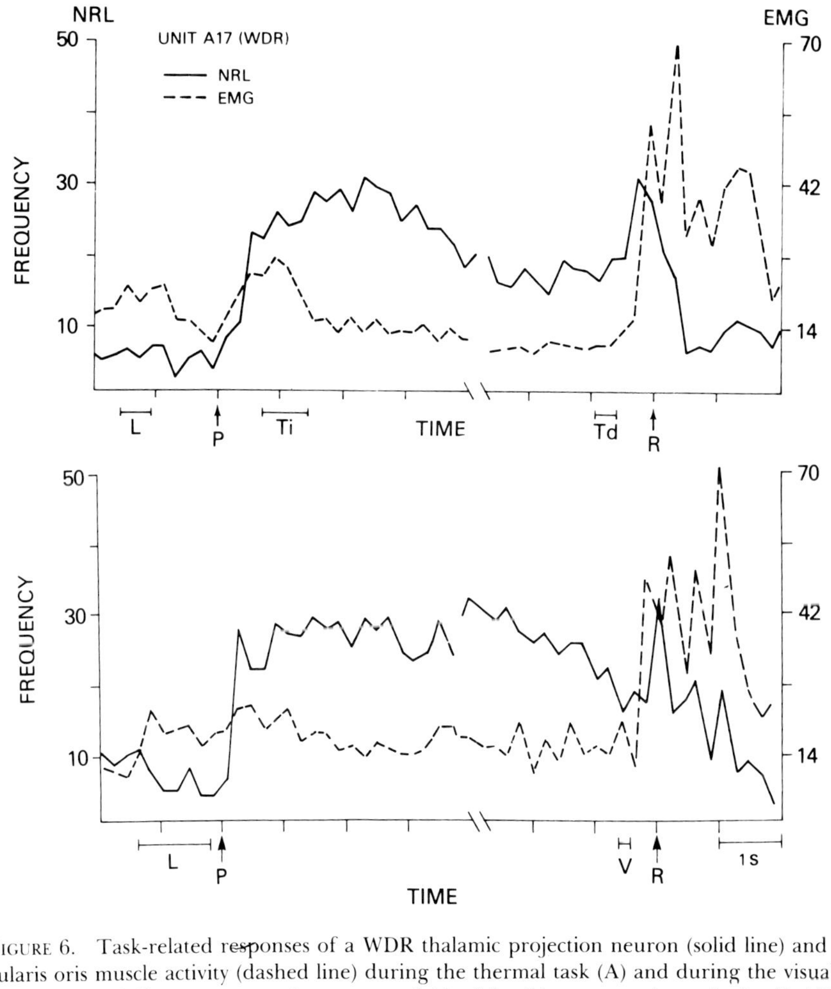

FIGURE 6. Task-related responses of a WDR thalamic projection neuron (solid line) and orbicularis oris muscle activity (dashed line) during the thermal task (A) and during the visual task (B). In A, each line represents the average of 11 trials of innocuous thermal stimuli. All temperatures were below thermal activation of the neuron. In B, each line represents the average of six trials with the thermode always at 35°C. Histograms are synchronized around button press (P) and button release (R). Brackets under the abscissa mark the time period of button light onset (L), temperature increase (Ti), temperature decrease (Td), and visual stimulus (V). (From Bushnell *et al.*, 1984.)

and visual (Figure 6B) tasks. Figure 6 also shows little correlation between lip EMG activity and neuronal frequency. Consequently, it is unlikely that this task-related activity was an artifact caused by mechanical stimulation of the face. Thermal nociceptive WDR and NS neurons also exhibited task-related responses to innocuous thermal and visual cues.

These findings indicate that specialized nociceptive pathways are subject to behavioral modulation unrelated to noxious stimulation. Their activation, therefore, does not always produce pain. The same nociceptive neuron that exhibits sensory-discriminative properties in response to noxious stimuli may also exhibit task-related responses independent of stimulus parameters.

G. *Summary and Conclusion*

The correlation of behavioral and physiological indices of pain is a powerful approach to the study of peripheral and central mechanisms of pain. Behavioral tasks that require animals to discriminate noxious stimuli indicate that peripheral nociceptors and dorsal horn nociceptive neurons code unique and specific information that is essential for performance of the tasks. These specialized nociceptive pathways are critical for signaling discriminative aspects of pain sensations and carry information about stimulus quality, intensity, location, and duration. A-δ heat nociceptors and C polymodal nociceptors provide information essential for fine discrimination in the noxious heat range. The monkey's fast reaction times in a noxious thermal escape task are dependent on activity in A-δ heat nociceptors. Response latencies in a thermal discrimination task correlate with the magnitude of discharge of WDR and NS medullary dorsal horn nociceptive neurons including those that project to the thalamus. These findings support the concept that specialized neural pathways are involved in coding pain sensations.

However, just as the experience of pain is modified by behavioral factors, these specialized nociceptive pathways are subject to descending control from multiple rostral brain sites such as the cerebral cortex and midline brainstem reticular nuclei. Behavioral variables alter the magnitude of response of nociceptive neurons in the dorsal horn. When monkeys use noxious thermal stimuli as discriminative cues in a task, thermal nociceptive neurons exhibit greater discharge frequencies than when the stimulus is unrelated to the monkey's behavior. These findings indicate that the behavioral relevance of a sensory stimulus and attentional factors enhance the response of nociceptive neurons.

Other findings suggest that activation of these specialized nociceptive pathways does not always produce pain. Some thermal nociceptive neurons in the medullary dorsal horn exhibit responses during behavior that are unrelated to pain discrimination and independent of stimulus modality or stimulus parameters. These task-related responses do not result in neuronal activity outside of the behavioral task and are associated with sensory cues that are components of the sequence of behavioral events leading to successful completion of the task. Thus, specialized nociceptive pathways are neither immutable nor exclusively related to the transmission of pain signals. These behavioral effects on neuronal activity likely involve multiple descending and segmental circuitry underlying the ability of an animal to extract useful information from its environment.

References

Adriaensen, H., Gybels, J., Handwerker, H. O., and van Hees, J. Response properties of thin myelinated (A-delta) fibers in human skin nerves. *J. Neurophysiol.* 49:111–122, 1983.

Basbaum, A. I., and Fields, H. L. Endogenous pain control mechanisms: Review and hypothesis. *Ann. Neurol.* 4:451–462, 1978.

Beitel, R. E., and Dubner, R. Response of unmyelinated (C) polymodal nociceptors to thermal stimuli applied to monkey's face. *J. Neurophysiol.* 39:1160–1175, 1976.

Burgess, P. R., and Perl, E. R. Cutaneous mechanoreceptors and nociceptors, in: *Handbook of Sensory Physiology, Somatosensory System,* Vol. 2 (A. Iggo, ed.), Springer, Heidelberg, 1973, pp. 29–78.

Bushnell, M. C., Jones, R. L., Duncan, G. H., and Dubner, R. Effects of attention on detection of noxious and innocuous thermal stimuli. *Soc. Neurosci. Abstr.* 9:473, 1983a.

Bushnell, M. C., Taylor, M. B., Duncan, G. H., and Dubner, R. Discrimination of innocuous and noxious thermal stimuli applied to the face in human and monkey. *Somatosens. Res.* 1:119–129, 1983b.

Bushnell, M. C., Duncan, G. H., Dubner, R., and He, L. F. Activity of trigeminothalamic neurons in medullary dorsal horn of awake monkeys trained in a thermal discrimination task. *J. Neurophysiol.* 52:170–187, 1984.

Dubner, R., and Bennett, G. J. Spinal and trigeminal mechanisms of nociception. *Annu. Rev. Neurosci.* 6:381–418, 1983.

Dubner, R., and Hu, J. W. Myelinated (A-delta) nociceptive afferent innervating the monkey's face. *J. Dent. Res.* 56:A167, 1977.

Dubner, R., Beitel, R. E., and Brown, F. J. A behavioral animal model for the study of pain mechanisms in primates, in: *Pain: New Perspectives in Therapy and Research,* (M. Weisenberg and B. Tursky, eds.), Plenum Press, New York, 1976, pp. 155–170.

Dubner, R., Price, D. D., Beitel, R. E., and Hu, J. W. Peripheral neural correlates of behavior in monkey and human related to sensory-discriminative aspects of pain, in: *Pain in the Trigeminal Region* (D. J. Anderson and B. Matthews, eds.), Elsevier, Amsterdam, 1977, pp. 57–66.

Dubner, R., Sessle, B. J., and Storey, A. T. *The Neural Basis of Oral and Facial Function,* Plenum Press, New York, 1978.

Dubner, R., Hoffman, D. S., and Hayes, R. L. Neuronal activity in medullary dorsal horn of awake monkeys trained in a thermal discrimination task. III. Task-related responses and their functional role. *J. Neurophysiol.* 46:444–464, 1981.

Dubner, R., Bushnell, M. C., and Duncan, G. H. Behavioral and neural correlates of nociception, in: *Current Topics in Pain Research and Therapy* (T. Yokota and R. Dubner, eds.), Excerpta Medica, Amsterdam, 1983, pp. 45–55.

Handwerker, H. O., Keck, F. S. and Neermann, G. Detection of temperature increases in the operating range of warm receptors and of nociceptors. *Pain* 14:11–20, 1982.

Hayes, R. L., Dubner, R., and Hoffman, D. S. Neuronal activity in medullary dorsal horn of awake monkeys trained in a thermal discrimination task. II. Behavioral modulation of responses to thermal and mechanical stimuli. *J. Neurophysiol.* 46:428–443, 1981.

Hoffman, D. S., Dubner, R., Hayes, R. L., and Medlin, T. P. Neuronal activity in medullary dorsal horn of awake monkeys trained in a thermal discrimination task. I. Responses to innocuous and noxious thermal stimuli. *J. Neurophysiol.* 46:409–427, 1981.

KOSTERLITZ, H. W. Opioid peptides and pain—an update. *Adv. Pain Res. Ther.* 5:199–208, 1983.

LAMOTTE, R. H., AND CAMPBELL, J. N. Comparison of responses of warm and nociceptive C-fiber afferents in monkey with human judgements of thermal pain. *J. Neurophysiol.* 41:509–528, 1978.

MAIXNER, W., BUSHNELL, M. C., OLIVERAS, J. L., DUNCAN, G. H., AND DUBNER, R. Thermal medullary dorsal horn neurons encode sensory intensity information in the noxious range. *Pain [Suppl.]* 2:5127, 1984.

MAYER, D. J., AND PRICE, D. D. Central nervous system mechanisms of analgesia. *Pain* 2:379–404, 1976.

MELZACK, R. *The Puzzle of Pain,* Basic Books, New York, 1973.

PERL, E. R. Is pain a specific sensation? *J. Psychiatr. Res.* 8:273–387, 1971.

PRICE, D. D., AND DUBNER, R. Neurons that subserve the sensory-discriminative aspects of pain. *Pain* 3:307–338, 1977.

PRICE, D. D., HU J. W., DUBNER, R., AND GRACELY, R. H. Peripheral suppression of first pain and central summation of second pain evoked by noxious heat pulses. *Pain* 3:57–68, 1977.

ROBINSON, C. J., TOREBJÖRK, H. E., AND LAMOTTE, R. H. Psychophysical detection and pain ratings of incremental thermal stimuli: A comparison with nociceptor responses in humans. *Brain Res.* 274:87–106, 1983.

SHERMAN, J. E., AND LIEBESKIND, J. C. An endorphinergic, centrifugal substrate of pain modulation: recent findings, current concepts, and complexities, in: *Pain* (J. J. Bonica, ed.), Raven Press, New York, 1980, pp. 191–204.

SUMINO, R., DUBNER, R., AND STARKMAN, S. Responses of small myelinated 'warm' fibers to noxious heat stimuli applied to the monkey's face. *Brain Res.* 62:260–263, 1973.

WILLIS, W. D. Control of nociceptive transmission in the spinal cord, in: *Progress in Sensory Physiology* (D. Ottoson, ed.), Springer-Verlag, Heidelberg, 1982, pp. 1–159.

WILLIS, W. D., AND COGGESHALL, R. E. *Sensory Mechanisms of the Spinal Cord.* Plenum Press, New York, 1978.

YAKSH, T. L., AND RUDY, T. A. Narcotic analgetics: CNS sites and mechanisms of action as revealed by intracerebral injection techniques. *Pain* 4:299–359, 1978.

14
Detection Thresholds of Cutaneous Sensations in Health and Disease in Man

PETER J. DYCK

A. Introduction

In considering the mechanisms by which spinal cord systems transfer, modulate, and integrate incoming sensory signals, it is necessary to know something about the location and structure (see Winklemann, Chapter 2) and the properties of the cutaneous and deep receptors that transduce physical and chemical events impinging on them from the external and internal environment (Light and Perl, 1981; Boyd and Smith, 1984; Crago, 1984). As crucial to our understanding of sensory transduction as are the physical and electrophysiological studies of receptors is the information obtained from psychophysical responses evoked by stimuli transduced by these receptors. Cutaneous sensory detection thresholds in man with respect to site, sex, age, and disease are thus the focus of this chapter.

B. Computer-Assisted Sensory Examination

1. System Characteristics

Each system was designed to provide stimuli with the same wave form but of various known magnitudes. Four types of stimuli were developed (Dyck

PETER J. DYCK • Peripheral Nerve Laboratory, Mayo Medical School and Foundation, Rochester, Minnesota 55905.

et al., 1984). The first stimulus consisted of a slow vertical indentation produced by the round end of a stylus at grid points on the surface of the skin. This was experienced by the subject as touch–pressure. The second stimulus, a sinusoidal wave form at 250 Hz produced by the round end of a stylus at grid points on the skin, was experienced as the sensation of flutter or vibration. For each of these tests, threshold was determined at each of nine (3×3) grid points separated from one another by 2 mm. The third stimulus, produced by a specially designed thermoelectric unit, provided ramps of cooling that reached a predetermined temperature in a given period of time. The fourth type of stimulus provided thermal warming.

2. *System Components*

The systems that deliver the stimuli are comprised of the following components: separate stimulator assemblies for each modality, electromechanical translator, electronic controller, computer, visual numerical display, observer or patient response key, and printer. The thermal stimulator does not employ the electromechanical translator.

In the touch–pressure system, a stimulating stylus is attached to the shaft of a jeweled-bearing galvanometer motor so that it can follow the up-and-down movement of the part being tested, which has been only partially restrained.

The vibratory transducer uses a cutter head designed for making vinyl records (Grampian cutter head, type B1/D, MOY, London, UK), with the stimulating stylus fastened at right angles to the heavy shaft of the cutter head.

The thermal transducer is a commercially available thermoelectric unit (TEU) with a surface area of approximately 3.5 cm^2. A thermocouple is attached to the surface in contact with the skin, and a temperature-controlled heat sink (an aluminum block, another thermoelectric unit, and air-cooled fins) is attached to the other side. The computer or microprocessor continuously monitors the TEU and solves heat flow equations (15 times per second) to provide corrected currents to the stimulating TEU.

Together, the computer and electronic components control the shape, magnitude, and time of appearance of the stimulus, the visual display of the numbers 1 and 2, the procedure of testing and scoring, the entry of responses from the observer response key, and the printer results. The computer also controls the elevation, setting down, and X and Y traverse of the touch–pressure and vibratory transducers. The electromechanical translator common to the touch–pressure and vibration transducers has an electric motor that can raise and move the stimulators in any desired direction. When normal values are available, the percentile response value is determined and printed.

3. Testing Procedures

A forced-choice testing paradigm was employed in these studies. In alternative forced-choice testing, stimulus and null-stimulus periods are presented in pairs (Sekular *et al.,* 1973). For a pair of events, one is a stimulus and the other a null stimulus. In our system, the numbers 1 and then 2 are displayed on the visual numerical display. They indicate the onset and duration of the first and second stimulus periods, respectively. Each period is 1.683 s in duration. On the basis of a rotating bank of random numbers, the stimulus is assigned to either stimulus period 1 or 2, and the null stimulus is assigned to the other. For each point tested, the stimuli will be presented first half of the time.

The wave forms employed for touch–pressure and for vibration are shown in Figure 1. For touch–pressure, a single mechanical wave form delivered twice and having the characteristics of a discharging capacitor is generated. The null stimulus is an unchanging static load. For vibration, the wave form is a sinusoidal wave at 250 Hz. The null stimulus consists of the slow mechanical deformation (the envelope) without the rapid deformation. For ther-

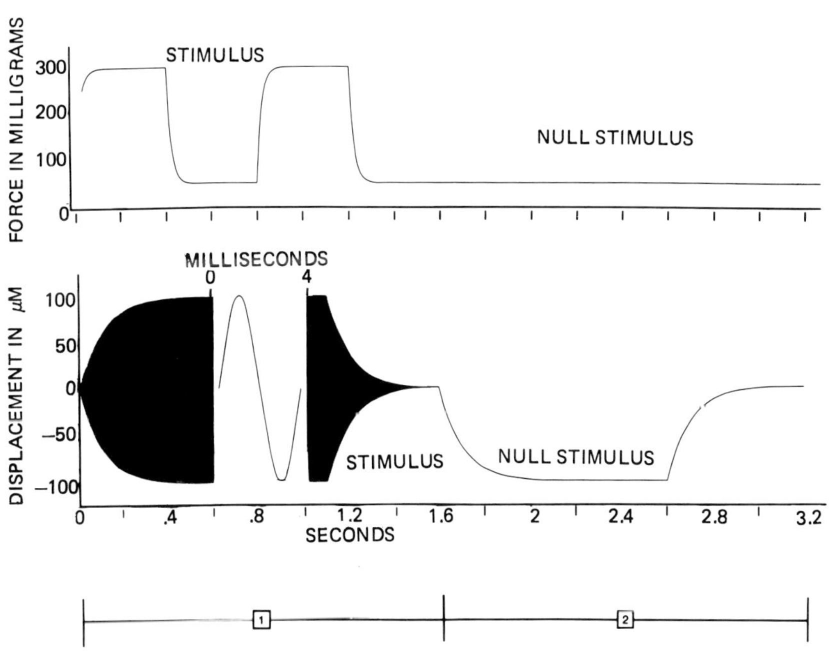

FIGURE 1. The wave form of the touch–pressure (upper) and vibratory (middle) stimuli delivered during forced-choice events marked 1 and 2 (lower) in computer-assisted sensory evaluation (CASE). (From Dyck *et al.,* 1978, with permission.)

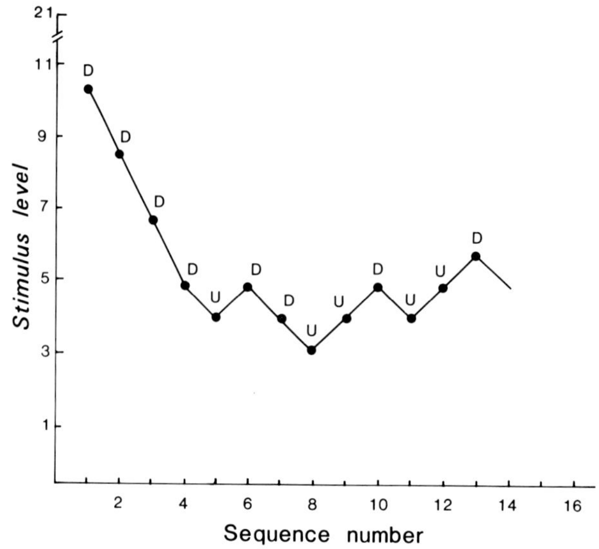

FIGURE 2. Illustrating the algorithm of testing used in CASE and as described in text. (From Dyck *et al.*, 1978, with permission.)

mal cooling or warming, linear ramps of thermal change for a fixed period of time are given.

In each system, 21 levels of stimulus magnitude are employed. The smallest stimulus level is coded L_1, and the largest L_{21}. Testing is initiated at L_{11} for touch–pressure and vibration, with the subject or patient exposed to a series of forced choices. If S represents a correct response and F an incorrect response to a forced-choice pair, an observed sequence of SSS or SSFS is judged as indicative of sensitivity and results in testing at L_9. Alternatively, an observed sequence of F, SF, or SSFF results in testing at L_{13}. The process is repeated at the new level and is continued until either (1) a step down from level 5 is reached, (2) a step up from level 17 is reached, or (3) three changes in direction (up versus down) occur, at which points changes in levels are single-spaced. On the occurrence of six changes in direction, the procedures terminate, and the mean of the six levels is used as the estimate of threshold. A typical sequence is shown in Figure 2.

For cooling and warming, testing is initiated at L_{15}. If responses at L_1 are SSS or SSFS, the response is judged too sensitive. Conversely, a response of F, SF, or SSFF at L_{21} is judged insensitive.

The objective of the described sequence of testing is to estimate the level at which the stimulus can be felt 50% of the time. This corresponds to a correct response rate of 75% in forced-choice testing.

If a threshold can be obtained, a point or site is called "sensitive." If a threshold cannot be obtained, it is either "supersensitive" or "insensitive." Sensory abnormality for touch–pressure or vibratory sensation (for which percentile responses have been obtained) is recognized, therefore, either by an increased number of insensitive grid points or by an elevated mean threshold of sensitive grid points or both.

C. Cutaneous Detection Thresholds in a Normal Human Population

1. Characteristics of Population

More than 300 persons at least 8 years of age were recruited from among laboratory, medical, and paramedical personnel, relatives and friends, responders to an advertisement in a news publication for Mayo Clinic employees, and members of a club consisting mainly of elderly people. Subjects excluded from this study included patients with diagnosed neurological disease, dementia, sciatica, diabetes mellitus, malignancy of various types, alcoholism, history of psychosis, known peripheral vascular disease, and neuromuscular disease. Of the group willing to participate, approximately one-third were excluded for these and other reasons.

For touch–pressure and vibratory sensation, the cutaneous sites tested included the forehead, upper lip, and dorsal surface at the base of the nail of the index finger and great toe. For thermal cooling, the sites included cheek, lip, hand, and foot.

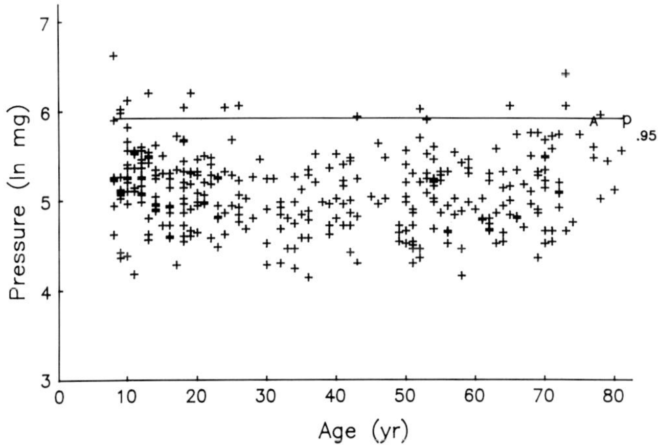

FIGURE 3. Detection threshold of force, plotted as the natural logarithm (ln mg) of pressure applied to the lip, against age of approximately 300 healthy subjects. The estimated 95th percentile value is shown. (From Dyck *et al.*, 1984 with permission.)

2. *Touch–Pressure Threshold*

a. Face

At the forehead and upper lip, all subjects had nine sensitive points (except for one subject with one insensitive point). Therefore, only mean values of the detection thresholds of pressure (ln mg) for the nine sensitive points need be considered. Although considerable variability was observed among subjects, the results (at both sites) were not statistically different between sexes or with age (Figure 3). On average, the threshold values for the forehead (not shown) were slightly higher (i.e., forehead is less sensitive) than those for the lip. No age or sex difference was seen.

b. Finger

Threshold values for the fingers of healthy subjects plotted against age are shown in Figure 4. All nine points were sensitive (except for one male with one insensitive point, represented by the letter A in the figure), permitting consideration of mean threshold alone. Whereas, on average, the thresholds were lower for the finger than for the face in the youngest subjects, this situation was reversed in the oldest subjects. The threshold values were not more variable with age. No sex difference was found.

c. Toe

The threshold values for sensitive points of the great toe of healthy subjects are shown in Figure 5. The threshold values rise with age. On average,

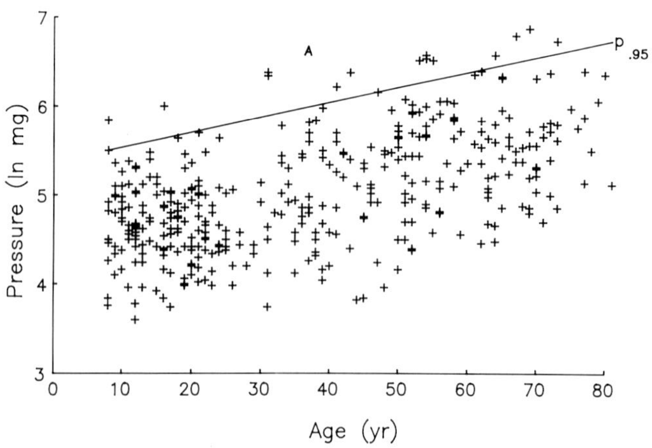

FIGURE 4. Detection threshold of force, plotted as the natural logarithm (ln mg) of pressure applied to the index finger, against age, showing an increase of threshold with age of healthy subjects. The estimated 95th percentile value is shown. (From Dyck *et al.*, 1984, with permission.)

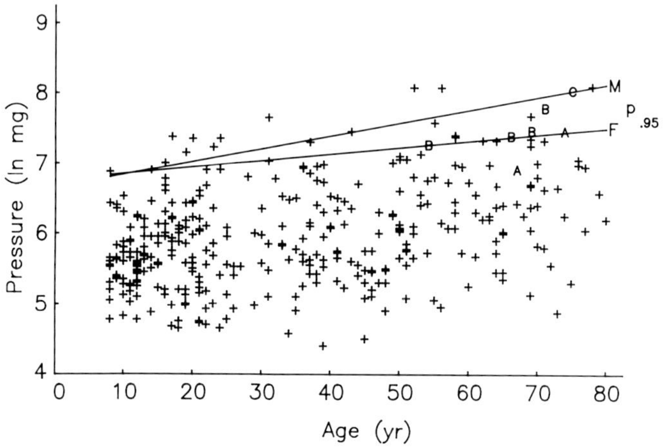

FIGURE 5. Detection threshold of force, plotted as the natural logarithm (ln mg) of pressure applied to the toe, against age, showing a higher threshold with age and a sex difference in healthy subjects. The estimated 95th percentile value is shown. (From Dyck *et al.*, 1984, with permission.)

thresholds were considerably higher than for the finger, and insensitive points were encountered. Patients <50 years old did not have insensitive points. For persons >50 years, the number of subjects having insensitive points, their median number of insensitive points, and the number of subjects tested were as follows: males 5, 2, and 50; females 2, 1.5, and 49. Males, especially those older than 50 years, have higher values than females. Seven subjects, all older than 50 years and represented by letters, had insensitive points. If testing had employed stimuli of even greater magnitude, the slope of the regression line for threshold on age might have been even steeper. The variability of threshold values increased with age. Some older people, however, were as sensitive as some younger people.

3. *Touch–Pressure Results as Displacement Rather Than as Force*

Because the effective stimulus for touch–pressure is a derivative of force (such as cutaneous displacement, shear modulus, or other derivative), it might have been desirable to express touch–pressure sensation in terms of displacement rather than force. It is possible to relate touch–pressure to displacement for the higher levels of force employed, since we had a device that could measure displacement. For small magnitudes of force, the measurement of displacement is inaccurate. Regression lines for displacement touch–pressure (force converted to displacement) against age for the four sites (Figure 6B) are markedly different from the lines for force touch–pressure against age (Figure 6A). For young persons, with displacement as criterion, the most

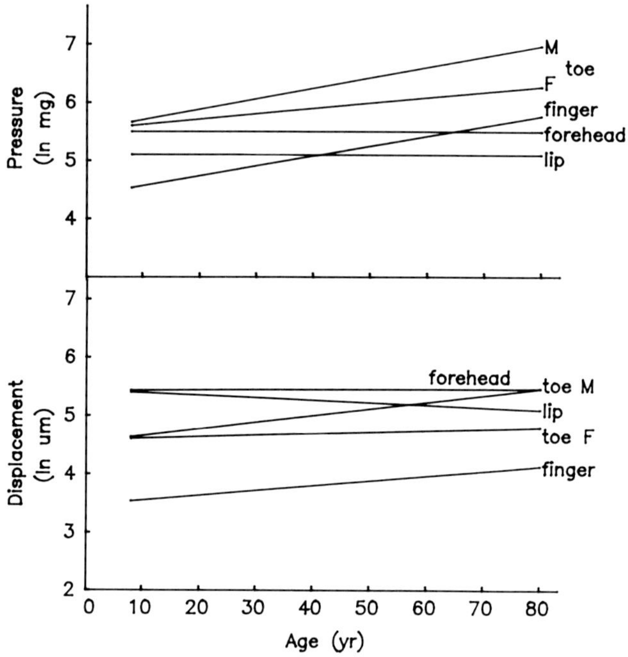

FIGURE 6. Comparison of touch–pressure thresholds displayed as pressure (top) or as displacement (bottom). The order of sensitivity is different for the two approaches, as discussed in text. (From Dyck *et al.*, 1984, with permission.)

sensitive sites in order of increasing thresholds are finger, toe, forehead, and lip. In older persons, the threshold for the toe rises so that it is similar to that of the forehead and lip. With force as the criterion, the order of sensitivity is finger, face, and toe for the young and face, finger, and toe for the old. It is evident that, for a given force, there is a greater displacement for face than for toe or finger.

4. Vibration Threshold

a. Face

The mean thresholds plotted against age are shown in Figure 7. As for touch–pressure at this site, no significant differences in thresholds were demonstrated between sexes or with age.

b. Finger

The mean thresholds plotted against age are shown in Figure 8. These thresholds are lower than those for the face in the young but rise with age.

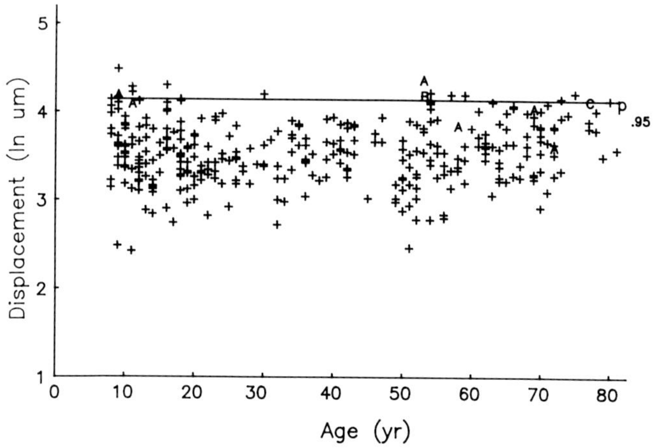

FIGURE 7. Vibratory threshold, plotted as the natural logarithm of displacement (ln μm) of the lip, against age of healthy subjects. The estimated 95th percentile value is shown. (From Dyck *et al.*, 1984, with permission.)

c. Toe

Occasionally in the young, but frequently in persons older than 50 years, insensitive points were encountered. The number of subjects with insensitive points, the median number of insensitive points, and the number of subjects tested were as follows: males <50 years 5, 1, and 100; females <50 years 2, 1, and 103; males ≥50 years 18, 2.5, and 51; females ≥50 years 22, 1, and

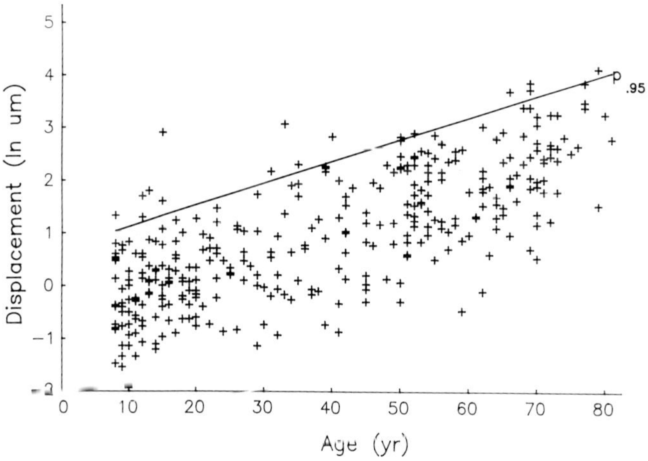

FIGURE 8. Vibratory threshold, plotted as the natural logarithm of displacement (ln μm) of the finger, against age of healthy subjects. The estimated 95th percentile value is shown. (From Dyck *et al.*, 1984, with permission.)

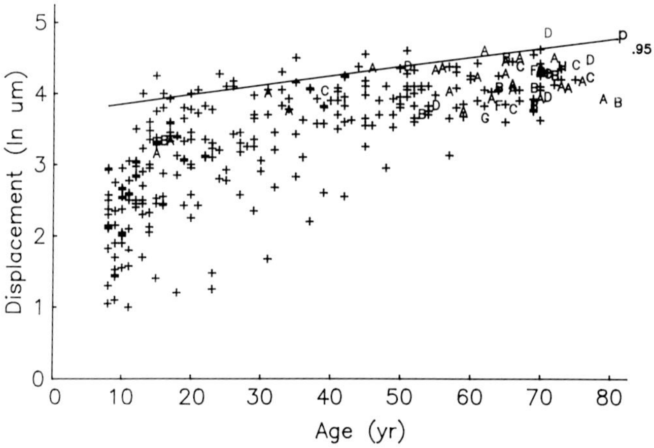

FIGURE 9. Vibratory threshold, plotted as the natural logarithm of displacement (ln μm) of the toe, against age of healthy subjects. The estimated 95th percentile value is shown. Where fewer than nine grid points are sensitive, capital letters have been placed at the threshold value of sensitive points to indicate the number of insensitive points; i.e., A = 1, B = 2. . . I = 9, respectively. (From Dyck *et al.*, 1984, with permission.)

51. There is a highly significant increase in the number of insensitive grid points with increasing age. No sex difference in the number of insensitive points is apparent. Because insensitive points are encountered in health and especially in disease, both the threshold of sensitive points and the number of insensitive points are needed for a description of the vibration threshold

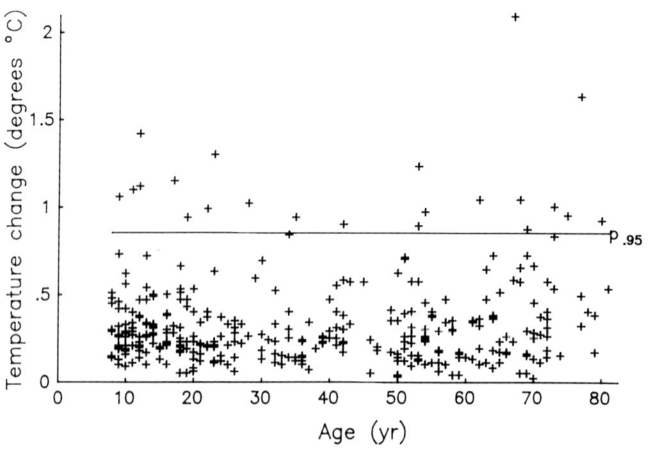

FIGURE 10. Thermal cooling, plotted as temperature change (degrees C) of the lip, against age of healthy subjects. The estimated 95th percentile value is shown. (From Dyck *et al.*, 1984, with permission.)

of the toe. For this reason also, the regression line of threshold on age (and the 95th percentile line, P_{95}) is less steep than it should be because points with higher but unknown thresholds were excluded. This also accounts for the diminished variability with older age. Therefore, it is not possible to compare the slope of the regression lines for different sites and sensory modalities. It is clear, however, that threshold rises with age. Threshold values of persons with the lowest threshold also rise with age. No sex difference was found (Figure 9).

5. *Cooling Threshold*

a. Cheek and Lip

No subject was insensitive, and thresholds did not differ with age or sex (Figure 10). The values for forehead are similar.

b. Hand

One person over 70 years of age was insensitive. Threshold was not significantly different between males and females. Both the mean threshold value and its variability increased with age (Figure 11).

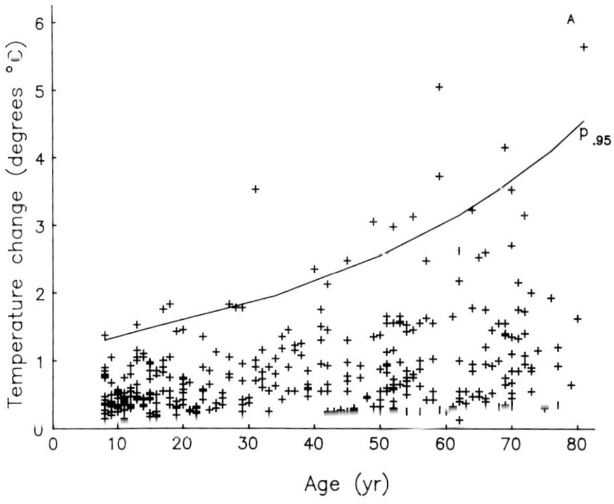

FIGURE 11. Thermal cooling, plotted as temperature change (degrees C) of the hand, against age of healthy subjects. The estimated 95th percentile value is shown. (From Dyck *et al.*, 1984, with permission.)

c. Foot

Whereas none of 203 subjects under the age of 50 years was insensitive, one of 100 subjects 50 years or older was insensitive (indicated by the letter A, Figure 12). On average, threshold and variability increased with age. Some older subjects were, however,, as sensitive as younger subjects.

6. *Comparison of Thresholds of Various Sensations at Different Sites*

For threshold of thermal cooling, the face (lip and forehead) was most sensitive, followed by the hand and, finally, the foot. For touch–pressure and vibration sensations, the hand is most sensitive, followed by the foot and then the face (Figure 13).

The observed variation in threshold with site, age, and sex may be caused by differences in (1) receptor type, (2) receptor density, (3) receptor location, (4) receptor properties, or (5) transmission and central processing. Differences in the topographic distribution of cutaneous receptors have been documented. To illustrate, Meissner's corpuscles are arranged regularly in rows in the superficial layers of the dermis early in life (Figure 14). With growth of the integument, the receptors become more widely spaced. In old age, the density of receptors is decreased, and they are focally situated (Figure 15). A difference in density of receptors with site and age may therefore account for some threshold differences (see Winkelmann, Chapter 2, for further discussion).

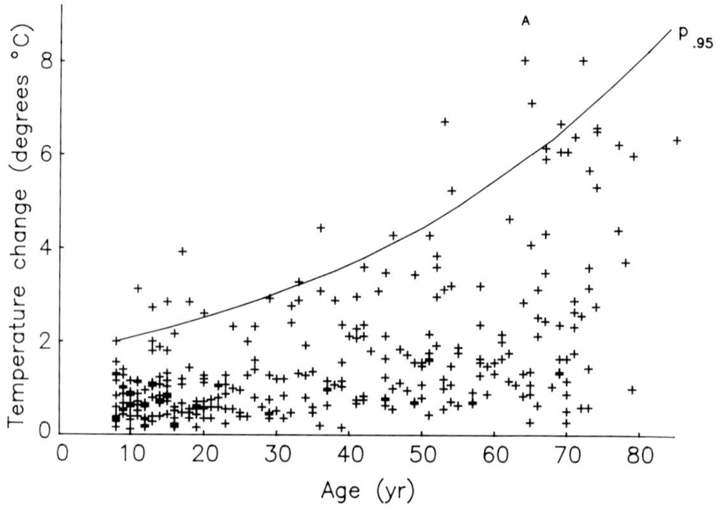

FIGURE 12. Thermal cooling, plotted as temperature change (degrees C) of the foot, against age of healthy subjects. The estimated 95th percentile value is shown. (From Dyck *et al.*, 1984, with permission.)

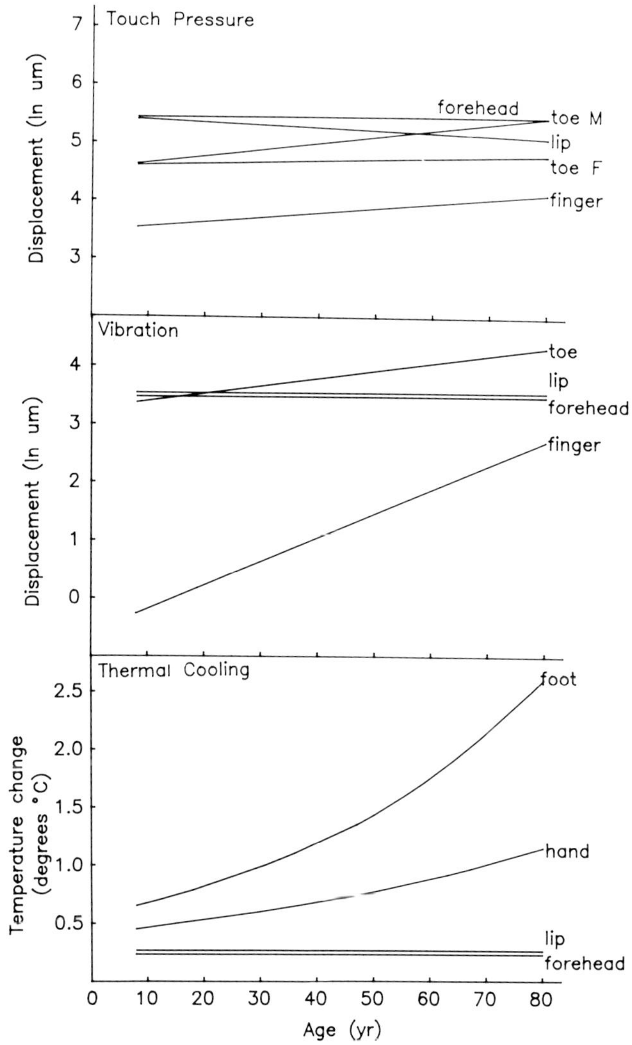

FIGURE 13. Comparison of average thresholds of various sensations for different sites and with age. (From Dyck *et al.*, 1984, with permission.)

D. Cutaneous Detection Thresholds in Several Neuropathies

Raised thresholds of sensation correspond to sensory loss or deficit as reported by the neurologist. Such a raised threshold is detected either by an increased number of insensitive points or by a raised threshold of sensitive points. The pattern of sensory loss among different sensory modalities predicts which receptors and afferent pathways are affected and is helpful in

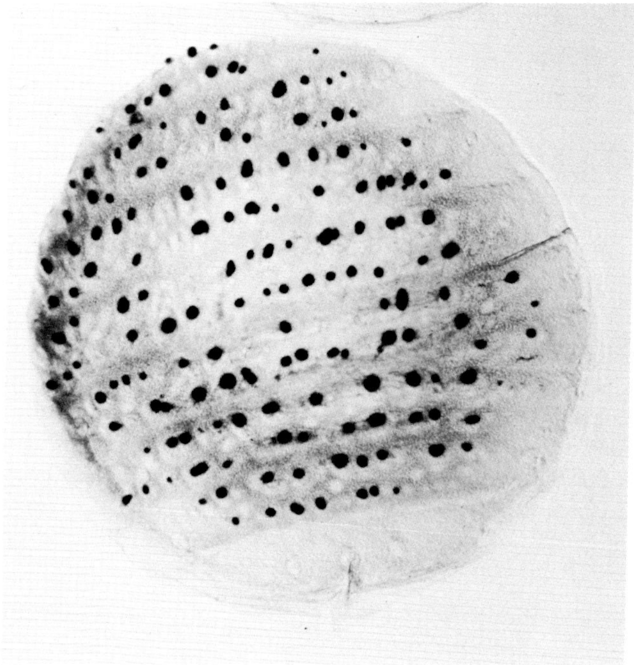

FIGURE 14. Three-millimeter full-thickness skin biopsy from the toe of a young child showing regularily spaced Meissner's corpuscles. (From Bolton *et al.*, 1966, with permission.)

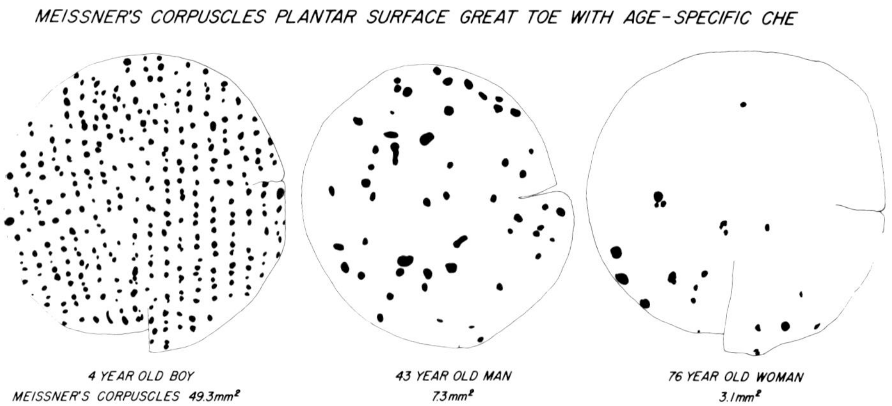

FIGURE 15. The distribution of Meissner's corpuscles in skin biopsies of healthy persons of increasing age. The effect of increasing integument area and age is apparent. (From Bolton *et al.*, 1966, with permission.)

diagnosis. In spinocerebellar degeneration, elevated touch–pressure and vibratory thresholds and a normal thermal cooling threshold are typical. In amyloidosis, an elevated threshold of thermal cooling with normal or elevated touch–pressure and vibratory thresholds is typical. These alterations in the pattern of sensory loss are related to changes in the compound action potential *in vitro* and in diameter histograms of myelinated and unmyelinated fibers of sural nerve. In cases of spinocerebellar degeneration, the A-α fibers appear to be preferentially affected. In dominantly inherited amyloidosis, unmyelinated and small myelinated fibers are preferentially affected.

1. Motor Neuron Disease

The threshold values of 80 patients diagnosed as having "motor neuron disease" or amyotrophic lateral sclerosis are shown in Figure 16. Of 80 patients, 14 had an abnormality of vibratory sensation (seven by elevated threshold, five by number of insensitive points, and two by a combination of these two criteria), five exhibited an abnormality of touch–pressure sensation, and

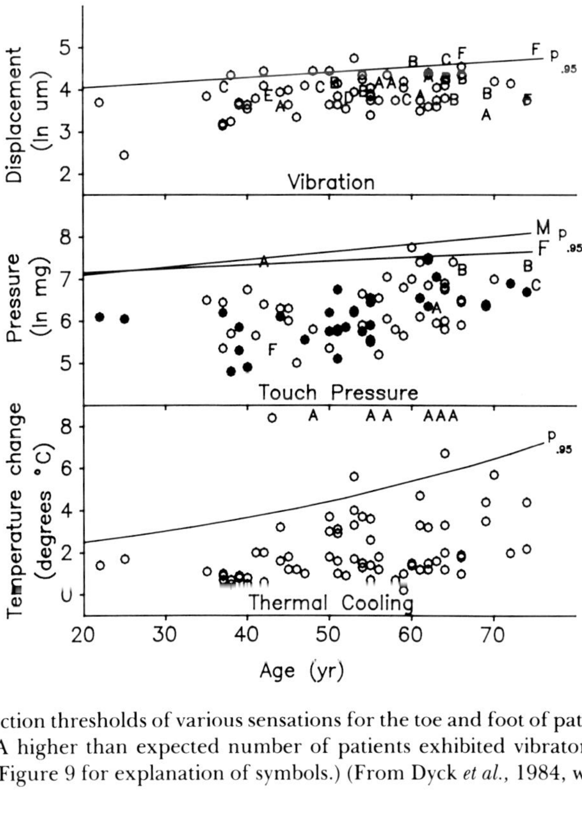

FIGURE 16. Detection thresholds of various sensations for the toe and foot of patients with motor neuron disease. A higher than expected number of patients exhibited vibratory threshold abnormalities. (See Figure 9 for explanation of symbols.) (From Dyck *et al.*, 1984, with permission.)

eight demonstrated an abnormality of thermal cooling. Touch–pressure and cooling thresholds appear to have a normal distribution, however. Vibratory thresholds were more frequently elevated than in controls ($P < 0.001$).

2. *Friedreich's Ataxia*

Thresholds for touch–pressure, vibration, and thermal cooling sensations with age are given for patients with Friedreich's ataxia (FA) in Figure 17. Eight of the ten patients tested had raised thresholds of vibratory sensation (upper). Nine of the ten had increased numbers of insensitive points, and raised thresholds of sensitive points were demonstrated in a similar number. All patients exhibited abnormalities of touch–pressure sensation—nine had excessive numbers of insensitive points, and most of these had raised thresholds of sensitive points (middle). Three of the eight patients tested had elevated thresholds of thermal cooling (lower). The greater involvement of touch–pressure and vibration sensations than of thermal cooling is consistent with what is known about the selective involvement of A-α afferent neurons in this disorder. Clinical evaluation of these patients and nerve conduction and electromyographic studies of muscle generally do not reveal any evidence of muscle involvement at this stage of the disease.

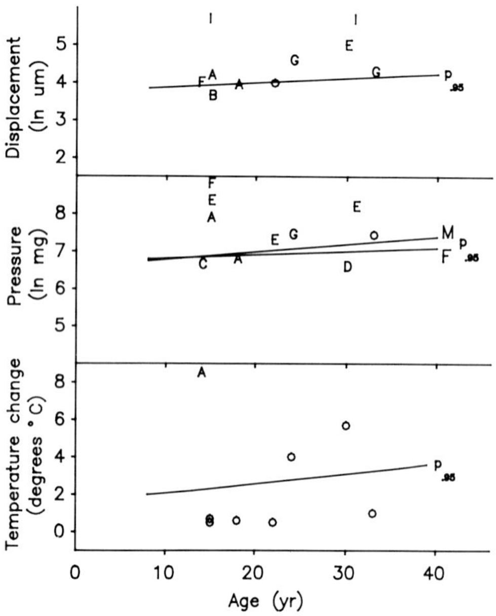

FIGURE 17. Range of detection thresholds in Friedreich's ataxia, as described in text. (See Figure 9 for explanation of symbols.) (From Dyck *et al.*, 1984, with permission.)

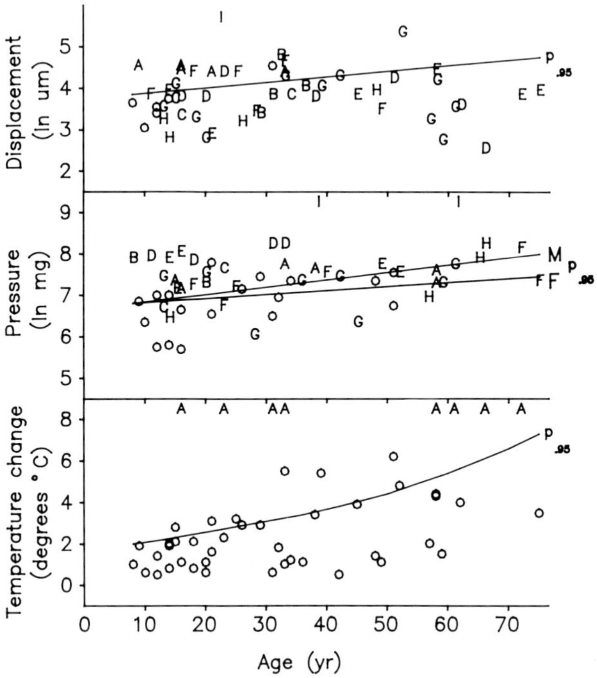

FIGURE 18. Range of detection thresholds in hereditary motor sensory neuropathy, type I, as described in text. (See Figure 9 for explanation of symbols.) (From Dyck *et al.*, 1984, with permission.)

3. *Hereditary Motor and Sensory Neuropathy, Type I*

Hereditary motor and sensory neuropathy (HMSN), type I, is a dominantly inherited disorder with foot and leg muscle weakness and insidious sensory loss generally beginning in the second and third decade. Detection thresholds of various sensations for the foot of patients with HMSN type I are shown in Figure 18. For vibration, 51 of 56 patients exhibited too many insensitive points, and another had elevated threshold of sensitive points. Only four patients had threshold values of vibration sensation within normal limits, and all of these were under the age of 15 years (upper). For touch–pressure sensation, 39 of 59 patients exhibited abnormal values (middle). By contrast, only 16 of 49 patients had abnormalities of thermal cooling thresholds (lower).

E. Summary

Using computer-assisted sensory examination at defined sites and in a large population of healthy subjects, we have demonstrated that thresholds vary with site, age, and sex. Whereas a significant age or sex effect was not found for the lip or forehead, threshold rose with age for the finger (hand) and the toe (foot).

For touch–pressure (as displacement) and vibration threshold in young subjects, the finger was most sensitive, followed by the toe and then the face. With old age, the hand approached the values for the face, and the toe became less sensitive. For touch–pressure and at older ages, males were less sensitive than females. For thermal cooling, the face was most sensitive, followed by the hand and then the foot.

Altered sensation with age and disease is recognized by an increased number of insensitive grid points and/or a raised threshold at sensitive points.

The pattern of loss among various sensory modalities predicts which receptors and afferent population of neurons (axons) are affected.

The approaches to test sensation and the normative values provided here will be useful in the study of patients with disease of receptors and sensory pathways.

ACKNOWLEDGMENTS. This investigation was supported in part by Peripheral Neuropathy Grants from NINCDS (NS14304 and NS18012), a Center Grant from MDA, and Mayo, Borchard, Upton, Herrick, and Leff Funds.

References

BOLTON, C. F., WINKELMANN, R. K., AND DYCK, P. J. A quantitative study of Meissner's corpuscles in man. *Neurology (Minneap.)* 16:1–9, 1966.

BOYD, I. A., AND SMITH, R. S. The muscle spindle, in: *Peripheral Neuropathy* (P. J. DYCK, P. K. THOMAS, E. H. LAMBERT, AND R. BUNGE, eds.), W. B. Saunders, Philadelphia, 1984, pp. 171–202.

CRAGO, P. E. Golgi tendon organs, in: *Peripheral Neuropathy* (P. J. DYCK, P. K. THOMAS, E. H. LAMBERT, AND R. BUNGE, eds.), W. B. Saunders, Philadelphia, 1984, pp. 203–209.

DYCK, P. J., ZIMMERMAN, I. R., O'BRIEN, P. C., NESS, A., CASKEY, P. E., KARNES, J., AND BUSHEK, W. Introduction of automated systems to evaluate touch-pressure, vibration and thermal cutaneous sensation in man. *Ann. Neurol.* 4:502–510, 1978.

DYCK, P. J., KARNES, J., O'BRIEN, P. C., AND ZIMMERMAN, I. R. Detection thresholds of cutaneous sensation in humans, in: *Peripheral Neuropathy* (P. J. DYCK, P. K. THOMAS, E. H. LAMBERT, AND R. BUNGE, eds.), W. B. Saunders, Philadelphia, 1984, pp. 1103–1138.

LIGHT, A. R., AND PERL, E. R. Peripheral sensory systems, in: *Peripheral Neuropathy* (P. J. DYCK, P. K. THOMAS, E. H. LAMBERT, AND R. BUNGE, eds.), W. B. Saunders, Philadelphia, 1984, pp. 210–230.

SEKULAR, R., NASH, D., AND ARMSTRONG, R. Sensitive objective procedure for evaluating response to light touch. *Neurology (Minneap.)* 23:1282–1289, 1973.

15
Control Systems for Nociceptive Afferent Processing
The Descending Inhibitory Pathways

DONNA L. HAMMOND

A. *Introduction*

Afferent transmission in the spinal cord is subject to regulation by supraspinally located neurons. This concept originated with Sherrington and Sowton's (1915) observation that transection of the spinal cord in decerebrate cats enhanced the flexion reflex and was developed further by Lundberg and associates in their studies of flexor reflex afferents (Eccles and Lundberg, 1959; Holmqvist and Lundberg, 1959, 1961). Although these early studies emphasized the effects of descending inhibitory control systems on motor function [see Willis (1982) and Lundberg (1982) for review], later studies demonstrated that this concept also applied to sensory function. Thus, Wall (1967) observed that cold block of the spinal cord in decerebrate cats not only enhanced the spontaneous activity of previously quiescent dorsal horn neurons but also augmented their response to peripheral stimuli. Similar observations were made by other laboratories with the additional finding that the inhibition appeared to be selective for the dorsal horn neurons' responses to noxious, as opposed to nonnoxious, stimuli (Besson *et al.*, 1975; Handwerker *et al.*, 1975; Duggan *et al.*, 1977a; Soja and Sinclair, 1983).

The neurons that comprise this descending inhibitory control system are contained not within any one specific nucleus but rather within many different nuclei. These include the nucleus raphe magnus, raphe dorsalis, reticularis

DONNA L. HAMMOND • Department of Biological Research, G.D. Searle and Co., Research and Development Division, Skokie, Illinois 60077.

paragigantocellularis, locus coeruleus, periaqueductal gray, mesencephalic reticular formation, hypothalamus, and somatosensory cortex. In reviewing the anatomy, physiology, and pharmacology of the centrifugal control systems, this chapter emphasizes their influence on nociceptive afferent transmission in the spinal cord. Further discussion on the anatomic substrates in the spinal cord that are affected by these spinopetal systems are found in the chapters by Ruda (Chapter 7) on the distribution of descending terminals at the electron microscopic level, Seybold (Chapter 6) on the distribution of neurotransmitter receptors in the dorsal gray, and LaMotte (Chapter 5) on the distribution of neurotransmitter terminal systems in the dorsal gray.

B. Descending Inhibitory Neuronal Pathways

1. Corticofugal

The control exerted by sensorimotor cortex on spinal afferent transmission was first recognized by Lloyd (1941) in his study of the effects of cortical stimulation on spinal cord neuronal activity. Stimulation of sensorimotor cortex was subsequently reported to affect the transmission of afferent volleys in the spinal cord (Hagbarth and Kerr, 1954), interneurons of spinal reflex pathways (Lundberg and Voorhoeve, 1962; Lundberg *et al.*, 1962), and primary afferent fibers (Carpenter *et al.*, 1963; Andersen *et al.*, 1964) as well.

More recently, the effect of cortical stimulation on spinothalamic tract neurons has been investigated (Coulter *et al.*, 1974; Yezierski *et al.*, 1983). Although stimulation of precentral motor cortex has a predominantly excitatory effect, stimulation of somatosensory cortex (SI) inhibits the spontaneous activity of wide-dynamic-range spinothalamic tract neurons. In addition, stimulation of SI cortex also inhibits these neurons' responses to nonnoxious and noxious stimuli. For a given stimulus strength, the response to the nonnoxious stimulus is inhibited to a greater extent than is the response to the noxious stimulus. However, stimulation of SI cortex clearly inhibits spinothalamic tract neurons' responses to C-fiber volleys in sural nerve and to noxious thermal and mechanical stimuli (Yezierski *et al.*, 1983). Sessle *et al.* (1981) similarly reported that stimulation of SI and SII somatosensory cortex inhibits wide-dynamic-range neurons of the pars caudalis of the spinal trigeminal nucleus. Although the inhibitory effects of SI and SII cortical stimulation appear to be preferential for these medullary dorsal horn neurons' responses to nonnoxious stimuli, inhibition of their responses to noxious stimuli clearly occurs (Sessle *et al.*, 1981).

Attempts to define the pathways that mediate the effects of cortical stimulation on spinal cord neurons have been limited to lesions of the pyramids or of the dorsal aspect of the lateral funiculus, in which the lateral corticospinal tract is located. Transection of the pyramids or of the dorsolateral funiculus either reduces or abolishes the effects of cortical stimulation, indicating that these effects are mediated by the corticospinal tract (Lundberg and Voorhoeve, 1962; Carpenter *et al.*, 1963; Hongo and Jankowska, 1967; Yezierski *et al.*, 1983). However, an involvement of extrapyramidal pathways is also indicated by the failure of these lesions to abolish fully the effects of cortical stimulation (Carpenter *et al.*, 1963; Yezierski *et al.*, 1983) and by the fact that similar effects can be obtained in acutely pyramidotomized animals (Hongo and Jankowska, 1967). The inhibitory influence of somatosensory cortex on spinothalamic tract neurons is similarly mediated by both pyramidal and extrapyramidal pathways (Yezierski *et al.*, 1983).

The pyramidally shaped neurons of SI and SII somatosensory cortex that project to the spinal cord or to the spinal trigeminal nucleus are situated in lamina V of the cortex and are somatotopically organized (Wise and Jones, 1977; Wise *et al.*, 1979; Murray and Coulter, 1981; Hayes and Rustioni, 1981). They are generally larger than the surrounding neuronal population, having a mean soma diameter between 19 and 22 μm in the rat (Wise and Jones, 1977) and between 19 and 30 μm in the monkey (Murray and Coulter, 1981). The SI and SII neurons that project to the spinal cord terminate principally in the nucleus proprius; few or no terminations are reported in the superficial laminae of the dorsal horn (Kuypers, 1960; Liu and Chambers, 1964; Coulter and Jones, 1977; Armand, 1982). A similar pattern of termination exists for projections of SI and SII neurons to the spinal trigeminal nucleus (Kuypers, 1960; Wise and Jones, 1977). The majority of axons in the corticospinal tract are less than 2 μm in diameter (Wiesendanger, 1969; Armand, 1982).

Neurons of the SI and SII somatosensory cortex also project to the striatum, the reticular, ventrobasal, posterior, and intralaminar nuclei of the thalamus, and to the mesencephalic and medullary reticular formation (Wise and Jones, 1977; Catsman-Berrevoets and Kuypers, 1981; Armand, 1982). Several of these nuclei have also been implicated in the centrifugal control of nociceptive transmission in the spinal cord. Therefore, the projections of SI and SII neurons to these nuclei may comprise the extrapyramidal pathway(s) that mediates the effects of somatosensory cortical stimulation. These relay nuclei are discussed individually in later sections of this review. However, because of their function as relay nuclei, a discussion of their properties would also apply to the extrapyramidal pathway(s).

2. *Diencephalic*

Several diencephalic nuclei participate in the centrifugal control of nociceptive transmission in the spinal cord. These include the periventricular gray, medial and lateral hypothalamus, medial preoptic/basal forebrain region, and somatosensory nuclei of the thalamus. Electrical stimulation of the periventricular gray, including the medial and lateral hypothalamus, and of the medial preoptic/basal forebrain region attenuates the response of wide-dynamic-range dorsal horn neurons to noxious radiant heating of the skin. This stimulation effectively reduces the slope of the temperature–response function of the dorsal horn neurons with little or no increase in their response threshold (Carstens, 1982; Carstens *et al.*, 1982, 1983a).

Stimulation of the ventral posterior medial and lateral nuclei of the thalamus also inhibits the evoked responses of identified wide-dynamic-range and high-threshold spinothalamic tract neurons (Gerhart *et al.*, 1981b, 1983). Although stimulation of these nuclei does not preferentially inhibit the responses to nonnoxious or noxious natural stimuli, the response to C-fiber volleys in the sural nerve is reduced to a greater extent than is the response to A-fiber volleys (Gerhart *et al.*, 1983).

Inhibition of dorsal horn neuronal responses to noxious stimuli is a mechanism consistent with an elevation in nociceptive threshold or the production of analgesia. In unanesthetized animals, electrical stimulation of the hypothalamus increases response latencies or thresholds to noxious stimuli (Black *et al.*, 1972; Yunger *et al.*, 1973; Rhodes and Liebeskind, 1978; Oleson *et al.*, 1980) and reduces escape responses to aversive stimuli (Oleson *et al.*, 1980; Cox and Valenstein, 1965). Similarly, response latencies or thresholds are increased (Schmidek *et al.*, 1971; Mayer and Liebeskind, 1974; Goodman and Holcombe, 1976; Rhodes and Liebeskind, 1978; Oleson *et al.*, 1980) and escape responses are reduced (Oleson *et al.*, 1980) by stimulation of thalamic nuclei. These results are supported by numerous clinical reports that electrical stimulation of these nuclei, and of the thalamus in particular, produces pain relief (Hosobuchi *et al.*, 1973; Gybels *et al.*, 1976; Richardson and Akil, 1977; Mazars *et al.*, 1979).

Preliminary studies suggest that the medial and lateral hypothalamic influence on nociceptive transmission in the spinal cord is mediated by a pathway in the dorsolateral quadrant of the spinal cord, because lesions of this area reduce or abolish the inhibitory effect of hypothalamic stimulation (Carstens, 1982; Carstens *et al.*, 1983a). A direct, predominantly ipsilateral projection of the medial and, to a lesser extent, lateral nuclei of the hypothalamus to the spinal cord is reported (Kuypers and Maisky, 1975, 1977; Saper *et al.*, 1976; Hancock, 1976; Kniesley *et al.*, 1978; Basbaum and Fields, 1979; Hosoya, 1980; Swanson and Kuypers, 1980; Watkins *et al.*, 1981). The spinal laminae in which these projections terminate are undefined as yet, although oxytocin- and vasopressin-containing neurons of the hypothalamus are known to terminate in laminae I–III of the spinal cord (Nilaver *et al.*, 1980). As the paraventricular nucleus of the medial hypothalamus projects principally in the dorsolateral funiculus, activation of this direct hypothalamospinal pathway may mediate the effects of medial hypothalamic stimulation. In contrast, the spinal projection of the lateral hypothalamus is less prominent and may descend in the ventral and ventrolateral funiculi as well. Precise definition of the funicular pathways that mediate the effects of medial and lateral hypothalamic stimulation awaits further studies of the relative involvement of contralateral and ipsilateral hypothalamospinal pathways in the dorsolateral and other funiculi.

Mediation of the hypothalamic influence by other than direct spinal projections is also feasible. Both the medial and lateral hypothalamus project to the periaqueductal gray and medullary reticular formation, including the nucleus raphe magnus (Conrad and Pfaff, 1976a,b; Grofova *et al.*, 1978; Hosoya and Matsushita, 1981; Abols and Basbaum, 1981; Berk and Finkelstein, 1982; Veazey *et al.*, 1982). As these areas are involved in the centrifugal control of noiception (see Sections B.3, B.4), they represent indirect pathways to the spinal cord by which hypothalamic nuclei may regulate nociceptive transmission.

There is little evidence for a significant direct projection of thalamic neurons to the spinal cord. Yet the inhibition of dorsal horn neurons produced by thalamic stimulation is antagonized when bilateral lesions of the dorsolateral funiculus are extended ipsilaterally to include the ventrolateral funiculus (Gerhart *et al.*, 1983). Because SI and SII somatosensory cortex receives projections from the ventrobasal thalamus (see references in Yaksh and Hammond, 1982), it is tempting to postulate that stimulation of the ventromedial and lateral thalamus results in the activation of corticofugal neurons of the pyramidal and extrapyramidal pathways discussed previously. However, in contrast to cortical stimulation, the inhibitory effect of thalamic stimulation is (1) not preferential for nonnoxious stimuli and (2) not antagonized by lesions of the dorsolateral funiculus. These observations make it unlikely that activation of corticofugal inhibitory pathways is responsible for the effects of thalamic stimulation.

Perhaps of greater importance is the potential for antidromic activation of spinothalamic tract neurons during stimulation of the ventrobasal thalamus (Gerhart *et al.*, 1983). As the axons of spinothalamic tract neurons ascend to the ventrobasal thalamus, collaterals are given off to the medullary reticular formation and periaqueductal gray (Price *et al.*, 1978; Giesler *et al.*, 1981b; Kevetter and Willis, 1982) as well as to other thalamic nuclei (Applebaum *et al.*, 1979; Giesler *et al.*, 1981b). Antidromic activation of these collaterals could activate neurons of the periaqueductal gray and medullary reticular formation that participate in centrifugal control of nociceptive transmission in the spinal cord. The recent demonstration by Tsubokawa *et al.* (1982) that stimulation of the ventrobasal thalamus activates spinally projecting neurons of the raphe magnus supports this postulate. Again, however, the failure of lesions of the dorsolateral funiculus to effectively attenuate the inhibitory effects of thalamic stimulation, as observed with stimulation of the raphe magnus and periaqueductal gray, (see Sections B.3, B.4) argues against this postulate. Thus, the pathways that mediate the effects of thalamic activation remain to be elucidated.

3. *Mesencephalic*

Within the mesencephalon, the periaqueductal gray (PAG), dorsal raphe nucleus (NRD), and adjacent mesencephalic reticular formation (MRF) have been identified as sources of centrifugal control. Electrical stimulation of these regions inhibits the evoked responses of medullary and spinal dorsal horn neurons; the response to noxious stimuli is inhibited to a greater extent than is the response to nonnoxious stimuli (Liebeskind *et al.*, 1973; Oliveras *et al.*, 1974; Bennett and Mayer, 1979; Hayes *et al.*, 1979; Sessle *et al.*, 1981; Carstens *et al.*, 1981a; Dostrovsky *et al.*, 1983; Duggan and Morton, 1983). Jurna (1980) has reported that stimulation of the PAG similarly inhibits Aγ- and C-fiber-evoked activity in ascending fibers of the spinal cord but does not affect the discharge evoked by activation of Aβ fibers.

This selective reduction of dorsal horn neuronal responsiveness to noxious stimuli predicts that stimulation of these sites in the unanesthetized animal would produce analgesia. Indeed, a multitude of studies have since demonstrated that activation of these regions, either by electrical stimulation or by microinjection of morphine or glutamate, increases response latencies and thresholds to noxious stimuli or decreases reflexive reactions to noxious stimuli (Liebeskind *et al.*, 1973; Oliveras *et al.*, 1974; Jacquet and Lajtha, 1974; Mayer and Liebeskind, 1974; Goodman and Holcombe, 1976; Soper, 1976; Yaksh *et al.*, 1976c; Lewis and Gebhart, 1977; Haigler and Mittleman, 1978; Rhodes and Liebeskind, 1978; Yaksh and Rudy, 1978; Hayes *et al.*, 1979; Soper and Melzack, 1982; Jensen and Yaksh, 1984). These studies are complemented by clinical reports of pain relief following stimulation of the PAG (Mazars *et al.*, 1979; Hosobuchi *et al.*, 1977).

The analgesia produced by stimulation of the PAG is attenuated or abolished by an ipsilateral lesion of the dorsolateral funiculus (Basbaum *et al.*, 1977), suggesting that the effect is mediated by a descending spinal projection. Yet, early anatomic studies failed to identify a significant projection of the PAG and NRD to the spinal cord (Kuypers and Maisky, 1975, 1977; Kneisley *et al.*, 1978; Leichnetz *et al.*, 1978). Consequently, discussions of the pathway(s) that mediates the effects of stimulation of the PAG and NRD emphasized the efferent projections of these nuclei to the nucleus raphe magnus (Gallager and Pert, 1978; Lovick *et al.*, 1978). The subsequent postulate that activation of raphe–spinal neurons mediated the effects of PAG stimulation was given widespread credence.

However, it is unfortunate that the results of recent retrograde and anterograde transport studies have been overlooked in the zeal to subscribe to this postulate. These studies, using much improved reaction methods and tracers, indicate that neurons of the PAG and NRD do project directly to the spinal cord and its medullary homologue, the spinal trigeminal nucleus; the projection is predominantly ipsilateral to the deeper laminae (Castiglioni *et al.*, 1978; Tohyama *et al.*, 1979b; Martin *et al.*, 1981; Watkins *et al.*, 1981; Mantyh and Peschanski, 1982; Beitz *et al.*, 1983; Mantyh, 1983). Basbaum and Fields (1979) and Watkins *et al.* (1981) have reported that the projection descends in the dorsolateral funiculus; the projection to the lumbar cord is much sparser than that to the cervical cord (Castiglioni *et al.*, 1978; Watkins *et al.*, 1981; Mantyh and Peschanski, 1982). A direct spinal projection that descends in the ventral and ventrolateral funiculi is described from the MRF as well (Castiglioni *et al.*, 1978; Tohyama *et al.*, 1979a; Basbaum and Fields, 1979; Hayes and Rustioni, 1981). Thus, a portion of the effects of PAG and

NRD stimulation may be mediated by activation of their direct projection to the spinal cord.*

As mentioned above, the effects of PAG stimulation are thought to be mediated by activation of raphe–spinal and reticulospinal neurons themselves involved in the regulation of nociception at the spinal level. There is ample anatomic and electrophysiological evidence to support this postulate. Retrograde and anterograde transport studies have documented a dense projection of PAG neurons (but not of dorsal raphe neurons) to the nucleus raphe magnus and closely adjacent medullary reticular formation (Gallager and Pert, 1978; Abols and Basbaum, 1981; Carlton *et al.*, 1983; Mantyh, 1983). Complementary electrophysiological studies report a direct, excitatory projection from the PAG to identified raphe–spinal neurons (Lovick *et al.*, 1978; Fields and Anderson, 1978; Pomeroy and Behbehani, 1979; Tsubokawa *et al.*, 1982). Estimates of conduction velocity indicate that a significant proportion of this projection is composed of myelinated fibers (Lovick *et al.*, 1978; Pomeroy and Behbehani, 1979; Shah and Dostrovsky, 1980). The projection from the PAG to the nucleus raphe magnus is distinct from its projection to the spinal cord (Shah and Dostrovsky, 1980; Mantyh, 1983). Furthermore, procedures that produce analgesia, such as focal electrical stimulation of or microinjection of morphine or glutamate into the PAG, are associated with an increase in the spontaneous activity of neurons of the nucleus raphe magnus (Behbehani and Fields, 1979; Fields and Anderson, 1978; Oleson *et al.*, 1978) and of the adjacent medullary reticular formation (Mohrland and Gebhart, 1980). Finally, the analgesia produced by activation of the PAG is attenuated by lesions of the nucleus raphe magnus and adjacent medullary reticular formation (Behbehani and Fields, 1979; Prieto *et al.*, 1983). Thus, the effects produced by stimulation of the PAG appear to be mediated by activation of neurons of the nucleus raphe magnus and adjacent medullary reticular formation that project to the spinal cord. However, in view of recent evidence for a direct spinal projection of the PAG to the spinal cord, studies of the relative contributions of these two pathways to the effects of stimulation will be required.

4. *Medullary*

Of the medullary nuclei involved in the centrifugal control of nociception at the spinal level, two have been examined quite extensively. These are the nucleus raphe magnus (NRM) and the closely adjacent reticular formation. In the cat, the portion of the reticular formation that lies immediately lateral to the NRM is termed the nucleus reticularis magnocellularis (Berman, 1968; Basbaum *et al.*, 1978). In the rodent, it is referred to as the nucleus reticularis

* It is notable that lesions of the dorsolateral funiculus are frequently made at the cervical and thoracic levels to which neurons of the PAG project. Transection of the PAG pathway to the spinal cord, as well as of the raphe–spinal pathway, may therefore contribute to the ability of such a lesion to abolish the effects of stimulation.

gigantocellularis pars alpha (Meessen and Olszewski, 1949) or as the nucleus reticularis paragigantocellularis (Fifkova and Marsala, 1967). In this review it is termed the nucleus reticularis paragigantocellularis (NRPG) and, as such, is not to be confused with the much more ventrolaterally situated nucleus reticularis paragigantocellularis lateralis or lateral reticular nucleus (Andrezik *et al.*, 1981).

In the unanesthetized animal, focal electrical stimulation of the NRM (Oliveras *et al.*, 1975, 1979; Proudfit and Anderson, 1975; Oleson *et al.*, 1980; Satoh *et al.*, 1980; Zorman *et al.*, 1981; Hammond and Yaksh, 1984) and of the NRPG (Akaike *et al.*, 1978; Satoh *et al.*, 1980; Zorman *et al.*, 1981; Hammond and Yaksh, 1984) increases response latencies and thresholds to noxious stimuli with little effect on responses to tactile stimuli. Analgesia is also produced by the microinjection of opiates (Takagi *et al.*, 1976; Akaike *et al.*, 1978; Fields and Anderson, 1978; Dickenson *et al.*, 1979; LeBars *et al.*, 1980), glutamate (Satoh *et al.*, 1983; Jensen and Yaksh, 1984), noradrenergic antagonists (Hammond *et al.*, 1980a; Sagen and Proudfit, 1985), and cholinergic agonists (Brodie and Proudfit, 1984) in these regions.

The neuronal correlate for stimulation-produced analgesia is thought to reside in the inhibitory effects of stimulation on the responses of spinal and medullary dorsal horn neurons to noxious and nonnoxious stimuli. These effects have been extensively examined for a wide variety of dorsal horn neurons including low-threshold mechanoreceptive neurons, nociceptive-specific and wide-dynamic-range neurons, and identified neurons of the spinothalamic and spinocervical tracts. In each study, focal electrical stimulation of the NRM profoundly inhibits the response of spinal and medullary dorsal horn neurons to noxious stimuli (Beall *et al.*, 1976; Fields *et al.*, 1977; Guilbaud *et al.*, 1977; Willis *et al.*, 1977; Belcher *et al.*, 1978; Duggan and Griersmith, 1979; McCreery *et al.*, 1979; Rivot *et al.*, 1980; Gerhart *et al.*, 1981a; Sessle *et al.*, 1981; Dostrovsky *et al.*, 1983; Edeson and Ryall, 1983; Gray and Dostrovsky, 1983). The response of these neurons to nonnoxious stimuli is either unaffected (Fields *et al.*, 1977; Guilbaud *et al.*, 1977; Duggan and Griersmith, 1979) or inhibited by stimulation of the NRM (Beall *et al.*, 1976; Willis *et al.*, 1977; Belcher *et al.*, 1978; McCreery *et al.*, 1979; Rivot *et al.*, 1980; Gerhart *et al.*, 1981a; Sessle *et al.*, 1981; Dostrovsky *et al.*, 1983; Gray and Dostrovsky, 1983; Kajander *et al.*, 1984).

Differences in interpretation of the latter effect may reflect the various types and intensities of stimuli used to activate dorsal horn neurons and the variety of methods used to express inhibition (i.e., calculation of current thresholds, incidence of inhibition, or percentage inhibition). Nevertheless, it is clear that the inhibition produced by stimulation of the NRM is not specific for the responses of dorsal horn neurons to noxious stimuli. It does appear, however, to be preferential for nociceptive responses (Fields *et al.*, 1977; Guilbaud *et al.*, 1977; Willis *et al.*, 1977; Belcher *et al.*, 1978; Duggan and Griersmith, 1979; Rivot *et al.*, 1980; Dostrovsky *et al.*, 1983), although alternate interpretations have been proffered (McCreery *et al.*, 1979; Gerhart *et al.*, 1981a; Gray and Dostrovsky, 1983).

Stimulation of the adjacent NRPG is also reported to inhibit the response of spinal and medullary dorsal horn neurons to noxious stimuli (McCreery and Bloedel, 1975; Fields *et al.*, 1977; Belcher *et al.*, 1978; Haber *et al.*, 1978; McCreery *et al.*, 1979; Rivot *et al.*, 1980; Dostrovsky *et al.*, 1983; Edeson and Ryall, 1983; Gray and Dostrovsky, 1983). The majority of studies that have compared the inhibitory effects of stimulation in the NRM and in the NRPG within the same preparation report that the NRM is the most effective site (Fields *et al.*, 1977; Belcher *et al.*, 1978; McCreery *et al.*, 1979; Rivot *et al.*, 1980; Sessle *et al.*, 1981; but see Dostrovsky *et al.*, 1983; Edeson and Ryall, 1983; Gray and Dostrovsky, 1983). The results of many of these studies indicate that the inhibitory effects of stimulation of these nuclei are attenuated by ipsilateral lesions of the dorsolateral funiculus and frequently are abolished by bilateral lesions of this funiculus (Fields *et al.*, 1977; Willis *et al.*, 1977; McCreery *et al.*, 1979).

The projection of neurons of the NRM to the spinal cord was initially identified in studies of retrograde degeneration (Brodal *et al.*, 1960). Since then, a multitude of retrograde transport studies have confirmed that neurons of the NRM and NRPG project directly to the spinal cord and spinal trigeminal nucleus (Kuypers and Maisky, 1975, 1977; Crutcher *et al.*, 1978; Kneisley *et al.*, 1978; Leichnetz *et al.*, 1978; Martin *et al.*, 1978; Basbaum and Fields, 1979; Tohyama *et al.*, 1979a,b; Watkins *et al.*, 1980; Martin *et al.*, 1981; Beitz *et al.*, 1983; Lovick and Wolstencroft, 1983); the projection to the lumbar cord is less dense that that to the cervical cord. The neurons that are retrogradely labeled range from 20 to 50 μm in diameter and are fusiform or polygonal in shape (Kneisley *et al.*, 1978; Leichnetz *et al.*, 1978; Martin *et al.*, 1978; Crutcher *et al.*, 1978; Tohyama *et al.*, 1979a,b; Lovick and Wolstencroft, 1983).

Studies of anterograde transport also identify a projection of neurons of the NRM and NRPG to the spinal cord and spinal trigeminal nucleus that terminate extensively in the superficial laminae; neurons of the NRPG also terminate in the ventral horn (Bobillier *et al.*, 1976; Basbaum *et al.*, 1978; Martin *et al.*, 1981; Holstege and Kuypers, 1982). The projection of neurons of the NRPG is predominantly ipsilateral to the spinal cord, descending in the dorsolateral and ventrolateral funiculi (Kuypers and Maisky, 1977; Basbaum *et al.*, 1978; Martin *et al.*, 1978; Basbaum and Fields, 1979; Tohyama *et al.*, 1979a; Martin *et al.*, 1981), and bilateral to the spinal trigeminal nucleus (Beitz *et al.*, 1983; Lovick and Wolstencroft, 1983). Predominantly ipsilateral projections are reported for neurons of the NRM following restricted injections of horseradish peroxidase in the spinal cord. However, the pattern of labeling following injections of tritiated leucine in this nucleus indicates a bilateral projection to the spinal cord (Basbaum *et al.*, 1978; Holstege and Kuypers, 1982). Nevertheless, the consensus of these studies is that the vast majority of NRM neurons that project to the spinal cord do so in the dorsolateral funiculus, although a small number appear to project in the ventrolateral funiculus as well (Kuypers and Maisky, 1977; Basbaum *et al.*, 1978; Crutcher *et al.*, 1978; Leichnetz *et al.*, 1978; Martin *et al.*, 1978; Basbaum and Fields, 1979; Tohyama *et al.*, 1979b; Watkins *et al.*, 1980; G. F. Martin *et al.*, 1981; Holstege and Kuypers, 1982). It should be noted that neurons of the NRM (Hayes and Rustioni, 1981) and of the NRPG (Martin *et al.*, 1981) innervate more than one level of the spinal cord.

The conduction velocity of neurons of the NRM that project to the spinal cord has been estimated following their antidromic activation from the spinal cord. In the cat, these estimates range between 5 and 67 m/s (Anderson *et al.*, 1977; West and Wolstencroft, 1977; Fields and Anderson, 1978; Lovick *et al.*, 1978). In the rat, the conduction velocity reportedly ranges from less than 1 to greater than 30 m/s (Wessendorf *et al.*, 1981). Failure to observe lower conduction velocities in earlier studies may be attributed to the characteristics of the recording micropipette and the intensity of the search stimulus used in the spinal cord. It is clear, however, that a significant proportion of the spinal projection of NRM neurons is composed of myelinated fibers. The short latencies to inhibition of dorsal horn neurons observed on stimulation of the NRM are consistent with this interpretation (Willis *et al.*, 1977; Belcher *et al.*, 1978; McCreery *et al.*, 1979; Rivot *et al.*, 1980; Giesler *et al.*, 1981a).

C. Pharmacology of the Descending Control Systems

Four avenues of approach have been pursued in studies of the pharmacology of the neuronal systems that modulate nociceptive afferent transmission at the level of the spinal cord. These are (1) immunohistochemical identification of neurons, (2) administration of antagonists, (3) depletion of neurotransmitters, and (4) documentation of the release of endogenous neurotransmitters during activation of the neuronal systems. Perhaps it has been the first approach, immunohistochemical identification, that has awakened us to the pharmacological complexity of the centrifugal control systems.

A list of neurotransmitters contained within neurons of the brain that project to the spinal cord would include serotonin (Dahlstrom and Fuxe, 1965; Bowker *et al.*, 1982a), norepinephrine (Dahlstrom and Fuxe, 1965; Westlund *et al.*, 1982), dopamine (Skagerberg *et al.*, 1982), enkephalin (Hökfelt *et al.*, 1979; Bowker *et al.*, 1983), substance P (Bowker *et al.*, 1983), thyrotropin-releasing hormone (Bowker *et al.*, 1983), and cholecystokinin (Skirboll *et al.*, 1983; Mantyh and Hunt, 1984). Furthermore, many of these neurotransmitters, such as enkephalin and serotonin (Glazer *et al.*, 1981) and substance P and serotonin (Hökfelt *et al.*, 1978; Chan-Palay, 1979) coexist within the same neurons. Finally, peptidergic neurons (enkephalin, dynorphin, substance P) contained within the spinal cord may function as interneurons in the bulbospinal pathways. Thus, more than one neurotransmitter is likely to mediate the effects produced by activation of the centrifugal neuronal pathways.

Identification of a substance as the neurotransmitter that mediates the effects of activation of a centrifugal pathway requires the demonstration that the effects of activation can be mimicked by exogenous administration of the substance. For example, the inhibition of dorsal horn neuronal responses produced by stimulation of the various nuclei discussed above can be mimicked by iontophoretic application of enkephalin (Duggan *et al.*, 1977b; Zieglgansberger and Tulloch, 1979), serotonin (Randic and Yu, 1976; Headley *et al.*, 1978; Jordan *et al.*, 1978), and norepinephrine (Headley *et al.*, 1978; Belcher *et al.*, 1978) to dorsal horn neurons. Similarly, administration of enkephalin (Yaksh *et al.*, 1977), serotonin (Yaksh and Wilson, 1979), and norepinephrine (Kuraishi *et al.*, 1979a; Reddy *et al.*, 1980) to the spinal cord subarachnoid space produces analgesia comparable to that produced by electrical stimulation of these nuclei. Additional requirements for identification, such as the ability of pharmacological antagonism to block the effects of activation, the presence of these neurotransmitters in the nuclei, and documentation of their release in the spinal cord on activation of these systems, is provided in the following sections. Because enkephalin, serotonin, and norepinephrine have been more amenable to pharmacological manipulation and, therefore, have been examined more extensively, the following section is restricted to an examination of their involvement.

1. *Pharmacology of Diencephalic Pathways*

The medial preoptic area, the anterior and lateral hypothalamus, and the paraventricular nucleus of the hypothalamus contain enkephalin-immunoreactive perikarya (Hökfelt *et al.*, 1977; Sar *et al.*, 1978; Wamsley *et al.*, 1980; Finley *et al.*, 1981; Williams and Dockray, 1983). However, a projection of these neurons to the spinal cord is as yet unidentified. Dynorphin-containing perikarya are also located in these nuclei (Vincent *et al.*, 1982; Khachaturian *et al.*, 1982). They do not appear to project to the spinal cord in significant numbers because no decrease in dynorphin content of the spinal cord occurs caudal to a thoracic transection (Goldstein and Ghazarossian, 1980). The vasopressin- and oxytocin-containing neurons of the paraventricular nucleus of the hypothalamus, however, do project to the superficial laminae of the spinal cord (Nilaver *et al.*, 1980; Sawchenko and Swanson, 1982). As yet, no studies have examined the involvement of enkephalin, dynorphin, or vasopressin in the inhibitory effects produced by stimulation of the hypothalamus or medial diencephalon.

In contrast, the possible mediation of these effects by serotonin has been explored. The inhibition of dorsal horn neurons produced by stimulation of the medial diencephalon and basal forebrain (Carstens *et al.*, 1983b) and of the lateral hypothalamus (Carstens *et al.*, 1983a) is antagonized by systemic administration of the serotonergic antagonist methysergide. Depletion of serotonin in the CNS by administration of *p*-chlorophenylalanine (PCPA) also attenuates the inhibitory effects of stimulation in the medial diencephalon and basal forebrain (Carstens *et al.*, 1983b). Although they afford no insight as to the site of action, these studies indicate that the inhibitory effect of stimulation of these regions is mediated by serotonin. Yet, no serotonergic perikarya have been identified in the hypothalamus, periventricular gray, or medial diencephalon (Steinbusch, 1981), although a small population of serotonin-containing perikarya has been reported in the dorsomedial nucleus of the hypothalamus (Frankfurt *et al.*, 1981). In addition, no serotonergic hypothalamospinal or diencephalospinal projections have been identified (Bowker *et al.*, 1982a). These observations imply that the serotonergically mediated effects produced by stimulation of these nuclei result from activation of the serotonergic relay nuclei to which they project, i.e., the nucleus raphe magnus, periaqueductal gray, or dorsal raphe nucleus.

2. *Pharmacology of Mesencephalic Pathways*

Many studies have examined the possible involvement of an endogenous opioid in the effects produced by stimulation of the PAG, NRD, and MRF. Systemically administered naloxone has been reported to antagonize the effects of activation of the PAG (Akil *et al.*, 1975; Hosobuchi *et al.*, 1977; Behbehani and Fields, 1979; Urca *et al.*, 1980) as frequently as it has been reported not to antagonize or to inconsistently antagonize these effects (Yaksh *et al.*, 1976b; Carstens *et al.*, 1979; Hayes *et al.*, 1979; Jurna, 1980; Sessle *et al.*, 1981). The contradictory nature of these results may arise from the systemic route of administration of naloxone. The effects of an antagonist at a supraspinal site may well oppose or negate its effects at the spinal level, as observed with noradrenergic antagonists (Hammond *et al.*, 1980a; Sagen and Proudfit, 1984, 1985). Thus, studies in which the pharmacological manipulation is indiscriminate often yield contradictory results and, worse, may fail to detect an involvement of the neurotransmitter.

Clearly, both enkephalin- and dynorphin-immunoreactive perikarya are contained within the PAG, NRD, and MRF (Hökfelt *et al.*, 1977; Uhl *et al.*, 1979; Finley *et al.*, 1981; Watson *et al.*, 1982; Moss *et al.*, 1983). However, the projections of these neurons have not been well characterized. In view of the postulate that activation of NRM neurons mediates the effects produced by stimulation of the PAG, it is notable that enkephalin-containing neurons of the PAG do not project to the NRM in significant numbers (Beitz, 1982a). The NRM does receive a significant projection from enkephalinergic neurons of the MRF (Beitz, 1982a). The effects of PAG stimulation may be mediated by activation of enkephalinergic neurons in the NRM and NRPG that project to the spinal cord or of enkephalinergic interneurons of the spinal cord.

The contradictory nature of the results obtained with naloxone may also arise from the likelihood that more than one neurotransmitter mediates the effects of stimulation of the mesencephalic nuclei. Serotonin is also implicated.

Serotonergic perikarya are located in the PAG, NRD, and ventral MRF (Dahlstrom and Fuxe, 1965; Schofield and Everitt, 1981; Steinbusch, 1981; Wiklund *et al.*, 1981), and a portion project to the spinal cord (Bowker *et al.*, 1981, 1982a) and spinal trigeminal nucleus (Beitz, 1982c). The effects produced by activation of the PAG and NRD are attenuated by depletion of serotonin (Akil and Mayer, 1972; Carstens *et al.*, 1981b) and by systemic administration of serotonergic antagonists (Guilbaud *et al.*, 1973; Liebeskind *et al.*, 1973; Yaksh *et al.*, 1976a; Hayes *et al.*, 1977; Carstens *et al.*, 1981b; Yezierski *et al.*, 1982b).

In studies in which antagonists are administered systemically or neurotransmitters are depleted indiscriminately, the site of action of the drug or neurotoxin has not been restricted to the spinal cord, the site at which the bulbospinal neurons terminate. Thus, such studies cannot determine whether the effect of stimulation is mediated by activation of neurons that project to the spinal cord. Following intrathecal injection, however, the action of a drug or neurotoxin is restricted to the spinal cord, as very little redistributes to peripheral or supraspinal sites, and then only after substantial delay (Yaksh and Rudy, 1976; LoPachin and Rudy, 1982; Schmauss *et al.*, 1983). Consequently, studies in which the drug or neurotoxin is administered intrathecally can directly evaluate whether activation of bulbospinal pathways mediates the effects of stimulation of supraspinal sites. Such studies represent a significant advance in studies of the pharmacology of the descending control systems.

Subsequent studies using this technique reported that the analgesia produced by microinjection or morphine or glutamate in the PAG is antagonized by intrathecal administration of a serotonergic antagonist (Yaksh, 1979; Jensen and Yaksh, 1985). These results suggested that the effects of activation of the PAG are mediated by a release of serotonin in the spinal cord. This was confirmed with the demonstration that microinjection of morphine in the PAG increased the release of endogenous serotonin from the spinal cord (Yaksh and Tyce, 1979). Together, these studies indicate that activation of bulbospinal serotonergic pathways mediates the actions of the PAG.

The ability of serotonergic antagonists to attenuate the effects produced by activation of the PAG and NRD cannot be attributed to antagonism of the spinal projection of the *serotonergic* neurons in these nuclei. This is based on the observations that (1) the serotonergic neurons of these nuclei project in sparse numbers no further than the cervical level of the spinal cord (Bowker *et al.*, 1981; 1982a), yet (2) intrathecal injection of serotonergic antagonists largely confined to the lumbar level effectively attenuates the effects of stimulation. Rather, it is thought that the effects of stimulation of the PAG are mediated by the subsequent activation of serotonergic neurons of the medulla that project to the lumbosacral level of the spinal cord (see Section C.3). Serotonergic neurons of the PAG also project to the NRM and NRPG (Yezierski *et al.*, 1982a; Beitz, 1982b). This serotonergic synapse on raphe–spinal and reticulospinal neurons therefore represents another site at which systemically administered serotonergic antagonists may act (Yezierski *et al.*, 1982a,b). In contrast to the wealth of studies that implicate serotonin in the actions of the PAG and NRD, the effects of activation of the adjacent MRF do not appear to be mediated by serotonin (Carstens *et al.*, 1981b). This region does not contain serotonergic perikarya (Steinbusch, 1981), although serotonergic perikarya are scattered more ventrally in the MRF (Bowker *et al.*, 1982a).

The effects produced by activation of the PAG are only partially antagonized by administration of serotonergic and opiate antagonists, suggesting that neurotransmitters other than serotonin and enkephalin may also mediate the effects of activation. This is supported by the observation that intrathecal administration of a noradrenergic antagonist also partially attenuates the analgesia produced by microinjection of morphine or glutamate in the PAG (Yaksh, 1979; Jensen and Yaksh, 1985). Intrathecal coadministration of methysergide and phentolamine, or depletion of serotonin and norepinephrine in the spinal cord, abolishes the analgesia, indicating that coactivation of both serotonergic and noradrenergic bulbospinal systems may mediate the analgesia (Yaksh, 1979; Johannessen *et al.*, 1982).

3. *Pharmacology of Medullary Pathways*

Enkephalin is also postulated to mediate the effects produced by activation of the NRM and NRPG. Enkephalin-immunoreactive perikarya are located in both of these nuclei (Hökfelt *et al.*, 1977; Uhl *et al.*, 1979; Finley *et al.*, 1981; Williams and Dockray, 1983), and a small number project to the spinal cord (Hökfelt *et al.*, 1979; Bowker *et al.*, 1983). However, enkephalin-containing neurons comprise only about 10% of the NRM and NRPG neurons that project to the spinal cord (Bowker *et al.*, 1982b). The effects produced by electrical stimulation of the NRM are attenuated by systemically administered naloxone (Oliveras *et al.*, 1977; Rivot *et al.*, 1979; Zorman *et al.*, 1981), although several investigators report no effect of naloxone (Duggan and Griersmith, 1979; Satoh *et al.*, 1980; Hammond and Yaksh, 1984). The analgesia produced by electrical stimulation of the NRPG is also attenuated by systemic administration of naloxone (Satoh *et al.*, 1980; Zorman *et al.*, 1981). Recently, Zorman *et al.*, (1982) reported that intrathecal administration of naloxone antagonizes the analgesia produced by electrical stimulation of the NRM and NRPG. This study, however, could not determine whether antagonism of enkephalinergic interneurons of the spinal cord (Sar *et al.*, 1978; Finley *et al.*, 1981) or of enkephalinergic neurons of the brainstem that project to the spinal cord was responsible for the attenuation.

In contrast to the effects reported using electrical stimulation of the NRM and NRPG, intrathecally administered naloxone does not attenuate the analgesia produced by microinjection of glutamate (Satoh *et al.*, 1983) or of phentolamine (Sagen and Proudfit, 1981) in the NRM and NRPG. Comparison of the results of these studies, in which two disparate means of activation were used, suggests that activation of fibers of passage by electrical stimulation in this region may be an important factor in the production of naloxone-reversible analgesia.

The NRM and NRPG also contain serotonergic perikarya (Dahlstrom and Fuxe, 1965; Schofield and Everitt, 1981; Steinbusch, 1981; Wiklund *et al.*, 1981). Greater than 70% of the neurons in the NRM and NRPG that project to the spinal cord or spinal trigeminal nucleus contain serotonin (Beitz, 1982c; Bowker *et al.*, 1982a,b, 1983). The inhibition of dorsal horn neurons produced by stimulation of the NRM is attenuated by depletion of serotonin (Rivot *et al.*, 1980) or by systemic administration of a serotonergic antagonist (Yezierski *et al.*, 1982b). The analgesia produced by electrical stimulation of the NRM is similary attenuated by systemic administration of a serotonergic antagonist (Satoh *et al.*, 1980). Intrathecal administration of a serotonergic antagonist or depletion of serotonin in the spinal cord also attenuates the analgesia produced by electrical stimulation or by microinjection of glutamate or a noradrenergic antagonist in the NRM (Hammond *et al.*, 1980b; Satoh *et al.*, 1983; Sagen *et al.*, 1983; Hammond and Yaksh, 1984; Jensen and Yaksh, 1985).

These studies indicate that the effects produced by activation of the NRM are mediated by serotonergic neurons of this region that project to the spinal cord. This is confirmed by the recent demonstration that electrical stimulation of the NRM, using current intensities comparable to those that produce analgesia in unanesthetized animals, increases the efflux of endogenous serotonin and 5-hydroxyindoleacetic acid into superfusates of the spinal cord (Hammond *et al.*, 1985). Other investigators have reached similar conclusions indirectly by measuring either the accumulation of 5-hydroxytryptophan (Bourgoin *et al.*, 1980) or the concentration of 5-hydroxyindoles (Rivot *et al.*, 1982) in the spinal cord following stimulation of the NRM.

The NRPG clearly contains serotonergic perikarya that project to the spinal cord and spinal trigeminal nucleus, albeit in smaller numbers than the NRM (Beitz, 1982c; Bowker *et al.*, 1982a,b). Yet, there is disagreement about the role of serotonin in mediating the effects produced by activation of this nucleus. Intrathecally administered methysergide attenuates the analgesia produced by electrical stimulation of or microinjection of glutamate in the NPRG (Hammond and Yaksh, 1984; Jensen and Yaksh, 1985). Satoh *et al.*, (1983), however, report that intrathecally administered methysergide does not attenuate the analgesia produced by microinjection of glutamate in the NRPG. These differences may result from the different antinociceptive tests utilized by the investigators.

The involvement of norepinephrine in the effects produced by activation of the NRM and NRPG has been less well examined, perhaps because these nuclei do not contain noradrenergic perikarya (Poitras and Parent, 1978; Westlund *et al.*, 1982). Nevertheless, there is evidence that the effects of activation of the NRM are mediated by noradrenergic neurons that project to the spinal cord. Intrathecal administration of a noradrenergic antagonist attenuates the analgesia produced by microinjection of glutamate (Jensen and Yaksh, 1985) or of a noradrenergic antagonist (Sagen and Proudfit, 1981) in, or by electrical stimulation (Hammond and Yaksh, 1984) of, the NRM. Depletion of spinal cord norepinephrine content also antagonizes the analgesia produced by microinjection of a noradrenergic antagonist in the NRM (Sagen *et al.*, 1983). Finally, electrical stimulation of the NRM increases the efflux of endogenous norepinephrine into superfusates of the spinal cord (Hammond *et al.*, 1985).

Although Satoh *et al.*, (1983) disagree on the involvement of norepinephrine in the effects produced by the NRM, they present evidence that norepinephrine mediates the effects produced by the NRPG. Microinjection of morphine in the NRPG increases the concentration of normetanephrine, a metabolite of norepinephrine, in the spinal cord (Kuraishi *et al.*, 1978). Intrathecal injection of a noradrenergic antagonist attenuates the analgesia produced by microinjection of morphine (Kuraishi *et al.*, 1979b), glutamate (Satoh *et al.*, 1983; Jensen and Yaksh, 1985), or a noradrenergic antagonist (Sagen and Proudfit, 1981) in the NRPG. Intrathecally administered phentolamine similarly attenuates the analgesia produced by electrical stimulation of the NRPG (Hammond and Yaksh, 1984).

The majority of pharmacological studies cited in this section are notable for their failure to examine the effects of more than one class of antagonist at any one stimulation site. This has fostered an overly circumscribed view that the effects of activation of the NRM are mediated by serotonin and that the effects of activation of the NRPG are mediated by norepinephrine. Yet, the effect of depletion or antagonism of either neurotransmitter is frequently merely partial. Furthermore, the number of neurotransmitters contained within these nuclei argues that more than one neurotransmitter mediates these effects. Recently, we examined the effects of intrathecally administered serotonergic and noradrenergic antagonists on the analgesia produced by stimulation at the same medullary sites and concluded that the effects of activation of the NRM and NRPG are mediated by coactivation of the descending serotonergic and noradrenergic projections (Hammond and Yaksh, 1984). We have since demonstrated that electrical stimulation of medullary sites, using current intensities comparable with those that produce analgesia in awake animals, increases the efflux of both serotonin and norepinephrine from the spinal cord (Hammond *et al.*, 1985). Coactivation of both serotonergic and noradrenergic bulbospinal systems has been demonstrated for the PAG as well (Yaksh, 1979).

D. *New Directions*

By virtue of its complexity, much remains to be determined about the pharmacology of the centrifugal control systems. The pharmacological tools for selectively altering the synthesis, metabolism, and disposition of classical neurotransmitters are readily available. Yet, such is not the case for the more recently identified peptidergic neurotransmitters. The paucity of selective antagonists and neurotoxins has hampered, and will continue to hamper for some time, our ability to evaluate the involvement of these peptides. It is anticipated that great strides will be made in our study of the pharmacology of the descending control systems on the introduction of antagonists and neurotoxins that are specific for the peptidergic neurotransmitters.

In the identification of a substance as the neurotransmitter of a neuronal system, it is crucial to demonstrate that activation of the system does indeed release the substance. In this manner, the behavioral or physiological effects of activation of the system can be correlated with alterations in the efflux of the endogenous neurotransmitter. Such studies are particularly challenging because (1) the sensitivity of methods for measurement of the endogenous neurotransmitter and its metabolites must be in the picomolar and femtomolar range and (2) most regions of the CNS are not easily accessed for measurement of neurotransmitter efflux. However, this approach is currently being pursued with respect to both the centrifugal and centripetal neuronal systems by measuring the efflux of endogenous monoamines and opioid peptides into *in vivo* superfusates of the spinal cord during activation of these systems (Yaksh and Tyce, 1979, 1981; Rivot *et al.*, 1982; Yaksh and Elde, 1981; Hammond *et al.*, 1985). The number of laboratories using this approach in studies of the pharmacology of the centrifugal control systems will surely increase in the future.

References

ABOLS, I. A., AND BASBAUM, A. I. Afferent connections of the rostral medulla of the cat: A neural substrate for midbrain–medullary interactions in the modulation of pain. *J. Comp. Neurol.* 201:285–297, 1981.

AKAIKE, A., SHIBATA, T., SATOH, M., AND TAKAGI, H. Analgesia induced by microinjection of morphine into, and electrical stimulation of, the nucleus reticularis paragigantocellularis of rat medulla oblongata. *Neuropharmacology* 17:775–778, 1978.

AKIL, H., AND MAYER, D. J. Antagonism of stimulation-produced analgesia by pCPA, a serotonin synthesis inhibitor. *Brain Res.* 44:692–697, 1972.

AKIL, H., MAYER, D. J., AND LIEBESKIND, J. C. Antagonism of stimulation-produced analgesia by naloxone, a narcotic antagonist. *Science* 191:961–962, 1975.

ANDERSEN, P., ECCLES, J. C., AND SEARS, T. A. Cortically evoked depolarization of primary afferent fibers in the spinal cord. *J. Neurophysiol.* 27:63–77, 1964.

ANDERSON, S. D., BASBAUM, A. I., AND FIELDS, H. L. Response of medullary raphe neurons to peripheral stimulation and to systemic administration. *Brain Res.* 123:363–368, 1977.

ANDREZIK, J. A., CHAN-PALAY, V., AND PALAY, S. L. The nucleus paragigantocellularis lateralis in the rat. Conformation and cytology. *Anat. Embryol.* 161:335–371, 1981.

APPLEBAUM, A. E., LEONARD, R. B., KENSHALO, D. R., JR., MARTIN, R. F., AND WILLIS, W. D. Nuclei in which functionally identified spinothalamic tract neurons terminate. *J. Comp. Neurol.* 188:575–586, 1979.

ARMAND, J. The origin, course and terminations of corticospinal fibers in various mammals. *Prog. Brain Res.* 57:329–360, 1982.

BASBAUM, A. I., AND FIELDS, H. L. The origin of descending pathways in the dorsolateral funiculus of the spinal cord of the cat and rat: Further studies on the anatomy of pain modulation. *J. Comp. Neurol.* 187:513–532, 1979.

BASBAUM, A. I., MARLEY, N. J. E., O'KEEFE, J., AND CLANTON, C. H. Reversal of morphine and stimulus-produced analgesia by subtotal spinal cord lesions. *Pain* 3:43–56, 1977.

BASBAUM, A. I., CLANTON, C. H., AND FIELDS, H. L. Three bulbospinal pathways from the rostral medulla of the cat: An autoradiographic study of pain modulating systems. *J. Comp. Neurol.* 178:209–224, 1978.

BEALL, J. E., MARTIN, R. F., APPLEBAUM, A. E., AND WILLIS, W. D. Inhibition of primate spinothalamic tract neurons by stimulation in the region of the nucleus raphe magnus. *Brain Res.* 114:328–333, 1976.

BEHBEHANI, M. M., AND FIELDS, H. L. Evidence that an excitatory connection between the periaqueductal gray and nucleus raphe magnus mediates stimulation-produced analgesia. *Brain Res.* 170:85–93, 1979.

BEITZ, A. J. The nuclei of origin of brain stem enkephalin and substance P projections to the rodent nucleus raphe magnus. *Neuroscience* 7:2753–2768, 1982a.

BEITZ, A. J. The sites of origin of brain stem neurotensin and serotonin projections to the rodent nucleus raphe magnus. *J. Neurosci.* 2:829–842, 1982b.

BEITZ, A. J. The nuclei of origin of brainstem serotonergic projections to the rodent spinal trigeminal nucleus. *Neurosci. Lett.* 32:223–228, 1982c.

BEITZ, A. J., WELLS, W. E., AND SHEPARD, R. D. The location of brainstem neurons which project bilaterally to the spinal trigeminal nuclei as demonstrated by the double fluorescent retrograde tracer technique. *Brain Res.* 258:305–312, 1983.

BELCHER, G., RYALL, R. W., AND SCHAFFNER, R. The differential effects of 5-hydroxytryptamine, noradrenaline and raphe stimulation on nociceptive and non-nociceptive dorsal horn interneurones in the cat. *Brain Res.* 151:307–321, 1978.

BENNETT, C. J., AND MAYER, D. J. Inhibition of spinal cord interneurons by narcotic microinjection and focal electrical stimulation in the periaqueductal central gray matter. *Brain Res.* 172:243–257, 1979.

BERK, M. L., AND FINKELSTEIN, J. A. Efferent connections of the lateral hypothalamic area of the rat: An autoradiographic investigation. *Brain Res. Bull.* 8:511–526, 1982.

BERMAN, A. L. *The Brain Stem of the Cat. A Cytoarchitectonic Atlas with Stereotaxic Coordinates,* University of Wisconsin Press, Madison, 1968.

BESSON, J. M., GUILBAUD, G., AND LEBARS, D. Descending inhibitory influences exerted by the brainstem upon the activities of dorsal horn lamina V cells induced by intra-arterial injection of bradykinin into the limbs. *J. Physiol. (Lond.)* 248:725–739, 1975.

BLACK, P., CIANCI, S. N., AND MARKOWITZ, R. S. Alleviation of pain by hypothalamic stimulation in the monkey. *Confin. Neurol.* 34:374–381, 1972.

BOBILLIER, P., SEGUIN, S., PETITJEAN, F., SALVERT, D., TOURET, M., AND JOUVET, M. The raphe nuclei of the cat brain stem: A topographical atlas of their efferent projections as revealed by autoradiography. *Brain Res.* 113:449–486, 1976.

BOURGOIN, S., OLIVERAS, J. L., BRUXELLE, J., HAMON, M., AND BESSON, J. M. Electrical stimulation of the nucleus raphe magnus in the rat. Effects on 5-HT metabolism in the spinal cord. *Brain Res.* 194:377–389, 1980.

BOWKER, R. M., WESTLUND, K. N., AND COULTER, J. D. Serotonergic projections to the spinal cord from the midbrain in the rat: An immunocytochemical and retrograde transport study. *Neurosci. Lett.* 24:221–226, 1981.

BOWKER, R. M., WESTLUND, K. N., SULLIVAN, M. C., AND COULTER, J. D. Organization of descending serotonergic projections to the spinal cord. *Prog. Brain Res.* 57:239–265, 1982a.

BOWKER, R. M., WESTLUND, K. N., SULLIVAN, M. C., WILBER, J. F., AND COULTER, J. D. Transmitters of the raphe–spinal complex: Immunocytochemical studies. *Peptides* 3:291–298, 1982b.

BOWKER, R. M., WESTLUND, K. N., SULLIVAN, M. C., WILBER, J. F., AND COULTER, J. D. Descending serotonergic, peptidergic and cholinergic pathways from the raphe nuclei: A multiple transmitter complex. *Brain Res.* 288:33–48, 1983.

BRODAL, A., TABER, E., AND WALBERG, F. The raphe nuclei of the brain stem in the cat. II. Efferent connections. *J. Comp. Neurol.* 114:239–259, 1960.

BRODIE, M. S., AND PROUDFIT, H. K. Hypoalgesia induced by the local injection of carbachol into the nucleus raphe magnus. *Brain Res.* 291:337–342, 1984.

CARLTON, S. M., LEICHNETZ, G. R., YOUNG, E. G., AND MAYER, D. J. Supramedullary afferents of the nucleus raphe magnus in the rat: A study using the transcannula HRP gel and autoradiographic techniques. *J. Comp. Neurol.* 214:43–58, 1983.

CARPENTER, D., LUNDBERG, A., AND NORRSELL, U. Primary afferent depolarization evoked from the sensorimotor cortex. *Acta Physiol. Scand.* 59:126–142, 1963.

CARSTENS, E. Inhibition of spinal dorsal horn neuronal responses to noxious skin heating by medial hypothalamic stimulation in the cat. *J. Neurophysiol.* 48:808–822, 1982.

CARSTENS, E., KLUMP, D., AND ZIMMERMAN, M. The opiate antagonist, naloxone, does not affect descending inhibition from midbrain of nociceptive spinal neuronal discharges in the cat. *Neurosci. Lett.* 11:323–327, 1979.

CARSTENS, E., BIHL, H., IRVINE, F., AND ZIMMERMANN, M. Descending inhibition from medial and lateral midbrain of spinal dorsal horn neuronal responses to noxious and nonnoxious cutaneous stimuli in the cat. *J. Neurophysiol.* 45:1029–1042, 1981a.

CARSTENS, E., FRAUNHOFFER, M., AND ZIMMERMAN, M. Serotonergic mediation of descending inhibition from midbrain periaqueductal gray, but not reticular formation, of spinal nociceptive transmission in the cat. *Pain* 10:149–167, 1981b.

CARSTENS, E., MACKINNON, J. D., AND GUINAN, M. J. Inhibition of spinal dorsal horn neuronal responses to noxious skin heating by medial preoptic and septal stimulation in the cat. *J. Neurophysiol.* 48:981–991, 1982.

CARSTENS, E., FRAUNHOFFER, M., AND SUBERG, S. N. Inhibition of spinal dorsal horn neuronal responses to noxious skin heating by lateral hypothalamus stimulation. *J. Neurophysiol.* 50:192–204, 1983a.

CARSTENS, E., MACKINNON, J. D., AND GUINAN, M. J. Serotonin involvement in descending inhibition of spinal nociceptive transmission produced by stimulation of medial diencephalon and basal forebrain. *J. Neurosci.* 3:2112–2120, 1983b.

CASTIGLIONI, A. J., GALLAWAY, M. C., AND COULTER, J. D. Spinal projections from the midbrain in monkey. *J. Comp. Neurol.* 178:329–346, 1978.

CATSMAN-BERREVOETS, C. E., AND KUYPERS, H. G. J. M. A search for corticospinal collaterals to thalamus and mescencephalon by means of multiple retrograde fluorescent tracers in cat and rat. *Brain Res.* 218:15–33, 1981.

CHAN-PALAY, V. Combined immunocytochemistry and autoradiography after *in vivo* injections of monoclonal antibody to substance P and ^{3}H-serotonin. *Anat. Embryol.* 156:241–255, 1979.

CONRAD, L. C. A., AND PFAFF, D. W. Efferents from medial basal forebrain and hypothalamus in the rat. I. An autoradiographic study of the medial preoptic area. *J. Comp. Neurol.* 169:185–220, 1976a.

CONRAD, L. C. A., AND PFAFF, D. W. Efferents from medial basal forebrain and hypothalamus in the rat. II. An autoradiographic study of the anterior hypothalamus. *J. Comp. Neurol.* 169:221–262, 1976b.

COULTER, J. D., AND JONES, E. G. Differential distribution of corticospinal projections from individual cytoarchitectonic fields in the monkey. *Brain Res.* 129:335–340, 1977.

COULTER, J. D., MAUNZ, R. A., AND WILLIS, W. D. Effects of stimulation of sensorimotor cortex on primate spinothalamic neurons. *Brain Res.* 65:351–356, 1974.

COX, V. C., AND VALENSTEIN, E. S. Attenuation of aversive properties of peripheral shock by hypothalamic stimulation. *Science* 149:323–325, 1965.

CRUTCHER, K. A., HUMBERTSON, A. D., JR., AND MARTIN, G. F. The origin of brainstem–spinal pathways in the North American opossum (*Didelphis virginiana*). Studies using the horseradish peroxidase method. *J. Comp. Neurol.* 179:169–194, 1978.

DAHLSTROM, A., AND FUXE, K. Evidence for the existence of monoamine neurons in the central nervous system. II. Experimentally induced changes in the intraneuronal amine levels of the bulbospinal neuron systems. *Acta Physiol. Scand.* [*Suppl.*] 247:1–36, 1965.

DICKENSON, A. H., OLIVERAS, J. L., AND BESSON, J. M. Role of the nucleus raphe magnus in opiate analgesia as studied by the microinjection technique in the rat. *Brain Res.* 170:95–111, 1979.

DOSTROVSKY, J. O., SHAH, Y., AND GRAY, B. G. Descending inhibitory influences from periaqueductal gray, nucleus raphe magnus, and adjacent reticular formation. II. Effects on medullary dorsal horn nociceptive and non-nociceptive neurons. *J. Neurophysiol.* 49:948–960, 1983.

DUGGAN, A. W., AND GRIERSMITH, B. T. Inhibition of the spinal transmission of nociceptive information by supraspinal stimulation in the cat. *Pain* 6:149–161, 1979.

DUGGAN, A. W., AND MORTON, C. R. Periaqueductal grey stimulation: An association between selective inhibition of dorsal horn neurones and changes in peripheral circulation. *Pain* 15:237–248, 1983.

DUGGAN, A. W., HALL, J. G., HEADLEY, P. M., AND GRIERSMITH, B. T. The effect of naloxone on the excitation of dorsal horn neurones of the cat by noxious and non-noxious cutaneous stimuli. *Brain Res.* 138:185–189, 1977a.

DUGGAN, A. W., HALL, J. G., AND HEADLEY, P. M. Enkephalins and dorsal horn neurones of the cat: Effects on responses to noxious and innocuous skin stimuli. *Br. J. Pharmacol.* 61:399–408, 1977b.

ECCLES, R. M., AND LUNDBERG, A. Supraspinal control of interneurons mediating spinal reflexes. *J. Physiol. (Lond.)* 147:565–584, 1959.

EDESON, R. O., AND RYALL, R. W. Systematic mapping of descending inhibitory control by the medulla of nociceptive spinal neurones in cats. *Brain Res.* 271:251–262, 1983.

FIELDS, H. L., AND ANDERSON, S. D. Evidence that raphe–spinal neurons mediate opiate and midbrain stimulation-produced analgesia. *Pain* 5:333–349, 1978.

FIELDS, H. L., BASBAUM, A. I., CLANTON, C. H., AND ANDERSON, S. D. Nucleus raphe magnus inhibition of spinal cord dorsal horn neurons. *Brain Res.* 126:441–453, 1977.

FIFKOVA, E., AND MARSALA, J. Stereotaxic atlases for the cat, rabbit and rat, in: *Electrophysiological Methods in Biological Research* (J. BURES, M. PETRAN, AND J. ZACHER, eds.), Academia, Prague, 1967, pp. 653–731.

FINLEY, J. C. W., MADERDRUT, J. L., AND PETRUSZ, P. The immunocytochemical localization of enkephalin in the central nervous system of the rat. *J. Comp. Neurol.* 198:541–565, 1981.

FRANKFURT, M., LAUDER, J. M., AND AZMITIA, E. C. The immunocytochemical localization of serotonergic neurons in the rat hypothalamus. *Neurosci. Lett.* 24:227–232, 1981.

GALLAGER, D. W., AND PERT, A. Afferents to brain stem nuclei (brain stem raphe, nucleus reticularis pontis caudalis and nucleus gigantocellularis) in the rat as demonstrated by microiontophoretically applied horseradish peroxidase. *Brain Res.* 144:257–275, 1978.

GERHART, K. D., WILCOX, T. K., CHUNG, J. M., AND WILLIS, W. D. Inhibition of nociceptive and non-nociceptive responses of primate spinothalamic cells by stimulation in medial brainstem. *J. Neurophysiol.* 45:121–136, 1981a.

GERHART, K. D., YEZIERSKI, R. P., WILCOX, T. K., GROSSMAN, A. E., AND WILLIS, W. D. Inhibition of primate spinothalamic tract neurons by stimulation in ipsilateral or contralateral ventral posterior lateral (VPL_c) thalamic nucleus. *Brain Res.* 229:514–519, 1981b.

GERHART, K. D., YEZIERSKI, R. P., FANG, Z. R., AND WILLIS, W. D. Inhibition of primate spinothalamic tract neurons by stimulation in the ventral posterior lateral (VPL_c) thalamic nucleus: Possible mechanisms. *J. Neurophysiol.* 49:406–423, 1983.

GIESLER, G. J., JR., GERHART, K. D., YEZIERSKI, R. P., WILCOX, T. K., AND WILLIS, W. D. Postsynaptic inhibition of primate spinothalamic neurons by stimulation in nucleus raphe magnus. *Brain Res.* 204:184–188, 1981a.

GIESLER, G. J., JR., YEZIERSKI, R. P., GERHART, K. D., AND WILLIS, W. D. Spinothalamic tract neurons that project to medial and/or lateral thalamic nuclei: Evidence for a physiologically novel population of spinal cord neurons. *J. Neurophysiol.* 46:1285–1308, 1981b.

GLAZER, E. J., STEINBUSCH, H., VERHOFSTAD, A., AND BASBAUM, A. I. Serotonin neurons in nucleus raphe dorsalis and paragigantocellularis of the cat contain enkephalin *J. Physiol. (Paris)* 77:241–245, 1981.

GOLDSTEIN, A., AND GHAZAROSSIAN, V. E. Immunoreactive dynorphin in pituitary and brain. *Proc. Natl. Acad. Sci. U.S.A.* 77:6207–6210, 1980.

GOODMAN, S. J., AND HOLCOMBE, V. Selective and prolonged analgesia in monkey resulting from brain stimulation. *Pain Res. Ther.* 1:495–502, 1976.

GRAY, B. G., AND DOSTROVSKY, J. O. Descending inhibitory influences from periaqueductal gray, nucleus raphe magnus, and adjacent reticular formation. I. Effects on lumbar spinal cord nociceptive and non-nociceptive neurons. *J. Neurophysiol.* 49:932–947, 1983.

GROFOVA, I., OTTERSEN, O. P., AND RINVIK, E. Mesencephalic and diencephalic afferents to the superior colliculus and periaqueductal gray substance demonstrated by retrograde axonal transport of horseradish peroxidase in the cat. *Brain Res.* 146:205–220, 1978.

GUILBAUD, G., BESSON, J. M., OLIVERAS, J. L., AND LIEBESKIND, J. C. Suppression by LSD of the inhibitory effect exerted by dorsal raphe stimulation on certain spinal cord interneurons in the cat. *Brain Res.* 61:417–422, 1973.

GUILBAUD, G., OLIVERAS, J. L., GIESLER, G., JR., AND BESSON, J. M. Effects induced by stimulation of the centralis inferior nucleus of the raphe on dorsal horn interneurons in cat's spinal cord. *Brain Res.* 126:355–360, 1977.

GYBELS, J., VANHEES, J., AND PELUSO, F. Modulation of experimentally produced pain in man by electrical stimulation of some cortical, thalamic and basal ganglia structures. *Pain Res. Ther.* 1:475–478, 1976.

HABER, L. H., MARTIN, R. F., CHATT, A. B., AND WILLIS, W. D. Effects of stimulation in nucleus reticularis gigantocellularis on the activity of spinothalamic tract neurons in the monkey. *Brain Res.* 153:163–168, 1978.

HAGBARTH, K.-E., AND KERR, D. I. B. Central influences on spinal afferent conduction. *J. Neurophysiol.* 17:295–307, 1954.

HAIGLER, H. J., AND MITTLEMAN, R. S. Analgesia produced by direct injection of morphine into the mesencephalic reticular formation. *Brain Res. Bull.* 3:655–662, 1978.

HAMMOND, D. L., AND YAKSH, T. L. Antagonism of stimulation-produced antinociception by intrathecal administration of methysergide or phentolamine. *Brain Res.* 298:329–337, 1984.

HAMMOND, D. L., LEVY, R. A., AND PROUDFIT, H. K. Hypoalgesia following microinjection of noradrenergic antagonists in the nucleus raphe magnus. *Pain* 9:85–101, 1980a.

HAMMOND, D. L., LEVY, R. A., AND PROUDFIT, H. K. Hypoalgesia induced by microinjection of a norepinephrine antagonist in the nucleus raphe magnus: Reversal by intrathecal administration of a serotonin antagonist. *Brain Res.* 201:475–479, 1980b.

HAMMOND, D. L., TYCE, G. M., AND YAKSH, T. L. Efflux of serotonin and noradrenaline into spinal cord superfusates during stimulation of the rat ventromedial medulla. *J. Physiol. (Lond.)* 359:151–162, 1985.

HANCOCK, M. B. Cells of origin of hypothalamo–spinal projections in the rat. *Neurosci. Lett.* 3:179–184, 1976.

HANDWERKER, H. O, IGGO, A., AND ZIMMERMAN, M. Segmental and supraspinal actions on dorsal horn neurons responding to noxious and non-noxious skin stimuli. *Pain* 1:147–165, 1975.

HAYES, N. L., AND RUSTIONI, A. Descending projections from brainstem and sensorimotor cortex to spinal enlargements in the cat. *Exp. Brain Res.* 41:89–107, 1981.

HAYES, R. L., NEWLON, P. G., ROSECRANS, J. A., AND MAYER, D. J. Reduction of stimulation-produced analgesia by lysergic acid diethylamide, a depressor of serotonergic neural activity. *Brain Res.* 122:367–372, 1977.

HAYES, R. L., PRICE, D. D., RUDA, M., AND DUBNER, R. Suppression of nociceptive responses in the primate by electrical stimulation of the brain or morphine administration: Behavioral and electrophysiological comparisons. *Brain Res.* 167:417–421, 1979.

HEADLEY, P. M., DUGGAN, A. W., AND GRIERSMITH, B. T. Selective reduction by noradrenaline and 5-hydroxytryptamine of nociceptive responses of cat dorsal horn neurones. *Brain Res.* 145:185–189, 1978.

HÖKFELT, T., ELDE, R., JOHANSSON, D., TERENIUS, L., AND STEIN, L. The distribution of enkephalin-immunoreacitve cell bodies in the rat central nervous system. *Neurosci. Lett.* 5:25–31, 1977.

HÖKFELT, T., LJUNGDAHL, A., STEINBUSCH, H., VERHOFSTAD, A., NILSSON, G., BRODIN, E., PERNOW, B., AND GOLDSTEIN, M. Immunohistochemical evidence of substance P-like immunoreactivity in some 5-hydroxytryptamine-containing neurons in the rat central nervous system. *Neuroscience* 3:517–538, 1978.

HÖKFELT, T., TERENIUS, L., KUYPERS, H. G. J. M., AND DANN, O. Evidence for enkephalin immunoreactive neurons in the medulla oblongata projecting to the spinal cord. *Neurosci. Lett.* 14:55–60, 1979.

HOLMQVIST, B., AND LUNDBERG, A. On the organization of the supraspinal inhibitory control of interneurons of various spinal reflex arcs. *Arch. Ital. Biol.* 97:340–356, 1959.

HOLMQVIST, B., AND LUNDBERG, A. Differential supraspinal control of synaptic actions evoked by volleys in the flexion afferents in alpha motoneurones. *Acta Physiol. Scand.* [*Suppl.*] 186:1–51, 1961.

HOLSTEGE, G., AND KUYPERS, H. G. J. M. The anatomy of brain stem pathways to the spinal cord in cat. A labeled amino acid tracing study. *Prog. Brain Res.* 57:145–175, 1982.

HONGO, T., AND JANKOWSKA, E. Effects from the sensorimotor cortex on the spinal cord in cats with transected pyramids. *Exp. Brain Res.* 3:117–134, 1967.

HOSOBUCHI, Y., ADAMS, J. E., AND RUTKIN, B. Chronic thalamic stimulation for the control of facial anesthesia dolorosa. *Arch. Neurol.* 29:158–161, 1973.

HOSOBUCHI, Y., ADAMS, J. E., AND LINCHITZ, R. Pain relief by electrical stimulation of the central gray matter in humans and its reversal by naloxone. *Science* 197:183–186, 1977.

HOSOYA, Y. The distribution of spinal projection neurons in the hypothalamus of the rat, studied with the HRP method. *Exp. Brain Res.* 40:79–87, 1980.

HOSOYA, Y., AND MATSUSHITA, M. Brainstem projections from the lateral hypothalamic area in the rat, as studied with autoradiography. *Neurosci. Lett.* 24:111–116, 1981.

JACQUET, Y. F., AND LAJTHA, A. Paradoxical effects after microinjection of morphine in the periaqueductal gray matter in the rat. *Science* 185:1055–1057, 1974.

JENSEN, T., AND YAKSH, T. L. Spinal monoamine and opiate systems partly mediate the antinociceptive effects produced by glutamate at brainstem sites. *Brain Res.* 321:287–297, 1985.

JORDAN, L. M., KENSHALO, D. R., JR., MARTIN, R. F., HABER, L. H., AND WILLIS, W. D. Depression of primate spinothalamic tract neurons by iontophoretic application of 5-hydroxytryptamine. *Pain* 5:135–142, 1978.

JURNA, I. Effect of stimulation in the periaqueductal grey matter on activity in ascending axons of the rat spinal cord: selective inhibition of activity evoked by afferent Aγ and C fibre stimulation and failure of naloxone to reduce inhibition. *Brain Res.* 196:33–42, 1980.

KAJANDER, K. C., EBNER, T. J., AND BLOEDEL, J. R. Effects of periaqueductal gray and raphe magnus stimulation on the responses of spinocervical and other ascending projection neurons to non-noxious inputs. *Brain Res.* 291:29–37, 1984.

KEVETTER, G. A., AND WILLIS, W. D. Spinothalamic cells in the rat lumbar cord with collaterals to the medullary reticular formation. *Brain Res.* 238:181–185, 1982.

KHACHATURIAN, H., WATSON, S. J., LEWIS, M. E., COY, D., GOLDSTEIN, A., AND AKIL, H. Dynorphin immunocytochemistry in the cat central nervous system. *Peptides* 3:941–954, 1982.

KNEISLEY, L. W., BIBER, M. P., AND LAVAIL, J. H. A study of the origin of brain stem projections to monkey spinal cord using the retrograde transport method. *Exp. Neurol.* 60:116–139, 1978.

KURAISHI, Y., FUKUI, K., SHIOMI, H., AKAIKE, A., AND TAKAGI, H. Microinjection of opioids into the nucleus reticularis gigantocellularis of the rat: Analgesia and increase in the normetanephrine level in the spinal cord *Biochem. Pharmacol.* 27:2756–2758, 1978.

KURAISHI, Y., HARADA, Y., AND TAKAGI, H. Noradrenaline regulation of pain-transmission in the spinal cord meidated by α-adrenoceptors. *Brain Res.* 174:333–336, 1979a.

KURAISHI, Y., HARADA, Y., SATOH, M., AND TAKAGI, H. Antagonism by phenoxybenzamine of the analgesic effect of morphine injected into the nucleus reticularis gigantocellularis of the rat. *Neuropharmacology* 18:107–110, 1979b.

KUYPERS, H. G. J. M. Central cortical projections to motor and somatosensory cell groups. *Brain* 83:161–187, 1960.

KUYPERS, H. G. J. M., AND MAISKY, V. A. Retrograde axonal transport of horseradish peroxidase from spinal cord to brain stem cell groups in the cat. *Neurosci. Lett.* 1:9–14, 1975.

KUYPERS, H. G. J. M., AND MAISKY, V. A. Funicular trajectories of descending brain stem pathways in cat. *Brain Res.* 136:159–165, 1977.

LEBARS, D., DICKENSON, A. H., AND BESSON, J. M. Microinjection of morphine within nucleus raphe magnus and dorsal horn neurone activities related to nociception in the rat. *Brain Res.* 189:476–481, 1980.

LEICHNETZ, G. R., WATKINS, L., GRIFFIN, G., MURFIN, R., AND MAYER, D. J. The projection from nucleus raphe magnus and other brainstem nuclei to the spinal cord in the rat: A study using the HRP blue-reaction. *Neurosci. Lett.* 8:119–124, 1978.

LEWIS, V. A., AND GEBHART, G. F. Evaluation of the periaqueductal central gray (PAG) as a morphine-specific locus of action and examination of morphine-induced and stimulation-produced analgesia at coincident PAG loci. *Brain Res.* 124:283–303, 1977.

LIEBESKIND, J. C., GUILBAUD, G., BESSON, J. M., AND OLIVERAS, J.-L. Analgesia from electrical stimulation of the periaqueductal gray matter in the cat: Behavioral observations and inhibitory effects on spinal cord interneurons. *Brain Res.* 50:441–446, 1973.

LIU, C. N., AND CHAMBERS, W. W. An experimental study of the corticospinal system in the monkey (*Macaca mulatta*). *J. Comp. Neurol.* 123:257–284, 1964.

LLOYD, D. P. C. The spinal mecahnism of the pyramidal system in cats. *J. Neurophysiol.* 4:525–546, 1941.

LOPACHIN, R. M., AND RUDY, T. A. The thermoregulatory effects of noradrenaline, serotonin and carbachol injected into the rat spinal subarachnoid space. *J. Physiol. (Lond.)* 333:511–529, 1982.

LOVICK, T. A., AND WOLSTENCROFT, J. H. Projections from brain stem nuclei to the spinal trigeminal nucleus in the cat. *Neuroscience* 9:411–420, 1983.

LOVICK, T. A., WEST, D. C., AND WOLSTENCROFT, J. H. Responses of raphespinal and other bulbar raphe neurones to stimulation of the periaqueductal gray in the cat. *Neurosci. Lett.* 8:45–49, 1978.

LUNDBERG, A. Inhibitory control from the brain stem of transmission from primary afferents to motoneurons, primary afferent terminals and ascending pathways. in: *Brain Stem Control of Spinal Mechanisms* (B. SJOLUND AND A. BJORKLUND, eds.) Elsevier, Amsterdam, 1982, pp. 179–224.

LUNDBERG, A., AND VOORHOEVE, P. Effects from the pyramidal tract on spinal reflex arcs. *Acta Physiol. Scand.* 56:201–219, 1962.

LUNDBERG, A., NORRSELL, U., AND VOORHOEVE, P. Pyramidal effects on lumbo-sacral interneurones activated by somatic afferents. *Acta Physiol. Scand.* 56:220–229, 1962.

MANTYH, P. W. Connections of midbrain periaqueductal gray in the monkey. II. Descending efferent projections. *J. Neurophysiol.* 49:582–594, 1983.

MANTYH, P. W., AND HUNT, S. P. Evidence for cholecystokinin-like imunoreactive neurons in the rat medulla oblongata which project to the spinal cord. *Brain Res.* 291:49–54, 1984.

MANTYH, P. W., AND PESCHANSKI, M. Spinal projections from the periaqueductal grey and dorsal raphe in the rat, cat and monkey. *Neuroscience* 7:2769–2776, 1982.

MARTIN, G. F., CABANA, T., HUMBERTSON, A. O., JR., LAXSON, L. C., AND PANNETON, W. M. Spinal projections from the medullary reticular formation of the North American opossum: Evidence for connectional heterogeneity. *J. Comp. Neurol.* 196:663–682, 1981.

MARTIN, R. F., JORDAN, L. M., AND WILLIS, W. D. Differential projections of cat medullary raphe neurons demonstrated by retrograde labelling following spinal cord lesions. *J. Comp. Neurol.* 182:77–88, 1978.

MAYER, D. J., AND LIEBESKIND, J. C. Pain reduction by focal electrical stimulation of the brain: An anatomical and behavioral analysis. *Brain Res.* 68:73–93, 1974.

MAZARS, G. J., MERIENNE, L., AND CIOLOLA, C. Comparative study of electrical stimulation of posterior thalamic nuclei, periaqueductal gray, and other midline mesencephalic structures in man. *Pain Res. Ther.* 3:541–546, 1979.

MCCREERY, D. B., AND BLOEDEL, J. R. Reduction of the response of cat spinothalamic neurons to graded mechanical stimuli by electrical stimulation of the lower brain stem. *Brain Res.* 97:151–156, 1975.

MCCREERY, D. B., BLOEDEL, J. R., AND HAMES, E. G. Effects of stimulating in raphe nuclei and in reticular formation on response of spinothalamic neurons to mechanical stimuli. *J. Neurophysiol.* 42:166–182, 1979.

MEESSEN, H., AND OLSZEWSKI, J. *A Cytoarchitectonic Atlas of the Rhombencephalon of the Rabbit,* S. Karger, Basel, 1949.

MOHRLAND, J. S., AND GEBHART, G. F. Effects of focal electrical stimulation and morphine microinjection in the periaqueductal gray of the rat mesencephalon on neuronal activity in the medullary reticular formation. *Brain Res.* 201:23–37, 1980.

MOSS, M. S., GLAZER, E. J., AND BASBAUM, A. I. The peptidergic organization of the cat periaqueductal gray. I. The distribution of immunoreactive enkephalin-containing neurons and terminals. *J. Neurosci.* 3:603–616. 1983.

MURRAY, E. A., AND COULTER, J. D., Organization of corticospinal neurons in the monkey. *J. Comp. Neurol.* 195:339–365, 1981.

NILAVER, G., ZIMMERMAN, E. A., WILKINS, J., MICHAELS, J., HOFFMAN, D., AND SILVERMAN, A. J. Magnocellular hypothalamic projections to the lower brain stem and spinal cord of the rat. *Neuroendocrinology* 30:150–158, 1980.

OLESON, T. D., TWOMBLY, D. A., AND LIEBESKIND, J. C. Effects of pain attenuating brain stimulation and morphine on electrical activity in the raphe nuclei of the awake rat. *Pain* 4:211–230, 1978.

OLESON, T. D., KIRKPATRICK, D. B., AND GOODMAN, S. J. Elevation of pain threshold to tooth shock by brain stimulation in primates. *Brain Res.* 194:79–95, 1980.

OLIVERAS, J. L., BESSON, J. M., GUILBAUD, G., AND LIEBESKIND, J. C. Behavioral and electrophysiological evidence of pain inhibition from midbrain stimulation in the cat. *Exp. Brain Res.* 20:32–44, 1974.

OLIVERAS, J. L., REDJEMI, F., GUILBAUD, G., AND BESSON, J. M. Analgesia induced by electrical stimulation of the inferior centralis nucleus of the raphe in the cat. *Pain* 1:139–145, 1975.

OLIVERAS, J. L., HOSOBUCHI, Y., REDJEMI, F., GUILBAUD, G., AND BESSON, J. M. Opiate antagonist, naloxone, strongly reduces analgesia induced by stimulation of a raphe nucleus (centralis inferior). *Brain Res.* 120:221–229, 1977.

OLIVERAS, J. L., GUILBAUD, G., AND BESSON, J. M. A map of serotonergic structures involved in stimulation producing analgesia in unrestrained freely moving cats. *Brain Res.* 164:317–322, 1979.

POITRAS, D., AND PARENT, A. Atlas of the distribution of monoamine-containing nerve cell bodies in the brain stem of the cat *J. Comp. Neurol.* 179:699–718, 1978.

POMEROY, S. L., AND BEHBEHANI, M. M. Physiological evidence for a projection from periaqueductal gray to nucleus raphe magnus in the rat. *Brain Res.* 176:143–147, 1979.

PRICE, D. D., HAYES, R. L., RUDA, M., AND DUBNER, R. Spatial and temporal transformations of input to spinothalamic tract neurons and their relation to somatic sensations. *J. Neurophysiol.* 41:933–947, 1978.

PRIETO, G. J., CANNON, J. T., AND LIEBESKIND, J. C. N. raphe magnus lesions disrupt stimulation-produced analgesia from ventral but not dorsal midbrain areas in the rat. *Brain Res.* 261:53–57, 1983.

PROUDFIT, H. K., AND ANDERSON, E. G. Morphine analgesia: Blockade by raphe magnus lesions. *Brain Res.* 98:612–618, 1975.

RANDIC, M., AND YU, H. H. Effects of 5-hydroxytryptamine and bradykinin in cat dorsal horn neurones activated by noxious stimuli. *Brain Res.* 111:197–203, 1976.

REDDY, S. V. R., MADERDRUT, J. L., AND YAKSH, T. L. Spinal cord pharmacology of adrenergic agonist-mediated antinociception. *J. Pharmacol. Exp. Ther.* 213:525–533, 1980.

RHODES, D. L., AND LIEBESKIND, J. C. Analgesia from rostral brain stem stimulation in the rat. *Brain Res.* 143:521–532,1978.

RICHARDSON, D. E., AND AKIL, H. Pain reduction by electrical brain stimulation in man. *J. Neurosurg.* 47:178–183, 1977.

RIVOT, J. P., CHAOUCH, A., AND BESSON, J. M. The influence of naloxone on the C fiber response of dorsal horn neurons and their inhibitory control by raphe magnus stimulation. *Brain Res.* 176:355–364, 1979.

RIVOT, J. P., CHAOUCH, A., AND BESSON, J. M. Nucleus raphe magnus modulation of response of rat dorsal horn neurons to unmyelinated fiber inputs: Partial involvement of serotonergic pathways. *J. Neurophysiol.* 44:1039–1057, 1980.

RIVOT, J. P., CHIANG, C. Y., AND BESSON, J. M. Increase of serotonin metabolism within the dorsal horn of the spinal cord during nucleus raphe magnus stimulation, as revealed by *in vivo* electrochemical detection. *Brain Res.* 238:117–126, 1982.

SAGEN, J., AND PROUDFIT, H. K. Hypoalgesia induced by blockade of noradrenergic projections to the raphe magnus: Reversal by blockade of noradrenergic projections to the spinal cord. *Brain Res.* 223:391–396, 1981.

SAGEN, J., AND PROUDFIT, H. K. Evidence for pain modulation by pre- and postsynaptic noradrenergic receptors in the medulla oblongata. *Brain Res.* 331:285–293, 1985.

SAGEN, J., AND PROUDFIT, H. K. Effect of intrathecally administered noradrenergic antagonists on nociception in the rat. *Brain Res.* 310:295–301, 1984.

SAGEN, J., WINKER, M. A., AND PROUDFIT, H. K. Hypoalgesia induced by the local injection of phentolamine in the nucleus raphe mangus: Blockade by depletion of spinal cord monoamines. *Pain* 16:253–263, 1983.

SAPER, C. B., LOEWY, A. D., SWANSON, L. W., AND COWAN, W. M. Direct hypothalamo–autonomic connections. *Brain Res.* 117:305–312, 1976.

SAR, M., STUMPF, W. E., MILLER, R. J., CHANG, K.-J., AND CUATRECASAS, P. Immunohistochemical localization of enkephalin in rat brain and spinal cord. *J. Comp. Neurol.* 182:17–38, 1978.

SATOH, M., AKAIKE, A., NAKAZAWA, T., AND TAKAGI, H. Evidence for involvement of separate mechanisms in the production of analgesia by electrical stimulation of the nucleus reticularis paragigantocellularis and nucleus raphe magnus in the rat. *Brain Res.* 194:525–529, 1980.

SATOH, M., OKU, P., AND AKAIKE, A. Analgesia produced by microinjection of L-glutamate into the rostral ventromedial bulbar nuclei of the rat and its inhibition by intrathecal alpha-adrenergic blocking agents. *Brain Res.* 261:361–364, 1983.

SAWCHENKO, P. E., AND SWANSON, L. W. Immunohistochemical identification of neurons in the paraventricular nucleus of the hypothalamus that project to the medulla or to the spinal cord in the rat. *J. Comp. Neurol.* 205:260–272, 1982.

SCHMAUSS, C., HAMMOND, D. L., OCHI, J. W., AND YAKSH, T. L. Pharmacological antagonism of the antinociceptive effects of serotonin in the rat spinal cord. *Eur. J. Pharmacol.* 90:349–357, 1983.

SCHMIDEK, H. H., FOHANNO, D., ERVIN, F. R., AND SWEET, W. H. Pain threshold alterations by brain stimulation in the monkey. *J. Neurosurg.* 35:715–722, 1971.

SCHOFIELD, S. P. M., AND EVERITT, B. J. The organization of indoleamine neurons in the brain of the rhesus monkey (*Macaca mulatta*). *J. Comp. Neurol.* 197:369–383, 1981.

SESSLE, B. J., HU, J. W., DUBNER, R., AND LUCIER, G. E. Functional properties of neurons in cat trigeminal caudalis (medullary dorsal horn). II. Modulation of responses to noxious and nonnoxious stimuli by periaqueductal gray, nucleus raphe magnus, cerebral cortex and afferent influences, and effect of naloxone. *J. Neurophysiol.* 45:193–207, 1981.

SHAH, Y., AND DOSTROVSKY, J. O. Electrophysiological evidence for a projection of the periaqueductal gray matter to nucleus raphe magnus in cat and rat. *Brain Res.* 193:534–538, 1980.

SHERRINGTON, C. S., AND SOWTON, S. C. M. Observations on reflex responses to single break shocks. *J. Physiol. (Lond.)* 49:331–348, 1915.

SKAGERBERG, G., BJORKLUND, A., LINDVALL, O., AND SCHMIDT, R. H. Origin and termination of the diencephalo–spinal dopamine system in the rat. *Brain Res. Bull.* 9:237–244, 1982.

SKIRBOLL, L., HÖKFELT, T., DOCKRAY, G., REHFELD, J., BROWNSTEIN, M., AND CUELLO, A. C. Evidence for periaqueductal cholecystokinin–substance P neurons projecting to the spinal cord. *J. Neurosci.* 3:1151–1157, 1983.

SOJA, P. J., AND SINCLAIR, J. G. Tonic descending influences on cat spinal cord dorsal horn neurons. *Somatosens. Res.* 1:83–93, 1983.

SOPER, W. Y. Effects of analgesic midbrain stimulation on reflex withdrawal and thermal escape in the rat. *J. Comp. Physiol. Psychol.* 90:91–101, 1976.

SOPER, W. Y., AND MELZACK, R. Stimulation-produced analgesia: Evidence for somatotopic organization in the midbrain. *Brain Res.* 251:301–311, 1982.

STEINBUSCH, H. W. M. Distribution of serotonin-immunoreactivity in the central nervous system of the rat—cell bodies and terminals. *Neuroscience* 6:557–618, 1981.

SWANSON, L. W., AND KUYPERS, H. G. J. M. The paraventricular nucleus of the hypothalamus: Cytoarchitectonic subdivisions and organization of projections to the pituitary, dorsal vagal complex, and spinal cord as demonstrated by retrograde fluorescence double-labeling methods. *J. Comp. Neurol.* 194:555–570, 1980.

TAKAGI, H., DOI, T., AND AKAIKE, A. Microinjection of morphine into the medial part of the bulbar reticular formation in rabbit and rat: Inhibitory effects on lamina V cells of spinal dorsal horn and behavioral analgesia, in: *Opiates and Endogenous Opioid Peptides* (H. W. KOSTERLITZ, ed.) Elsevier, Amsterdam, 1976, pp. 191–197.

TOHYAMA, M., SAKAI, K., SALVERT, D., TOURET, M., AND JOUVET, M. Spinal projections from the lower brain stem in the cat as demonstrated by the horseradish peroxidase technique. I. Origins of the reticulospinal tracts and their funicular trajectories. *Brain Res.* 173:383–403, 1979a.

TOHYAMA, M., SAKAI, K., TOURET, M., SALVERT, D., AND JOUVET, M. Spinal projections from the lower brainstem in the cat as demonstrated by the horseradish peroxidase technique. II. Projections from the dorsolateral pontine tegmentum and raphe nuclei. *Brain Res.* 176:215–231, 1979b.

TSUBOKAWA, T., YAMAMOTO, T., KATAYAMA, Y., AND MORIYAU, N. Clinical results and physiological basis of thalamic relay nucleus stimulation for relief of intractable pain with morphine tolerance. *Appl. Neurophysiol.* 45:143–155, 1982.

UHL, G. R., GOODMAN, R. R. KUHAR, M. J., CHILDERS, S. R., AND SNYDER, S. H. Immunohistochemical mapping of enkephalin containing cell bodies, fibers and nerve terminals in the brain stem of the rat. *Brain Res.* 166:75–94, 1979.

URCA, G., NAHIN, R. L., AND LIEBESKIND, J. C. Glutamate-induced analgesia: Blockade and potentiation by naloxone. *Brain Res.* 192:523–530, 1980.

VEAZEY, R. B., AMARAL, D. G., AND COWAN, W. M. The morphology and connections of the posterior hypothalamus in the cynomolgus monkey (*Macaca fascicularis*). II. Efferent connections. *J. Comp. Neurol.* 207:135–156, 1982.

VINCENT, S. R., HÖKFELT, T., CHRISTENSSON, I., AND TERENIUS, L. Dynorphin-immunoreactive neurons in the central nervous system of the rat. *Neurosci. Lett.* 33:185–190, 1982.

WALL, P. D. The laminar organization of dorsal horn and effects of descending impulses. *J. Physiol. (Lond.)* 188:403–423, 1967.

WAMSLEY, J. K., YOUNG, W. S. III, AND KUHAR, M. J. Immunohistochemical localization of enkephalin in rat forebrain. *Brain Res.* 190:153–174, 1980.

WATKINS, L. R., GRIFFIN, G., LEICHNETZ, G. R., AND MAYER, D. J. The somatotopic organization of the nucleus raphe magnus and surrounding brain stem structures as revealed by HRP slow-release gels. *Brain Res.* 181:1–15, 1980.

WATKINS, L. R., GRIFFIN, G., LEICHNETZ, G. R., AND MAYER, D. J. Identification and somatotopic organization of nuclei projecting via the dorsolateral funiculus in rats: A retrograde tracing study using HRP slow-release gels. *Brain Res.* 223:237–255, 1981.

WATSON, S. J., KHACHATURIAN, H., AKIL, H., COY, D. H., AND GOLDSTEIN, A. Comparison of the distribution of dynorphin systems and enkephalin systems in brain. *Science* 218:1134–1136, 1982.

WESSENDORF, M. W., PROUDFIT, H. K, AND ANDERSON, E. G. The identification of serotonergic neurons in the nucleus raphe magnus by conduction velocity. *Brain Res.* 214:168–173, 1981.

WEST, D. C., AND WOLSTENCROFT, J. H. Location and conduction velocity of raphe spinal neurones in nucleus raphe magnus and raphe pallidus in the cat. *Neurosci. Lett.* 5:147–151, 1977.

WESTLUND, K. N., BOWKER, R. M., ZIEGLER, M. G., AND COULTER, J. D. Descending noradrenergic projections and their spinal terminations. *Prog. Brain Res.* 57:219–238, 1982.

WIESENDANGER, M. The pyramidal tract. Recent investigations on its morphology and function. *Ergeb. Physiol. Biol. Chem. Exp. Pharmakol.* 61:72–136, 1969.

WIKLUND, L., LEGER, L., AND PERSSON, M. Monoamine cell distribution in the cat brain stem. A fluorescence histochemical study with quantification of indolaminergic and locus coeruleus cell groups. *J. Comp. Neurol.* 203:613–647, 1981.

WILLIAMS, R. G., AND DOCKRAY, G. J. Distribution of enkephalin-related peptides in rat brain: Immunohistochemical studies using antisera to met-enkephalin and met-enkephalin Arg^6Phe^7. *Neuroscience* 9:563–586, 1983.

WILLIS, W. D. Control of nociceptive transmission in the spinal cord, in: *Progress in Sensory Physiology*, Vol. 3 (H. AUTRUM, D. OTTOSON, E. R. PERL, AND R. F. SCHMIDT, eds.), Springer-Verlag, New York, 1982, pp. 54–75.

WILLIS, W. D., HABER, L. H., AND MARTIN, R. F. Inhibition of spinothalamic tract cells and interneurons by brain stem stimulation in the monkey. *J. Neurophysiol.* 40:968–981, 1977.

WISE, S. P., AND JONES, E. G. Cells of origin and terminal distribution of decending projections of the rat somatic sensory cortex. *J. Comp. Neurol.* 175:129–158, 1977.

WISE, S. P., MURRAY, E. A., AND COULTER, J. D. Somatotopic organization of corticospinal and corticotrigeminal neurons in the rat. *Neuroscience* 4:65–78, 1979.

YAKSH, T. L. Direct evidence that spinal serotonin and noradrenaline terminals mediate the spinal antinociceptive effects of morphine in the periaqueductal gray. *Brain Res.* 160:180–185, 1979.

YAKSH, T. L., AND ELDE, R. E. Factors governing the release of methionine enkephalin-like immunoreactivity from the mesencephalon and spinal cord of the cat *in vivo*. *J. Neurophysiol.* 46:1056–1075, 1981.

YAKSH, T. L., AND HAMMOND, D. L. Peripheral and central substrates involved in the rostrad transmission of nociceptive information. *Pain* 13:1–85, 1982.

YAKSH, T. L., AND RUDY, T. A. Chronic catheterization of the spinal subarachnoid space. *Physiol. Behav.* 17:1031–1036, 1976.

YAKSH, T. L., AND RUDY, T. A. Narcotic analgetics: CNS sites and mechanisms of action as revealed by intracerebral injection techniques. *Pain* 4:299–359, 1978.

YAKSH, T. L., AND TYCE, G. M. Microinjection of morphine into the periaqueductal gray evokes the release of serotonin from spinal cord. *Brain Res.* 171:176–181, 1979.

YAKSH, T. L., AND TYCE, G. M. Monoamine release from cat spinal cord by somatic stimuli: An intrinsic modulatory system. *J. Physiol. (Lond.)* 314:513–529, 1981.

YAKSH, T. L., AND WILSON, P. R. Spinal serotonin terminal system mediates antinociception. *J. Pharmacol. Exp. Ther.* 208:446–453,1979.

YAKSH, T. L., DUCHATEAU, J. C., AND RUDY, T. A. Antagonism by methysergide and cinanserin of the antinociceptive action of morphine administered into the periaqueductal gray. *Brain Res.* 104:367–372, 1976a.

YAKSH, T. L., YEUNG, J. C., AND RUDY, T. A. An inability to antagonize with naloxone the elevated thresholds resulting from electrical stimulation of the mesencephalic central gray. *Life Sci.* 18:1193–1198, 1976b.

YAKSH, T. L., YEUNG, J. C., AND RUDY, T. A. Systematic examination in the rat of brain sites sensitive to the direct application of morphine: Observation of differential effects within the periaqueductal gray. *Brain Res.* 114:83–103, 1976c.

YAKSH, T. L., HUANG, S. P., AND RUDY, T. A. The direct and specific opiate-like effect of met^5 enkephalin and analogues on the spinal cord. *Neuroscience* 2:593–598, 1977.

YEZIERSKI, R. P., BOWKER, R. M., KEVETTER, G. A., WESTLUND, K. N. COULTER, J. D., AND WILLIS, W. D. Serotonergic projections to the caudal brainstem: A double label study using horseradish peroxidase and serotonin immunoreactivity. *Brain Res.* 239:258–264, 1982a.

YEZIERSKI, R. P., WILCOX, T. K., AND WILLIS, W. D. The effects of serotonin antagonists on the inhibition of primate spinothalamic tract cells produced by stimulation in nucleus raphe magnus or periaqueductal gray. *J. Pharmacol. Exp. Ther.* 220:266–277, 1982b.

YEZIERSKI, R. P., GERHART, K. D., SCHROCK, B. J., AND WILLIS, W. D. A further examination of effects of cortical stimulation on primate spinothalamic tract cells. *J. Neurophysiol.* 49:424–441, 1983.

YUNGER, L. M., HARVEY, J. A., AND LORENS, S. A. Dissociation of the analgesic and rewarding effects of brain stimulation in the rat. *Physiol. Behav.* 10:909–913, 1973.

ZIEGLGANSBERGER, W., AND TULLOCH, I. F. The effects of methionine-and leucine-enkephalin on spinal neurones of the cat. *Brain Res.* 167:53–64, 1979.

ZORMAN, G., HENTALL, I. D., ADAMS, J. E., AND FIELDS, H. L. Naloxone-reversible analgesia produced by microstimulation in the rat medulla. *Brain Res.* 219:137–148, 1981.

ZORMAN, G., BELCHER, G., ADAMS, J. E., AND FIELDS, H. L. Lumbar intrathecal naloxone blocks analgesia produced by microstimulation of the ventromedial medulla in the rat. *Brain Res.* 236:77–84, 1982.

16
Modulatory Effects of Descending Systems on Spinal Dorsal Horn Neurons

G. F. GEBHART

A. *Introduction*

It is well established that suprasegmental modulation of spinal reflexes and spinal neuronal responses can be demonstrated from widespread areas of the brain, including the brainstem, diencephalon, and cortex. Indeed, many of these spinal reflexes and neurons are tonically modulated from supraspinal sites. Early investigators employed lesions and intracerebral electrical stimulation to locate the site(s) of origin of descending control of flexion reflexes. Although these efforts were directed primarily toward understanding mechanisms of motor control, they also contributed significantly to our knowledge of sensory mechanisms and the suprasegmental modulation of nociception. Focal electrical brain stimulation and intracerebral drug microinjections are widely employed today to examine descending modulatory influences on spinal dorsal horn neurons and nociceptive reflexes, focusing often on "intrinsic" systems of pain control. This chapter considers descending *inhibitory* modulation of nociceptive transmission in the spinal cord, but it is important to recognize that centrifugal influences on somatosensory pathways can be either inhibitory *or* excitatory. The substrates for these spinopetal effects have been discussed further in the chapters by Hammond (Chapter 15), Ruda (Chapter 7), and LaMotte (Chapter 5).

G. F. GEBHART • Department of Pharmacology, College of Medicine, University of Iowa, Iowa City, Iowa 52242.

B. Descending Control of Flexor Withdrawal Reflexes

Willis (1982) has recently summarized and reviewed the descending control of flexion reflexes; the important historical antecedents to the focus of this chapter thus are not reviewed here. His commendable treatise is a valuable source of information for the student of pain and its control. It is important here only to reemphasize the likely relationship between flexor withdrawal reflexes (e.g., the widely used nociceptive tail-flick reflex) and nociceptive interneurons in the spinal cord dorsal horn.

The cutaneous afferent classes of fibers that evoke flexion reflexes and activity in wide-dynamic-range (WDR) neurons include both large-diameter myelinated fibers (e.g., flexor reflex afferents originating from mechanoreceptors) and small-diameter Aδ and C fibers (e.g., long-lasting flexion reflexes). Both the duration and intensity of the responses increase as smaller diameter fibers are activated by cutaneous stimulation (e.g., Chung *et al.*, 1983).

The location of nociceptive interneurons in the spinal cord dorsal horn that are excited by stimuli evoking flexor withdrawal reflexes is similar to that of WDR cells. Although it is uncertain whether dorsal horn neurons participate in both motor and sensory mechanisms, WDR (class 2) interneurons have recently been demonstrated to be intercalated in the flexion reflex pathway responsible for a C-fiber-evoked late reflex discharge in the rat (Schouenborg and Sjolund, 1983). Both flexion reflexes and dorsal horn interneurons are under tonic descending inhibitory control, and, as Willis (1984) suggests, this must in part result from inhibition of dorsal horn interneurons that are part of flexion reflex pathways.

Inhibition of flexion reflexes is produced by opioid microinjection and stimulation in brainstem areas that also inhibit dorsal horn neuronal responses to noxious stimulation and attenuate responses to noxious cutaneous stimulation in awake animals (see below).

The foregoing discussion is important inasmuch as flexor withdrawal reflexes, particularly the rodent nociceptive tail-flick reflex, are widely and increasingly employed in studies on pathways, neurotransmitters, and mechanisms of descending control of spinal nociceptive transmission. Thus, although space limits this chapter to consideration of centrifugal modulation of spinal dorsal horn neurons, the study of descending influences on flexor withdrawal reflexes also has contributed significantly to our understanding of the organization and pathways of the centrifugal modulation of pain.

C. Descending Control of Dorsal Horn Interneurons

Before the mid-1970s, there were relatively few reports in the literature of descending influences on spinal dorsal horn neuronal responses to noxious stimuli. Many reports have since established the inhibitory influence of centrifugal systems (activated by focal electrical brain stimulation) on spinal dorsal horn nociceptors. Focal electrical stimulation in the sensorimotor cortex (Coulter *et al.*, 1974; Yezierski *et al.*, 1983), ventrobasal thalamus (Gerhart *et al.*, 1983), hypothalamus (Carstens, 1982; Carstens *et al.*, 1983), midbrain periaqueductal gray (PAG) and lateral midbrain reticular formation (Carstens *et al.*, 1980; Gebhart *et al.*, 1983b; Gerhart *et al.*, 1984), medullary nucleus raphe magnus (NRM) and areas adjacent in the rostral ventral medulla (Fields *et al.*, 1977; Gebhart *et al.*, 1983b; Gerhart *et al.*, 1981; Gray and Dostrovsky, 1983), and the caudal medullary lateral reticular nucleus (Morton *et al.*, 1984) all have been demonstrated to inhibit spinal dorsal horn neuronal excitation evoked by noxious stimuli (see Hammond, Chapter 15, for further discussion).

Most such studies have been performed in the cat, but the monkey and, increasingly, the rat are also used. With some exceptions, the results obtained in different species are consistent qualitatively. It is not easy to compare results quantitatively with respect to thresholds for inhibition of neuronal responses, intensities of stimulation required to inhibit responses, etc. Aside from differences in the parameters of intracerebral stimulation (e.g., frequency, duration, pulse width), electrodes (size and whether mono- or bipolar), anesthetic agent, stimuli employed to evoke spinal neuronal responses (e.g., mechanical pinch, radiant or contact heat, electrical peripheral nerve stimulation), the neurons in the dorsal horn sampled and studied may be different. With the exception of Willis' studies of WDR and high-threshold (class 2 and 3, respectively; Handwerker *et al.*, 1975; Menétrey *et al.*, 1977; Price and Dubner, 1977) spinothalamic tract neurons in the primate, most studies have examined dorsal horn neurons characterized only by their receptive fields and response properties to peripheral stimuli and not on the basis of whether they could be antidromically activated from supraspinal sites. Although this is an important consideration insofar as identification of spinal neurons as projection or spinothalamic tract cells is concerned (since these cells are believed to be directly involved in the transmission and signaling of nociceptive information to supraspinal sensory centers), it is likely that many, if not most, of the "unidentified" cells examined in other studies were also spinothalamic tract cells and/or important in nociceptive transmission. This assumption is supported by (1) comparison of results of studies on descending control of spinothalamic tract cells with similar studies on unidentified spinal dorsal horn cells and (2) examination of the locations in the dorsal horn of the recording sites in these studies; they are essentially the same.

That the descending inhibition of spinal nociceptors is functionally significant is supported by reports that electrical stimulation in many of these same areas is antinociceptive or antinocisponsive in awake, behaving animals. That is, stimulation produces an analgesia. The term analgesia (without pain) is used in this chapter, but it bears emphasizing that such use to describe drug- or stimulation-produced effects in nonhuman animals is neither accurate nor strictly appropriate.

Stimulation-produced analgesia from the midbrain PAG was first reported by Reynolds (1969). Others confirmed his results in the rat and extended them to the cat and primate (Mayer and Price, 1976; Willis, 1982), including man (e.g., Hosobuchi *et al.,* 1977; Richardson and Akil, 1977). Further support is provided by reports establishing that opioids are analgetic (Yaksh and Rudy, 1978) and inhibit spinal nociceptors (e.g., Bennett and Mayer, 1979; Du *et al.,* 1984; Gebhart *et al.,* 1984) when microinjected into some of the same brainstem areas from which stimulation-produced analgesia can be evoked. It is generally considered that the analgesias evoked from the PAG (or NRM, etc.) in awake, behaving animals are a consequence of descending inhibitory influences on spinal and medullary dorsal horn nociceptors (Basbaum and Fields, 1978; Mayer and Price, 1976). However, this remains to be resolved, since it has long been recognized that dorsal horn neuronal responses evoked by noxious stimuli can also be inhibited by stimulation in supraspinal sites that do not produce an analgesia or produce aversive effects in awake animals. Liebeskind *et al.* (1973) reported that the distribution of stimulation sites in the midbrain that inhibited spinal nociceptors in the cat was wider than the distribution of sites from which an analgesia could be produced, extending into the adjacent reticular formation and including sites that produced aversive responses when stimulated in the waking animal. Thus, whereas stimulation in the dorsal PAG inhibits spinal dorsal horn nociceptive transmission, stimulation at similar sites in the waking cat (Besson *et al.,* 1981) and rat (Oliveras *et al.,* 1983) is not analgetic and, moreover, is often aversive.

It also has been generally accepted that stimulation-produced inhibition is selective, if not specific, for nociceptive transmission in the spinal cord, leaving the transmission of innocuous information relatively unaffected (Basbaum and Fields, 1978). Similarly, stimulation-produced analgesia in awake animals is generally considered not to be associated with overt changes in motor control, responses to other sensory stimuli, or attentional or motivational deficits (Besson *et al.,* 1981; Mayer, 1979; Oliveras *et al.,* 1983). The selectivity of the production of analgesia by supraspinal stimulation is supported by reports that stimulation-produced analgesia is often expressed as a restricted field of hypoalgesia (Mayer and Liebeskind, 1974; Soper, 1976; Soper and Melzack, 1982) and also that animals are capable of performing motivated behaviors during stimulation (e.g., Soper, 1976).

In summary, stimulation-produced analgesia has been demonstrated from many supraspinal sites. That these systems may be tonically active is suggested by the hypoalgesia observed when spinal lesions involving these descending tracts are made (see Vierck *et al.,* Chapter 12, for further discussion). It is generally held that the analgesia is a consequence of selective descending inhibitory influences on spinal nociceptors. However, descending inhibitory effects are also produced from sites that do not produce an analgesia or produce aversive effects when stimulated in the waking animal. Both the specificity of descending inhibition for nociceptive tranmission and its relevance to analgesic mechanisms require clarification.

D. Descending Inhibition of Nociceptive Transmission

Quantitative studies of supraspinal modulation of dorsal horn neurons require that controllable, reproducible, and quantifiable stimuli be used. Commonly, feedback-controlled heat and direct peripheral nerve electrical stimulation have been employed. The responses of a dorsal horn interneuron to radiant heating of the cat's hind-limb footpad and its modulation from supraspinal sites are shown in Figure 1. Typically, the number of discharges per unit time or the maximum frequency of response to the applied stimulus is employed to quantify spinal neuronal responses to natural, mechanical, or heat stimuli. The efficacy of supraspinal inhibition is easily determined by

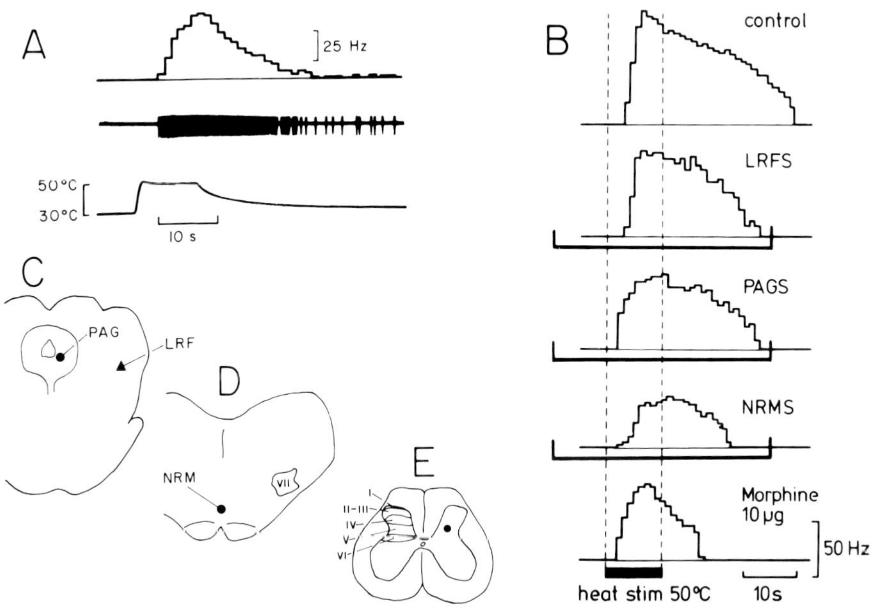

FIGURE 1. Inhibition of heat-evoked neuronal excitation by focal electrical stimulation and morphine in the brainstem. A: Record of a class 2 (WDR) dorsal horn neuronal response to noxious heating of a cat's hind-limb footpad (50°C, 10 s). Skin temperature, recorded by a thermocouple, is shown below; the oscilloscope record of the unit's response and its peristimulus time histogram (PSTH, 1-s bin width) are shown above. To quantify a unit's response, the total number of discharges were counted for 20 s beginning with the onset of the heat stimulus. B: Examples (PSTHs) of inhibition of another class 2 dorsal horn unit by focal electrical stimulation and morphine administered intracerebrally (10 μg in 1 μl). Focal electrical brain stimulation was started 10 s before the onset of the heat stimulus and lasted for 35 s (illustrated beneath each PSTH). The control response to noxious heating of the skin is shown uppermost; the period of heating of the skin (50°C, 10 s) is shown below. C,D: Sites of stimulation in the midbrain (periaqueductal gray, PAG; lateral reticular formation, LRF) and medulla (nucleus raphe magnus, NRM) drawn on representation coronal sections of the cat brainstem. Morphine was administered in the same site as stimulation in the PAG. E: Recording locus of the class 2 neuron represented in B. (Adapted from Gebhart *et al.*, 1984, with permission.)

comparison of responses to cutaneous stimuli before (or after) and during stimulation (Fig. 1B; see also Gebhart *et al.,* 1983a,b). Responses of dorsal horn WDRs to repeated, controlled (duration and intensity) radiant heating of the footpad have been established to be reproducible and quantifiable (e.g., Beck *et al.,* 1974; Carstens *et al.,* 1979). Adaptation and sensitization of the responses to noxious heat can result from repetitive heat stimuli, however, particularly as both duration and intensity of the heat stimulus increase (e.g., Kenshalo *et al.,* 1979). Sensitization of responses of high-threshold Aδ mechanoreceptors is well established (Fitzgerald and Lynn, 1977), but class 2 dorsal horn interneurons (i.e., WDRs) respond reproducibly to repetitive heat stimuli of limited duration and intensity (e.g., Beck *et al.,* 1974; Carstens *et al.,* 1979; Gebhart *et al.,* 1983a,b).

The modulation of dorsal horn nociceptors by supraspinal stimulation is characterized by increased inhibition and duration of inhibition as the intensity of supraspinal electrical stimulation is incremented (e.g., Gebhart *et al.,* 1983a,b; Gerhart *et al.,* 1984). Examples are given in Figure 2. The recruitment of

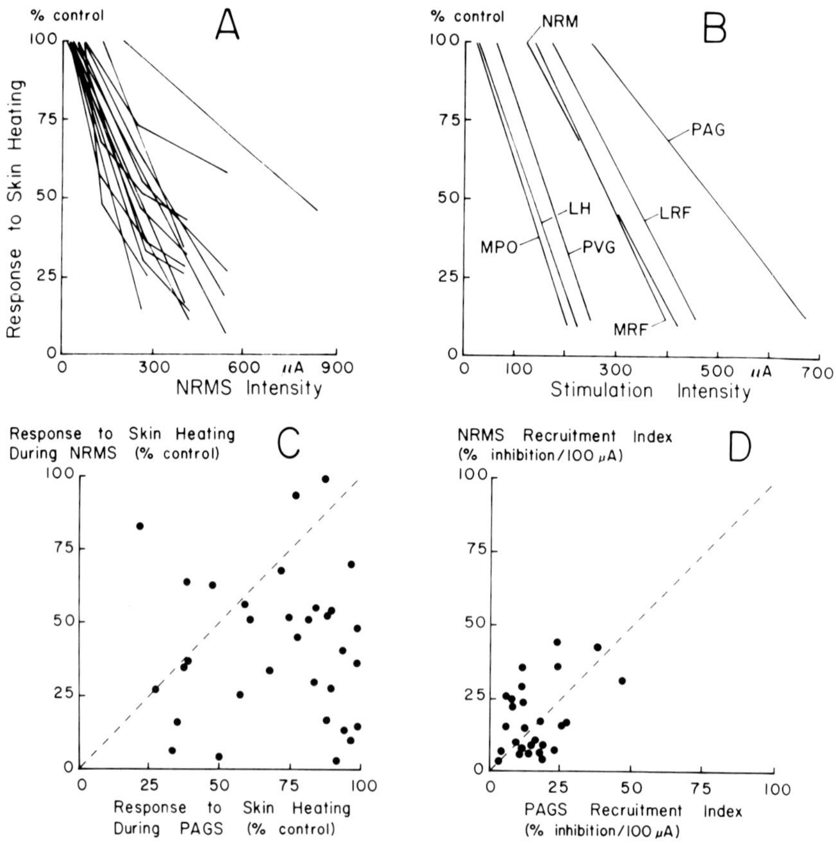

dorsal horn neuronal inhibition of nociceptive transmission by increasing intensities of supraspinal stimulation (Figure 2A) permits estimation of thresholds for neuronal inhibition, determination of stimulating currents producing significant (e.g., 50%) inhibition, and calculation of a recruitment index from the slopes of the lines of recruitment of inhibition, all of which allow quantitative comparison of the efficacy of stimulation-produced inhibition evoked from different supraspinal sites (Figure 2B). The comparison of inhibition of spinal dorsal horn nociceptors from different supraspinal sites is strengthened when inhibition from several supraspinal sites is examined on the same dorsal horn neuron (Figure 2C,D).

A note of caution, however, is appropriate. It is not likely that in every experiment the stimulation sites producing inhibition at the lowest intensity of stimulation in the NRM, PAG, etc. will be studied. Thus, one must rely on the accumulated weight of many experiments. The results of several studies are summarized in Table I and Figure 2B. The studies summarized were performed using the same animal preparation, anesthetic, peripheral noxious heat stimulus, intracerebral electrodes and stimulation parameters, and experimental paradigm examining class 2 and 3 dorsal horn neurons (primarily WDRs).

It is clear from the data presented that descending modulation of heat-

FIGURE 2. Quantitative evaluation of centrifugal control of spinal neuronal responses evoked by noxious heating of the skin. A: Descending inhibition produced by stimulation in the NRM (NRMS) as a function of the intensity of stimulation. In A and B, responses to heating of the skin (50°C, 10 s) are represented on ordinates as precentage of the control response (total number of discharges in 20 s) against the intensity (μA) of stimulation on abscissas. Lines of recruitment of inhibition in A connect data points for at least three different intensities of NRMS. The lines of recruitment of inhibition in B portray the thresholds of inhibition and recruitment indices as determined from individual experiments (as shown in A) and summarized in Table I (abbreviations as in Table I). C,D: Quantitative comparison between descending inhibition produced by stimulation in the PAG (PAGS) and by NRMS. C: Inhibition of the spinal neuronal response to heating of the skin (50°, 10 s) is expressed as percentage of the control 50°C heat-evoked response (total number of discharges in 20 s) for each of 33 spinal units; inhibition of the heat-evoked response by NRMS (ordinate) is plotted against the inhibition produced by PAGS (abscissa) at the same intensity of stimulation. The broken diagonal line indicates equal inhibition from both stimulation sites. The mean magnitude of inhibition produced by NRMS (to 46% of control) was significantly greater than that produced on the same spinal units by the same intensity of PAGS (to 72% of control; Gebhart *et al.*, 1983a). D: Comparison of the recruitment indices for NRMS and PAGS. The increase in inhibition produced by a 100-μA increase in PAGS or NRMS was determined from slopes of lines of recruitment of inhibition (e.g., see A) for 27 spinal units. These recruitment indices, expressed as the percentage inhibition/100 μA for NRMS (ordinate) and PAGS (abscissa), are plotted against each other for each spinal unit. The broken diagonal line indicates equality in the recruitment indices for PAGS and NRMS. Stimulation in the NRM and PAG produced the same mean percentage change in inhibition per 100-μA increase in the intensity of stimulation. Thus, the slopes of the recruitment of descending inhibition from the PAG and the NRM as a function of increasing intensities of stimulation are the same; the lines of recruitment of inhibition are parallel (see B). (Adapted from Gebhart *et al.*, 1984a, with permission.)

TABLE I
Summary of Inhibition in the Spinal Dorsal Horn of Nociceptive Information by Supraspinal Stimulation in the Cat[a]

Site of stimulation[b]	Threshold of inhibition (μA)	Stimulation current (μA) producing inhibition to 50% of control	Recruitment index (% inhibition/100 μA)	Stimulus–response function[c]	Reference
PVG	67 ± 17	170 ± 20	46 ± 12	Slope change	Carstens *et al.* (1982)
LH	30 ± 8	135 ± 29	54 ± 14	Slope change	Carstens *et al.* (1983)
MPO/VMS	25 ± 7	126 ± 14	41 ± 7	Slope change	Carstens *et al.* (1982)
PAG	252 ± 30	497 ± 91	16.5 ± 2.3	Slope change	Gebhart *et al.* (1983a)
PAG	275	502	21	Slope change	Carstens *et al.* (1980)
LRF	175	334	56	Threshold change	Carstens *et al.* (1980)
NRM	178 ± 43	374 ± 24	18.7 ± 2.2	Threshold change	Gebhart *et al.* (1983a)
NRM	147 ± 32	288 ± 46	20.1 ± 2.9	Threshold change	Gebhart *et al.* (1983b)
MRF	165 ± 37	289 ± 65	22.7 ± 3.6	Threshold change	Gebhart *et al.* (1983b)
PAG (morphine)				Slope change	Gebhart *et al.* (1984)

[a] All data were accumulated in the anesthetized, paralyzed cat; the spinal units studied were class 2 and 3 type (Hankwerker *et al.*, 1975; Price and Dubner, 1977), and radiant heat (typically 50°C, 10 s) was the noxious stimulus applied to the glabrous skin of the hind-limb footpad. Values reported are mean ± S.E.M. Details of the derivation and interpretation of the measures of inhibition contained in this table are available in the sources identified.

[b] Abbreviations: PVG, periventricular gray; LH, lateral hypothalamus; MPO/VMS, medial preoptic/ventromedial septal areas; PAG, periaqueductal gray; LRF, midbrain reticular formation 4 mm lateral to the PAG; NRM, nucleus raphe magnus; MRF, medullary retiular formation 2 mm lateral to the NRM.

[c] The responses of class 2 and 3 spinal units are a monotonic linear function of skin temperatures in the range 40–50°C (e.g., Zimmermann, 1977). Stimulation in the brainstem shifts the stimulus response function (SRF) to the right (threshold change) or decreases the slope of the SRF (slope change). See Figure 5 for examples.

evoked spinal neuronal responses can be demonstrated from many and widespread supraspinal sites. However, the thresholds of stimulation producing inhibition differ significantly among the supraspinal sites investigated, as does the amount of inhibition produced per unit increment in the intensity of stimulation (i.e., recruitment indices). Not shown in the table are data establishing, for example, that the magnitude of inhibition produced by stimulation in the NRM at a given intensity of stimulation is significantly greater than that produced on the same spinal units by the same intensity of stimulation in the PAG (Figure 2C; Gebhart *et al.,* 1983a). Similarly, the magnitude of inhibiton by stimulation in the midbrain reticular formation lateral to the PAG is significantly greater than is the magnitude of inhibition of the same spinal units produced by the same intensity of stimulation in the PAG (Carstens *et al.,* 1980). In the rostral ventral medulla, however, stimulation in the NRM produced the same magnitude of inhibition of the same spinal units as did stimulation at the same intensity in the medullary reticular formation lateral to the NRM (Gebhart *et al.,* 1983b).

Such quantitative comparisons reveal that supraspinal stimulation is more easily produced at some sites than others and could be interpreted to support the existence of separate systems of descending modulation of nociceptive transmission in the spinal cord. This interpretation also is supported by reports establishing that lower intensities of stimulation are required for inhibition of nociceptive reflexes in cats (oral–facial) and rats (tail flick) from outside the PAG (Dostrovsky *et al.,* 1982; Sandkühler and Gebhart, 1984a).

The effects of supraspinal stimulation on the responses of spinal nociceptors to graded increments of peripheral noxious stimulation (i.e., stimulus–response functions) also reveal that significant differences exist in the character of inhibiton of spinal nociceptive transmission (see below). Thus, it remains to be clarified whether there exists a single modulatory system composed of several components or several independent pathways in the brainstem, each important to centrifugal modulation of spinal nociceptive transmission. Experimental results discussed later in this chapter and elsewhere in this book increasingly suggest the existence of multiple and separate systems of descending modulation.

The effects of opioids administered systemically, applied topically onto the exposed spinal cord, or by microinjection into supraspinal sites also have been examined on spinal neuronal responses evoked by peripheral noxious stimuli (Gebhart *et al.,* 1984). It is well documented that opioids microinjected supraspinally produce an analgesia in waking animals (Yaksh and Rudy, 1978). When administered systemically, opioids attenuate significantly noxious-evoked responses of spinal nociceptive neurons (Gebhart *et al.,* 1984), but it is unknown where this action arises, since opioids have direct and indepenedent spinal and supraspinal sites of action (Yaksh, 1981). When applied topically to the exposed spinal cord (Homma *et al.,* 1983) or microinjected into the PAG (Gebhart *et al.,* 1984) or NRM (Du *et al.,* 1984), morphine attenuates significantly spinal neuronal responses evoked by noxious heating of the footpad of the cat (e.g., see Figure 1B).

That opioids directly activate centrifugal systems of spinal inhibition when administered supraspinally has not always been observed. Bennett and Mayer (1979) reported that the intra-PAG microinjection of morphine inhibited by 25% or more fewer than half of the WDR units examined in rat spinal cord, whereas Le Bars *et al.* (1976) failed to observe any influence of morphine on C-fiber-evoked spinal neuronal responses in the rat. A relatively modest inhibition of heat-evoked spinal neuronal discharges in the cat produced by large doses of morphine microinjected into the PAG (>90 μg) led Clark *et al.* (1983) to suggest that the effects observed might have occurred after morphine redistributed to the systemic circulation from its intracerebral site of administration (see also Clark and Ryall, 1983). When administered in much lower doses in the PAG (10–20 μg), morphine produced a greater than 50% reduction of noxious heat-evoked spinal neuronal responses, an effect antagonized by naloxone given either intravenously or intra-PAG but not reproduced by 100 μg of morphine given intravenously (Gebhart *et al.*, 1984). When morphine is administered into the NRM, there is a similar inconsistency in its effect on spinal neuronal responses. Le Bars *et al.* (1980) failed in the rat and Du *et al.* (1984) succeeded in the cat to observe a significant inhibition of spinal nociceptors following the microinjection of morphine into the NRM. In addition to differences in the animal species employed in these studies, the type and level of anesthesia may likely be responsible for the mixed results observed. Ossipov and Gebhart (1984) recently observed that morphine was significantly less potent an analgetic when microinjected into the PAG of lightly pentobarbital-anesthetized rats than when similarly examined in waking rats.

In summary, the efficacy of supraspinal manipulations such as focal electrical stimulation and opioid microinjection in the descending modulation of spinal nociceptive transmission has clearly been established. Quantitative comparisons of inhibition of spinal nociceptors by stimulation in the brainstem have revealed that simulation in the NRM or midbrain lateral reticular formation is more efficacious than is stimulation in the PAG. Stimulation in the medullary reticular formation produces inhibition as efficacious as that produced from the NRM. Such results may indicate the convergence of midbrain neurons onto medullary relay neurons or, alternatively, the existence of multiple descending inhibitory pathways in the brainstem. Whether these descending inhibitory influences are nociceptive specific remains to be considered.

E. Descending Inhibition of Nonnociceptive Transmission

As indicated earlier, the descending inhibition of spinal dorsal horn neurons generally has been considered to be selective or specific for nociceptive transmission. It is clear, however, that supraspinal stimulation also significantly affects spinal neuronal responses evoked by innocuous brush or mechanical stimuli and electrical nerve stimulation at intensities that activate only Aα,β fibers. An example is presented in Figure 3; data from several reports are summarized in Table II. In Figure 3, focal electrical stimulation in the NRM is shown to attenuate the responses of the same dorsal horn WDR neuron to both Aα,β- and C-fiber electrical activation. In this study (Gebhart *et al.*, 1983a), it was determined that the same intensities of supraspinal stimulation

TABLE II
Comparison of Supraspinal Inhibitory Effects on Noxious- and Nonnoxious-Evoked Spinal Neuronal Activity[a]

CNS stimulation		Peripheral stimulus	Dorsal horn neurons	Inhibitory modulation	Reference
Site	Animal				
Cortex	Macaque	Brush, squeeze,	WDR (STT)	Brush > squeeze	Yezierski *et al.* (1983)
		elec. A and C	WDR (STT)	A fiber > C fiber	
VPL	Macaque	Elec. A and C	WDR (STT)	C fiber > A fiber	Gerhart *et al.* (1983)
PAG	Rat	Innoc. mech., nox. heat	WDR and LTM	WDR only	Bennett and Mayer (1979)
PAG	Macaque	Elec. A and C,	WDR (STT)	C fiber > A fiber	Gerhart *et al.* (1984)
		brush, squeeze	WDR (STT)	Brush = squeeze	
PAG/NRM	Cat	Elec. and tactile	LTM (SCT)	>80% LTMs inhibited	Dostrovsky (1984)
PAG/NRM	Cat	Just-suprathreshold elec.	LTM, WDR, and HT	Noci. > nonnoci.	Gray and Dostrovsky (1983)
PAG/NRM	Cat	Elec. Aα,β and C	WDR	C fiber > A fiber	Gebhart *et al.* (1983a)
NRM	Cat	Light touch, pinch	LTM and WDR	WDR only	Guilbaud *et al.* (1977)
NRM	Cat	Cutaneous	LTM and WDR	WDR only	Fields *et al.* (1977)
NRM	Macaque	Elec. Aα,β and Aδ	STT	Aδ > Aα,β	Willis *et al.* (1977)
NRM	Cat	Light touch, DLH	Noci. > nonnoci.	Noci. > nonnoci.	Belcher *et al.* (1978)
NRM	Rat	Elec. Aα, Aδ, and C	LTM & WDR	WDR > LTM	Rivot *et al.* (1980)
NRM	Macaque	Elec. A and C	WDR (STT)	C fiber > Aα,β fiber	Gerhart *et al.* (1981)
NRM	Cat	Elec. Aα,β and C	WDR	C fiber = Aα,β fiber	Du *et al.* (1984)
NGC	Macaque	Elec. Aα,β and Aδ	WDR (STT)	Aδ > Aα,B	Haber *et al.* (1980)

[a]Abbreviations: First column: NGC, n. reticularis gigantocellularis; NRM, n. raphe magnus; PAG, midbrain periaqueductal gray; VPL, thalamic ventral posterior lateral n. Second column: DLH, DL-homosysteic acid; elec., electrical; innoc. mech., innocuous mechanical; nox., noxious. Third column: HT, high threshold; LTM, low-threshold mechanoreceptor; noci. and nonnoci., nociceptive and nonnociceptive; SCT, spinocervical thalamic; STT, spinothalamic tract; WDR, wide dynamic range (class 2).

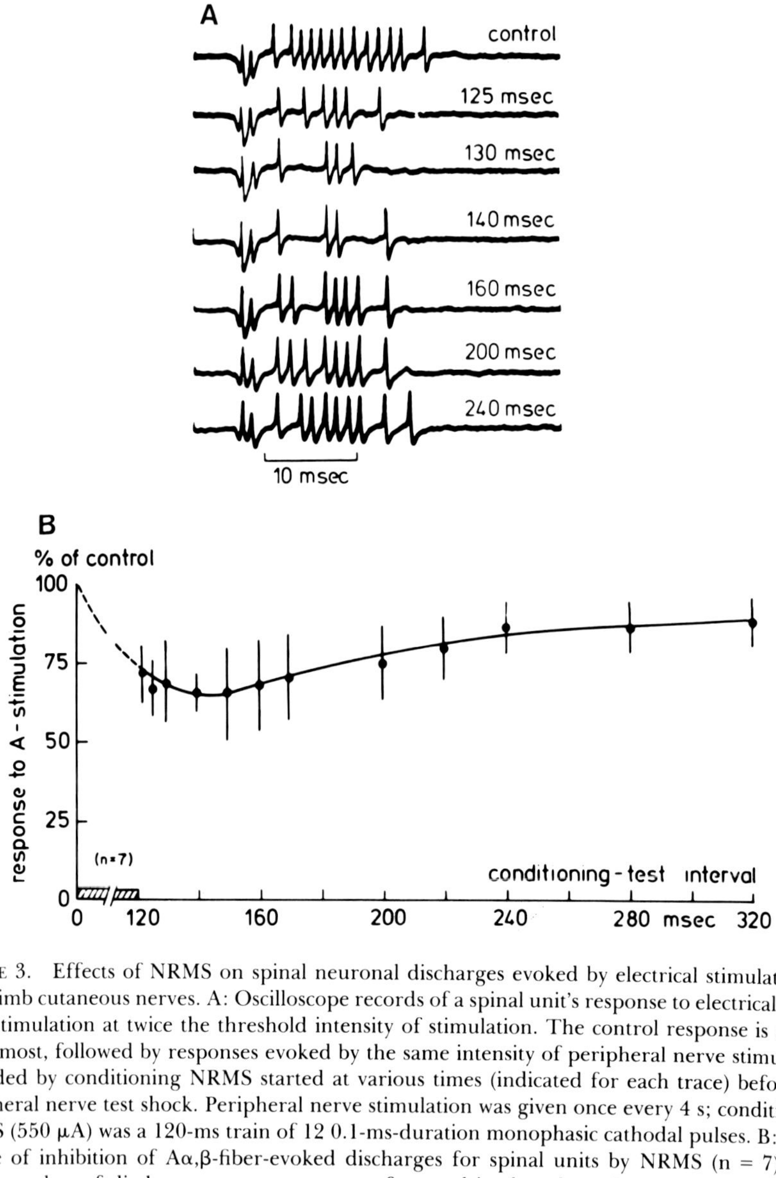

FIGURE 3. Effects of NRMS on spinal neuronal discharges evoked by electrical stimulation of hind-limb cutaneous nerves. A: Oscilloscope records of a spinal unit's response to electrical Aα,β-fiber stimulation at twice the threshold intensity of stimulation. The control response is shown uppermost, followed by responses evoked by the same intensity of peripheral nerve stimulation preceded by conditioning NRMS started at various times (indicated for each trace) before the peripheral nerve test shock. Peripheral nerve stimulation was given once every 4 s; conditioning NRMS (550 μA) was a 120-ms train of 12 0.1-ms-duration monophasic cathodal pulses. B: Time course of inhibition of Aα,β-fiber-evoked discharges for spinal units by NRMS (n = 7). The mean number of discharges as a percentage of control is plotted on the ordinate against the

in the NRM attenuated responses of dorsal horn neurons to C-fiber activation to a greater extent than responses of the same neurons to Aα,β-fiber activation (36% versus 66% of control, respectively). Similarly, Willis' laboratory has examined the selectivity of supraspinal inhibition of evoked responses of spinothalamic tract WDR neurons to C- and A-fiber volleys; stimulation in the PAG attenuated the response of spinothalamic tract cells to C-fiber volleys to

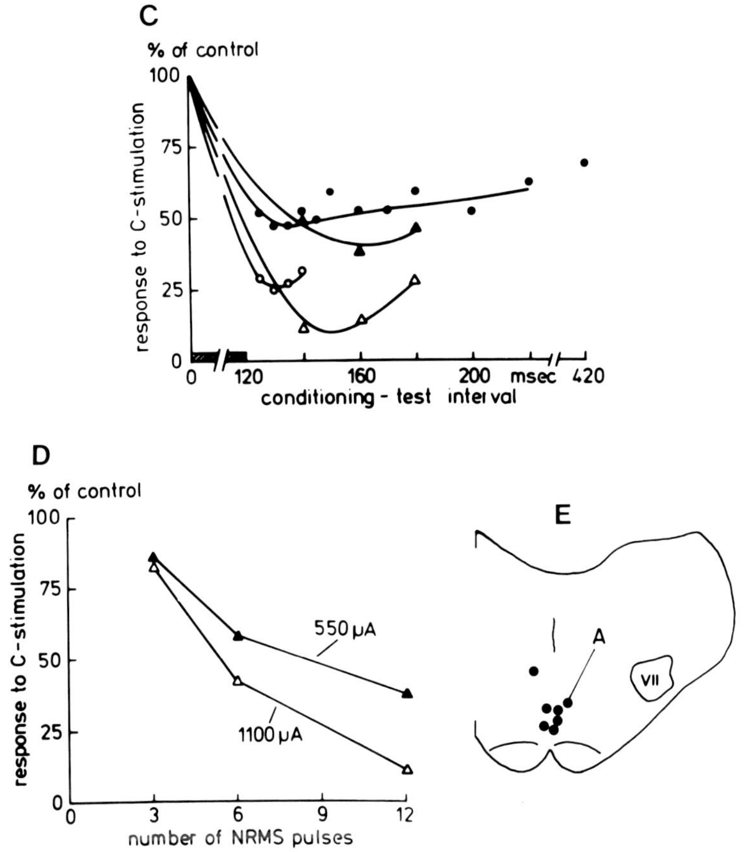

conditioning–test interval on the abscissa. Peripheral nerve stimulation and NRMS were as described for A. C: Time courses of inhibition of C-fiber-evoked discharges of spinal units by NRMS. The number of discharges as a percentage of control is plotted on the ordinate against the conditioning–test interval on the abscissa for different spinal neurons. Peripheral nerve stimulation was given once every 10 s; NRMS was as described for A. D: Effect of different intensities of NRMS and numbers of conditioning pulses of NRMS on C-fiber-evoked discharges. The number of C-fiber-evoked discharges as a percentage of control is given on the ordinate; the number of pulses of NRMS is given on the abscissa. E: Stimulation sites diagrammed on a representative coronal section through the medulla. The stimulation site producing the inhibition presented in A is indicated. (Adapted from Gebhart *et al.*, 1983a, with permission.)

27% of control and responses to A-fiber volleys to 65% of control (Gerhart *et al.*, 1984). Stimulation in the NRM similarly attenuated spinothalamic tract cell responses to C-fiber volleys to a significantly greater extent (to 8% of control) than responses to Aα,β-fiber volleys (49% of control; Gerhart *et al.*, 1981). In contrast, Du *et al.* (1984) recently reported that stimulation in the NRM inhibited WDR responses to A-fiber volleys to the same extent as C-fiber volleys (to 60% and 65% of control, respectively).

In an examination of the effects of supraspinal stimulation on brush-evoked responses of class 1 and 2 dorsal horn neurons (i.e., low-threshold mechanoreceptors and WDRs, respectively), Carstens *et al.* (1981) observed the responses to be attenuated by stimulation in both the PAG and midbrain lateral reticular formation. Class 1 and 2 spinal neuronal responses to brushing of the skin were affected similarly by stimulation in either site (i.e., to 70–80% of control). However, the magnitude of inhibition of the noxious heat-evoked response was significantly greater than the magnitude of inhibiton of the brush-evoked response of the same class 2 dorsal horn cells at the same intensity of stimulation in the PAG (55% versus 81% of control) or midbrain lateral reticular formation (54% versus 73% of control). Midbrain stimulation also has been recently reported to inhibit the background discharges and responses of WDR spinothalamic tract cells evoked by innocuous and noxious cutaneous stimuli (Gerhart *et al.,* 1984). Whereas the responses of all WDR cells to squeezing of the skin of the receptive field were inhibited by midbrain stimulation, the responses of only 78% of the spinal units to innocuous brushing of the skin were similarly inhibited.

Thus, there appears to be some descending inhibitory selectivity for nociceptive C-fiber as opposed to nonnociceptive Aα,β-fiber input, but there is no clear specificity of descending modulatory inhibition of nociceptive transmission produced by focal electrical brain stimulation. Most investigations have examined spinal WDR interneurons; fewer studies have examined low-threshold mechanoreceptors (class 1). Perhaps it is not surprising that WDR dorsal horn interneurons that respond to both innocuous and noxious input should be inhibited by supraspinal stimulation across their dynamic range of responses to cutaneous or electrical stimulation. Indeed, one may question why noxious-evoked responses of WDR interneurons are inhibited to a greater extent than their responses to nonnoxious stimuli. Factors such as the parameters of intracerebral stimulation (e.g., pulse width, frequency, and train duration in addition to electrode size and configuration and the intensity of stimulation) and of peripheral cutaneous and electrical nerve stimulation have not been thoroughly evaluated.

Supraspinal inhibitory effects are generally examined against peripheral nerve stimulation at intensities significantly above threshold for activation (e.g., twice or three times threshold). When supraspinal stimulation is examined on spinal neuronal responses evoked by just suprathreshold electrical activation of a peripheral nerve, the intensity of stimulation in the PAG or medulla required to inhibit nociceptive interneurons may not differ significantly from that required to inhibit nonnociceptive spinal interneurons (Gray and Dostrovsky, 1983). In regard to low-threshold mechanoreceptors, fewer studies have examined their descending modulation by supraspinal stimulation, but it is clear that they too can be inhibited (e.g., Carstens *et al.,* 1981; Gray and Dostrovsky, 1983). Such considerations question the specificity of supraspinal manipulations such as stimulation and drug microinjection as well as the relationship between descending inhibitory systems and analgesia.

In summary, centrifugal modulatory influences are not specific for spinal nociceptive transmission. Nonnociceptive transmission of class 1 and 2 dorsal horn neurons has been demonstrated to be attenuated significantly by supraspinal focal electrical stimulation. Effects on nonnociceptive transmission, however, are less marked than effects on nociceptive transmission.

F. Descending Modulation of Intensity Coding of Nociceptive Transmission

An important characteristic of supraspinal modulation of spinal nociceptive transmission is its influence on the stimulus–response function of dorsal horn neurons to graded intensities to nociceptive stimuli. Studies of the effects of supraspinal inhibition of dorsal horn neurons discussed above characterize centrifugal control of responses to relatively fixed, static peripheral stimuli (e.g., 50°C radiant heat, 10 s). Studies of supraspinal influences on stimulus–response functions of dorsal horn neurons further characterize centrifugal control over a dynamic range of neuronal responses, providing important insight into modulation of the encoding of spinal dorsal horn nociceptive transmission.

Wide-dynamic-range neurons respond to graded intensities of innocuous and noxious stimuli in an accelerating, monotonic manner (Kenshalo *et al.*, 1979; Price and Browe, 1975; Zimmermann, 1977), generating typical stimulus–response functions. This indicates that these neurons not only signal the presence of a stimulus but, moreover, convey information about the intensity of the stimulus encoded in the discharge frequency. An example of the linear relationship between the magnitude of spinal WDR neuronal responses and the temperature of heating of the skin is given in Figure 4.

Whereas focal electrical stimulation and morphine administered systemically, applied directly onto the exposed spinal cord, or microinjected intracerebrally produce qualitatively similar effects (i.e., inhibition of spinal dorsal horn neuronal responses to noxious heating of the skin), stimulation in different supraspinal sites affects the characteristic stimulus–response functions of the same neurons differently. Zimmermann (1977; see also Carstens *et al.*, 1980) has discussed these centrifugal effects in terms of alteration in the gain control of spinal nociceptive transmission (without a change in neuronal response threshold) and changes in the response threshold/set point (without a change in the slope of the stimulus–response function), proposing that the effects may be considered as multiplicative and additive interactions, respectively.

Example of the effects of supraspinal focal electrical stimulation on the stimulus–response functions of dorsal horn neuronal responses to graded increments in radiant heating of the cat's hind-limb footpad are shown in Figure 5. Focal electrical stimulation in the lateral hypothalamus, periventri-

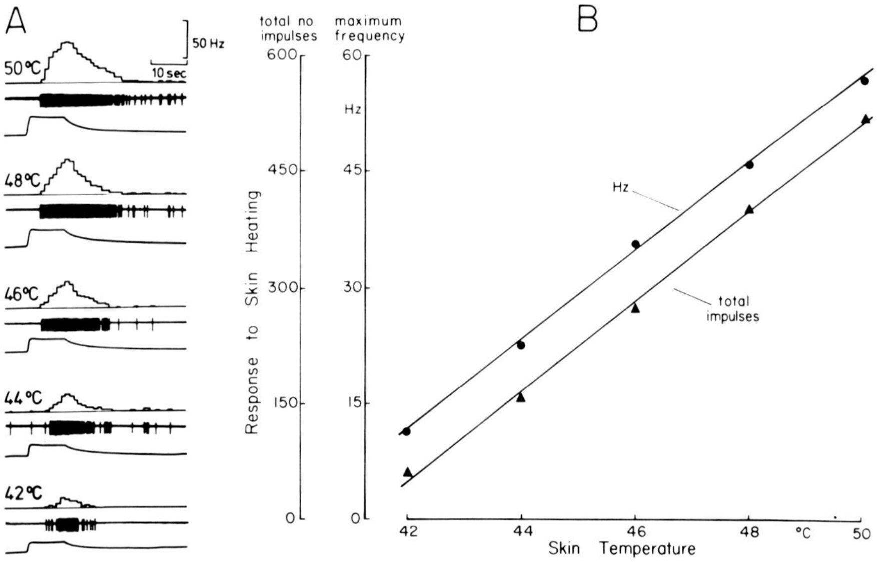

FIGURE 4. Responses of a class 2 (WDR) spinal dorsal horn neuron to noxious heating of the glabrous skin of a cat's hind-limb footpad. A: Oscilloscope records and peristimulus time histograms (1-s bin width) of the unit's response to heating of the footpad for 10 s. Skin temperature (42–50°C) was recorded with a thermocouple and is shown beneath each tracing. B: Relationship between skin temperature and the response to heating of the skin. Whether the responses are quantified as the maximum frequency (Hz) or the total number of discharges in 20 s, the stimulus–response function is shown to be a linear monotonic relationship over the temperatures tested.

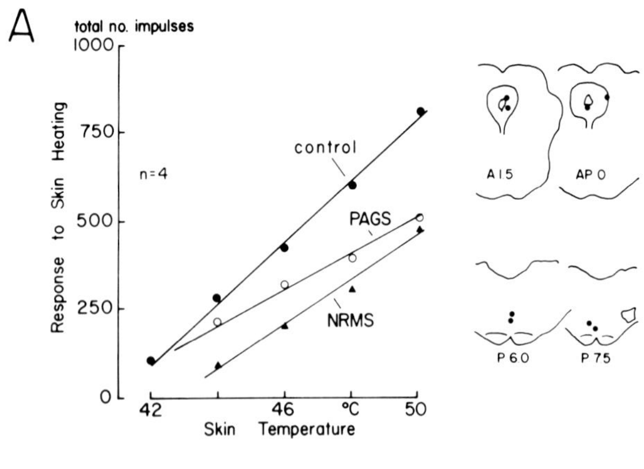

FIGURE 5. Centrifugal control of responses to graded noxious heating of the cat's hind-limb footpad. A: Differential effect of PAGS and NRMS on the stimulus–response functions of the same four dorsal horn neurons. Mean responses (total number of discharges in 20 s) are plotted against skin temperature. Control heat stimulation (10 s) at any given temperature was followed

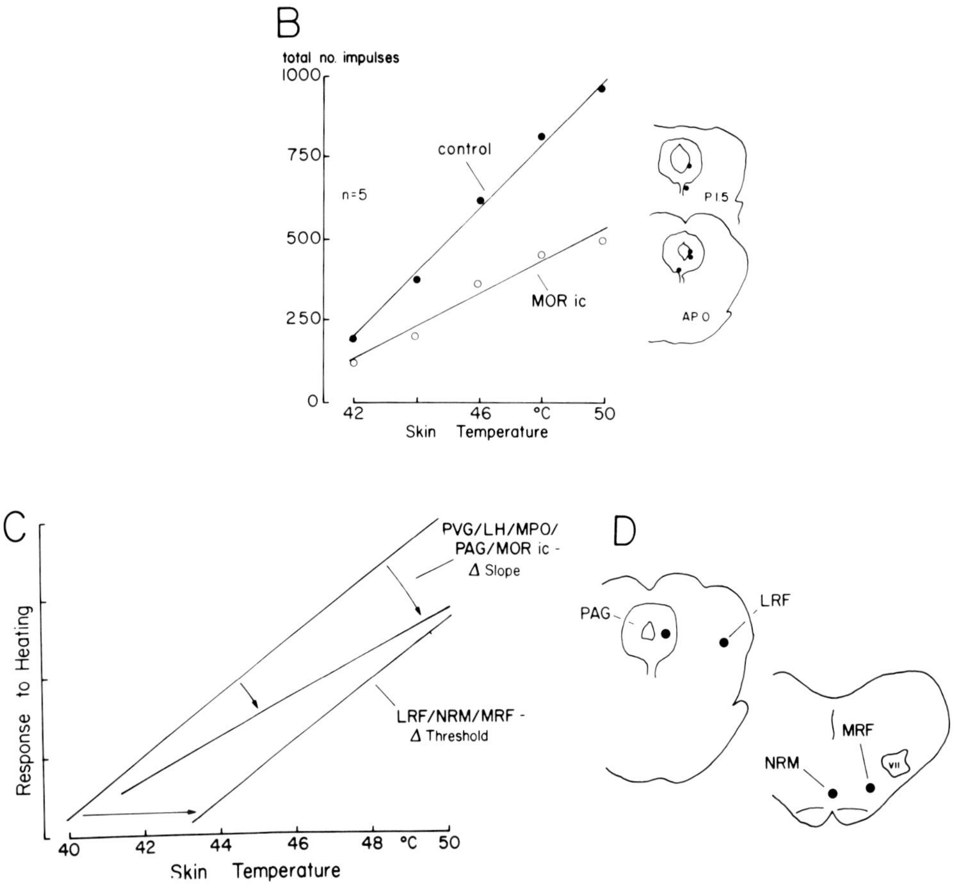

by heat stimulation during either PAGS or NRMS, and this procedure was repeated for subsequent randomly selected temperatures of heating of the skin. At the conclusion of this series, the same procedure was followed in testing effects of stimulation at the other brainstem site (either NRM or PAG). Each data point represents the mean of responses for different dorsal horn neurons in four different experiments. Histological localization of the four stimulation sites in the PAG and NRM are diagrammed on representative sections through the brainstem. B: Mean responses (total number of discharges in 20 s) of five dorsal horn neurons are plotted against temperatures of heating the skin. In all five experiments, control responses to graded heating of the skin were determined prior to the intra-PAG administration of morphine (MOR, 10–15 μg). Effects of morphine on the stimulus–response functions were assessed when morphine's effect was maximum and stable (see Figure 5 in Gebhart *et al.*, 1984). Each data point represents the mean response of five dorsal horn units from five different experiments. Histological localization of the five sites of administration of morphine in the PAG is diagrammed on representative sections of the midbrain. C: Summary of centrifugal control of spinal nociceptive transmission (see Table I for abbreviations and references). Centrifugal control is exercised as a significant reduction in the slope of the stimulus–response function without alteration in the response threshold (i.e., a gain control mechanism) or as a rightward parallel shift of the stimulus–response function with a significant increase in the response threshold/set point. D: Representative sites of focal electrical stimulation drawn on coronal sections through the midbrain and medulla. (Adapted from Gebhart *et al.*, 1983a, 1984, with permission.)

cular gray, medial preoptic area, and PAG and morphine administered systemically or into the PAG reduce significantly the slope of the stimulus–response function to noxious heating of the skin without affecting the threshold of the response (see Table I for references). Parallel shifts to the right of stimulus–response functions to noxious heating of the skin, on the other hand, are produced by focal electrical stimulation in the midbrain lateral reticular formation and rostral ventral medulla (see Table I for references). These centrifugal controls of spinal nociceptive transmission are graphically summarized in Figure 5C. As portrayed in this figure and as indicated in Table I, stimulation in periventricular and PAG sites decreases significantly the slope of the stimulus–response function without affecting the neuronal threshold of response to heating of the skin. This result has been taken to suggest the existence of a functionally homogeneous system of centrifugal modulation of spinal nociceptive transmission located medially in the brainstem. Since stimulation laterally in the midbrain lateral reticular formation (LRF; see Figure 5D) produces a very different effect on the stimulus–response function, namely, a change in response threshold and a rightward parallel shift in the stimulus–response function, another, separate descending system of inhibition is thought to exist (e.g., see Carstens *et al.*, 1980).

However, it is difficult to reconcile these proposals with observations that focal electrical stimulation in the medial or lateral rostral ventral medulla (NRM and MRF; see Figure 5D) produces both threshold increases and rightward parallel shifts in WDR stimulus–response functions to heating of the skin. Recall that there exist relatively few direct spinopetal afferents that arise from the PAG; a bulbar relay is thus believed to mediate descending inhibitory influences evoked from the PAG (Gebhart, 1982; Willis, 1982). It is not clear at present how changes in the slope of the stimulus–response function produced by stimulation or morphine given in the midbrain PAG are consistent with the existence of a descending functionally homogeneous system of spinal inhibition when stimulation medially or laterally in the rostral ventral medulla produces threshold changes in the stimulus–response functions to heating of the skin. The functional organization of these descending inhibitory systems has recently been established to be more complex than previously believed (see below).

In summary, although examination of the effects of supraspinal stimulation on spinal neuronal stimulus–response functions to heating of the skin characterizes centrifugal modulation of the encoding of nociceptive transmission, the data do not provide clear evidence for a functional homogeneity of descending systems. Rather, the data are best interpreted to suggest that there exist functionally separate descending systems of inhibition, likely involving presently undertermined pre- and/or postsynaptic excitatory and/or inhibitory influences on spinal dorsal horn neurons mediated by descending and perhaps local spinal neurotransmitter systems.

G. Supraspinal Organization of Descending Systems of Inhibition

Until recently, it was generally considered that descending inhibitory and analgesic effects of stimulation or morphine given in the midbrain relied on a bulbar relay in the rostral ventral medullary NRM (Basbaum and Fields, 1978; Fields and Basbaum, 1978). Recent studies, however, have revealed that the medial and lateral rostral ventral medulla can both serve as functionally important relays for descending inhibitory effects evoked from the midbrain. It has been demonstrated that the inhibition of spinal dorsal horn nociceptors produced by stimulation in the midbrain PAG (or midbrain lateral reticular formation) was unaffected when either the NRM or reticular formation lateral in the rostral ventral medulla (MRF) was reversably blocked by lidocaine (Figure 6; Gebhart *et al.*, 1983b). Similarly, Morton *et al.* (1984) demonstrated that the descending inhibitory effects of stimulation in the PAG were not affected by electrolytic destruction of the NRM. Descending inhibition of spinal nociceptors by stimulation in the midbrain is not affected until both the medial NRM and MRF are simultaneously blocked by lidocaine (Gebhart *et al.*, 1983b). Confirmation of this result has been provided in a study of the descending inhibition of the spinal nociceptive tail-flick reflex in the rat produced by focal electrical stimulation in the PAG. Reversible lidocaine blockade of either the NRM or MRF alone failed to increase significantly the stimulation threshold in the PAG required to inhibit the tail-flick reflex. Only after the NRM and MRF bilaterally were simultaneously blocked by lidocaine was the threshold in the PAG required to inhibit the tail-flick reflex increased significantly (Figure 7; Sandkühler and Gebhart, 1984b).

Anatomic support has recently been provided by Beitz *et al.* (1983). Microinjection of two different retrogradely transported fluorescent dyes into the NRM and MRF lateral in the rat rostral ventral medulla showed the midbrain PAG neurons of origin to be adjacent and mixed but not the same. These rostral ventral medullary areas considered important to analgesic mechanisms and descending spinal modulation are thus innervated by separate neuronal populations within the PAG. Stimulation in the midbrain PAG must certainly affect neurons that project to both the NRM and MRF, and it is clear that NRM and MRF concurrently serve as relays between the midbrain PAG and spinal cord.

The chemical identity of the terminals of the PAG neurons in the rostral ventral medulla is unknown at present, but the chemical modulators of spinal nociceptive transmission arising from the NRM and MRF are considered to be different (see Hammond, Chapter 15). Indeed, whether the neurons in the rostral ventral medulla that receive efferents from the PAG are spinopetal projection neurons is unknown. It is generally accepted that they are, and a recent report provides experimental support (Maciewicz *et al.*, 1984). Thus, the descending modulatory effects of stimulation in the brain rostral to the medulla may require significant interaction with and convergence onto neu-

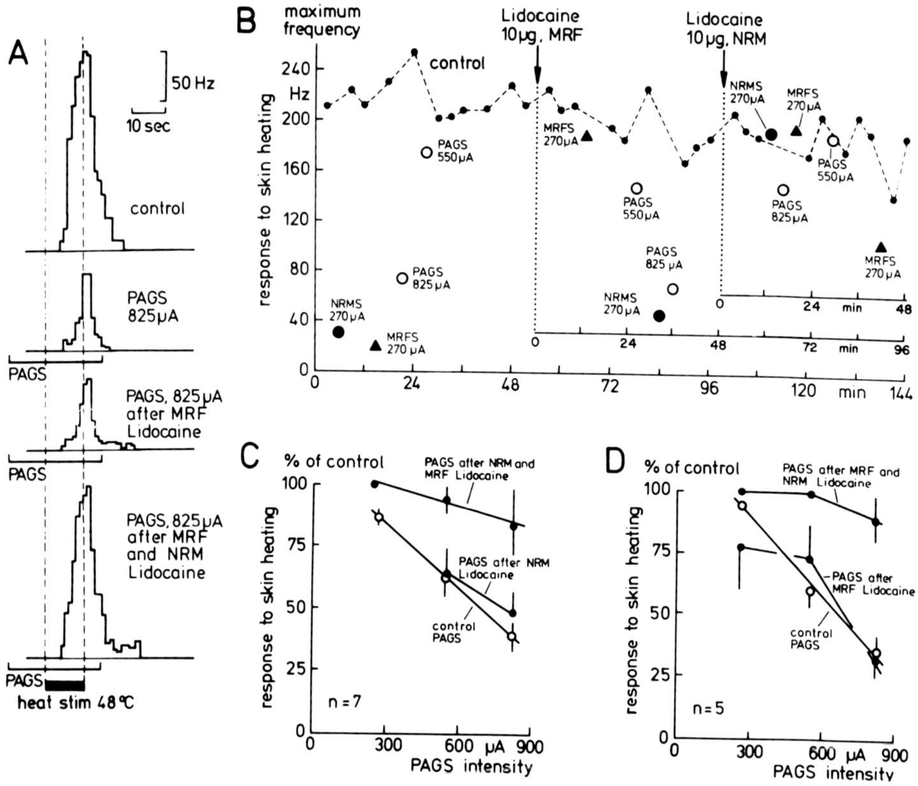

FIGURE 6. Effect of lidocaine microinjected into the medulla on the inhibition of spinal nociceptive transmission produced by stimulation in the PAG. A: Peristimulus time histograms (1-s bin width) of a spinal unit's response to noxious heating of the skin. The period of heating of the skin (48°C, 10 s) is shown below the histograms; the unit's control response is shown uppermost. The PAGS was started 10 s before the onset of the heat stimulus and lasted 25 s. Lidocaine (10 μg/1 μl) was administered first in the medullary reticular formation (MRF; third histogram) and later in the NRM (bottom histogram); see Figure 5D for representative sites of lidocaine microinjection in the medulla. The experiment is portrayed in B, where the response (maximum frequency, Hz) to heating of the skin (48° C, 10 s) is plotted against time on the abscissa. The control responses to 48°C heating of the skin are connected by the broken line. The spinal inhibition produced by NRMS, MRFS, and PAGS at the given intensities of stimulation is indicated, as is the administration of lidocaine (10 μg/1 μl) in the MRF and NRM. C,D: Responses to noxious heating of the skin (total number of discharges in 20 s) are expressed as a percentage of the control heat-evoked response on ordinates. The intensity (μA) of PAGS is shown on abscissas. Each data point represents the mean of the heat-evoked responses of five to seven spinal neurons; the vertical bars represent the S.E.M. The recruitment of inhibition by PAGS was determined before the administration of lidocaine (○). Lidocaine was microinjected in single doses of 10 μg/1 μl and repeated once (five of the 12 experiments) if its local anesthetic action was incomplete. The PAGS was tested again when the local anesthetic block produced by lidocaine was complete (see B for an example). Lidocaine microinjected first in the NRM (C) or first in the MRF (D) did not attenuate the spinal inhibition produced by PAGS. The spinal inhibition produced by PAGS was blocked only after lidocaine had been microinjected in both the NRM and MRF. (Adapted from Gebhart *et al.*, 1983b, with permission.)

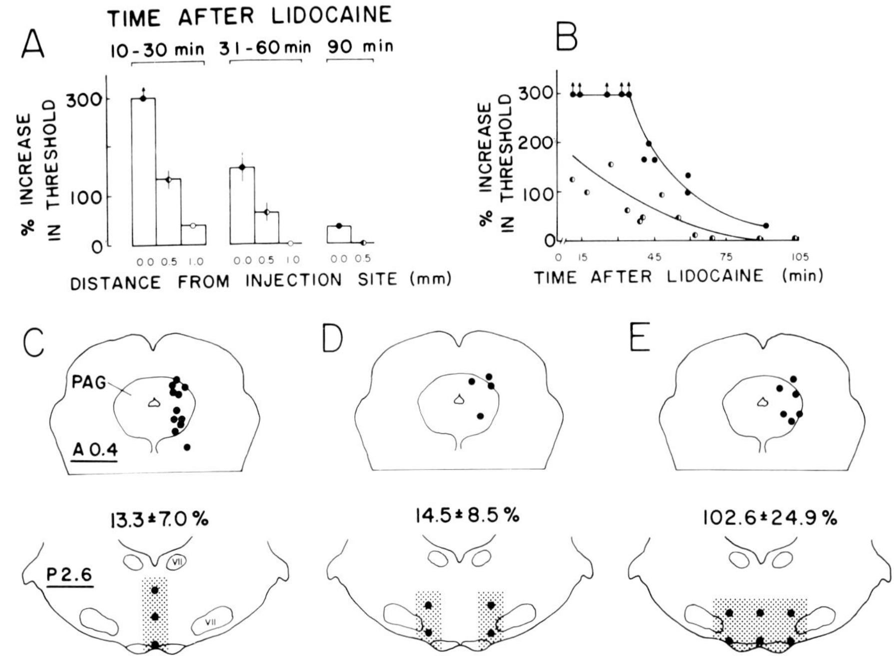

FIGURE 7. Effect of lidocaine microinjected into the medulla on inhibition of the spinal nociceptive tail-flick reflex produced by focal electrical stimulation in the PAG. A: The time course of the effect and extent of the functional block produced by lidocaine (0.5 μl, 4%) in the rat medulla is summarized for three periods of time after the microinjection of lidocaine. The blockade produced by lidocaine was tested at each of three positions 0.5 mm apart and is plotted against the percentage increase in the threshold of stimulation required to inhibit the tail flick reflex (mean ± S.E.M.). B: Percentage increase in the threshold for inhibition of the tail-flick reflex for stimulation at the intramedullary site of microinjection of lidocaine (●) and 0.5 mm lateral (◐) at various times. ↑, > 300%. The area of the functional block and its duration produced by 0.5 μl of 4% lidocaine were estimated to be 1 mm and 30 min, respectively. C–E: Effects of the intramedullary microinjection of lidocaine on stimulation thresholds in the PAG for inhibition of the tail-flick reflex. Stimulation sites in the PAG and sites of lidocaine microinjection in the medulla are portrayed on representative coronal brain sections. The estimated area of the functional block produced by lidocaine in the medulla is indicated by the stippled area. The mean percentage increase ± S.E.M. in the midbrain stimulation threshold for inhibition of the tail-flick reflex produced by lidocaine is indicated for each set of experiments. Only when the rostral ventral medulla medially and laterally was simultaneously blocked by lidocaine was the stimulation threshold in the PAG for inhibition of the tail-flick reflex elevated significantly. (Adapted from Sandkühler and Gebhart, 1984b, with permission.)

rons in the rostral ventral medulla. It remains to be determined, however, how qualitatively and quantitatively different effects on spinal nociceptive transmission are produced by stimulation in these sites. More is presently known about the spinal neurotransmitters involved, but relatively little is known about the brainstem neurotransmitters functionally important to the expression of either stimulation-produced analgesia or the inhibition of spinal nociceptive transmission.

In summary, it is now apparent that the medial NRM and reticular formation lateral in the rostral ventral medulla are functionally important bulbar relays between the midbrain and spinal cord. There are, however, also direct projections from forebrain, hypothalamus, midbrain, and pons to the spinal cord, and the organization of these pathways and their possible interactions remain to be elucidated.

H. Conclusions and Remaining Questions

It is clear that descending inhibition of spinal dorsal horn neurons can be evoked from widespread supraspinal sites. The inhibition is not restricted to modulation of spinal nociceptive transmission; nonnociceptive transmission of both class 1 and 2 dorsal horn neurons also is attenuated by supraspinal stimulation, although generally to a lesser extent. Thus, there exists some inhibitory selectivity but no specificity for spinal nociceptors. Moreover, although it is generally considered that the analgesias produced by drugs or stimulation in the brain rely on activation of descending systems of inhibition, centrifugal modulatory influences on flexor withdrawal reflexes and dorsal horn neurons can be powerfully produced from sites that are aversive in the awake, behaving animal or fail to produce an analgesia. Indeed, as others also have suggested (e.g., Duggan, 1982), the number and distribution in brain of sites from which descending inhibition can be demonstrated are so great that one is obligated to question the relevance of such inhibition to mechanisms of analgesia. Further, there is a large body of literature establishing that these systems of descending nociceptive modulation presently of interest also likely affect sympathetic and motor function. Thus, important questions remain as to whether analgesia-producing systems can be distinguished from systems of descending inhibition and are nociceptive specific and free of nonselective effects on sympathetic and motor systems. Whether they exist independently and can be anatomically or neurochemically differentiated is uncertain at present.

Although examination of the centrifugal modulation of stimulus–response functions to noxious heating of the skin suggests that both pre- and postsynaptic influences on supraspinal stimulation exist, at present there exists no anatomic support for the existence of presynaptic modulation of dorsal horn neurons by descending systems of inhibition (see Dubner *et al.*, 1984, and Ruda, Chapter 7, for further discussion). There are reports that suggest that such presynaptic modulation of primary afferents is functionally important (e.g., Carpenter *et al.*, 1966; Hentall and Fields, 1979; Martin *et al.*, 1979; Proudfit and Anderson, 1974); there also exists evidence suggesting that the centrifugal modulation of spinal nociceptors is postsynaptic (e.g., Giesler *et al.*, 1981; Willis, 1984). As Hammond (Chapter 15) discusses and Ruda (Chapter 7) notes, there are significant noradrenergic and serotonergic descending influences that likely play important roles in both analgesia and spinal neuronal inhibition. It remains to be demonstrated, however, whether there are functionally important presynaptic noradrenergic or serotonergic influences on, for example, spinothalamic tract neurons in the dorsal horn.

ACKNOWLEDGMENTS. Lack of space prohibits inclusion of all relevant literature, and I regret not being able to cite contributions of many colleagues. This manuscript and the author's data reported in it were supported by USPHS awards NS 19912 and DA 02879, the Alexander von Humboldt Stiftung, and the Deutsche Forschungsgemeinschaft.

References

BASBAUM, A. I., AND FIELDS, H. L. Endogenous pain control mechanisms: Review and hypothesis. *Ann. Neurol.* 4:451–461, 1978.

BECK, P. W., HANDWERKER, H. O., AND ZIMMERMANN, M. Nervous outflow from the cat's foot during noxious heat stimulation. *Brain Res.* 67:373–386, 1974.

BEITZ, A. J., MULLETT, M. A., AND WEINER, L. L. The periaqueductal gray projections to the rat spinal trigeminal, raphe magnus, gigantocellular pars alpha and paragigantocellular nuclei arise from separate neurons. *Brain Res.* 288:307–314, 1983.

BELCHER, G., RYALL, R. W., AND SCHAFFNER, R. The differential effects of 5-hydroxytryptamine, noradrenaline and raphe stimulation on nociceptive and nonnociceptive dorsal horn interneurones in the cat. *Brain Res.* 151:307–321, 1978.

BENNETT, G. J., AND MAYER, D. J. Inhibition of spinal cord interneurons by narcotic microinjection and focal electrical stimulation in the periaqueductal central gray matter. *Brain Res.* 172:243–257, 1979.

BESSON, J. M., OLIVERAS, J. C., CHAOUCH, A., AND RIVOT, J. P. Role of the raphe nuclei in stimulation producing analgesia. *Adv. Exp. Biol. Med.* 133:153–176, 1981.

CARPENTER, C. J., ENGBERG, I., AND LUNDBERG, A. Primary afferent depolarization evoked from the brain stem and cerebellum. *Arch. Ital. Biol.* 104:73–85, 1966.

CARSTENS, E. Inhibition of spinal dorsal horn neuronal responses to noxious skin heating by medial hypothalamic stimulation in the cat. *J. Neurophysiol.* 41:808–822, 1982.

CARSTENS, E., YOKOTA, T., AND ZIMMERMANN, M. Inhibition of spinal responses to noxious skin heating by stimulation of mesencephalic periaqueductal gray in the cat. *J. Neurophysiol.* 42.558–568, 1979.

CARSTENS, E., KLUMPP, D., AND ZIMMERMANN, M. Differential inhibitory effects of medial and lateral midbrain stimulation on spinal neuronal discharges to noxious skin heating in the cat. *J. Neurophysiol.* 43:332–342, 1980.

CARSTENS, E., BIHL, H., IRVINE, D. R. F., AND ZIMMERMANN, M. Descending inhibition from medial and lateral midbrain of spinal dorsal horn neuronal responses to noxious and nonnoxious cutaneous stimuli in the cat. *J. Neurophysiol.* 45:1029–1042, 1981.

CARSTENS, E., MACKINNON, J. D., AND GUINAN, M. J. Inhibition of spinal dorsal horn neuronal responses to noxious skin heating by medial preoptic and septal stimulation in the cat. *J. Neurophysiol.* 48:981–991, 1982.

CARSTENS, E., FRAUNHOFFER, M., AND SUBERG, S. N. Inhibition of spinal dorsal horn neuronal responses to noxious skin heating by lateral hypothalamic stimulation in the cat. *J. Neurophysiol.* 50:192–204, 1983.

CHUNG, J. M., FANG, Z. E., CARGILL, C. L., AND WILLIS, W. D. Prolonged, naloxone-reversible inhibition of the flexion reflex in the cat. *Pain* 15:35–53, 1983.

CLARK, S. L., AND RYALL, R. W. The antinociceptive action of etorphine in the dorsal horn is due to direct spinal action and not to activation of descending inhibition. *Br. J. Pharmacol.* 78:307–319, 1983.

CLARK, S. L., EDESON, R. O., AND RYALL, R. W. The relative significance of spinal and supraspinal actions in the antinociceptive effect of morphine in the dorsal horn: An evaluation of the microinjection technique. *Br. J. Pharmacol.* 79:807–818, 1983.

COULTER, J. D., MAUNZ, R. A., AND WILLIS, W. D. Effect of stimulation of sensorimotor cortex on primate spinothalamic neurons. *Brain Res.* 65:351–356, 1974.

DOSTROVSKY, J. O. Brain stem influences on transmission of somatosensory information in the spinocervicothalamic pathway. *Brain Res.* 292:229–238, 1984.

DOSTROVSKY, J. O., HU, J. W., SESSLE, B. J., AND SUMINO, R. Stimulation sites in periaqueductal gray, nucleus raphe magnus and adjacent regions effective in suppressing oral–facial reflexes. *Brain Res.* 252:287–297, 1982.

DU, H.-J., KITAHATA, L. M., THALHAMMER, J. G., AND ZIMMERMANN, M. Inhibition of nociceptive neuronal responses in the cat's spinal dorsal horn by electrical stimulation and morphine microinjection in nucleus raphe magnus. *Pain* 19:249–257, 1984.

DUBNER, R., RUDA, M. A., MILETIC, V., HOFFERT, M. J., BENNETT, G. J., NISHIKAWA, N., AND COFFIELD, J. Neural circuitry mediating nociception in the medullary and spinal dorsal horns *Adv. Pain Res. Ther.* 6:151–166, 1984.

DUGGAN, A. W. Brain stem inhibition of the spinal transmission of nociceptive information—pharmacologic studies of tonic and stimulation-induced inhibition, in: *Brain Stem Control of Spinal Mechanisms,* (B. SJOLUND AND A. BJORKLUND, eds.), Elsevier, Amsterdam, 1982, pp. 439–450.

FIELDS, H. L., AND BASBAUM, A. I. Brain stem control of spinal pain-transmission neurons. *Annu. Rev. Physiol.* 40:217–248, 1978.

FIELDS, H. L., BASBAUM, A. I., CLANTON, C. H., AND ANDERSON, S. D. Nucleus raphe magnus inhibition of spinal cord dorsal horn neurons. *Brain Res.* 126:441–453, 1977.

FITZGERALD, M., AND LYNN, B. The sensitization of high threshold mechanoreceptors with myelinated axons by repeated heating. *J. Physiol. (Lond.)* 365:549–563, 1977.

GEBHART, G. F. Opioid and opioid peptide effects on brain stem neurons: Relevance to nociception and antinociceptive mechanisms. *Pain* 12:93–140, 1982.

GEBHART, G. F., SANDKÜHLER, J., THALHAMMER, J. G., AND ZIMMERMANN, M. Quantitative comparison of inhibition in spinal cord of nociceptive information by stimulation in periaqueductal gray or nucleus raphe magnus of the cat. *J. Neurophysiol.* 50:1433–1445, 1983a.

GEBHART, G. F., SANDKÜHLER, J., THALHAMMER, J. G., AND ZIMMERMANN, M. Inhibition of spinal nociceptive information by stimulation in midbrain of the cat is blocked by lidocaine microinjected in nucleus raphe magnus and medullary reticular formation. *J. Neurophysiol.* 50:1446–1459, 1983b.

GEBHART, G., SANDKÜHLER, J., THALHAMMER, J. G., AND ZIMMERMANN, M. Inhibition in spinal cord of nociceptive information by electrical stimulation and morphine microinjection at identical sites in midbrain of the cat. *J. Neurophysiol.* 51:75–89, 1984.

GERHART, K. D., WILCOX, T. K., CHUNG, J. M., AND WILLIS, W. D. Inhibition of nociceptive and nonnociceptive responses of primate spinothalamic cells by stimulation in the medial brain stem. *J. Neurophysiol.* 45:121–136, 1981.

GERHART, K. D., YEZIERSKI, R. P., FANG, Z. R., AND WILLIS, W. D. Inhibition of primate spinothalamic tract neurons by stimulation in ventral posterior lateral (VPL_c) thalamic nucleus: Possible mechanisms. *J. Neurophysiol.* 49:406–423, 1983.

GERHART, K. D., YEZIERSKI, R. P., WILCOX, T. K., AND WILLIS, W. D. Inhibition of primate spinothalamic tract neurons by stimulation in periaqueductal gray or adjacent midbrain reticular formation. *J. Neurophysiol.* 51:450–466, 1984.

GIESLER, G. J., JR., GERHART, K. D., YEZIERSKI, R. P., WILCOX, T. K., AND WILLIS, W. D. Postsynaptic inhibition of primate spinothalamic neurons by stimulation in nucleus raphe magnus. *Brain Res.* 204:184–188, 1981.

GRAY, B. G., AND DOSTROVSKY, J. O. Descending inhibitory influences from periaqueductal gray, nucleus raphe magnus, and adjacent reticular formation. I. Effects on lumbar spinal cord nociceptive and nonnociceptive neurons. *J. Neurophysiol.* 49:932–947, 1983.

GUILBAUD, G., OLIVERAS, J. L., GIESLER, G., JR., AND BESSON, J. M. Effects induced by stimulation of the centralis inferior nucleus of the raphe on dorsal horn interneurons in cat's spinal cord. *Brain Res.* 126:355–360, 1977.

HABER, L. H., MARTIN, F. R., CHUNG, J. M., AND WILLIS, W. D. Inhibition and excitation of primate spinothalamic tract neurons by stimulation in region of nucleus reticularis gigan-ocellularis. *J. Neurophysiol.* 43:1578–1593, 1980.

HANDWERKER, H. O., IIGGO, A., AND ZIMMERMANN, M. Segmental and supraspinal actions on dorsal horn neurons responding to noxious and non-noxious skin stimuli. *Pain* 1:147–165, 1975.

HENTALL, I. D., AND FIELDS, H. L. Segmental and descending influences on intraspinal thresholds of single C-fibers. *J. Neurophysiol.* 42:1527–1537, 1979.

HOMMA, E., COLLINS, J. G., KITAHATA, L. M., MATSUMOTO, M., AND KAWAHARA, M. Suppression of noxiously evoked WDR dorsal horn neuronal activity by spinally administered morphine. *Anesthesiology* 58:232–236, 1983.

HOSOBUCHI, Y., ADAMS, J. E., AND LINCHINTZ, R. Pain relief by electrical stimulation of the central gray matter in humans and its reversal by naloxone. *Science* 197:183–186, 1977.

KENSHALO, D. R., JR., LEONARD, R. B., CHUNG, J. M., AND WILLIS, W. D. Responses of primate spinothalamic neurons to graded and to repeated noxious heat stimuli. *J. Neurophysiol.* 42:1370–1389, 1979.

LE BARS, D., MENETREY, D., AND BESSON, J. M. Effects of morphine upon the laminae V type cells activities in the dorsal horn on the decerebrate cat. *Brain Res.* 113:293–310, 1976.

LE BARS, D., DICKENSON, A. H., AND BESSON, J. M. Microinjection of morphine within nucleus raphe magnus and dorsal horn neuron activities related to nociception in the rat. *Brain Res.* 189:467–481, 1980.

LIEBESKIND, J. C., GUILBAUD, G., BESSON, J. M., AND OLIVERAS, J. L. Analgesia from electrical stimulation of the periaqueductal gray matter in the cat: Behavioral observations and inhibitory effects on spinal cord interneurons. *Brain Res.* 50:441–446, 1973.

MACIEWICZ, R., SANDREW, B. B., PHIPPS, B. S., POLETTI, C. E., AND FOOTE, W. E. Pontomedullary raphe neurons: Intracellular responses to central and peripheral electrical stimulation. *Brain Res.* 293:17–33, 1984.

MARTIN, R. F., HABER, L. H., AND WILLIS, W. D. Primary afferent depolarization of identified cutaneous fibers following stimulation in medial brain stem. *J. Neurophysiol.* 42:779–790, 1979.

MAYER, D. J. Endogenous analgesia systems: Neural and behavioral mechanisms. *Adv. Pain Res. Ther.* 1:385–410, 1979.

MAYER, D. J., AND LIEBESKIND, J. C. Pain reduction by focal electrical stimulation of the brain: An anatomical and behavioral analysis. *Brain Res.* 68:73–93, 1974.

MAYER, D. J., AND PRICE, D. D. Central nervous system mechanisms of analgesia. *Pain* 2:379–404, 1976.

MENÉTREY, D., GIESLER, G. J., AND BESSON, J. M. An analysis of response properties of spinal cord dorsal horn neurons to nonnoxious and noxious stimuli in the spinal rat. *Exp. Brain Res.* 27:15–33, 1977.

MORTON, C. R., DUGGAN, A. W., AND ZHAQ, Z. Q. The effects of lesions of medullary midline and lateral reticular areas on inhibition in the dorsal horn produced by periaqueductal gray stimulation in the cat. *Brain Res.* 301:121–130, 1984.

OLIVERAS, J. L., FARDIN, V. AND BESSON, J. M. Stimulation produced analgesia in animals: A review based on behavioral investigations, in: *Current Topics in Pain Research and Therapy* (T. YOKOTA AND R. DUBNER, eds.), Excerpta Medica, Amsterdam, 1983, pp. 95–105.

OSSIPOV, M. H., AND GEBHART, G. F. Light pentobarbital anesthesia diminishes the antinociceptive potency of morphine administered intracranially but not intrathecally in the rat. *Eur. J. Pharmacol.* 97:137–140, 1984.

PRICE, D. D., AND BROWE, A. C. Spinal cord coding of graded nonnoxious and noxious temperature increases. *Exp. Neurol.* 48:201–221, 1975.

PRICE, D. D., AND DUBNER, R. Neurons that subserve the sensory-discriminative aspects of pain. *Pain* 3:307–338, 1977.

PROUDFIT, H. K., AND ANDERSON, E. G. New long latency bulbospinal evoked potential blocked by serotonin antagonists. *Brain Res.* 65:542–546, 1974.

REYNOLDS, D. V. Surgery in the rat during electrical analgesia induced by focal brain stimulation. *Science* 164:444–445, 1969.

RICHARDSON, D. E., AND AKIL, H. Pain reduction by electrical brain stimulation in man: Part 1: Acute administration in periaqueductal and periventricular sites. *J. Neurosurg.* 47:178–183, 1977.

RIVOT, J. P., CHAOUCH, A., AND BESSON, J. M. Nucleus raphe magnus modulation of response of rat dorsal horn neurons to unmyelinated fiber inputs: Partial involvement of serotonergic pathways. *J. Neurophysiol.* 44:1039–1057, 1980.

SANDKÜHLER, J., AND GEBHART, G. F. Characterization of inhibition of a spinal nociceptive reflex by stimulation medially and laterally in the midbrain and medulla in the pentobarbital-anesthetized rat. *Brain Res.* 305:67–76, 1984a.

SANDKÜHLER, J., AND GEBHART, G. F. Relative contributions of the nucleus raphe magnus and adjacent medullary reticular formation to the inhibition by stimulation in the periaqueductal gray of a spinal nociceptive reflex in the pentobarbital-anesthetized rat. *Brain Res.* 305:77–87, 1984b.

SCHOUENBORG, J., AND SJOLUND, B. G. Activity evoked by A- and C-afferent fibers in rat dorsal horn neurons and its relation to a flexion reflex. *J. Neurophysiol.* 50:1108–1121, 1983.

SOPER, W. Y. Effects of analgesic midbrain stimulation on reflex withdrawal and thermal escape in the rat. *J. Comp. Physiol. Psychol.* 90:91–101, 1976.

SOPER, W. Y., AND MELZACK, R. Stimulation-produced analgesia: Evidence for somatotopic organization in the midbrain. *Brain Res.* 251:301–311, 1982.

WILLIS, W. D. Control of nociceptive transmission in the spinal cord. *Progress in Sensory Physiology 3*. Springer-Verlag, Heidelberg, 1982, 159 pp.

WILLIS, W. D. The raphe–spinal system, in: *Brain Stem Control of Spinal Cord Function (C. D. BARNES*, ed.), Academic Press, Orlando, 1984, pp. 141–214.

WILLIS, W. D., HABER, L. D., AND MARTIN, R. F. Inhibition of spinothalamic tract cells and interneurons by brain stem stimulation in the monkey. *J. Neurophysiol.* 40:968–981, 1977.

YAKSH, T. L. Spinal opiate analgesia: Characteristics and principles of action. *Pain* 11:293–346, 1981.

YAKSH, T. L., AND RUDY, T. A. Narcotic analgetics: CNS sites and mechanisms of action as revealed by intracerebral injection techniques. *Pain* 4:299–359, 1978.

YEZIERSKI, R. P., GERHART, K. D., SCHROCK, B. J., AND WILLIS, W. D. A further examination of effects of cortical stimulation on primate spinothalamic tract cells. *J. Neurophysiol.* 49:424–441, 1983.

ZIMMERMANN, M. Encoding in dorsal horn interneurons receiving noxious and nonnoxious afferents. *J. Physiol. (Paris)* 73:221–232, 1977.

17
The Controversial Nature of the Evidence for Neuroplasticity of Afferent Axons in the Spinal Cord

PAUL E. MICEVYCH, BARBARA E. RODIN, AND LAWRENCE KRUGER

A. Introduction

The failure to obtain recovery of function following lesions of the spinal cord has long been one of the more discouraging features of the practice of clinical neurosurgery. Few neurosurgeons would actively pursue the study of patients presenting the frequently devastating effects of spinal injuries, and even fewer would approach the problem with laboratory experiments in the hope of eventually achieving therapeutic benefits. Frederick Kerr was the most energetic individual who could hope to fill this void, and because he pursued this subject with such fervor and presented his polemic views with such passion, a current appraisal of the validity of Kerr's thesis concerning sprouting (Kerr, 1972, 1975) would seem a particularly fitting memorial, especially in this era in which the tide of evidence may be turning. It is the aim of this chapter to reexamine Kerr's views and experimental findings in the context of current information, for there is good reason to believe that there was keen insight and wisdom in Kerr's skepticism concerning the potential of neuro-

---

PAUL E. MICEVYCH, BARBARA E. RODIN, AND LAWRENCE KRUGER • Departments of Anatomy and Anesthesiology and the Brain Research Center, UCLA Center for Health Sciences, Los Angeles, California 90024.

plasticity and restructuring of function pathways in the adult mammalian central nervous system.

From personal conversations, it was clear that Kerr supported the parsimonious principle that all axons possess the capacity to grow or sprout and that this might be a permanent continuous process, as espoused by Ramon y Cajal (1928). Esteem for the Spanish master was exceptional, for Kerr was reared and medically trained in Argentina and read the works of Cajal in their original language with special care and affection. Thus, it was perhaps inevitable that his bias was to share Cajal's opinion—and evidence—that abortive sprouting of cut primary afferent axons was a generalized phenomenon but that failure of long expanses of axonal growth and formation of new functional connections was also a consistent corollary for axons interrupted in the mature central nervous system.

The possibility of central axonal sprouting of intact primary afferent axons adjoining zones of denervation seemed attractive for explaining some functional recovery and was supported by the evidence reported by Liu and Chambers (1958) of intraspinal dorsal root axon sprouting following adjacent dorsal rhizotomy. There was also evidence that neural destruction induced in the cerebral cortex by ionizing particle irradiation could reveal a luxurious increase in axonal silver impregnation if the dose for destruction was below the level inducing frank vascular damage and glial cell proliferation (Rose *et al.*, 1960); with higher doses, a glial scar formed through which axonal penetration failed. Thus, the inference was strong that axons interrupted within the central nervous system could exhibit nothing more than abortive sprouting, whereas intact axons near a zone of damage might display a detectable change resulting from enhanced normal growth by a mechanism analogous to plant growth induced by pruning. There was essentially no conflict with Cajal's opinion that the absence of physical barriers caused by scarring and early stages of development were key factors conducive to optimizing the study of axonal growth.

In addition to age and physical barriers, Kerr was impressed by the functional specificity expressed by most mature neurons and found it difficult to imagine how growth in a somatotopically organized zone of sensory neuropil could be functionally useful. He was undoubtedly biased by his consistent clinical observations of sensory deficits accompanied by little reorganization following neural injury. The model system he chose for testing the efficacy of sensory axon sprouting was the sensory trigeminal nucleus, which he and his co-workers had shown to be precisely somatotopically organized (Kerr *et al.*, 1968) and to receive more diverse sources of input than the spinal cord dorsal horn (Kerr *et al.*, 1968; Kerr, 1972). Failing to demonstrate cervical root sprouting after trigeminal denervation of the spinal V nucleus in mature animals (Kerr, 1972), he proceeded to develop new surgical approaches to testing the potential for plasticity by doing the same experiment in the neonatal condition (Kerr, 1975). When the same negative result became evident after the first postnatal week, he ultimately argued that afferent sprouting in cats and kittens was not appreciable and, further, that "maladaptive regeneration following injuries might result in gross disorders of motor or sensory function" if collateral growth actually occurred (Kerr, 1975). A further electrophysiological evaluation of this problem (Beckerman and Kerr, 1976) enabled him to firmly reject the sprouting hypothesis and its functional implications.

The issue of whether axonal sprouting occurs in the spinal cord has continued to attract considerable attention, and evidence has been adduced to support compensatory growth following interruption of primary afferents (Murray and Goldberger, 1974; Goldberger and Murray, 1978), descending axons (Goldberger and Murray, 1974; Prendergast and Misantone, 1980), and interneuronal systems (Bernstein and Bernstein, 1971; Bernstein *et al.*, 1978; Tessler *et al.*, 1981). There is also a body of evidence suggesting that neurons deprived of their normal input may respond to a novel input by a variety of mechanisms, not necessarily invoking sprouting (Merrill and Wall, 1978). The following account attempts to evaluate the available recent evidence for intraspinal afferent axon sprouting derived from anatomic tracing methods, electrophysiological studies, and the recent application of pharmacological and immunochemical techniques, thereby extending Kerr's (1975) views into the current context. It seems that despite increased controversy and much experimental activity, his views on this subject may well endure the test of time.

B. Anatomic Studies Assessing Postlesion Regrowth

Three methods have been used to study sprouting in dorsal root axons (DRAs): (1) impregnating degenerating primary afferent axons with silver, (2) counting axons in dorsal roots in the electron microscope, and (3) labeling primary afferents with transport tracers. Unfortunately, the various techniques yielded different results concerning the presence of sprouting, and thus the relative strengths and weaknesses of each method should be considered before any conclusions are drawn.

1. Silver Methods

One of the earliest studies of collateral growth in DRAs in mature animals was that of Liu and Chambers (1958). Using their now classic spared-root paradigm (Figure 1) and one of the suppressive silver stains in cats, they found that following long-term dorsal rhizotomies, an intervening spared dorsal root both expanded its rostrocaudal trajectory within the spinal cord and increased its projection to normal terminal regions. This work was later expanded by Goldberger and Murray (Goldberger and Murray, 1978, 1982; Murray and Goldberger, 1974; see also McCough *et al.*, 1958), who more

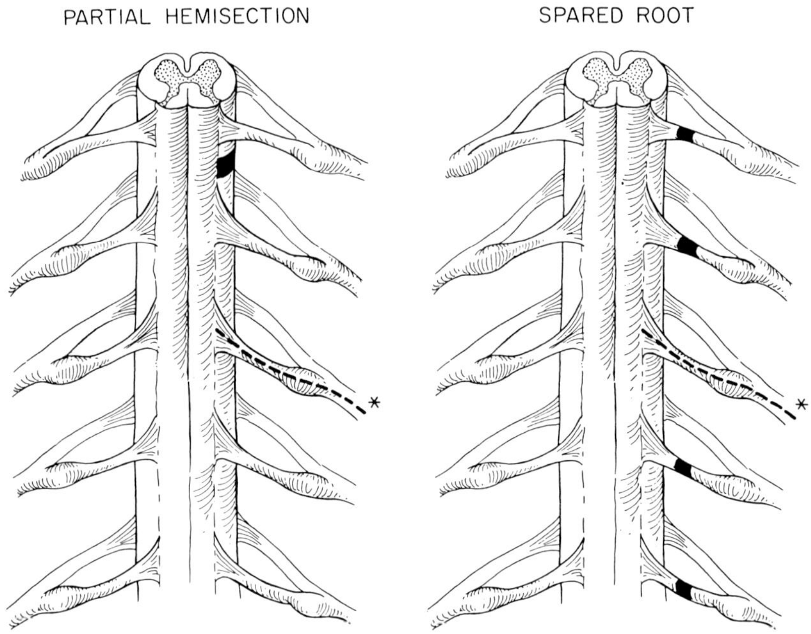

FIGURE 1. Diagrams summarizing the partially hemisected and spared-root preparations. A partial hemisection is performed rostral to the dorsal root in question (*) and spares all or part of the dorsal column, avoiding damage to the ascending collaterals of root afferents. In the spared-root preparation, primary afferent input to the spinal cord is removed by dorsal rhizotomy or dorsal root ganglionectomy, and an intervening root (*) is left intact. Lesioned roots or spinal tissue are indicated with a heavy dark line. (From Rodin and Kruger, 1984.)

recently reported that following either dorsal rhizotomy or a rostral partial spinal hemisection (Figure 1), spared DRAs do not invade aberrant terminal regions but rather increase their projection to normal zones of trajectory, particularly those heavily denervated by the long-term lesion and normally receiving a relatively sparse primary afferent projection. Both sets of conclusions were derived from comparisons of the pattern of silver impregnation resulting from surgical interruption of a spared dorsal root (after the degeneration products from the long-term rhizotomy or hemisection disappeared) to that resulting from surgical interruption of the contralateral homologous root on the intact side of the cord.

Although the use of silver impregnation for demonstrating axonal populations is of uncontested value in many anatomic studies, particular problems arise with their use in the study of DRAs and in chronically denervated tissue. Different populations of DRAs degenerate at different rates following rhizotomy (LaMotte, 1977), and thus growth in major groups of large- or small-diameter afferents cannot be demonstrated unless a range of survival times following an acute rhizotomy is studied. For practical reasons, long-term lesions were not inflicted on control tissue in sprouting studies, yet such lesions may elicit staining that could be spuriously interpreted. For example, nonaxonal profiles may be revealed by silver impregnation. Glial cells and processes in any neuropil displaying degeneration contain electron-dense cytoplasmic inclusions (e.g., lysosomes) susceptible to heavy-metal impregnation (Matthews and Kruger, 1973). Further silver staining of degenerating dendrites can occur (De Olmos *et al.*, 1981), and it is possible that some spinal neurons that have survived substantial chronic denervation may undergo degeneration following a subsequent acute deafferentation. An additional problem is that the impregnation properties of residual axons in chronically deafferented areas may be altered in ways that result in increased resistance to "suppressive" impregnation. This was indicated by the recent report (Goldberger and Murray, 1982) that under conditions of reduced histological "suppression," a descending spinal pathway to Clarke's nucleus, previously thought to be an aberrant consequence of denervation (Goldberger and Murray, 1974), was found in both chronically denervated and control spinal cord.

In view of the above problems, unequivocal statements concerning collateral sprouting on the basis of silver studies alone seem precarious. Kerr was one of the first to report an absence of consistent evidence for intraspinal sprouting in silver-impregnated cervical DRAs following long-term trigeminal rhizotomy in adult cats (Kerr, 1972) and a large series of kittens (Kerr, 1975), although the choice of a model that required sprouting interaction between cervical and trigeminal systems has been criticized on the grounds that sprouting does not occur into inappropriate levels (Goldberger and Murray, 1978). Thus, reorganization may be precluded in topographically organized regions such as between cervical and trigeminal levels. It is noteworthy that much of the evidence for intraspinal sprouting in fiber systems other than DRAs in adult animals is similarly derived from the use of silver techniques (e.g., Goldberger and Murray, 1974; Prendergast and Misantone, 1980).

2. *Electron Microscopy*

Hulsebosch and Coggeshall (1981a,b) counted axons in adult rat dorsal roots and found that the number of unmyelinated axons in roots ipsilateral and contiguous to a rostral spinal hemisection performed at birth or interposed between roots lesioned when the animals were 30 days of age was 13–22% greater than in homologous roots on the nonlesioned side of the cord. Further, the putative axonal proliferation was not found in rats in which spinal hemisection was performed at 1 year of age (Hulsebosch and Coggeshall, 1983). One might conclude that the potential for collateral growth is present only in immature rats, but that is also uncertain because early lesions might merely arrest fiber death in ipsilateral and contiguous roots. Cell death (Finlay and Slattery, 1983; Rager, 1981) and fiber loss (Innocenti, 1981; Land

and Lund, 1979; Stanfield *et al.*, 1982) occur normally during development and can be impeded by early lesions (Sengelaub and Finlay, 1981). The failure to find increased numbers of DRAs in animals lesioned as adults may simply reflect the completion of the fiber loss epoch of development when maturity is reached. In any event, even if unmyelinated axons grow new collaterals at the root level following spinal deafferentation, the sprouts probably do not penetrate the central nervous system and form synapses. Regenerating dorsal root axons enter the dorsal column but then grow in whorls and apparently fail to penetrate the spinal gray matter (Cajal, 1928; Messenger and Kingsley, 1982).

3. Transported Tracers

These offer an advantage over the other two methods described in their use provides the opportunity to selectively label the fiber populations of interest and to trace their trajectory within the cord. A number of techniques have been used to study primary afferent sprouting, including the injection of dorsal root ganglia with tritiated amino acids (Murray and Goldberger, 1974) and labeling dorsal roots (Beattie *et al.*, 1981) or peripheral nerves (Rodin *et al.*, 1982, 1983; Rodin and Kruger, 1984) with horseradish peroxidase (HRP). Intraganglionic injections have not proved to be especially useful, as it is difficult to secure homogeneous, consistent, or complete labeling, mandatory prerequisites for valid comparisons between chronically denervated and control preparations. Labeling dorsal roots with HRP has the disadvantage that the enzyme diffuses through the axoplasm for a limited distance rather than being incorporated into cytoskeletal components and transported to terminals, producing an incomplete picture of the intraspinal projection. Beattie *et al.*, (1981) reported that following spinal hemisection in adult cats, DRAs labeled by direct HRP application may display an apparently aberrant course within the cord, but this may not constitute evidence for terminal field reorganization.

When a peripheral nerve is labeled with HRP, the enzyme is transported transganglionically to the spinal cord, resulting in labeling of the full intraspinal trajectory (Koerber and Brown, 1980, 1982; Mesulam and Brushart, 1979; Mesulam, 1982). Rodin *et al.*, (1983; Rodin and Kruger, 1984) demonstrated that the distribution pattern of intraspinal labeling following HRP application to the sciatic nerve is remarkably consistent in different rats. They used this technique to study the sprouting potential of spared sciatic DRAs following either dorsal root ganglionectomies (dorsal and ventral root afferents removed) or a rostral partial spinal hemisection (all or part of the dorsal column containing the ascending collaterals of sciatic axons spared). Following either lesion, DRAs do not apparently (1) invade aberrant segments (Figure 2), (2) expand their distribution within normal segments of entry (Figure 3), or (3) increase their projection to their normal terminal regions (Figure 4).

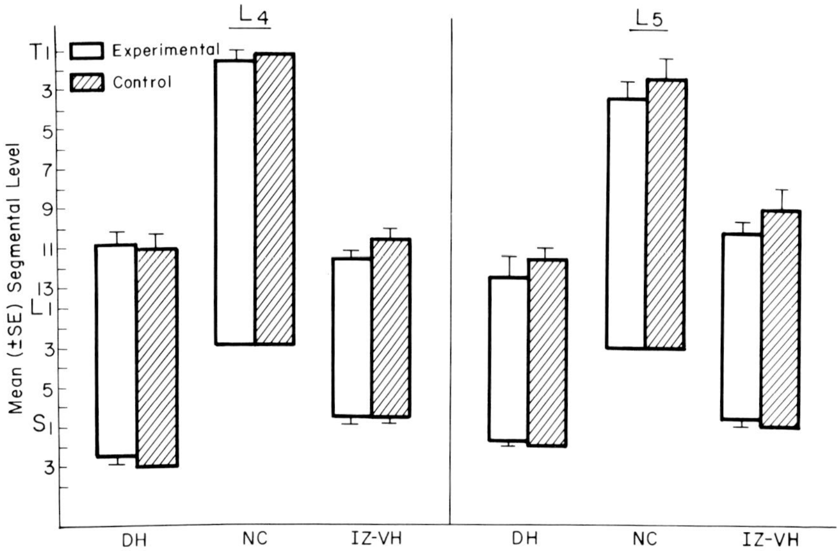

FIGURE 2. The average rostral and caudal boundaries (+S.E. where it was greater than zero) of the sciatic nerve projection to the rat dorsal horn (DH) (excluding the nucleus of Clarke), nucleus of Clarke (NC), and intermediate zone–ventral horn (IZ–VH) in experimental and control spared-root preparations with the L_4 or L_5 dorsal roots spared. The sciatic nerve, which projects to the cord in the rat through the L_4, L_5, and L_6 roots, was labeled with HRP at long-term (2 weeks to 3 months) or short-term (same day) intervals following dorsal root ganglionectomies (two to five lumbar ganglia removed) with the L_4 or L_5 ganglion spared. (From Rodin *et al.*, 1983.)

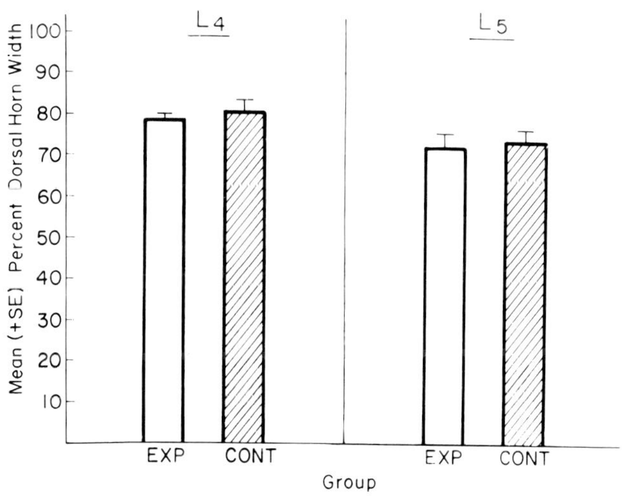

FIGURE 3. The maximal mediolateral extent of HRP reaction product (lamina III) within the spared L_4 or L_5 dorsal horn in experimental (EXP) and control (CONT) preparations. The extent of reaction product is expressed as a percentage of the maximal width of the dorsal horn in laminae II–III. (From Rodin *et al.*, 1983.)

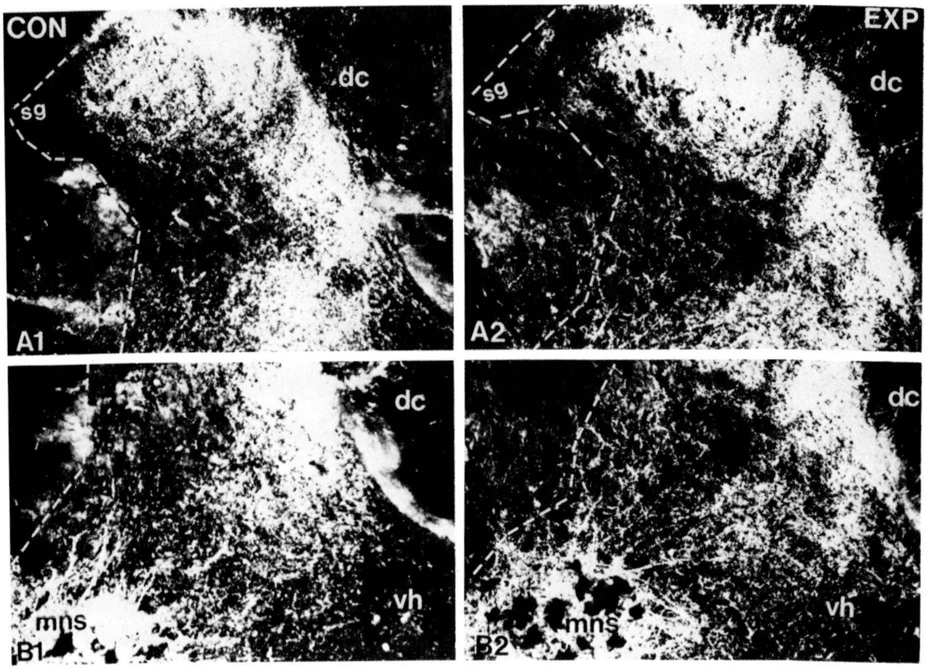

FIGURE 4. A: Dark-field photomicrographs of HRP reaction product in transverse sections of the dorsal column (dc), marginal zone, substantia gelatinosa (sg), and deeper laminae of L_4 spinal gray matter following sciatic nerve labeling in a nonlesioned control (CON; 1) animal, and in an experimental (EXP; 2) rat with an ipsilateral partial spinal hemisection at T_{13}, performed 2 months earlier, involving all but the most medial dorsal column. Most of the corticospinal tract was transected. Dotted lines outline the lateral border of the spinal gray matter. ×140. (Reproduced at 68%.) B: Photomicrographs of the intermediate zone and ventral horn (vh) at L_4 in the rat described in A. Note the labeled motoneurons (mns) in the lower corner of each micrograph. ×160. (Reproduced at 68%.) (Both from Rodin and Kruger, 1984.)

These results occurred regardless of the magnitude of denervation of a region or the relative density of its normal sciatic projection.

Although these data support the Kerr (1972, 1975) thesis that anatomic plasticity in the central connections of noninjured spinal afferents in mature animals is considerably more limited than often believed, if it exists at all, several alternatives warrant examination.

There may be species-related differences in plasticity between adult rats (HRP and electron microscopic studies) and cats (silver studies). One silver study (Stelzner *et al.*, 1979) indicated that the potential for DRA sprouting in rats with hemisected spinal cords is limited to the neonatal period, but the older group of animals used in this study included long-term lesions invading the control side of the cord, and other possible interpretations of these findings (Stelzner and Weber, 1974; Rodin and Kruger, 1984) compromise confidence in the ease with which the putative sprouting can be detected. The demonstration of intraspinal sprouting in nonprimary afferent axons in adult rats with silver methods (Bernstein and Bernstein, 1971; Bernstein *et al.*, 1978; Prendergast and Misantone, 1980) provides evidence that a species difference in plasticity need not be invoked, although this is a limited result, as emphasized by earlier workers (e.g., Cajal, 1928; Kerr, 1975).

Visceral afferents may sprout (Thor *et al.*, 1982). Most investigators studied the projection of one or more dorsal roots containing both visceral and somatic afferents. Data derived from labeling somatic nerves (e.g., sciatic), may not apply to visceral afferents.

Limited growth, not readily discernable with optical microscopy, may occur. Minute increases in the density of intraspinal HRP reaction product might be detected with more sensitive, quantifiable histochemical techniques or with quantitative electron microscopy.

Collateral pruning (Schneider, 1973; Schneider and Jhaveri, 1974) may occur. A recent preliminary report (Thor *et al.*, 1982) indicated that the projection of HRP-labeled pudendal nerve afferent axons to the sacral dorsal horn was enhanced following spinal transection in adult cats. As the ascending collaterals of the pudendal axons were severed by the lesion, it is possible that both terminal field denervation and collateral injury are necessary for the incitement of sprouting. However, this study did not include acutely lesions controls, and, as the rate of axonal transport and/or the amount of material transported might be greater in injured than noninjured axons (Grafstein and McQuarrie, 1978), it is not certain whether increased densities of reaction product in lesioned versus intact preparations were attributable to a difference in transport of label or to new growth.

C. Electrophysiological Evidence for Postlesion Reorganization

1. Altered Somatotopic Maps

A highly controversial literature has emerged from attempts to measure the reorganization believed to result from various forms of partial deafferentation of central neurons. The pioneer finding of Wall and Egger (1971), presented only in a brief report, suggested that a shift of less than 200 μm in the forelimb and hindlimb digit representation in the rat ventrobasal thalamus could be mapped with a series of parallel microelectrode penetrations for which multiunit receptive fields (RFs) were determined throughout the electrode traverse. There is some uncertainty as to whether the method is amenable to the resolutuion required for the summary figurine drawings. A series of papers, largely by Wall and his colleagues (Basbaum and Wall, 1976; Mendell *et al.*, 1978; Devor and Wall, 1981a,b, Markus *et al.*, 1981; Lisney, 1983), has presented more detailed accounts of somatotopic reorganization in the dorsal horn following partial peripheral deafferentation, but there are several reports from other laboratories that demur from confirming these findings and conclusions (P. B. Brown *et al.*, 1979; Pubols and Goldberger, 1980; Pubols and Brenowitz, 1981; Brinkus and Zimmermann, 1983; A. G. Brown *et al.*, 1983 a,b; Pubols, 1984) without satisfactorily accounting for the apparent discrepancy.

2. *Sources of Discrepancies*

There are several methodological features worthy of consideration if this controversy is to be resolved, for in the absence of a credible explanation, positive results often outweigh negative findings. Some points of consensus can be found in recognizing that the acute effect of partial deafferentation (by dorsal rhizotomy or peripheral nerve section) is to render neurons in a sector of dorsal horn unresponsive to peripheral tactile stimulation. This provides a condition that facilitates the recognition of far-ranging effects demonstrable with electrical stimulation via distant dorsal roots but not with low-threshold mechanical stimulation (Wall and Werman, 1976; Devor *et al.*, 1977; Mendell *et al.*, 1978). Although there is little evidence of increased excitability in partially deafferented neurons (Brinkus and Zimmermann, 1983), it seems reasonable to hypothesize the unmasking of inactive synapses (Merrill and Wall, 1978) to explain expanded receptive field domains. The time required for "mature reorganization" of approximately 1 month may be consistent with axonal growth and synaptic reorganization (Merrill and Wall, 1978), but the acquisition of receptive field reorganization within only 4 or 5 days in rats (Devor and Wall, 1981a,b) would best be explained by the strengthening of preexisting relatively ineffective synapses.

The major problem appears to be the accuracy with which the border of a deafferented zone of dorsal horn can be determined with a series of electrode penetrations. The spacing of electrodes is limited by shaft width, surface vasculature, and a tendency for penetrations to veer off at slightly different angles despite fixed micromanipulator orientation. With shifts caused by denervation-induced reorganization of less than 0.5 mm and often ~200 μm, this can be an imprecise exercise that is difficult to evaluate without knowing the exact number and spacing of electrode tracks. The number of sampling tracks can be increased by mapping across several transverse rows, but this also requires a means of compensation for rostrocaudal position because of mediolateral shifts in representation along this axis (Brown and Fuchs, 1975; Rethelyi *et al.*, 1979; Koerber and Brown, 1982).

In a recent attempt to resolve the discrepant findings despite serious efforts at replication, Pubols (1984) suggested that the method of anatomic reconstruction is the most likely source of significant error. Most of the "positive" findings concerning somatotopic reorganization are apparently based on estimating electrode track position with respect to a single reference pipette fixed *in situ* and traced from a thick, cleared, unstained section of the cord. With a substantial sampling of neurons in numerous electrode tracks and use of a second marker electrode for the border of the denervated zone (Devor and Wall, 1981a,b), the predominance of units in the deep dorsal horn (laminae IV and V) still might introduce a substantial spatial error. Even when all electrode tracks were reconstructed, variations in dorsal horn width resulting from a variety of technical factors (e.g., shrinkage, cutting compression) were of sufficient magnitude to require computation, rather than direct drawings, of relative electrode track positions (Pubols, 1984). Although Pubols offers the opinion that anatomic reconstruction probably constitutes the largest error, her findings also indicate that other factors such as the choice of anesthetic may also contribute significantly to the efficacy of exciting dorsal horn neurons.

When natural cutaneous stimuli are employed for mapping RFs, their boundaries can be determined with reasonable accuracy within a wide range of anesthetic conditions when delicate tactile stimuli are employed. It should be noted that claims of somatotopic rearrangement or shift are generally based on new RFs with several distinctive features: (1) reliance on excitation of high-threshold mechanoreceptors, (2) RF enlargement in the proximal direction only, although if tactile stimuli are used, average RFs are smaller (Brinkus and Zimmermann, 1983), and (3) increased variability in neuronal responsiveness and resultant difficulty in accurately delimiting RFs. Reliance on pinching, crushing, or needling is inherently susceptible to error because the number of stimulus trials is usually smaller and the problems of receptor "sensitization" or damage "inactivation" are not measurable. Evidence for a somatotopic shift based on large-diameter afferent input would largely dispel the argument based on a required shift to high-threshold mechanoreceptors. Basbaum and Wall (1976) report an asymmetric distribution of the N-wave amplitude (believed to reflect the A-fiber-induced postsynaptic currents of dorsal horn cells) comparing normal and deafferented sides, but this finding has also been contested (Brinkus and Zimmermann, 1983).

An additional source of uncertainty in all of the studies reported is the limited sampling of neuronal activity. It is unnecessary to single out a given report to note that most electrode tracks yield no more than a handful of isolated neuronal records at best and that much of the mapping is based on multiunit recording, thus rendering RF delimitation a factor skewed by the undetermined number of neurons sampled. The key factor that remains unexplained is that despite the numerous error factors, the reported shift in somatotopy is consistently in the same direction—lateral to medial, with RFs shifting proximally. The controversy could be resolved by denervating the proximal representation in lateral dorsal horn (see Pubols and Goldberger, 1980) and determining whether distal RFs appear in that zone. This might also clarify the significance of the putative shift to high-threshold mechanoreceptors and the extensive RF enlargement, but the experiment is somewhat more difficult for some practical reasons.

In summary, the electrophysiological evidence on which plasticity in dorsal horn somatotopic reorganization is based might be questioned on several reasonable grounds. A sufficient number of error factors has been identified to explain some of the controversial results and to impose an inconclusive status on the evidence to date. Improved accuracy will ultimately resolve this issue, and this might be achieved with intracellular labeling of afferent units, including the thin-fiber population.

D. Immunochemical Studies

It has become clear in the past few years that primary afferents in general and small-diameter afferent fibers specifically are heterogeneous populations of neurons, both in terms of electrophysiological properties and neurotransmitter content (See LaMotte, Chapter 5; Cervero, Chapter 9). Recent investigators have approached the problem of intraspinal sprouting of primary afferents by determining how specific, chemically identified populations of neurons respond to deafferentation.

1. Substance P and Cholecystokinin as Putative Primary Afferent Transmitters

The undecapeptide substance P is the best-studied primary afferent transmitter candidate (Pernow, 1983). Substance P immunoreactivity (SP-IR) has been localized in the spinal cord of rat, cat, monkey, and human using both immunohistochemical (Hökfelt *et al.*, 1977a,b; Hunt *et al.*, 1981; Difiglia *et al.*, 1982; Barber *et al.*, 1979; Nilsson *et al.*, 1974; Ljungdahl *et al.*, 1978; LaMotte and de Lancrolle, 1981; de Lanerolle and LeMotte, 1982a,b, 1983; Massari *et al.*, 1983) and radioimmunoassay (RIA; Brownstein *et al.*, 1976; Homma *et al.*, 1979; Mroz *et al.*, 1977) techniques.

Substance-P-immunoreactive fibers have been visualized throughout the spinal gray matter but are most densely concentrated in the dorsal horn, especially in laminae I–II and the lateral spinal nucleus of the lateral funiculus. Immunocytochemistry at the electron microscopic level has localized SP-IR in unmyelinated and thinly myelinated small-diameter fibers that form axodendritic synapses with dorsal horn cells (Difiglia *et al.*, 1982; Barber *et al.*, 1979; Pickel *et al.*, 1977). Takahashi and Otsuka (1975) demonstrated that dorsal rhizotomy in the cat reduced SP in the dorsal horn, and this loss of SP-IR was confirmed both immunohistochemically and with RIA (Barbut *et al.*, 1981; Jessel *et al.*, 1979; Hökfelt *et al.*, 1975a,b, 1977a,b; Micevych *et al.*, 1985; Tessler *et al.*, 1980). Examination of the dorsal root ganglia (DRG) revealed SP-IR localized in small type B neurons, which are associated with small-diameter Aδ and C fibers. Electrical stimulation of the sciatic nerve at intensities activating Aδ and C but not large-diameter fibers causes a release of SP-IR from spinal cord (Yaksh *et al.*, 1980). Further, SP-IR has been shown to be depleted by the neurotoxin capsaicin, which exerts a somewhat selective action on primary sensory neurons (Bucsics and Lembeck, 1981; Gamse *et al.*, 1979; Jansco *et al.*, 1981; Micevych *et al.*, 1983; Therialt *et al.*, 1979; Yaksh *et al.*, 1979). Although these data indicate that most SP-IR in the spinal cord is of primary afferent origin, immunohistochemistry has revealed a population of SP-IR-containing neurons in laminae I–III (Ljungdahl *et al.*, 1978; Senba *et al.*, 1981). Another source of spinal cord SP-IR is derived from raphe neurons that project to the ventral horn (Helke *et al.*, 1982) (see Yaksh, Chapter 8 for further discussion).

As discussed by LaMotte (see Chapter 5), within the spinal cord, cholecystokinin immunoreactivity (CCK-IR) has been localized in layer I and the outer part of lamina II (Innis *et al.*, 1979; Rehfeld *et al.*, 1979; Schultzberg *et al.*, 1982; Vanderhaegen *et al.*, 1980, 1982). Although the distribution of CCK-IR is similar to that of SP-IR, it does not overlap exactly. Recently, Dalsgaard *et al.* (1982b) reported that a population of SP-IR neurons in the DRG may contain yet another neurotransmitter candidate, cholecystokinin octapeptide (CCK). Resembling SP-IR, CCK-IR is profoundly depleted from the dorsal horn by dorsal rhizotomy (Maderdrut *et al.*, 1982, but see Marley *et al.*, 1982). Capsaicin has been shown to deplete CCK-IR (Schultzberg *et al.*, 1982) from dorsal horn in parallel with SP-IR (Jansco *et al.*, 1981; Micevych *et al.*, 1983; but see Marley *et al.*, 1982; Yaksh *et al.*, 1982). Micevych *et al.*, 1983 have correlated the capsaicin-induced depletion of SP-IR and CCK-IR with alterations in responsiveness to noxious thermal stimuli. Interestingly, piperine, the active ingredient in black pepper, evokes the release and eventual depletion of SP-IR from the substantia gelatinosa but does not deplete CCK-IR or elevate the thermal sensory threshold. These data imply a possible synergistic action between these neurotransmitters in signaling different nociceptive information. Further, these data indicating that SP and CCK "neurotransmitter" pools can be preferentially released imply separate regulatory mechanisms. Cholecystokinin IR has been localized in neurons of lamina X (Gibson *et al.*, 1981; Vanderhaegen *et al.*, 1982) and a descending system originating in the raphe (Mantyh and Hunt, 1984).

2. *Changes in Peptide Immunoreactivity Postlesion*

The partial recovery of motor function in cats after extensive lumbosacral deafferentation (Goldberger, 1977; Goldberger and Murray, 1974, 1978) has prompted the investigation of how chemically identified neurons respond to such lesions. This phenomenon of recovery suggests that some type of reorganization of the spinal cord sensory system may follow deafferentation. Since SP asnd CCK are associated with primary afferent fibers, the study of these neurotransmitters may provide clues about the nature of the observed motor recovery of cats.

Trauma to peripheral nerves in a variety of species, including man, reduces the levels of SP-IR in the dorsal horn. The most profound depletion is observed after all primary afferent input to the spinal cord is interrupted by either combined dorsal and ventral rhizotomy or dorsal root ganglionectomy. Tessler and colleagues (1980) observed that after dorsal rhizotomy in the cat, SP-IR in the spinal cord is partially depleted. The lowest density of staining was observed between 9 and 11 days after deafferentation. The depletion is followed by a partial recovery, which was noted on day 14 or 15. Micevych and co-workers (Stroink *et al.*, 1982a,b, 1983a,b; Micevych *et al.*, 1985) confirmed the time course of SP-IR depletion but observed a parallel depletion and recovery of CCK-IR after ganglionectomy (Figures 5, 6). Further, the recovery of SP-IR and CCK-IR proceeded so rapidly that by day 21 after deafferentation, it was difficult to distinguish between the control and lesioned sides (Figure 7).

These studies in the cat are in direct contrast to studies using rat and to observations of human material that indicate that there is no recovery of SP-IR and, by implication, CCK-IR in these species. Cuello *et al.* (1978) demonstrated that SP-IR is reduced in the spinal nucleus of the trigeminal nerve in the rat after 10 days following electrolytic lesions of the trigeminal ganglion or intracranial rhizotomy. In a parallel study, sciatic nerve section in the rat reduced SP-IR in the dorsal horn by 75–80% (Jessel *et al.*, 1979). This reduction is similar to that achieved with dorsal rhizotomy, in which the SP-IR level declined from postoperative day 7 to a nadir at day 28 and remained unchanged until day 57. Although the findings could indicate species differences between rat and cat, it seems more likely that the variety of deafferentation may also account for the discrepancy. Barbut *et al.* (1981) observed a maximal depletion of SP-IR from rat substantia gelatinosa by day 15 after section and ligation of the sciatic nerve, and no recovery was observed even after 31 days. However, these authors noted that a crush injury to the sciatic nerve diminished the spinal cord SP-IR and that this loss of SP-IR was reversed with time. Hunt *et al.* (1982) examined the spinal cords of amputees and observed a profound reduction of SP-IR staining in the substantia gelatinosa in two patients that was still evident after 25 months.

Studies in both rat and human indicate that ligation of peripheral nerve does not elicit the same depletion of spinal cord SP as observed after rhizotomy, and in both species the recovery of SP is not observed. In contrast, studies in the cat report a depletion followed by recovery of SP-IR (Micevych, 1985; Stroink *et al.*, 1982a,b, 1983a,b; Tessler *et al.*, 1980, 1981). Csillak and Knyihar (1978) have indicated that in the rat, the 2-month survival may not provide sufficient time for recovery. In the cat, the recovery is much more rapid. Are the cat experiments with recovery of SP-IR evidence for primary afferent sprouting?

To answer this question, Tessler *et al.*, (1981) and Micevych *et al.* 1985) used combinations of midline myelotomies (to interrupt crossing fibers), hemisections (descending or ascending primary afferents), and dorsal and ventral rhizotomies (primary afferent fibers traveling in the ventral roots; Coggeshall *et al.*, 1974; Dalsgaard *et al.*, 1982a; Stroink *et al.*, 1983a,b) in order to deaf-

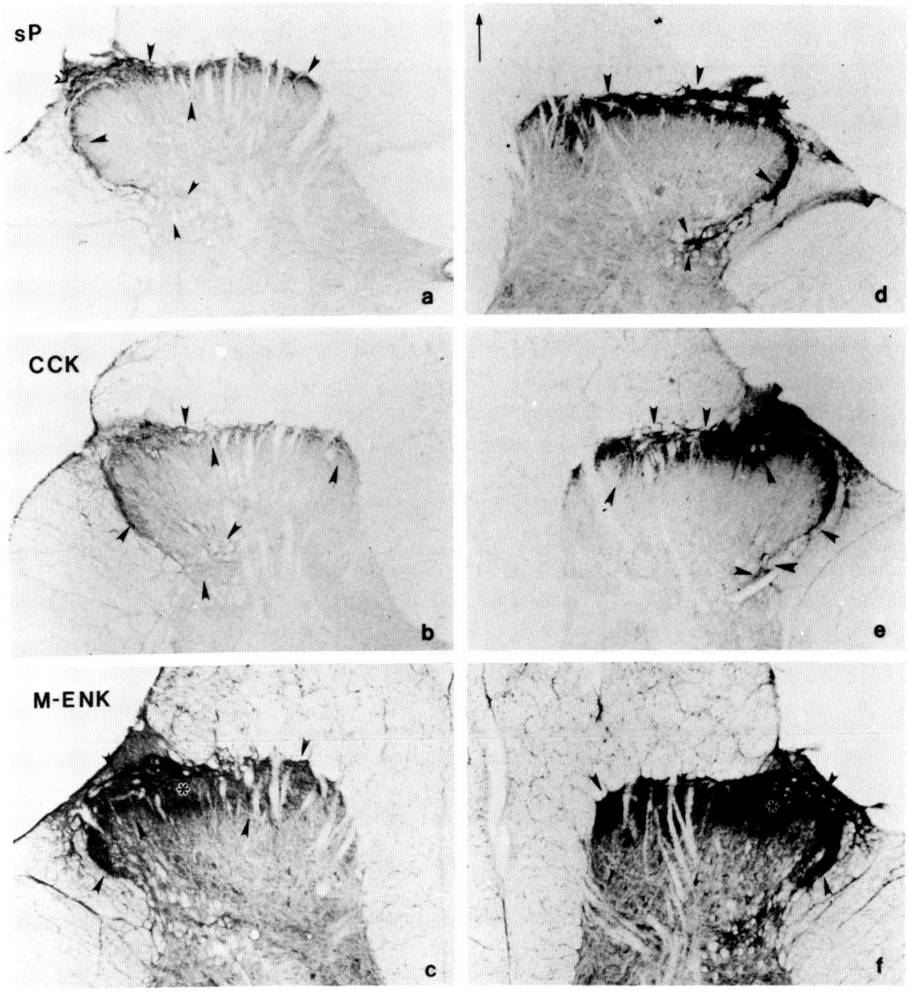

FIGURE 5. Transverse sections of spinal cord from a cat unilaterally ganglionectomized 11 days before sacrifice, incubated with antisera directred against SP (a,d), CCK-8 (b,e), and M-ENK (c,f). The sections on the left (a,b,c) were obtained from the ganglionectomized side, and the sections on the right (d,e,f) were from the contralateral side. The side contralateral to the ganglionectomy had a typical distribution of SP-, CCK-8-, and M-ENK-immunoreactive staining and was used as the control. The ganglionectomized side was observed to have a significantly lower intensity and decreased distribution of SP and CCK staining compared to the control side. Both the SP- and CCK-immunoreactive staining patterns on the deafferented side were restricted to lamina I. The enkephalin staining was not affected. This 11-day survival period represents the nadir of the staining density on the ganglionectomized side (a,b,c). The arrowheads in all photomicrographs outline the staining in the superficial laminae of the dorsal horn and the reticular portion of lamina V. The asterisks in c and f indicate an area of decreased M-ENK-immunoreactive staining in outer lamina II. Arrow in d points dorsally. × 100. (Reproduced at 69%.) (From Micevych *et al.*,1985.)

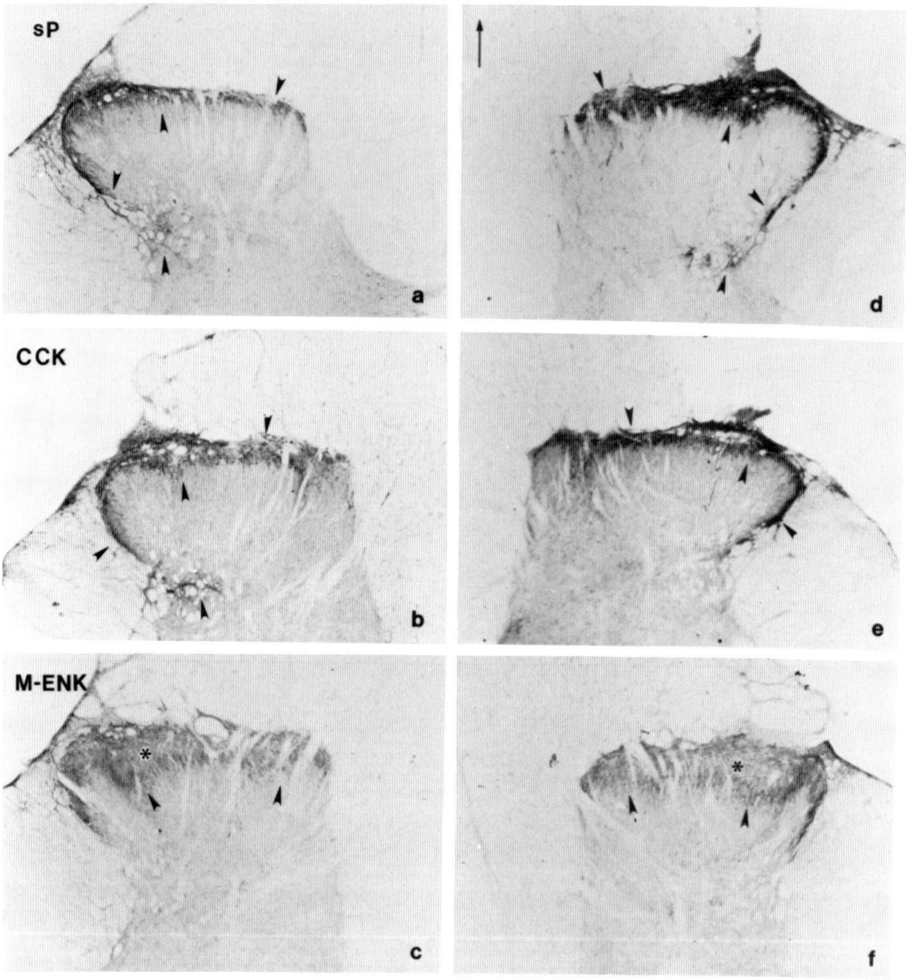

FIGURE 6. Transverse sections of dorsal horn from a cat unilaterally ganglionectomized 14 days prior to sacrifice, incubated with antisera directed against SP (a,d,), CCK-8 (b,e), and M-ENK (c,f). The sections on the left (a,b,c) were unilateral to the ganglionectomy; those on the right (d,e,f) were contralateral to the deafferentation. As in Figure 5, the contralateral side was observed to have a typical distribution, density, and staining intensity in the superficial laminae of the dorsal horn. The ganglionectomized side, however, had a decreased intensity of staining in sections incubated with SP (a) and CCK (b) when compared to the control contralateral side (d and e, respectively). The staining on the ganglionectomized side was more robust in these animals than in the 11-day survival cats. Moreover, the distribution of CCI-8-immunoreactive staining was more extensive than in Figure 5b, extending into lamina II. This increase in intensity and distribution of staining compared to Figure 5a,b appears to indicate a recovery of immunoreactive SP and CCK-8 distributions in the dorsal horn of the ganglionectomized side. The arrowheads outline the staining in the dorsal horn of the respective antisera. The asterisks in c and d indicate the M-ENK-poor region between the highly stained laminae I and inner II. The arrow in b points dorsally. ×100. (Reproduced at 69%.) (From Micevych et al., 1985.)

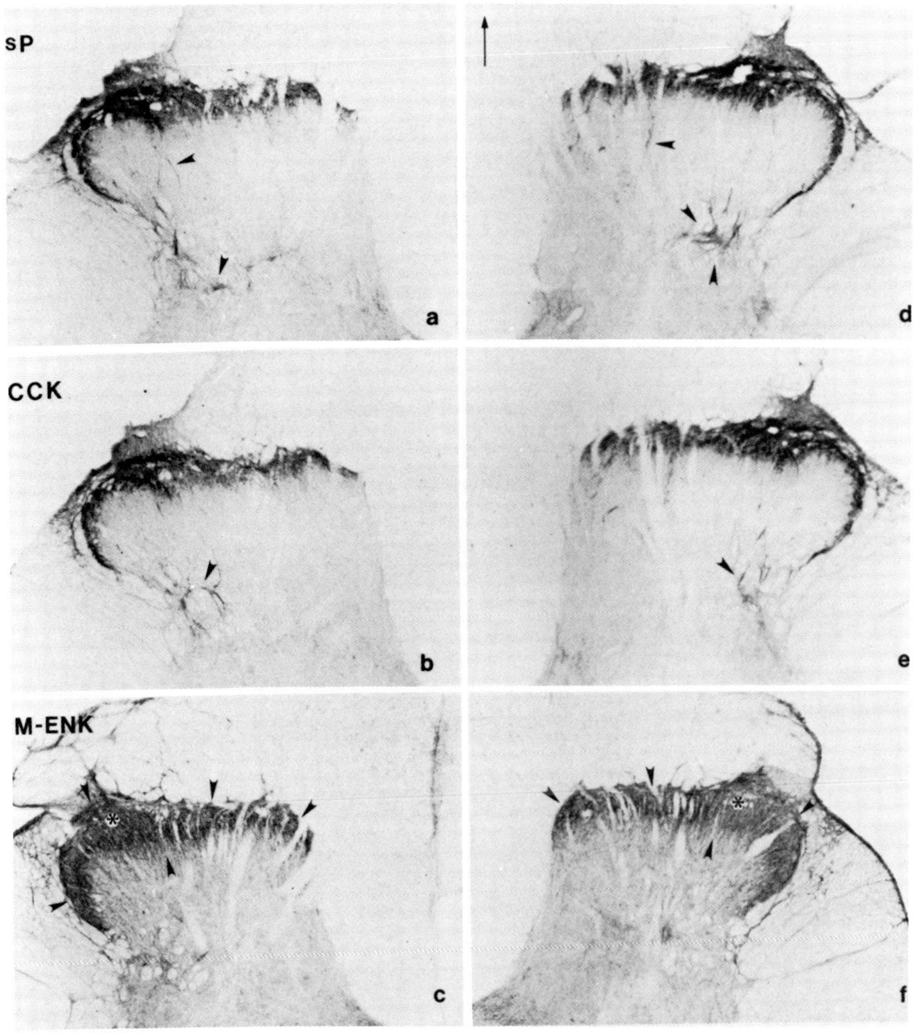

FIGURE 7. Transverse section of dorsal horn obtained from a cat unilaterally ganglionectomized 21 days prior to sacrifice, incubated with antisera directed against SP (a,d), CCK-8 (b,e), and M-ENK (c,f). As in Figures 5 and 6, the left side of the figure shows sections unilateral to the ganglionectomy, and the right side sections from the contralateral side. The contralateral side had a typical distribution and was used as an internal control. The two sides were compared for staining density, intensity, and reaction product distribution. There was little difference in the staining of SP, CCK, and M-ENK in the above parameters between the deafferented and intact sides (arrowheads). The deafferented side had a less dense accumulation of reaction product in the superficial laminae of the dorsal horn. The distribution of SP and CCK on the deafferented side is not as intense as that on the control side. The observations suggest a partial recovery of SP and CCK immunoreactivity in the dorsal horn following a 21-day survival after ganglionectomy. The asterisks in c and f indicate the relative paucity of M-ENK immunostaining in outer lamina II. The arrow in b points dorsally. ×100. (Reproduced at 69%.) (From Micevych *et al.*, 1985.)

ferent a series of segments in the lumbosacral spinal cord. It was observed that none of these deafferentations disrupted the recovery of SP-IR or CCK-IR. To control for nonspecific degeneration or vascular damage to the spinal cord segments, Micevych *et al.* (1985) measured and stained for methionine-enkephalin immunoreactivity. Most methionine-enkephalin was present in spinal neurons and was not affected by the several ablative manipulations. That the recovery of SP-IR was blocked by the injection of the neural cell body toxin kainic acid into the deafferented, isolated segments was interpreted as evidence that the observed SP-IR recovery was mediated not by primary afferents but by intrinsic SP-containing neurons (Tessler *et al.*, 1981). Moreover, intrathecal injection of capsaicin into a ganglionectomized cat (L_1–S_3) 20 days postoperatively followed by an additional 7-day recovery failed to deplete SP-IR on the ganglionectomized side (Micevych *et al.*, 1985), indicating that the recovered SP-IR is not associated with primary afferent terminals.

All of the deafferentation studies point to the same conclusion: immunochemical evidence for the hypothesized intraspinal sprouting of primary afferent fibers is lacking. However, whether the nature of the SP-IR and CCK-IR recovery is the consequence of interneuronal sprouting or an increase in the accumulation of SP and CCK in remaining terminals remains undetermined. Although immunohistochemistry has allowed visualization of the morphological aspects of this recovery, radioimmunoassay (RIA) analysis has allowed quantification of the recovery of SP-IR following deafferentation. Deafferentation by dorsal rhizotomy or ganglionectomy yielded similar immunohistochemical results, but a significant difference is apparent between these deafferentations when analyzed by RIA (Table I). It has been demonstrated (Stroink *et al.*, 1983a,b) that dorsal rhizotomy produces 54 ± 3% depletion of SP-IR, whereas ganglionectomy produces 69 ± 13% loss. However, ventral rhizotomy causes a 35 ± 4% depletion of dorsal horn primary afferent SP-IR. These data support the proposition that a significant proportion of

TABLE I
RIA Determined Levels of SP and M-ENK at Various Times following Unilateral Ganglionectomy

	SP	M-ENK
Days survival[a]	Percent of nonlesioned side[b]	Percent of nonlesioned side[b]
0	94 ± 16	120 ± 8
7	65 ± 16*	100 ± 8
11	55 ± 17*	100 ± 16
21	30 ± 12*	98 ± 16
28	58 ± 14*	92 ± 12

[a] $n = 3$.

[b] Each value $\frac{\text{lesioned}}{\text{nonlesioned}}$ ± S.E.M. %.

* $P < 0.05$.

dorsal horn primary afferent SP-IR reaches the spinal cord through the ventral roots (Dalsgaard *et al.*, 1982a). We have observed that the time course of SP-IR recovery measured by RIA is different from that described with immunohistochemistry. Deafferentation of the dorsal horn by ganglionectomy caused a depletion of SP-IR that was maximum at 21 days. Some recovery of SP-IR in the deafferented dorsal horn is apparent at 30 days post-ganglionectomy. These data are in general agreement with those of Tessler *et al.* (1983), who, while using RIA, described a loss of SP-IR at 10 days and recovery at 30 days post-ganglionectomy; however, they did not measure the dorsal horn at 21 days, which may be the point of maximum depletion.

The difference between the time course of depletion and recovery of SP-IR measured by RIA and visualized by immunohistochemistry may reflect a discrepancy between these techniques or may indicate the possible nature of the observed recovery. It is important to remember that these antibody-dependent techniques depend on the recognition of an antigenic site, which may not always be the peptide of interest. Thus, it is probable that the two methods recognize different, albeit antigenically similar, molecules. High-performance liquid chromatographic analysis of spinal cord reveals only 87% of the SP-IR to be SP (Harmar and Keen, 1981). This difference may not be apparent immunohistochemically or by RIA, when the antigenically similar molecules are present in large quantities such as in normal dorsal horn or on the contralaterial nonganglionectomized side. However, after ganglionectomy, the concentrations of these molecules may be altered.

This hypothesis was made more likely, by the recent discovery of Maggio *et al.* (1983) and Kimura *et al.* (1983), who independently described two novel peptides with carboxy-terminal sequence homologies to SP that cross reacted with the antisera generated against SP. Both peptides belong to the tachykinin family, of which only SP had previously been recognized. One of these novel peptides has been named substance K (Maggio *et al.*, 1983) because of its affinity for a subclass of SP receptors, the SP-K receptor, which preferentially binds eledoisin and kassinin. Nawa *et al.*, (1983), using cDNA hybridization, have described two precursor molecules to SP, λ- and β-preprotachykinin. The structure of β-preprotachykinin contains the sequence for substance K. This may imply either the existence of separate groups of SP- and SP/substance-K-containing neurons or the existence of a neuron that could modulate its pattern of biosynthesis between SP and substance K in response to a stimulus such as deafferentation. After ganglionectomy, each tachykinin may decrease and recover at different rates. Thus, the synthesis of SP in dorsal horn neurons after ganglionectomy may be changed intially only to substance K and subsequently to both SP and substance K. Such putative posttranslational changes would alter the biosynthetic pattern, making a "new SP" (possibly substance K) that is not recognized by the antibodies in the SP-RIA; after fixation, a SP-like antigenic site (C-terminus) might be exposed and visualized by immunohistochemistry.

The discrepancy between immunoreactive staining at day 14 and day 21 thus may reveal the weakness of analyzing tissue with single immunochemical technique. If, however, both methods are recognizing the same molecule, then the difference in the time course and recovery of SP-IR in the dorsal horn following ganglionectomy may reveal the nature of the recovery. Since there is a continued depletion of SP-IR measured by RIA even after the immunohistochemistry reveals recovery (day 14 post-ganglionectomy), this discrepancy may indicate that there is an initial redistribution of SP-IR in dorsal horn neurons from the cell bodies to the processes without an increase in the concentration of SP. Thus, the actual concentration of SP-IR in the spinal cord decreases as measured by RIA, but redistribution of SP is revealed by immunohistochemistry, implying an SP recovery. The compensatory synthesis of SP may not begin until day 21 post-ganglionectomy, and it is then revealed by RIA as elevated tissue concentration of SP-IR.

The results of these immunochemical experiments do not support the concept of intraspinal sprouting of primary afferents, and this is consistent with the views expressed by Kerr (1971, 1975). The recovery of SP-IR following dorsal rhizotomy and ganglionectomy in cats may reflect the remodeling and possible sprouting of local spinal interneurons containing these substances. The failure to demonstrate recovery of SP-IR and CCK-IR in either rats or humans after deafferentation poses an additional unexplained problem. Interneuronal sprouting, if present, may not be a specific SP and/or CCK response but rather a generalized spinal cord reaction to denervation. Indeed, Hunt *et al.* (1982) report an apparent increase in M-ENK-immunoreactive staining on the deafferented side, and we have observed an apparent increased number of 5-HT fibers (in laminae II–V) following ganglionectomy in the cat spinal cord. It is perhaps these responses to deafferentation that underlie some aspects of causalgia and the partial recovery of motor function following deafferentation of the spinal cord.

E. Conclusion

These findings do not preclude the possibility that intraspinal primary afferent sprouting may occur under special circumstances, but they do indicate that there is still deficient evidence for sprouting of sensory fibers in the spinal cord under ordinary conditions. Negative observations lack persuasiveness, and the fundamental issue should not be reduced to a simple affirmation or denial of sprouting. Kerr's failure to demonstrate substantial anatomic sprouting in a large series of experiments and our supportive findings with axonal transport labeling methods are perhaps less compelling than the cogent arguments concerning somatotopic reorganization. There is a body of evidence for reorganization of the somatosensory cortex following peripheral nerve injury (Kaas *et al.*, 1983), and it would be valuable to understand the nature and extent of the subcortical contributions to this phenomenon, especially in light of the current immunochemical evidence for reorganization in the spinal cord following deafferentation. The unmasking of undetected connections and the formation of new connections may both contribute to "plasticity." The imprecision in determining the magnitude of each factor and the uncertainties concerning their functional significance continue to merit homage to Kerr's skepticism.

ACKNOWLEDGMENTS. The original research reported in this article was partially supported by grants from the National Institutes of Health, NS-21220 and 05685. The authors are indebted to Ms. Anita Roff for assistance in manuscript preparation.

References

BARBER, R. P., VAUGHN, J. E., SLEMMON, J. R., SALVATERRA, P. M., ROBERTS, E., AND LEEMAN, S. E. The origin, distribution and synaptic relationships of substance P axons in rat spinal cord. *J. Comp. Neurol.* 184:331–352, 1979.

BARBUT, D., POLAK, J. M., AND WALL, P. Substance P in spinal cord dorsal horn decreases following peripheral nerve injury. *Brain Res.* 205:289–298, 1981.

BASBAUM, J. I., AND WALL, P. D. Chronic changes in the response of cells in adult cat dorsal horn following partial deafferentation: The appearance of responding cells in a previously non-responsive region. *Brain Res.* 116:181–204, 1976.

BEATTIE, J. S., BRESNAHAN, J. C., AND LIUZZI, F. J. Aberrant axons from the dorsal roots after chronic spinal hemisection in the cat: The dorsal horn. *Soc. Neurosci. Abstr.* 7:626, 1981.

BECKERMAN, S. B., AND KERR, F. W. L. Electrophysiologic evidence that neither sprouting nor neuronal hyperactivity occur following long term trigeminal or cervical primary deafferentation. *Exp. Neurol.* 50:427–438, 1976.

BERNSTEIN, J. J., AND BERNSTEIN, M. E. Axonal regeneration and formation of synapses proximal to the site of lesion following hemisection of the rat spinal cord. *Exp. Neurol.* 30:336–351, 1971.

BERNSTEIN, J. J., WELLS, M. R., AND BERNSTEIN, M. E. Spinal cord regeneration: Synaptic renewal and neurochemistry, in: *Neuronal Plasticity* (C. W. COTMAN, ed.), Raven Press, New York, 1978, pp. 49–72.

BRINKHUS, H. B., AND ZIMMERMANN, M. Characteristics of spinal dorsal horn neurons after partial chronic deafferentation by dorsal root transection. *Pain* 15:221–236, 1983.

BROWN, A. G., BROWN, P. B., FYFFE, R. E. W., AND PUBOLS, L. M. Effects of dorsal root section on spinocervical tract neurones in the cat. *J. Physiol. (Lond.)* 337:589–608, 1983a.

BROWN, A. G., FYFFE, R. E. W., AND ROWE, M. Effects of peripheral nerve section on dorsal horn somatotopy in the cat. *J. Physiol. (Lond.)* 339:36–37P, 1983b.

BROWN, P. B., AND FUCHS, J. L. Somatotopic representation of hindlimb skin in cat dorsal horn. *J. Neurophysiol.* 38:1–9, 1975.

BROWN, P. B., KOERBER, H. R., AND YEZIERSKI, R. P. Absence of alterations of dorsal horn somatotopy after unilaterial L Section in cat. *Neurosci. Abstr.* 5:704, 1979.

BROWNSTEIN, M. J., MROZ, E. A., KIZER, S., PALKOVITS, M., AND LEEMAN, S. E. Regional distribution of substance P in the brain of the rat. *Brain Res.* 116:299–305, 1976.

BUCSICS, A., AND LEMBECK, F. *In vitro* release of substance P from spinal cord slices by capsaicin congeners. *Eur. J. Pharmacol.* 71:71–77, 1981.

CAJAL RAMON Y, S. *Degeneration and Regeneration of the Nervous System,* Oxford University Press, Oxford, 1928.

COGGESHALL, R., COULTER, J., AND WILLIS, W. D. Unmyelinated axons in the ventral roots of the cat lumbosacral enlargement. *J. Comp. Neurol.* 139:39–58, 1974.

CSILLAK, B., AND KNYIHAR, E. Biodynamic plasticity in the Rolando substance. *Prog. Neurobiol.* 10:203–230, 1978.

CUELLO, C. A., DEL FIACCO, M., AND PAXINOS, G. The central and peripheral ends of the substance P-containing neurones in the rat trigeminal system. *Brain Res.* 152:499–509, 1978.

DALSGAARD, C.-J., RISLING, M., AND CUELLO, C. Immunohistochemical localization of substance P in the lumbosacral spinal pia mater and ventral roots of the cat. *Brain Res.* 246:168–171, 1982a.

DALSGAARD, C.-J., VINCENT, S., HÖKFELT, T., DOCKRAY, G., AND CUELLO, C. Immunohistochemical evidence for coexistence of cholecystokinin- and substance P-like peptides in primary sensory neurons. *Neurosci. Abstr.* 8:474, 1982b.

DE LANEROLLE, N., AND LAMOTTE, C. The human spinal cord: Substance P and methionine enkephaline immunoreactivity. *J. Neurosci. 2:1369–1386, 1982a.*

DE LANEROLLE, N., AND LAMOTTE, C. The morphological relationships between substance P immunoreactive processes and ventral horn neurons in human and monkey spinal cord. *J. Comp. Neurol.* 207:305–313, 1982b.

DE LANEROLLE, N., AND LAMOTTE, C. Ultrastructure of chemically defined neuron-systems in the dorsal horn of the monkey. I. Substance P immunoreactivity. *Brain Res.* 274:31–49, 1983.

DE OLMOS, J. S., EBBESSON, S. O. E., AND HEIMER, L. Silver methods for the impregnation of degenerating axoplasm, in: *Neuroanatomical Tract-Tracing Methods* (L. HEIMER AND M. J. ROBARDS, eds.), Plenum Press, New York, 1981, pp. 117–170.

DEVOR, M., AND WALL, P.D. Effect of peripheral nerve injury on receptive fields of cells in the cat spinal cord. *J. Comp. Neurol.* 199:277–291, 1981a.

DEVOR, M., AND WALL, P. D. Plasticity in the spinal cord sensory map following peripheral nerve injury in rats. *J. Neurosci.* 1:679–684, 1981b.

DEVOR, M., MERRILL, E. G., AND WALL, P. D. Dorsal horn cells that respond to stimulation of distant dorsal roots. *J. Physiol. (Lond.)* 270:519–531, 1977.

DIFIGLIA, M. ARONIN, N., AND LEEMAN, S. E. Light microscopic and ultrastructural localization of immunoreactive substance P in the dorsal horn of monkey spinal cord. *Neuroscience* 233:381–388, 1982.

FINLAY, B. L., AND SLATTERY, M. Local differences in the amount of early cell death in neocortex predict adult local specializations. *Science* 219:1349–1351, 1983.

GAMSE, R., MOLNAR, A., AND LEMBECK, F. Substance P release from spinal cord slices by capsaicin. *Life Sci.* 25:629–636, 1979.

GIBSON, S., POLAK, J., BLOOM, S., AND WALL, P. Distribution of nine peptides in rat spinal cord with special emphasis on the substantia gelatinosa and on the area around the central canal (lamina X). *J. Comp. Neurol.* 201:65–79, 1981.

GOLDBERGER, M. E. Locomotor recovery after hindlimb deafferentation in cats. *Brain Res.* 123:59–74, 1977.

GOLDBERGER, M. E., AND MURRAY, M. Restitution of function and collateral sprouting in the cat spinal cord: The deafferented animal. *J. Comp. Neurol.* 158:37–54, 1974.

GOLDBERGER, M. E., AND MURRAY, M. Recovery of movement and axonal sprouting may obey some of the same laws, in: *Neuronal Plasticity* (C. W. Cotman, ed.), Raven Press, New York, 1978, pp. 73–96.

GOLDBERGER, M. E., AND MURRAY, M. Lack of sprouting and its presence after lesions of the cat spinal cord. *Brain Res.* 241:227–239, 1982.

GRAFSTEIN, B., AND MCQUARRIE, I. G. Role of nerve cell body in axonal regeneration, in: *Neuronal Plasticity* (C. W. Cotman, ed.), Raven Press, New York, 1978, pp. 155–195.

HARMAR, A., AND KEEN, P. Chemical characterization of substance P-like immunoreactivity in primary afferent neurons. *Brain Res.* 220:203–207, 1981.

HELKE, C., NEIL, J., MASSARI, J., AND LOEWY, A. Substance P neurons project from ventral medulla to the intermediolateral cell column and ventral horn in the rat. *Brain Res.* 243:147–152, 1982.

HÖKFELT, T., KELLERTH, J.-O., NILSSON, G., AND PERNOW, B. Experimental immunohistochemical studies on the localization and distribution of substance P in cat primary sensory neurons. *Brain Res.* 100:235–252. 1975a.

HÖKFELT, T., KELLERTH, J.-O., NILSSON, G., AND PERNOW, B. Substance P: Localization in the central nervous system and in some primary sensory neurons. *Science* 190:889–890, 1975b.

HÖKFELT, T., JOHANSSON, O., KELLERTH, J.-O., LJUNGDAHL, A., NILSSON, G., NYGÅRDS, A., AND PERNOW, B. Immunohistochemical distribution of substance P, in: *Substance P, Nobel Symposium 37* (U. S. VON EULER AND B. PERNOW, eds.), Raven Press, New York, 1977a, pp. 117–145.

HÖKFELT, T., LJUNGDAHL, A., TERENIUS, L., ELDE, R., AND NILSSON, G., Immunohistochemical analysis of peptide pathways possibly related to pain and analgesia: Enkephalin and substance P. *Proc. Natl. Acad. Sci. U.S.A.* 74:3081–3085, 1977b.

HOMMA, S., SUZUKI, T., MURAYAMA, S., AND OTSUKA, M. Amino acid and substance P contents in the spinal cord of cats with experimental hind-limb rigidity produced by occlusion of spinal cord blood supply. *J. Neurochem.* 32:691–698, 1979.

HULSEBOSCH, C. E., AND COGGESHALL, R. E. Quantitation of sprouting of dorsal root axons. *Science* 213:1020–1021, 1981a.

HULSEBOSCH, C. E., AND COGGESHALL, R. E. Sprouting of dorsal root axons. *Brain Res.* 224:170–174, 1981b.

HULSEBOSCH, C. E., AND COGGESHALL, R. E. A comparison of axonal numbers in dorsal roots following spinal cord hemisection in neonate and adult rats. *Brain Res.* 265:187–197, 1983.

HUNT, S. P., KELLEY, J. S., EMSON, C., KIMMEL, J. R., MILLER, R. J., AND WU, J.-Y. An immunohistochemical study of neuronal populations containing neuropeptides or δ-amino-butyrate within superficial layers of the rat dorsal horn. *Neuroscience* 6:1883–1898, 1981.

HUNT, S. P., ROSSOR, M., EMSON, P., AND CLEMENT-JONES, V. Substance P and enkephalins in spinal cord after limb amputation. *Lancet* 1:1023, 1982.

INNIS, R., CORREA, F. M., UHL, G., SCHNEIDER, B., AND SNYDER, S. H. Cholecystokinin octapeptide-like immunoreactivity: Histochemical localization in rat brain. *Proc. Natl. Acad. Sci. U.S.A.* 76:521–525, 1979.

INNOCENTI, G. M. Growth and reshaping of axons in the establishment of visual collosal connections. *Science* 212:824–827, 1981.

JANSCO, G., HÖKFELT, T., LUNDBERG, M., KIRALY, E., HALÁSZ, N., NILSSON, G., TERENIUS, L., REHFELD, J. STEINBUSCH, H., VERHOFSTAD, A., ELDE, R., SAID, S., AND BROWN, M. Immunohistochemical studies on the effect of capsaicin on spinal and medullary peptide and monoamine neurons using antisera to substance P, gastrin/CCK, somatostatin, VIP, enkephalin, neurotensin and 5-hydroxytryptamine. *J. Neurocytol.* 10:963–980, 1981.

JESSEL, TSUMOO, A., KANAZAWA, I., AND OTSUKA, M. Depletion in the dorsal horn of the rat spinal cord after section of the peripheral processes of primary sensory neurons. *Brain Res.* 168:247–259, 1979.

KAAS, J. H. MERZENICH, M. M., AND KILLACKEY, H. P. The reorganization of somatosensory cortex following peripheral nerve damage in adult and developing mammals. *Annu. Rev. Neurosci.* 6:325–356, 1983.

KERR, F. W. L. A study of potential sprouting of primary cervical afferents into the chronically denervated trigeminal nuclei. *Anat. Rec.* 169:355, 1971.

KERR, F. W. L. The potential of cervical primary afferents to sprout in the spinal nucleus of V following long term trigeminal denervation. *Brain Res.* 43:547–560, 1972.

KERR, F. W. L. Neuroplasticity of primary afferents in the neo-natal cat and some results of early deafferentation of the trigeminal spinal nucleus. *J. Comp. Neurol.* 163:305–328, 1975.

KERR, F. W. L., KRUGER, L. SCHWASSMANN, H. O., AND STERN, R. Somatotopic organization of mechanoreceptor units in the trigeminal nuclear complex of the macaque. *J. Comp. Neurol.* 134:127–144, 1968.

KIMURA, S., OKADA, M., SUGITA, Y., KANAZAWA, I., AND MUNEKATA, E. Novel neuropeptides, neurokinin α and β, isolated from porcine spinal cord. *Proc. Jpn. Acad. [B]* 59:101–104, 1983.

KOERBER, H. R., AND BROWN, P. B. Projections of two hindlimb cutaneous nerves to cat dorsal horn. *J. Neurophysiol.* 44:259–269, 1980.

KOERBER, H. R., AND BROWN, P. B. Somatotopic organization of hindlimb cutaneous nerve projections to cat dorsal horn. *J. Neurophysiol.* 48:481–489, 1982.

LAMOTTE, C. C. Distribution of the tract of Lissauer and the dorsal root fibers in the primate spinal cord. *J. Comp. Neurol.* 172:529–561, 1977.

LAMOTTE, C. AND DE LANEROLLE, M. Substance P, Enkephaline and serotinin: Ultrastructural basis of pain transmission in primate spinal cord. *Pain [Suppl.]* 1:19, 1981.

LAND P. W. AND LUND, R. D. Development of rat's uncrossed retinotectal pathway and its relation to plasticity studies. *Science* 205:698–700, 1979.

LISNEY, S. J. W. Changes in the somatotopic organization of the cat lumbar spinal cord following peripheral nerve transection and regeneration. *Brain Res.* 259:31–39, 1983.

LIU, C. N., AND CHAMBERS, W. W. Intraspinal sprouting of dorsal root axions. *Arch. Neurol. Psychiatry* 79:46–61, 1958.

LJUNGDAHL, Å., HÖKFELT, T., AND NILSSON, G., Distribution of substance P-like immunoreactivity in the central nervous system of the rat. I. Cell bodies and nerve terminals. *Neuroscience* 3:945–976, 1978.

MADERDRUT, J., YAKSH, T., PETRUSZ, P., AND GO, V. L. W. Origin and distribution of cholecystokinin-containing nerve terminals in the lumbar dorsal horn and nucleus caudalis of the cat. *Brain Res.* 243:363–368, 1982.

MAGGIO, J. E., SANDBERG, B., BRADLEY, C., IVERSON, L., SANTIKARN, S., WILLIAMS, D., HUNTER, J. C., AND HANLEY, M. Substance K: A novel tachykinin in mammalian spinal cord, in: *Substance P* (P. SKRABANEK AND D. POWELL, eds.), Boole, Dublin, 1983, pp. 20–21.

MANTYH, P., AND HUNT, S. P. Evidence for cholecystokinin-like immunoreactive neurons in the rat medulla oblongata which project to the spinal cord. *Brain Res.* 291:49–54, 1984.

MARKUS, H., KRUSHELNKY, D., AND POMERANZ, The effect of acute and chronic denervation on the rat spinal cord. *Soc. Neurosci. Abstr.* 7:472, 1981.

MARLEY, P., NAGY, J. I., EMSON, P., AND REHFELD, J. Cholecystokinin in the rat spinal cord: Distribution and lack of effect of neonatal capsaicin treatment and rhizotomy. *Brain Res.* 238:494–498, 1982.

MASSARI, J. Y., TIZABI, Y., PARK, C., MOODY, T., HELKE, C., AND O'DONOHUE, T. Distribution and origin of bombesin, substance P and somatostatin in cat spinal cord. *Peptides* 4:673–681, 1983.

MATTHEWS, M. A., AND KRUGER, L. Electron microscopy of non-neuronal cellular changes accompanying neural degeneration in thalamic nuclei of the rabbit. II. Reactive elements within the neuropil. *J. Comp. Neurol.* 148:313–346, 1973.

MCCOUCH, G. P., AUSTIN, G. M., LIU, C. N. AND LIU, C. Y. Sprouting as a cause of spasticity. *J. Neurophysiol.* 21:205–216, 1958.

MENDELL, L. M., SASSOON, E. M., AND WALL, P. D. Properties of synaptic linkage from long ranging afferents onto dorsal horn neurones in normal and deafferented cats. *J. Physiol. (Lond.)* 285:299–310, 1978.

MERRILL, E. G., AND WALL, P. D. Plasticity of connection in the adult nervous system, in: *Neuronal Plasticity* (C. W. Cotman, ed.), Raven Press, New York, 1978, pp. 94–111.

MESSENGER, K. K., AND KINGSLEY, R. E. A horseradish peroxidase study of peripheral nerve reinnervation into the spinal cord. *Soc. Neurosci. Abstr.* 8:869, 1982.

MESULAM, M.-M. Principles of horseradish peroxidase neurohistochemistry and their applications for tracing neural pathways—axonal transport, enzyme histochemistry and light microscopic analysis, in: *Tracing Neural Connections with Horseradish Peroxidase* (M.-M. MESULAM, ed.), John Wiley & Sons, New York, 1982, pp. 1–152.

MESULAM, M.-M., AND BRUSHART, T. M. Transganglionic and anterograde transport of horseradish peroxidase across dorsal root ganglia: A tetramethylbenzidine method for tracing central sensory connections of muscles and peripheral nerves. *Neuroscience* 4:1107–1117, 1979.

MICEVYCH, P. E., YAKSH, T. L., AND SZOLCSANYI, J. Effect of intrathecal capsaicin analogues on the immunofluorescence of peptides and serotonin in the dorsal horn in rats. *Neuroscience* 8:123–131, 1983.

MICEVYCH, P., STROINK, A., GO, V. L. W., AND YAKSH, T. L., Immunohistochemical and radioimmunoassay studies of substance P and cholecystokinin recovery in the dorsal horn following lumbosacral ganglionectomy. *Somatosens. Res.* (in press), 1985.

MROZ, E. A., BROWNSTEIN, M. J., AND LEEMAN, S. E. Distribution of immunoassayable substance P in the rat brain: Evidence of substance P-containing tracts, in: *Substance P, Nobel Symposium 37* (U. S. VON EULER AND B. PERNOW, eds.), Raven Press, New York, 1977, pp. 147–154.

MURRAY, M., AND GOLDBERGER, M. E. Restitution of function and collateral sprouting in the cat spinal cord: The partially hemisected animal. *J. Comp. Neurol.* 158:19–36, 1974.

NAWA, H., HIROSE, T., TAKASHIMA, H., INAYAMA, S., AND NAKAMISHI, S. Nucleotide sequences of cloned cDNAs for two types of bovine brain substance P precursor. *Nature* 306:32–36, 1983.

NILSSON, G., HÖKFELT, T., AND PERNOW, B. Distribution of substance P-like immunoreactivity in the rat central nervous system as revealed by immunohistochemistry. *Med. Biol.* 52:424–427, 1974.

PERNOW, B. Substance P. *Pharmacol. Rev.* 35:85–141, 1983.

PICKEL, V. REIS, D., AND LEEMAN, S. Ultrastructural localization of substance P in neurons of the rat spinal cord. *Brain Res.* 122:534–540, 1977.

PRENDERGAST, J., AND MISANTONE, L. J. Sprouting by tracts descending from the midbrain to the spinal cord: The result of thoracic funiculotomy in the newborn, 21-day-old and adult rat. *Exp. Neurol.* 69:458–480, 1980.

PUBOLS, L. M. The boundary of proximal hindlimb representation in the dorsal horn following peripheral nerve lesions in cats: A re-evaluation of plasticity in the somatotopic map. *Somatosens. Res.* 2:19–32, 1984.

PUBOLS, L. M., AND BRENOWITZ, G. L. Maintenance of dorsal horn somatotopic organization and increased high threshold response after single root or spared root deafferentation in cats. *J. Neurophysiol.* 47:103–112, 1981.

PUBOLS, L. M. AND GOLDBERGER, M. E. Recovery of function in the dorsal horn following partial deafferentation. *J. Neurophysiol.* 43:102–117, 1980.

RAGER, G. The significance of neuronal cell death during the development of the nervous system, in: *Lesion-Induced Neuronal Plasticity in Sensorimotor Systems* (H. FLOHR AND W. PRECHT, eds.), Springer-Verlag, New York, 1981, pp. 3–12.

REHFELD, J. F., GOLTERMANN, N., LARSSON, L., EMSON, P. M., AND LEE, C. M. Gastrin and cholecystokinin in central and peripheral neurons. *Fed. Proc.* 28:2325–2329, 1979.

RETHELYI, M., TREVINO, D. L., AND PERL, E. R. Distribution of primary afferent fibers within the sacrococcygeal dorsal horn: An autoradiographic study. *J. Comp. Neurol.* 185:603–622, 1979.

RODIN, B. E., AND KRUGER, L. Absence of evidence for intraspinal sprouting in dorsal root axons caudal to a partial spinal hemisection: A horseradish peroxidase transport study. *Somatosens. Res.* 2:171–192, 1984.

RODIN, B. E., SAMPOGNA, S., AND KRUGER, L. Intraspinal sprouting in dorsal root afferents (DRAs) following partial spinal hemisection: A re-appraisal with the tracer horseradish peroxidase. *Soc. Neurosci. Abstr.* 8:748, 1982.

RODIN, B. E., SAMPOGNA, S., AND KRUGER, L. An examination of intraspinal sprouting in dorsal root axons with the tracer horseradish peroxidase. *J. Comp. Neurol.* 215:187–198, 1983.

ROSE, J. E., MALIS, L., KRUGER, L., AND BAKER, C. P. Effects to heavy ionizing monoenergetic particles on the cerebral cortex. II. Histological appearance of laminar lesions and growth of nerve fibers after laminar destruction. *J. Comp. Neurol.* 115:243–296, 1960.

SCHNEIDER, G. E. Early lesions of superior colliculus: Factors affecting the formation of abnormal retinal projections. *Brain Behav. Evol.* 8:73–109, 1973.

SCHNEIDER, G. E., AND JHAVERI, S. R. Neuroanatomical correlates of spared or altered function after brain lesions in the newborn hamster, in: *Plasticity and Recovery of Function in the Central Nervous System* (J. J. ROSEN AND N. BUTTERS, eds.), Academic Press, New York, 1974, pp. 65–109.

SCHULTZBERG, M., DOCKRAY, G., AND WILLIAMS, R. Capsaicin depletes CCK-like immunoreactivity detected by immunohistochemistry, but not that measured by radioimmunoassay in rat dorsal spinal cord. *Brain Res.* 235:198–204, 1982.

SENBA, E., SHIOSAKA, S., INAGAKI, S., TAKAGI, H., TAKATUSUKI, K., SAKANAKA, M., KAWAI, Y., TOHYAMA, M., AND SHIOTANI, Y. Peptidergic neuron systems in the rat spinal cord. I. Experimental immunohistocheminal study. *Neurosci. Lett. [Suppl.]* 6:77, 1981.

SENGELAUB, D. R., AND FINLAY, B. L. Early removal of one eye reduces normally occurring cell death in the remaining eye. *Science* 213:573–574, 1981.

STANFIELD, B. B., O'LEARY, D. D. M., AND FRICKE, C. Selective collateral elimination in early postnatal development restricts cortical distribution of rat pyramidal tract neurones. *Nature* 298:371–373, 1982.

STELZNER, D. J., AND WEBER, E. D. A lack of dorsal root sprouting found after spinal hemisection in neonatal or weanling rats. *Soc. Neurosci. Abstr.* 1:437, 1974.

STELZNER, D. J., WEBER, E. D., AND PRENDERGAST, J. A comparison of the effect of mid-thoracic spinal hemisection in the neonatal or weanling rat on the distribution and density of dorsal root axons in the lumbosacral spinal cord of the adult. *Brain Res.* 172:407–426, 1979.

STROINK, A., MICEVYCH, P., GO, V. L. W., AND YAKSH, T. Immunohistochemical and radioimmunoassay studies of substance P in dorsal horn following ganglionectomy. *Soc. Neurosci. Abstr.* 8:583, 1982a.

STROINK, A., MICEVYCH, P., AND YAKSH, T. Immunohistochemical studies of substance P and cholecystokinin recovery after ganglionectomy. *Anat. Rec.* 202:183a, 1982b.

STROINK, A., MICEVYCH, P., AND YAKSH, T. Radioimmunoassay studies of substance P in the dorsal horn following ganglionectomy and ventral root rhizotomy. *Am. Assoc. Neurol. Surg. Abstr.* 30:19–20, 1983a.

STROINK, A., MICEVYCH, P., GO, V. L. W., AND YAKSH, T. Immunohistochemical studies of substance P in the dorsal horn following ventral root rhizotomy. *Anat. Rec.* 205:192A, 1983b.

STROINK, A., MICEVYCH, P., YAKSH, T., AND GO, V. L. W., Biochemical evidence of SP containing nerve fibers in the ventral spinal roots: Peptides. (submitted for publication), 1985.

TAKAHASHI, T., AND OTSUKA, M. Regional distribution of substance P in spinal cord and nerve roots of the cat and the effect of dorsal root section. *Brain Res.* 87:1–11, 1975.

TESSLER, A., GLAZER, E., ARTYMYSHYN, R., MURRAY, M., AND GOLDBERGER, M. Recovery of substance P in the cat spinal cord after unilateral lumbosacral deafferentation. *Brain Res.* 191:459–470, 1980.

TESSLER, A., HIMES, B. T., ARTYMYSHYN, R., MURRAY, M., AND GOLDBERGER, M. E. Spinal neurons mediate return of substance P following deafferentation of cat spinal cord. *Brain Res.* 230:263–281, 1981.

TESSLER, A., HIMES, B., MURRAY, M., AND GOLDBERGER, M. Recovery of intraspinal substance P after section of the cat sciatic nerve. *Soc. Neurosci. Abstr.* 9:987, 1983.

THERIALT, E., OTSUKA M., AND JESSEL, T. Capsaicin-evoked release of substance P from primary sensory neurons. *Brain Res.* 170:209–213, 1979.

THOR, K. B., KUO, D. C., DE GROAT, W. C., BLAIS, D., AND BACKES, M. Alterations of HRP-labelled pudendal nerve afferent projections in the sacral spinal cord of the cat during neonatal development and after spinal cord transection: Correlation with physiological plasticity of a spinal somatovesical reflex. *Soc. Neurosci. Abstr.* 8:305, 1982.

VANDERHAEGEN, J. J. LOTSTRA, F., DE MAY, J., AND GILLES, C. Immunohistochemical localization of cholecystokinin- and gastrin-like peptides in the brain and hypophysis of the rat. *Proc. Natl. Acad. Sci. U.S.A.* 77:1190–1194, 1980.

VANDERHAEGEN, J. J. DESCHEPPER, C., LOTSTRA, F., VIERENDEELS, G., AND SCHOENEN, J. Immunohistochemical evidence for cholecystokinin-like peptides in neural cell bodies of the rat spinal cord. *Cell Tissue Res.* 223:463–467, 1982.

WALL, P. D., AND EGGER, M. D. Formation of new connections in adult rat brains after partial deafferentation. *Nature* 232:542–545, 1971.

WALL, P. D., AND WERMAN, R. The physiology and anatomy of long-ranging afferent fibers with the spinal cord. *J. Physiol. (Lond.)* 255:321–334, 1976.

YAKSH, T., FARB, D., LEEMAN S., AND JESSEL, T. Intrathecal capsaicin depletes substance P in the rat spinal cord and prolongs thermal analgesia. *Science* 206:481–483, 1979.

YAKSH, T., JESSEL, T., GAMSE, R., MUDGE, A. W., AND LEEMAN, S. E. Intrathecal morphine inhibits substance P release from mammalian spinal cord *in vivo*. *Nature* 286:155–157, 1980.

YAKSH, T. L., ABAY, E. O., AND GO, V. L. W. Studies on the location and release of cholecystokinin and vasoactive intestinal peptide in rat and cat spinal cord. *Brain Res.* 242:279–290, 1982.

18
The Question of How the Dorsal Horn Encodes Sensory Information

DONALD D. PRICE

A. Introduction

The dorsal gray matter of the mammalian spinal cord is the origin of ascending somatosensory pathways. Impulses from thermoreceptive, nociceptive, and mechanoreceptive afferents excite various types of second-order neurons of the dorsal horn. Radical transformations are made of these inputs in such a manner that responses to somatosensory stimuli do not simply passively reflect the responses of cutaneous receptors. These transformations have important implications for perception of somatosensory sensations. The dorsal horn also is the central focal point for autonomic and somatomotor reflexes initiated by stimulation of body tissues. This region clearly does not function autonomously but is under the influence of several descending control mechanisms. For these reasons and others, it is important to characterize these afferent input–output relationships in terms of their role in encoding sensory information.

This chapter focuses on afferent input–output relationships of the dorsal horn and how such relationships help to explain the encoding of sensory information. It first summarizes the microanatomic organization of the dorsal horn and how such organization accounts for the physiological characteristics of interneurons and sensory projection neurons of this region. For other comments on the dorsal horn response characteristics, see chapters by Cervero

DONALD D. PRICE • Department of Anesthesiology, Medical College of Virginia, Richmond, Virginia 23298.

(Chapter 9) and Willis (Chapter 11). The physiological characteristics of sensory dorsal horn neurons are then related to their possible roles in various factors that underlie sensory coding mechanisms. Finally, the question of functional characterization of ascending afferent systems is addressed.

B. Microanatomic Organization of the Dorsal Horn

The microanatomic organization of the dorsal horn helps to explain the physiological types of neurons that exist in different laminae. The convergent input of dorsal horn sensory projection neurons and local circuit interneurons appears to be determined by three general factors: (1) the termination of various types of primary afferents within different dorsal horn laminae, (2) the location of dendritic arbors of different types of dorsal horn neurons, and (3) the axonal interconnections within the dorsal horn. Figure 1 is a schematic that can be used to help explain these factors.

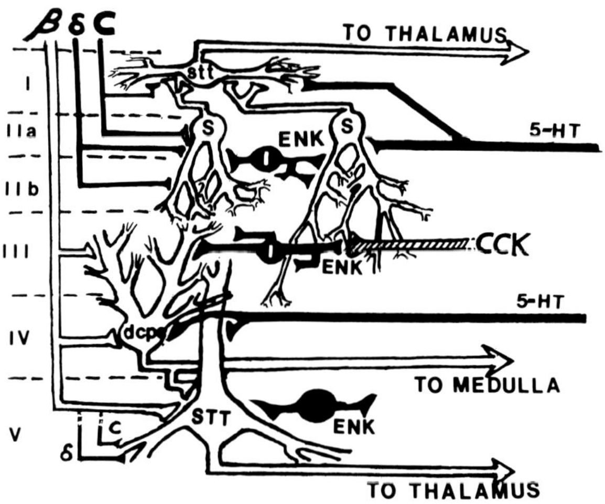

FIGURE 1. Schematic diagram illustrating the major morphological–functional characteristics of neurons within dorsal horn layers I–V. Projection neurons are indicated in layers I, IV, and V. These include nociceptive-specific (NS) and wide-dynamic-range (WDR) spinothalamic tract (STT) neurons as well as dorsal column postsynaptic neurons (DCPS). These neurons directly receive primary afferent excitatory input through synapses on their dendritic spines. In addition, layer I projection neurons are likely to receive excitatory input from stalked cells in layer IIa. Stalked cells are either NS (left neuron in IIa) or WDR (right neuron in IIa). Nociceptive-specific stalked cells receive their input via axodendritic synapses on their spines in layers IIa and IIb. The WDR stalked cells receive nociceptive afferent input in layers IIa and IIb as well as low-threshold mechanoreceptive input in layers III–IV. Layer V projection neurons receive interneuronal excitatory input from layer IV neurons. Several types of inhibitory interneurons, some of which are enkephalinergic (ENK), are shown and are designated in black. The layer IIa NS islet cell receives exclusive input from nociceptive afferents, and it inhibits the output of stalked cells via axoaxonic, axodendritic, dendrodendritic, and dendroaxonic synapses. The more ventral islet cell in IIb and III receives input from low-threshold mechanoreceptive afferents and inhibits the output of stalked cells via axodendritic and dendrodendritic synapses. Other inhibitory interneurons exist in layers III and IV. These are mostly low-threshold mechanoreceptive neurons.

1. Distribution and Termination of Primary Afferents

It has been proposed that the dorsoventral progression of physiological types of neurons in the dorsal horn is at least partially explicable in terms of the dorsoventral progression of the terminal arbors of the various functional categories of primary afferents (Dubner *et al.*, 1976; Gobel, 1979; see Cervero, Chapter 9). In general, primary nociceptive afferents have been shown to terminate in layers I and II (Light and Perl, 1979; Gobel, 1979; Gobel *et al.*, 1985). Some of these afferents have collaterals that arborize in lamina V. Unmyelinated polymodal nociceptive afferents are considered to terminate in layer I (Gobel *et al.*, 1981) and possibly also in layers IIa and V (see Dubner and Bennett, 1983, for review). Direct evidence for termination of Aδ high-threshold mechanoreceptive afferents in layers I and IIa come from horseradish peroxidase (HRP) injections (from the recording microelectrode) into axons of functionally identified afferents (Light and Perl, 1979). Horseradish peroxidase filled the terminal arbors of these afferents, and its reaction product was identified in layers I and IIa with both light and electron microscopic analysis.

In contrast, low-threshold mechanoreceptive primary afferents, also identified morphologically by HRP injections of their axons, terminate heavily in layers III–IV and sparsely in layer IIb (Brown *et al.*, 1977b, 1978). This differential distribution of nociceptive and nonnociceptive afferents at least partially accounts for the predominance of second-order nociceptive neurons in layers I and IIa and the predominance of low-threshold mechanoreceptive interneurons in layers III–IV (Dubner and Bennett, 1983; Gobel, 1979).

2. Distribution of Dendritic Arbors

The location and distribution of dendritic arbors of the various types of dorsal horn neurons further explain their physiological characteristics (see Gobel, 1979, for review). The dendrites of lamina I neurons are mostly confined to this layer and are distributed in a mediolateral fashion (Figure 1). Since both the terminal arborizations of primary afferents in layers I–III and the dendrites of lamina I cells occupy mediolaterally flattened territories, this organization helps account for the mediolateral somatotopic organization found among neurons of this lamina (Gobel, 1979). In contrast, the dendrites of stalked cells extend ventrally to varying extents. Some stalked cells have dendrites confined to lamina II, a site of termination of nociceptive input, whereas others have dendrites that extend as far ventrally as lamina III or IV, a site of termination of low-threshold mechanoreceptive afferents (Bennett *et al.*, 1979, 1980; Gobel, 1979; Price *et al.*, 1979). This differential extension of dendritic arbors helps to explain why the former have only nociceptive afferent input whereas the latter have both low-threshold mechanoreceptive and nociceptive afferent input (Bennett *et al.*, 1979, 1980; Gobel, 1979). Similarly, islet cells whose dendrites extend mediolaterally in lamina II have only nociceptive afferent input, whereas islet cells of lamina III and other local circuit interneurons of layers III and IV have predominantly low-threshold mechanoreceptive input (Bennett *et al.*, 1979; Dubner and Bennett, 1983). Finally, some lamina IV and V pyramidal neurons have dendrites that extend dorsally into laminae I through III (Willis, 1979; Willis *et al.*, 1979). These dendritic extensions may provide part of the basis for lamina IV and V neurons that receive both low-threshold mechanoreceptive and nociceptive afferent input.

3. Distribution of Axonal Arbors

The distribution of axonal terminals of dorsal horn interneurons also helps to explain the convergence of input on some types of dorsal horn neurons. Indeed, there appear to be two major sites within the dorsal horn where axonal interconnections provide a basis for a "cascading" or progressive increase in somatosensory input. The first site is within laminae IV–VI, and the second is within laminae I–II.

A progression of somatosensory convergence within laminae IV–VI was conceptualized in terms of a cascade model several years ago (Wall, 1967). A major tenet of this model was that lamina IV neurons excited lamina V neurons, which in turn converged on neurons of lamina VI. This model served to explain three important observations. The first was that within a given vertical microelectrode trajectory, the receptive field locations were similar among laminae IV–VI neurons. The second was that receptive field areas increased as microelectrode recordings progressed from layer IV to VI. Receptive fields of layer IV neurons were usually small and had sharply defined borders. Layer V neurons had larger receptive fields with gradients of sensitivity. Layer VI neuron receptive fields were even larger, often encompassing a major portion of a limb. Finally, excitatory convergence from different types of primary afferents increased as recordings progressed from layer IV to VI. These general findings have been corroborated in several studies of dorsal horn neurons (Price and Browe, 1975; Price *et al.*, 1976; Price and Mayer, 1975; Willis, 1979). Major consequences of this type of vertical organization include somatotopic representation and functional columns of neurons wherein the dorsal neurons tend to have modality specificity and the ventral neurons have greater convergence of input.

Propriospinal interconnections, some of which extend over several spinal cord segments, are likely to provide at least part of the anatomic basis for the model described above, especially the extensive convergence on lamina V and VI neurons (Matsushita *et al.*, 1979). The longest propriospinal connections extend from cervical to lumbar levels and originate largely from lamina V (Matsushita *et al.*, 1979; Yezierski *et al.*, 1980). Since this lamina also is a major site of origin of spinothalamic tract neurons, it seems reasonable that lamina V spinothalamic neurons are influenced by extensive intersegmental connections. This influence is consistent with the extensive receptive fields of some spinothalamic neurons.

A second and similar progression of somatosensory convergence appears to occur in laminae I–II (Gobel, 1979; Price *et al.*, 1979; Bennett *et al.*, 1980). A major excitatory interconnection is likely to exist between layer II stalked cells and layer I projection neurons (Figure 1). The evidence for this connection, like those of dorsoventrally directed connections in layers IV–VI, is indirect and is based on several anatomic and physiological studies. In one study, extracellular recordings were made of dorsoventrally adjacent pairs of neurons in layers I and II (Price *et al.*, 1979). The dorsal cell of each pair was antidromically activated from the thalamus and therefore was almost certainly a layer I neuron. The ventral cell of each pair was a histologically confirmed layer II neuron; many of these were likely to be stalked cells. It was found that the layer II neurons' pattern of primary afferent convergence was the same as or a subset of the pattern of input of the layer I neuron above it and that both neurons had very similar receptive field locations and gradients of sensitivity. It was also found that the layer II neurons usually had a smaller receptive field than did the layer I neuron above it. The layer II neuron also had a shorter first-spike latency.

A second reason that many stalked cells are likely to be excitatory begins with the observation that many layer I projection neurons are excited by activation of nociceptive afferents and by activation of low-threshold mechanoreceptive afferents (Price *et al.*, 1979; Willis, 1979). Since low-threshold mechanoreceptive afferents do not terminate directly in layer I (Gobel, 1979; Brown *et al.*, 1977b, 1978), this input must get relayed to layer I through an interneuron. The only interneuron whose axon extensively arborizes in layer I is the stalked cell. In direct corroboration of this hypothesis, stalked cells stained intracellulary with HRP have been characterized physiologically as having both nociceptive and low-threshold primary afferent inputs (Bennett *et al.*, 1979, 1980).

Finally, stalked cells but not islet cells are heavily innervated by serotonergic inhibitory synapses (Dubner *et al.*, 1983). If stalked cells were predominantly inhibitory, an effect of stimulation of serotonergic inputs to laminae I–II would be disinhibition of lamina I cells. Since only inhibition of lamina I neurons results from stimulation of descending serotonergic pathways, most stalked cells are more likely to be excitatory than inhibitory. Indeed, part of the inhibition of lamina I neurons by stimulation of serotonin pathways is likely to be indirectly mediated through inhibition of stalked cells. However, a small minority of stalked cells contain enkephalin and therefore may be inhibitory (Dubner *et al.*, 1983).

The microanatomic organization of input–output relationships described above for the spinal cord dorsal horn accounts for some of the physiological characteristics of sensory projection neurons of this region. Although these characteristics have been discussed by Cervero (Chapter 12) and in previous reviews (Price and Dubner, 1977; Dubner and Bennett, 1983; Willis, 1979), they are briefly summarized below to provide a basis for discussion of possible sensory coding mechanisms.

C. Functional Classes of Dorsal Horn Sensory Projection Neurons

There is now general agreement about major functional classes of dorsal horn sensory neurons. Although slightly different classifications are made and different names are sometimes used for the same class, dorsal horn sensory projection neurons can be divided into the following four classes.

1. Wide-Dynamic-Range Neurons

These neurons have been more extensively studied that any other class of dorsal horn neuron (see Price and Dubner, 1977; Dubner and Bennett, 1983, for reviews). Their potential involvement in pain is a critical aspect of the gate control theory (Melzack and Wall, 1965). This theory proposed that both large-diameter afferents and small-diameter afferents converged on central cells of this type and that the final output of these neurons (called T cells) was controlled by interactions between large and small fiber input and by descending pathways from the brain. Since the proposal of the gate control theory, a large body of evidence has accumulated that indicates that wide-dynamic-range (WDR) neurons contribute to the perception of pain (see Price and Dubner, 1977, for review). Most important, there is evidence that selective activation of human WDR neurons is sufficient to produce pain (Mayer *et al.*, 1975; Price and Mayer, 1975).

Wide-dynamic-range neurons exist in high concentrations in lamina V of the dorsal horn and to a lesser extent in laminae I, II, IV, and VI. Many WDR neurons in laminae I and V are spinothalamic tract neurons. Wide-dynamic-range neurons comprise approximately two-thirds of all neurons in the spinothalamic tract and are the main if not exclusive source of low-threshold mechanoreceptive input to this pathway (Price and Dubner, 1977; Giesler *et al.*, 1981; Willis, 1979). Some WDR neurons in laminae III and IV are dorsal column postsynaptic neurons and/or spinocervical tract neurons (Dubner and Bennett, 1983). The WDR neurons receive excitatory effects from impulses in both large-diameter (Aβ) sensitive mechanoreceptive afferents and in small-diameter (Aδ and C) nociceptive afferents. Receptive fields of these neurons range considerably in size but are usually much larger than those of primary afferents. They are often organized into central zones in which the neuron responds with increasingly higher frequencies of impulse discharge to gentle touch, firm pressure, and pinch and much larger zones wherein only nociceptive stimulation is effective in evoking impulse discharges

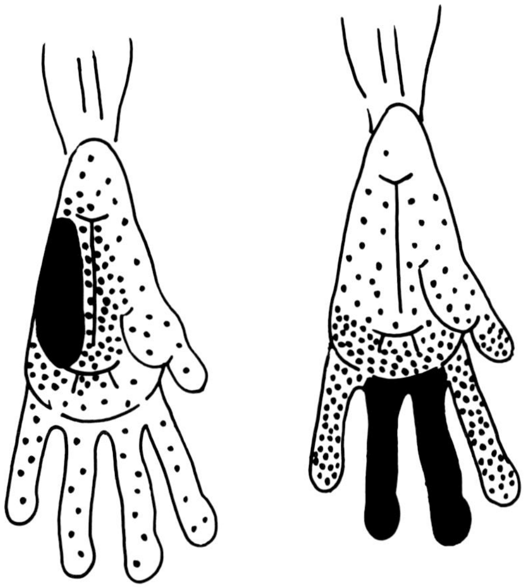

FIGURE 2. Illustration of the gradient of responsivity recorded from two different WDR neurons (left and right) observed in anesthetized monkey (Price *et al.*, 1978). The central portions of their receptive fields (darkly shaded) are most sensitive and respond with increasing frequency as the intensity of mechanical stimulation is increased from touch to pressure to pinch with toothed forceps. The more peripheral regions of the receptive fields are systematically less sensitive, responding differentially only to pressure and pinch (heavily stippled) or to pinch only (lightly stippled).

(Figure 2). Consistent with the cascade models described above (Wall, 1967), the total receptive field sizes of WDR neurons are smallest in laminae I and II, larger in lamina V, and largest in lamina VI. For example, those in laminae I and II often include a portion of a monkey's foot, those in lamina V often include most of the foot, and those in lamina VI often include the foot and a major portion of the rest of the limb (Price and Mayer, 1975; Willis, 1979).

2. *Nociceptive-Specific Neurons*

Spinal cord neurons that respond exclusively or nearly exclusively to nociceptive stimuli exist in high concentrations in the superficial layers of the dorsal horn (laminae I–II) and to a lesser extent in layers IV–V. The existence of nociceptive-specific (NS) neurons supports the specificity theory of pain, which states that pain is dependent on central neurons and pathways activated exclusively by nociceptive stimulation. Nociceptive-nspecific neurons, which comprise 20–25% of spinothalamic neurons, originate mainly in lamina I and to a lesser extent layers IV and V (Willis, 1979). The NS neurons receive exclusive excitatory effects from impulses in nociceptive afferents, most of which are slowly conducting. A major source of input to these neurons is from high-threshold Aδ mechanosensitive afferents, Aδ heat nociceptive afferents, and C polymodal nociceptive afferents. Receptive fields of these cells are usually smaller than those of WDR neurons and sometimes show a gradient of sensitivity similar to that of WDR neurons. There is a somatotopic organization of these cells within the marginal layer. For example, monkey L-7 spinothalamic neurons whose receptive fields are located on the ventral surface of the foot exist in the medial part of the dorsal horn, whereas spinothalamic cells with dorsal receptive fields are in the lateral part of the dorsal horn (Willis, 1979).

3. *Low-Threshold Mechanoreceptive Neurons*

A third general category of central neurons in the dorsal horn responds to light touch, pressure, or hair movement and appears to receive input exclusively from sensitive mechanoreceptive afferents (Price and Dubner, 1977; Dubner and Bennett, 1983). Most of these primary afferents are large myelinated Aβ afferents. Low-threshold mechanoreceptive (LTM) neurons do not respond to noxious heat or exhibit higher discharge rates to noxious than to innocuous stimuli. The LTM neurons are concentrated in laminae III–IV. Very few if any LTM neurons project in the spinothalamic tract (Giesler *et al.*, 1981; Price and Dubner, 1977; Willis, 1979), but many project in spinocervical and dorsal column postsynaptic tract pathways (Dubner and Bennett, 1983).

4. *Thermoreceptive Neurons*

Second-order neurons responding exclusively to either warming (35–43°C) or cooling (35–20°C) stimuli exist in layer I and to a lesser extent in layers III–V (Price and Dubner, 1977). They have small receptive fields and often respond as if they received exclusive input from one type of primary thermoreceptive afferent, either cold afferents or warm afferents. These neurons are likely to form an important thermoreceptive afferent system involved in perception of warmth or cooling.

D. Possible Factors in Dorsal Horn Sensory Coding Mechanisms

Given the complex neural circuitry and variety of functional types of neurons described above, it seems very unlikely that all of the messages transmitted by dorsal horn sensory projection neurons are simple analogue functions of impulse frequencies in primary afferent neurons. Indeed, anatomic and physiological studies of the last 15 years have shown that radical spatial and temporal transformations take place between inputs from primary afferent somatosensory neurons and outputs of dorsal horn sensory neurons (Melzack, 1973; Hayes *et al.*, 1979b; Price and Dubner, 1977; Price *et al.*, 1978). Moreover, it has become increasingly apparent that one must consider the profile of responses contained in populations of different types of dorsal horn neurons as well as the input–output relationships that exist for each functional type of sensory neuron. Finally, one must take into account the role of descending modulation in sensory processing.

With these considerations in mind, the following discussion represents an attempt to explain the roles of various factors in providing somatosensory messages that are interpretable by supraspinal centers. These factors include the possible roles of modality-specific neurons, composition of centrally activated neurons, spatial factors, temporal factors, and descending modulation. Finally, the question of the functional roles of ascending afferent systems is considered.

1. *Role of Modality-Specific Neurons*

There is no question that there exist sensory relay neurons within the dorsal horn that respond to a specific form of somatic stimulation and not to other types of stimulation. Thus, a single class of afferents excites a given spinal neuron. Most sensitive thermoreceptive neurons (i.e., warm- or cold-sensitive neurons), most low-threshold mechanoreceptive, and some of the nociceptive-specific neurons appear to receive input from one or only a few types of primary somatosensory afferent neurons and to have response characteristics that closely reflect restricted convergence from primary afferents. Such types of neurons thus preserve to some extent the modality specificity of the primary afferents themselves.

It is not difficult to understand how the physiological characteristics of modality-specific neurons serve to encode sensory information. Stimulus location is likely to be encoded by small receptive field areas and retained by the somatotopic organization that is known to exist within the dorsal horn (Willis, 1979). Stimulus intensity would be encoded by impulse frequencies, which are in turn closely dependent on stimulus–response relationships of the primary afferents. Finally, the recognition of different types of somatic stimuli, such as warmth, cold, touch, or nociceptive stimulation, would be served by the different central destinations of modality-specific neurons, a concept often termed "labeled lines."

Modality-specific neurons play an important role in encoding somatosensory information, and yet such a factor taken by itself would be an oversimplification of sensory coding mechanisms. As is true for other sensory modalities such as taste and smell, the variety of sensory experiences evoked by somatosensory stimuli far exceeds the limited number of possible labeled lines that could account for them. Furthermore, as is discussed below, there are many perplexing features of some somatosensory phenomena, such as painful or pleasurable body sensations, that would be very difficult to explain exclusively on the basis of modality-specific neurons or labeled lines.

2. Role of Composition of Activated Central Neurons

Although the modality-selective neurons discussed above clearly provide a straightforward method of coding, such simplicity is the exception rather than the rule. It is clear from the above discussions and the comments of Cervero (Chapter 9) that the model must be considerably more complex. Thus, electrophysiological data show that several types of afferents can innervate a given neuron. Alternatively, activation of a single type of primary afferent can simultaneously activate different classes of dorsal horn sensory projection neurons. For example, as discussed, guard hair movement activates both WDR and some LTM neurons. It is equally true that activation of different types of somatosensory primary afferent neurons can activate the same type of dorsal horn neuron. Thus, the central (supraspinal) representation of different somatosensory events may well depend largely on the coactivation of different proportions and combinations of classes of sensory projection neurons. The unique composition of centrally activated neurons could be an integral factor in distinguishing between different qualities of somatic sensations. The concept of central composition as a code for sensory qualities has been discussed extensively by Erickson (1972) and seems especially applicable to sensory coding in the dorsal horn. Indeed, Le Bars and colleagues (see Chapter 19) suggest that the content of the projected message is indeed one of the central elements.

A compelling example of why composition is an important factor is the distinction between heat-induced and mechanically induced pain. The two types of pain obviously are perceived differently. Radiant heat that raises skin temperature above 45°C activates WDR, some heat-responsive NS neurons, and thermoreceptive neurons. Needle penetration applied to the same site would activate many of the same WDR and NS neurons because spinothalamic tract neurons that respond to 45–51°C temperatures also respond to nociceptive mechanical stimulation (Kenshalo *et al.*, 1979; Price *et al.*, 1976, 1978). Thermal pain is subserved, at least in part, by a subset of sensory neurons that respond to both mechanical and thermal stimuli. On the other hand, needle penetration would additionally activate low-threshold mechanoreceptive neurons and those NS neurons that receive exclusive input from high-threshold mechanoreceptive primary afferents. Activation of WDR, LTM, and the two types of NS neurons in different proportions or combinations may be necessary for distinguishing between the unique qualities of sensations that are evoked by radiant heat and needle penetration. Even low-threshold mechanoreceptive afferents would be involved in this discrimination, because sensations evoked by needle penetration have a more burning quality after selective impulse blockade in low-threshold mechanoreceptive afferents (Price, 1972).

Another example is the distinction between first and second pain evoked by synchronous stimulation of Aδ and C nociceptive afferents (Price, 1972; Price *et al.*, 1980). The two pains have somewhat different qualities and durations and are differentially responsive to temporal parameters of stimulation. One might propose that the two pains have two separate central pathways. However, such is not the case, since Aδ and C nociceptive afferents often converge on the same dorsal horn sensory projection neurons (Chung *et al.*, 1979; Price and Browe, 1975; Price *et al.*, 1978, 1979). Although neurons with only Aδ nociceptive afferent input exist (Price *et al.*, 1976), those with only C nociceptive afferent input are extremely rare (Kumazawa and Perl, 1978). Thus, second pain is likely to be subserved by dorsal horn neurons that are also involved in first pain. However, the composition of activated dorsal horn neurons would be different for the two types of pain.

It may be evident from the foregoing two examples that the roles of central composition and modality-specific neurons are not mutually exclusive. Modality-specific neurons are likely to play an integral role in "fine tuning" sensory discriminative information. However, the diverse number of possible qualities of somatosensory sensations appears much more consistent with the possible number of unique compositions of central activated neurons than with the limited number of available labeled lines or types of sensory neurons.

3. Spatial Factors in Sensory Coding

Closely related to the concept of composition of centrally activated neurons is the idea that different somatosensory events are represented in part by different spatial distributions of centrally activated neurons. Radical spatial transformations take place between inputs from primary somatosensory afferents and outputs of dorsal horn sensory projection neurons. As described above, these transformations are related to the manner in which primary afferent input is dispersed within the dorsal horn and to the extensive axonal interconnections within the spinal gray matter. On the basis of these anatomic facts, it is not difficult to infer that different types of somatic stimuli activate different numbers of central neurons in different distributions throughout the spinal gray matter.

Spatial factors seem especially critical for the distinction between nociceptive and nonnociceptive somatosensory events. These spatial factors become evident when one considers the fact that most spinothalamic tract neurons have receptive fields that are very large compared to those of primary afferent neurons and that the receptive fields have extensive gradients of sensitivity. Consider the receptive fields of WDR neurons shown in Figure 2. They have large gradients of sensitivity wherein the area mapped by touch is much smaller than that mapped by nociceptive stimuli. Although the highest frequencies of impulse discharge are evoked by nociceptive stimulation within the most sensitive zone, a single WDR neuron may respond to touch in the most sensitive region and to pinch in the least sensitive region with the same impulse frequency. If that is the case, how can a single WDR neuron provide messages that discriminate between nociceptive and nonnociceptive events?

The answer may well be that single WDR neurons are not capable of discriminating between nociceptive and nonnociceptive events but that populations of WDR neurons can make that discrimination. The vast majority of WDR neurons have receptive fields of the type shown in Figure 2, and there is at least a general rostral–caudal somatotopic arrangement of such neurons within the dorsal horn. Given these facts, there is one simple inference that one can make about the role of spatial summation: the total number of dorsal horn sensory projection neurons activated by a nociceptive stimulus inevitably would be larger than that activated by a tactile stimulus. Touch applied to a given body site would activate only the smaller, more sensitive zones of WDR neurons receiving low-threshold mechanoreceptive input from that site. As stimulus intensities increased into the noxious range, more WDR neurons would be recruited, since this same body site lies within the less sensitive zones of other WDR neurons. For example, a gentle tactile stimulus applied to the third toe would activate the neuron whose receptive field is shown at the right in Figure 2. A mildly noxious stimulus (e.g., 45°C or pinch with fine-toothed forceps) would evoke a higher frequency impulse discharge in this neuron but would not activate the neuron whose receptive field is shown at the left (Figure 2). If the stimulus intensity extended to even higher levels (e.g., 47°C or heavy pinch), the neuron whose receptive field is shown at the left also would be recruited. This recruitment would increase the total number of central sensory neurons activated. Both the frequency of impulse discharge and the total number of central sensory neurons activated could contribute to the overall perceived intensity of somatic sensations and could provide part of the basis for discriminating between nociceptive and nonnociceptive events.

A second implication of this spatial factor in sensory coding is that painful sensations would radiate when stimulus intensities extend above pain threshold. At pain threshold, only neurons would be activated whose most sensitive receptive field regions contain the site of the stimulus. As stimulation intensity increased within the noxious range, more nociceptive neurons would be activated, since the stimulus would activate WDR neurons with very extensive receptive fields and whose most sensitive receptive field regions are remote from the actual stimulus. Such neurons would be located a few spinal segments distal to the main flow of primary afferent input. Since such neurons within the nucleus caudalis and the spinal cord dorsal horn are somatotopically organized, one might expect sensation to radiate to surrounding zones as stimulus intensities increase within the noxious range. This prediction is supported by the observation that radiation is a salient feature of suprathreshold pain. If one pinches a fold of skin on the forearm with increasing intensities, it is quite clear that the painful sensation spreads as the pinch becomes more painful. Similarly, suprathreshold heat-induced pain radiates to surrounding areas whose temperatures are in fact not elevated (Price *et al.*, 1978). Finally, radiation is a common feature of many types of clinical pain (Noordenbos, 1959; Melzack, 1973).

The work of Denny-Brown and co-workers (1972) has shown that pain is more vulnerable to a loss of central spatial summation than is touch or temperature sense. In particular, the authors showed that interruption of the descending tract of the fifth nerve or section of dorsal roots results in zones of sensory loss that are greater for pain than for touch. These analgesic zones are not constant but can be contracted by subconvulsive doses of strychnine or by small lesions of the medial portion of Lissauer's tract. They can be expanded by picrotoxin or by lesions of the lateral portion of Lissauer's tract. Thus, pain sensibility is under the control of intrinsic facilitatory and inhibitory interconnections within the spinal cord. The facilitatory connections may provide part of the basis for the widespread receptive fields with extensive gradients of sensitivity. This idea has been partly confirmed by Yokota *et al.* (1979), who found that subconvulsive doses of strychnine greatly expanded the nociceptive portions of wide-dynamic-range neuron receptive fields and that picrotoxin contracted them. Interestingly, picrotoxin expanded the tactile portion of the receptive fields (Yokota and Nishika, 1979).

Studies of pain evoked by stimulation of the cervical anterolateral quadrant (ALQ) in humans also support the idea that central spatial summation is important for the distinction between pain and tactile sensations (Mayer *et al.*, 1975). When the frequency was held constant (50 Hz), it was found that the perception of ALQ-evoked pain invariably required larger stimulus intensities and presumably activation of a larger number of ALQ axons than were required for perceptions of tingle, warmth, or cooling. The amount of spatial summation was critical, since stimulus intensities just sufficient to evoke tingle would only evoke nonpainful sensations even when stimulus frequencies extended up to 500 Hz. In contrast, when stimulus intensities were increased to activate a critical number of axons, much lower frequencies (5 to 25 Hz) evoked pain.

Therefore, different types of anatomic, physiological, neurological, and psychophysical observations converge to indicate that pain is critically dependent on central spatial summation and that this factor is also critical in encoding the distinction between nonnociceptive and nociceptive somatosensory events. Whether similar spatial factors are important for distinguishing among other somatosensory events is quite an open question.

E. Temporal Factors in Sensory Coding

1. Frequency Coding

The simplest and most obvious temporal factor in sensory coding is the encoding of stimulus intensity by impulse frequency. Dorsal horn sensory neurons have some stimulus intensity–impulse frequency relationships that are similar to those of the primary afferents that converge on them. To take one example, the relationship between 45–51°C skin temperatures and WDR neuron impulse frequency is that of a positively accelerating function that is similar to that observed for Aδ heat nociceptive and C polymodal nociceptive afferents (Price *et al.*, 1976; Price and Dubner, 1977). This temperature–WDR neuron impulse frequency relationship also is very similar to the positively accelerating power function relating 45–51°C to perceived sensation (Hoffman *et al.*, 1981; Price *et al.*, 1978, 1980, 1983). Although impulse frequencies of NS neurons also increase monotonically over 45–51°C, their responses to these stimuli do not parallel the responses of primary nociceptive afferents and human psychophysical responses (Hoffman *et al.*, 1981; Price and Mayer, 1975; Price *et al.*, 1978, 1980, 1983). Other stimulus intensity–primary afferent impulse frequency relationships undoubtedly are preserved among dorsal horn sensory neurons and could be related to human psychophysical data.

2. *Temporal Transformations*

Beyond the simple coding of stimulus intensity by impulse frequency, there are somatosensory phenomena that are dependent on radical temporal transformations of primary afferent input. These phenomena include tactile sensations and pain sensations that persist well beyond the duration of the stimulus and beyond the arrival of primary afferent impulses that evoke them (Melzack and Eisenberg, 1968; Melzack, 1973). They also include slow temporal summation of certain types of pain.

Some nonnoxious stimuli evoke prolonged afterresponses in spinothalamic neurons and aftersensations. For example, a very gentle moving tactile stimulus applied to glabrous skin of a monkey's foot will evoke 20 to 60-s afterdischarges in WDR spinothalamic neurons (Price *et al.*, 1978). These afterdischarges can be abruptly terminated by rubbing the stimulated region. Likewise, a similar stimulus applied to humans evokes a long-lasting aftersensation, which can be terminated by rubbing the stimulated area (Melzack and Eisenberg, 1968). Since low-threshold mechanoreceptive primary afferents do not have long-duration afterresponses, these responses must be generated within the dorsal horn. Interestingly, WDR neurons are the only class of dorsal horn neurons that exhibit tactile-evoked afterresponses. Second-order LTM neurons, although activated by the same primary afferents that trigger aftersensations, do not have prolonged evoked afterresponses. Thus, there may be an intriguing relationship between tactile-evoked afterresponses and pain mechanisms. Such a relationship may also partly account for certain pathological pain syndromes such as tic doloureux, wherein very gentle stimulation can evoke intense paroxysmal pain (Melzack, 1973).

Vaginal stimulation, which evokes behavioral afterresponses in cats, also evokes prolonged afterdischarges in cat dorsal horn neurons that persist long after the responses of primary afferent neurons (Price *et al.*, 1981). As for tactile-evoked afterresponses, WDR neurons are the only class of dorsal horn neurons that respond with afterdischarges to vaginal probing.

Another series of studies has shown that slow temporal summation of second pain is the result of dorsal horn summation mechanisms (Price, 1972; Price *et al.*, 1977, 1978, 1979). Controlled brief heat pulses were used to compare human psychophysical responses to first and second pain with primary afferents and spinothalamic tract neuronal responses. Peripherally, first and second pain are a consequence of synchronous activation of Aδ and C nociceptive afferents, both of which directly excite spinothalamic tract neurons. A single heat pulse (peak temp 51°C) to the skin reliably evokes first and second pain in humans and early and long-latency impulse discharges in monkey WDR and NS spinothalamic neurons (Price, 1972; Price *et al.*, 1977, 1978, 1979). The early neuronal response, like first pain, decreases in magnitude with each successive heat pulse. The late neuronal response, like second pain, increases in magnitude with each successive heat pulse. Summation of the late neuronal response and of second pain occur only with interstimulus intervals of 3 or less. Since responses of C primary nociceptive afferent neurons do not temporally summate with identical types of heat pulses, such summation must take place within the dorsal horn.

Temporal summation and extension of somatosensory signals beyond stimulus duration may be important for certain somatic sensations, especially those that have sensory, arousal, and emotional significance. Certainly, the types of afterresponses and summation described above are most often experienced as unpleasant or pleasant. That spinothalamic tract neurons participate in these different functions also is indirectly supported by the observation that interrupting the spinoreticular and spinothalamic pathways at cervical levels (i.e., anterolateral chordotomy) results in a loss not only of pain but also of other types of pleasant and unpleasant somatosensory sensations, including sexual sensations (White and Sweet, 1971). The electrophysiological observation that spinothalamic neurons have collateral axons to reticular formation nuclei and central gray (Price *et al.*, 1978) lends support to this idea, since these regions participate in arousal and autonomic nervous system functions that strongly influence affect and hence motivation.

3. *Role of Impulse Interval Patterning*

Another possible temporal factor in dorsal horn sensory coding is the coding of different types of somatosensory events by impulse interval patterning. There are two kinds of observations that tend to rule out this factor. The first is that the distribution of interspike intervals evoked in different types of dorsal horn sensory neurons does not appear to be systematically different for different types of stimuli (Brown and Franz, 1970). Thus, although the average impulse frequencies of WDR and NS neurons increase monotonically with stimulus intensity, different types of somatic stimuli such as touch, heat, or pinch do not evoke different or unique patterns of interspike intervals.

Another reason impulse-interval coding can be ruled out is based on results of studies of human sensations evoked by anterolateral quadrant (ALQ) stimulation (Mayer *et al.,* 1975). First, it is of considerable significance that sensations evoked by stimulation of the cervical ALQ were somewhat similar to those evoked by naturally occurring stimuli. Most of the reports were burning pain, but descriptions of dull aching pain, cramping, and sharp pain were also given. All of these types of pain were evoked by 50-Hz trains of regularly spaced pulses, a pattern that is not likely to be generated by natural stimuli. Therefore, these results indicate that pain is not subserved by some special temporal pattern that depends on the exact intervals of impulses in spinal cord nociceptive neurons. However, the intensity of burning, aching, or cramping pain was found to be dependent on the overall frequency in ALQ neurons over a range of 5 to 100 Hz. Tactile sensations could be evoked by lower current strengths and by trains of regularly spaced pulses of 50–500 Hz.

Although the exact interspike intervals of dorsal horn sensory neurons may not be critical in sensory coding, the overall poststimulus impulse response profiles may contribute to the distinctions among different somatosensory events. For example, the poststimulus response profiles of individual spinothalamic neurons are different for Aδ-afferent-mediated and C-afferent-mediated responses (Price *et al.,* 1978, 1979). The two responses have different latencies, durations, and peak frequencies. The brief and sharper quality of first pain as compared to second pain may well be related to the briefer and higher-frequency discharge responses of dorsal horn neurons to synchronous Aδ afferent stimulation as compared to C afferent stimulation.

F. Role of Intrinsic Modulatory Influences

Each of the sensory coding factors discussed so far is probably influenced by ongoing modulation from active controlling processes. Moreover, this modulation is based not on a single entity but rather represents a multitude of anatomically and functionally distinguishable systems that can be differentially activated. For example, as illustrated in Figure 1, descending serotonergic inputs directly contact sensory relay neurons of the dorsal horn and appear anatomically and functionally independent from segmental enkephalinergic neurons and mechanisms (Dubner *et al.,* 1983). Finally, modulation from diverse sources is not constant but shows ongoing changes that are part of the "reflex" adjustment of the gain and modality responsiveness of spinal afferent processing systems. The role of modulation in sensory coding is discussed here in light of these general considerations.

It has become evident that different types of dorsal horn sensory neurons and even different parts of the response ranges of these neurons are differentially controlled by supraspinal centers. For example, as discussed at length in Chapter 15 by Hammond, electrical stimulation of brain structures involved in stimulation-produced analgesia (midbrain central gray, raphe magnus) inhibits dorsal horn nociceptive neurons much more frequently than low-threshold mechanoreceptive neurons (Hayes *et al.*, 1979a; Willis, 1979). Similarly, systemic morphine reduces nociceptive responses of NS and WDR neurons without greatly reducing nonnociceptive responses of WDR neurons and LTM neurons (Hayes *et al.*, 1979a). On the other hand, electrical stimulation of cat sensorimotor cortex appears to inhibit low-intensity mechanoreceptive responses of LTM and WDR neurons without reducing nociceptive responses of these same neurons (Coulter *et al.*, 1974, 1976). Thus, these studies indicate that the types of somatosensory stimuli to which different classes of dorsal horn sensory neurons are sensitive are not constant but are under differential control from various supraspinal structures.

One of the limitations of studies supporting this concept is that they are based on artificial activation of endogenous systems by either electrical or pharmacological means. This raises the question of how descending modulation is manifested in awake, behaving organisms.

Perhaps the most illuminating series of studies that begin to help answer this question are those carried out by Hayes *et al.* (1981) and Hoffman *et al.* (1981). They showed that responses of medullary dorsal horn WDR and NS neurons in awake, behaving monkeys could be modulated by different attentional sets and conditions of different stimulus relevance. Receptive field zones of WDR and NS neurons expanded or contracted depending on the attentional set of the animal (Hayes *et al.*, 1981). The receptive field areas from which neural responses could be evoked by nociceptive temperatures (45–49°C) expanded during a thermal discrimination task and contracted during a visual discrimination task. In light of the role of spatial factors in sensory encoding, this result indicates that a stimulus-relevant attentional set (i.e., thermal discrimination) would have the effect of recruiting more dorsal horn sensory projection neurons. This effect, in turn, would increase the perceived intensities of 45–49°C thermal stimuli if the total number of sensory neurons activated has a role in coding nociceptive intensity.

The impulse frequencies evoked in WDR and NS by 45–49°C also can be modulated by attentional set and stimulus relevance. Their evoked impulse frequencies were found to be higher when these nociceptive thermal stimuli were preceded by a warning light as opposed when they occurred unexpectedly. Therefore, the gain of stimulus–response relationships, the number of sensory neurons activated, and hence the composition of centrally activated neurons are all under dynamic modulatory control and may have as much to do with the somatosensory perceptions of organisms as the peripheral sensory events themselves.

The psychological factors that modulate somatosensory processing at the first synapse need to be further related to their neuroanatomic and neurophysiological substrates. Likewise, the anatomic structures that have been implicated in modulation of dorsal horn neural responses need to be related to the psychological contexts under which they are activated. Clearly, much further work needs to be done in the area of descending modulation and its role in somatosensory processing.

G. *Functional Specificity of the Characteristics Associated with Outputs of the Dorsal Horn*

From the above discussion and the comments made by other contributors to this volume, it appeares certain that somatosensory events are encoded by unique spatiotemporal profiles of activated dorsal horn neurons. The number, types, and patterning of this output and subsequently the patterning of the central neurons that receive this spinal outflow are controlled by segmental and supraspinally organized modulation.

A question that remains is whether the different functional consequences of somatosensory events are represented in different outputs of the dorsal horn or whether the same coded outputs are transmitted simultaneously to different supraspinal centers. For example, it is now understood that pain is not just a sensory experience but one in which there are sensory-discriminative, arousal, and affective–motivational dimensions (Melzack and Wall, 1965; Melzack, 1973; Price and Dubner, 1977). Are these different dimensions of the experience of pain differentially represented in distinguishable outputs from the spinal cord? A similar question could be asked about other types of somatosensory events that have multiple functional consequences.

The idea of a functional separation of spinopetal systems is strongly indicated by the popular assertion that the paleospinothalamic pathway is more important for affective–motivational aspects of pain and the neospinothalamic pathway carries mainly sensory-discriminative information (Melzack, 1973). The idea is based partly on Mehler's anatomic observation (Mehler *et al.*, 1960) that anterolateral quadrant axons appear to ascend in two components in the brainstem. The medial component of this system (paleospinothalamic tract) gives off numerous collaterals to brainstem structures now thought to be involved in arousal (e.g., reticular formation structures) or affect (dorsal portion of periaqueductal gray). The lateral component (neospinothalamic tract) is said to have fewer collaterals to medial brainstem structures and to project mainly to thalamic nuclei that are involved in processing sensory-discriminative information.

Although the question of different functional subdivisions of the spinothalamic tract is still open, quite different kinds of anatomic and physiological information tend to show that different functional consequences of somatosensory input are triggered by the same types of spinothalamic neurons. First, individual spinothalamic tract WDR and NS neurons whose terminals end within medial and/or lateral somatosensory thalamic relay nuclei commonly have collateral axons to medial brainstem structures including central gray and reticular formation nuclei (Price *et al.*, 1978; Giesler *et al.*, 1981;

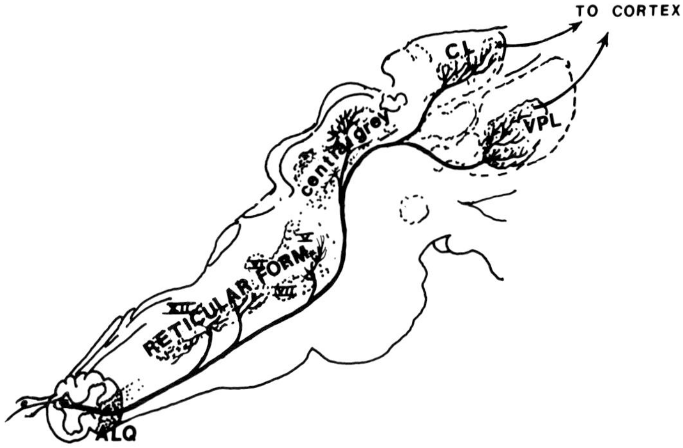

FIGURE 3. Schematic illustration of collateralization in the spinothalamic tract. This diagram is based partly on Mehler's anatomic studies (Mehler *et al.*, 1960) but emphasizes present knowledge that individual spinothalamic tract axons have collateral axons to one or more of the brainstem structures shown. VPL, N. ventroposteriolateralis; C.L., N. centralis–lateralis; Reticular form, reticular formation nuclei.

Willis, 1979). Likewise, some WDR and NS spinothalamic neurons project to both medial and lateral thalamic nuclei and are functionally similar to those that project only to lateral thalamic nuclei (Giesler *et al.*, 1981). These various patterns of spinothalamic terminations indicate that individual spinothalamic tract neurons may participate in multiple functions.

Studies of human sensations evoked by anterolateral quadrant stimulation also support the concept that spinothalamic neurons participate in multiple functions (Mayer *et al.*, 1975). First, stimulation of spinothalamic tract axons within the cervical spinal cord was shown to give rise to pain that had both sensory-discriminative and affective components. The pains evoked by ALQ stimulation were clearly aversive, although certainly tolerable. Behavioral responses and reports indicating that the pain was unpleasant (i.e., "bad," "hurts") were given without provocation or suggestion. Since the currents and frequencies were adjusted so as to activate the axons of wide-dynamic-range neurons, these indications of aversion are significant. They lead to the inference that wide-dynamic-range neurons activate central mechanisms related to the affective–motivational dimension of pain as well as the central mechanisms related to sensory discrimination.

It also has become evident that different somatosensory modalities such as touch, temperature sensibility, and nociception are uniformly represented throughout the spinothalamic system and are not represented in separate pathways. First, small lesions of the anterolateral quadrant immediately result in a restricted body zone in which all components of pain and temperature sensibility are absent and, contrary to popular notions, some aspects of tactile sensibility are altered (White and Sweet, 1971; Nathan and Smith, 1979). Second, tactile sensations can be evoked by electrical stimulation at the same anterolateral quadrant loci from which pain sensations can be evoked (Mayer *et al.*, 1975). Third, NS and WDR neuron axons are intermingled in the anterolateral quadrant in a somatotopic fashion (Applebaum *et al.*, 1975). Since these WDR neurons are the main if not exclusive source of low-threshold mechanoreceptive input to the spinothalamic system (Giesler *et al.*, 1981; Willis, 1979; Price *et al.*, 1978), such neurons are likely to be critical for nonnociceptive as well as nociceptive sensations. This inference, of course, requires the assumption that input over the spinothalamic pathway alone is sufficient to provide both tactile and nociceptive sensations. This assumption is supported by the observation that pain, temperature, and tactile sensibility (including the ability to discretely localize the site of stimulation) were preserved in a patient whose entire spinal cord was transected except for portion of the anterolateral quadrant (Noordenbos and Wall, 1976).

It is clear that one cannot easily label dorsal horn neurons or afferent systems of the dorsal horn in terms of simple functions or dichotomies. It also is evident that the spinothalamic system is not a simple sensory pathway. Rather, it is a functionally heterogeneous system that mediates sensory, arousal, and affective motivational consequences of both nociceptive and nonnociceptive somatosensory events. Other ascending output systems of the dorsal horn, including the spinocervical and dorsal column postsynaptic systems, have yet to be characterized in terms of their functional roles in primates. How different functional output messages from the dorsal horn are processed and decoded at supraspinal centers is the subject for several years of future research.

References

APPLEBAUM, A. E., BEALL, J. E., FOREMAN, R. D., AND WILLIS, W. D. Organization and receptive fields of primate spinothalamic tract neurons. *J. Neurophysiol.* 38:572–586, 1975.

BENNETT, G. J., HAYASHI, H., ABDELMOUMENE, M., AND DUBNER, R. Physiological properties of stalked cells of the substantia gelatinosa intracellularly stained with horseradish peroxidase. *Brain Res.* 164:285–289, 1979.

BENNETT, G. J., ABDELMOUMENE, M., HAYASHI, H., AND DUBNER, R. Physiology and morphology of substantia gelatinosa neurons intracellularly stained with horseradish peroxidase. *J. Comp. Neurol.* 194:809–827, 1980.

BROWN, A. G., AND FRANZ, D. N. Patterns of response in spinocervical tract neurons to different stimuli of long duration. *Brain Res.* 17:156–160, 1970.

BROWN, A. G., ROSE, P. K., AND SNOW, A. J. The morphology of spinocervical tract neurons revealed by intracellular injection of horseradish peroxidase. *J. Physiol. (Lond.)* 270:747–764, 1977a.

BROWN, A. G., ROSE, P. K., AND SNOW, P. J. The morphology of hair follicle afferent fiber collaterals in the spinal cord of the cat. *J. Physiol. (Lond.)* 272:779–797, 1977b.

BROWN, A. G., ROSE, P. K., AND SNOW, P. J. Morphology and organization of axon collaterals from afferent fibers of slowly adapting type I units in cat spinal cord. *J. Physiol. (Lond.)* 277:15–27, 1978.

CHUNG, J. M., KENSHALO, D. R., JR., GERHART, K. D., AND WILLIS, W. D. Excitation of primate spinothalamic neurons by cutaneous C-fiber volleys. *J. Neurophysiol.* 42:1354–1369, 1979.

COULTER, J. D., MAUNZ, R. A., AND WILLIS, W. D. Effects of stimulation of sensorimotor cortex on primate spinothalamic neurons. *Brain Res.* 65:351–356, 1974.

COULTER, J. D., FOREMAN, R. D., BEALL, J. E., AND WILLIS, W. D. Cerebral cortical modulation of primate spinothalamic neurons. *Adv. Pain Res. Ther.* 1:271–277, 1976.

DENNY-BROWN, D., KIRK, E. J., AND YANAGISAWA, N. The tract of Lissauer in relation to sensory transmission in the dorsal horn of the spinal cord in the macaque monkey. *J. Comp. Neurol.* 151:175–200, 1972.

DUBNER, R., AND BENNETT, G. J. Spinal and trigeminal mechanisms of nociception. *Annu. Rev. Neurosci.* 6:381–418, 1983.

DUBNER, R., GOBEL, S., AND PRICE, D. D. Peripheral and central "pain" pathways. *Adv. Pain Res. Ther.* 1:137–248, 1976.

DUBNER, R., RUDA, M. A., MILETIC, V., HOFFERT, M. J., BENNETT, G. J., NISHIKAWA, N., AND DOFFIELD, J. Neural circuitry mediating nociception in the medullary and spinal dorsal horns. *Adv. Pain Res. Ther.* 6:151–166, 1983.

ERICKSON, R. P. Parallel "population" neural coding in feature extraction, in: *The Neurosciences*, Vol. III (F. O. SCHMITT AND F. G. WORDEN, eds.), MIT Press, Cambridge, 1972, pp. 155–169.

GIESLER, G. J., JR., YEZIERSKI, R. P., GERHART, K. D., WILLIS, W. D. Spinothalamic tract neurons that project to medial and/or lateral thalamic nuclei: Evidence for a physiologically novel population of spinal cord neurons. *J. Neurophysiol.* 46:1285–1308, 1981.

GOBEL, S. Neural circuitry in the substantia gelatinosa of Rolando: Anatomical insights. *Adv. Pain Res. Ther.* 3:175–195, 1979.

GOBEL, S., FALLS, W. M., BENNETT, G. J., ABDELMOUMENE, M., HAYASHI, H., AND HUMPHREY, E. An EM analysis of the synaptic connections of horseradish peroxidase-filled stalked cells and islet cells in the substantia gelatinosa of the adult cat spinal cord. *J. Comp. Neurol.* 194:781–807, 1980.

GOBEL, S., FALLS, W. M., AND HUMPHREY, E. Morphology of ultrafine primary axons in lamina I of the spinal dorsal horn: Candidates for the terminal axonal arbors with unmyelinated (C) axons. *J. Neurosci.* 1:1163–1179, 1981.

HAYES, R. L., PRICE, D. D., RUDA, M. A., AND DUBNER, R. Suppression of nociceptive reflexes in the primate by electrical stimulation of the brain or morphine administration: Behavioral and electrophysiological comparisons. *Brain Res.* 167:417–421, 1979a.

HAYES, R. L., PRICE, D. D., AND DUBNER, R. Behavioral and physiological studies of sensory coding and modulation of trigeminal nociceptive input. *Adv. Pain Res. Ther.* 3:219–243, 1979b.

HAYES, R. L., DUBNER, R., AND HOFFMAN, D. S., Neuronal activity in medullary dorsal horn of awake monkeys trained in a thermal discrimination task II: Behavioral modulation of responses to thermal and mechanical stimuli. *J. Neurophysiol.* 46:428–443, 1981.

HOFFMAN, D. S., DUBNER, R., HAYES, R. L., AND MEDLIN, T. P. Neuronal activity in medullary dorsal horn of awake monkeys trained in a thermal discrimination task I: Responses to innocuous and noxious thermal stimuli. *J. Neurophysiol.* 46:409–427, 1981.

KENSHALO, D. R., JR., LEONARD, R. B., CHUNG, J. M., AND WILLIS, W. D. Responses of primate spinothalamic neurons to graded and to repeated noxious heat stimuli. *J. Neurophysiol.* 42:1370–1389, 1979.

KUMAZAWA, T., AND PERL, E. R. Excitation of marginal and substantia gelatinosa neurons in the primate spinal cord: Indications of their place in dorsal horn functional organization. *J. Comp. Neurol.* 177:417–434, 1978.

LIGHT, A. R., AND PERL, E. R. Differential termination of large-diameter and small-diameter primary afferent fibers in the spinal dorsal grey matter as indicated by labelling with horseradish peroxidase. *J. Comp. Neurol.* 186:117–139, 1979.

MATSUSHITA, M., MICHIKO, I., AND HOSODA, Y., The location of spinal neurons with long descending axons in the cat: A study with the horseradish peroxidase technique. *J. Comp. Neurol.* 184:63–80, 1979.

MAYER, D. J., PRICE, D. D., AND BECKER, D. P. Neurophysiological characterization of the anterolateral spinal cord neurons contributing to pain perception in man. *Pain* 1:51–58, 1975.

MEHLER, W. R., FETERMAN, M. E., AND NAUTA, W. J. H. Ascending axon degeneration following anterolateral cordotomy. An experimental study in the monkey. *Brain* 83:718–750, 1960.

MELZACK, R. *The Puzzle of Pain,* Basic Books, New York, 1973.

MELZACK, R., AND EISENBERG, H. Skin sensory afterflows. *Science* 351:445–449, 1968.

MELZACK, R., AND WALL, P. D. Pain mechanisms: A new theory. *Science* 150:971–979, 1965.

NATHAN, P. W., AND SMITH, M. C. Clinico-anatomical correlation in anterolateral cordotomy. *Adv. Pain Res. Ther.* 3:921–926, 1979.

NOORDENBOS, W. *Pain,* Elsevier, Amsterdam, 1959.

NOORDENBOS, W. AND WALL, P. D. Diverse sensory functions with an almost totally divided spinal cord. A case of spinal cord transection with preservation of part of one anterolateral quadrant. *Pain* 2:185–195, 1976.

PRICE, D. D. Characteristics of second pain and flexion reflexes indicative of prolonged central summation. *Exp. Neurol.* 37:371–391, 1972.

PRICE, D. D., AND BROWE, A. C. Responses of spinal cord neurons to graded noxious and non-noxious stimuli. *Exp. Neurol.* 48:201–221, 1975.

PRICE, D. D., AND DUBNER, R. Neurons that subserve the sensory-discriminative aspects of pain. *Pain* 3:307–338, 1977.

PRICE, D. D., AND MAYER, D. J. Neurophysiological characterization of the anterolateral quadrant neurons subserving pain in *M. Mulatta. Pain* 1:59–72, 1975.

PRICE, D. D., DUBNER, R., AND HU, J. W. Trigeminothalamic neurons in nucleus caudalis responsive to tactile, thermal, and nociceptive stimulation of monkey's face. *J. Neurophysiol.* 39:936–953, 1976.

PRICE, D. D., HU, J. W., DUBNER, R., AND GRACELY, R. H. Peripheral suppression of first pain and central summation of second pain evoked by noxious heat pulses. *Pain* 3:57–68, 1977.

PRICE, D. D., HAYES, R. L., RUDA, M. A., AND DUBNER, R. Spatial and temporal transformations of input to spinothalamic tract neurons and their relation to somatic sensation. *J. Neurophysiol.* 41:933–947, 1978.

PRICE, D. D., HAYASHI, H., DUBNER, R., AND RUDA, M. A. Functional relationships between neurons of marginal and substantia gelatinosa layers of primate dorsal horn. *J. Neurophysiol.* 42:1590–1608, 1979.

PRICE, D. D., BARRELL, J. J., AND GRACELY, R. H. A psychological analysis of experiential factors that selectively influence the affective dimension of pain. *Pain* 8:137–150, 1980.

PRICE, D. D., BUSHNELL, M. C., AND IADAROLA, M. J. Responses of primary afferents and sacral spinal cord neurons to vaginal probing in the cat. *Neurosci. Lett.* 26:67–73, 1981.

PRICE, D. D., MCGRATH, P. A., RAFII, A., AND BUCKINGHAM, B. The validation of visual analogue scales as ratio scale measures for chronic and experimental pain. *Pain* 17:45–56, 1983.

WALL, P. D. The physiological laminar organization of the dorsal horn. *J. Physiol. (Lond.)* 188:403–425, 1967.

WHITE, A. R., AND SWEET, W. C. *Pain and the Neurosurgeon: A Forty Year Experience,* Charles C. Thomas, Springfield, IL, 1971, p. 333.

WILLIS, W. D. Physiology of dorsal horn and spinal cord pathways related to pain, in: *Mechanisms of Pain and Analgesia Compounds* (R. F. BEERS, JR. AND E. G. BASSETT, eds.), Raven Press, New York, 1979, pp. 143–156.

WILLIS, W. D., KENSHALO, D. R., JR., AND LEONARD, R. B. The cells of origin of the spinothalamic tract. *J. Comp. Neurol.* 188:543–574, 1979.

YEZIERSKI, R. P., CULBERSON, J. L., AND BROWN, P. B. Cells of origin of propriospinal connections to cat lumbosacral grey as determined with horseradish peroxidase. *Exp. Neurol.* 69:493–512, 1980.

YOKOTA, T., AND NISHIKAWA, Y. Action of picrotoxin upon trigeminal subnucleus caudalis in the monkey. *Brain. Res.* 171:369–373, 1979.

YOKOTA, T., NISHIKAWA, N., AND NISHIKAWA, Y. Effects of strychnine upon different classes of trigeminal subnucleus caudalis neurons. *Brain Res.* 168:430–434, 1979.

19
Aspects of Sensory Processing through Convergent Neurons

DANIEL LE BARS, ANTHONY H. DICKENSON, JEAN MARIE BESSON, AND LUIS VILLANUEVA

A. *Introduction*

The spinal mechanisms of nociception are generally interpreted in terms of a single-channel transmission system, the gain of which can be modulated by inhibitory processes from both spinal and supraspinal origins. This interpretation is based on the intuitive supposition that neurons putatively involved in a sensory-discriminative nociceptive system might exhibit, in nonpathological conditions, their highest frequencies of firing when noxious stimuli are applied to their receptive fields.

Several criteria appear necessary to be fulfilled before a spinal neuron can be implicated in the processes that lead to the recognition of a nociceptive stimulus as being painful (Table I): (1) the discrimination of nociceptive from nonnociceptive information, (2) the encoding of the intensity of nociceptive stimuli, (3) the transmission of nociceptive information towards the brain, and (4) that any reduction in neuronal activity might be associated or correlated with hypoalgesia phenomena.

These criteria are rather more complex than would seem at first sight. The interpretation of the first two could be altered by the activation of modulatory mechanisms at any time. The third criterion, although satisfied by the demonstration that the particular neuron sends axons toward the higher

DANIEL LE BARS, JEAN MARIE BESSON, AND LUIS VILLANUEVA • Research Unit of Pharmacological Neurophysiology of Inserm (U. 161), Paris 75014, France. ANTHONY H. DICKENSON • Department of Pharmacology, University College, London WC1E 6BT, England.

TABLE I
Criteria That a Dorsal Horn Neuron Should Fulfill to Be a Candidate for a Role in Nociception

Criteria	Nociceptive-specific neurons	Convergent neurons
Main criteria		
Discrimination between nociceptive and nonnociceptive information (criterion 1)	+ +	− −
Encoding of the the intensity of nociceptive stimuli (criterion 2)	±[a]	+ +[b]
Transmission towards the brain (criterion 3)	+ +	+ +
Reduction in activity correlated with hypoalgesia phenomena (criterion 4)	+[a]	+ +[b]
Supplementary criteria		
Visceral convergence	+[a]	+ +[b]
Muscular convergence	?	+ +
Activation by algogenic agents	?	+ +
Correlation with psychophysical observations (e.g., "wind up")	?	+ +

[a] Poorly documented.
[b] Heavily documented.

centers of the CNS, cannot exclude the involvement of polysynaptic pathways in nociceptive transmission; electrophysiological and anatomic techniques cannot resolve the existence of these latter pathways even when they consist of the simplest pathways with a single synapse.

B. Classes of Spinal Nociceptive Neurons

Two main categories of neuron responding to nociceptive stimuli have been characterized by the many electrophysiological studies on the dorsal horn of the spinal cord and the nucleus caudalis of the trigeminal complex: the first class are specifically activated by nociceptive stimuli (Christensen and Perl, 1970); the second respond in a nonexclusive way (Wall, 1960).

1. Nociceptive-Specific Neurons

This class of neuron, initially described in lamina I of the cat, has been further confirmed in several species. Cells of this type have been reported in the substantia gelatinosa and, to a lesser degree, in the deeper laminae. These cells are exclusively activated by noxious cutaneous mechanical and/or thermal stimuli activating A and/or C fibers. In general, nociceptive-specific neurons have discrete receptive fields that often have gradients of sensitivity (Price and Mayer, 1974; Willis *et al.*, 1974). At the level of lamina I, a somatotopic organization of the receptive fields exists both in the spinal cord (Price and Mayer, 1974; Willis *et al.*, 1974; Cervero *et al.*, 1976) and the nucleus caudalis of the trigeminal complex (see Dubner *et al.*, Chapter 13).

This class of neuron, by merit of its exclusive activation by intense or nociceptive peripheral stimuli (criterion 1), is a cornerstone of theories of specificity. The single modality of input, restricted receptive fields, and, furthermore, the somatotopic organization indicate that these neurons are suitable for signaling spatial and temporal indices of nociceptive information. Recent results from the awake, unrestrained monkey are in general agreement with a role for these cells in the analysis of location of noxious stimuli (Hayes *et al.*, 1979a; Hoffman *et al.*, 1981). However, it is essential to stress that despite this exclusive nociceptive input to these cells, their ability to code the intensity of stimuli (criterion 2), particularly thermal stimuli (Hoffman *et al.*, 1981), seems weak. Consequently, these neurons only partially fulfill criterion 2.

By contrast, the neurons in this class meet criterion 3, as it is well established that information emanating from these cells passes in several ascending tracts, particularly those that terminate in the ventrobasal thalamus (see Willis, Chapter 11).

Evidence for the fourth criterion is less extensive for this neuronal type. However, there is evidence for a reduction in the responses of certain of these nociceptive specific cells by maneuvers that reduce reactions to a noxious stimulus: transcutaneous electrical stimulation (Cervero *et al.*, 1976), dorsal column stimulation (Foreman *et al.*, 1976), brainstem stimulation (Hayes *et al.*, 1979b; Gerhart *et al.*, 1981a; Yezierski *et al.*, 1982), and systemic morphine (Hayes *et al.*, 1979b; Le Bars *et al.*, 1980) all reduce the activity of some of these cells.

It seems clear from these studies that the functional role of these neurons is related to the discriminative aspects of pain intensity but probably more to the location and nature of the stimulus. Their exclusive responsivity to noxious cutaneous stimuli makes a role in processes other than nociception unlikely. The recent report of a visceral convergence onto a few of these neurons is further evidence of their importance (see Foreman, Chapter 10; Foreman *et al.*, 1981; Milne *et al.*, 1981), although as yet there is no evidence for nociceptive muscle afferents onto these cells.

2. *Convergent Neurons*

These cells form a high proportion of the neurons recorded in the dorsal horn and in the nucleus caudalis of the trigeminal complex. They are characterized above all by their capacity to respond to various nociceptive stimuli and also to mechanical stimuli of weak intensity. Various authors have classified these cells as common carriers (Wall, 1960), trigger cells (Melzack and Wall, 1965), wide-dynamic-range cells (Mendell, 1966), lamina V type (Wall,

1967), class 2 cells (Iggo, 1974), polymodal cells (Zimmermann, 1977), and multireceptive cells (see Brown and Réthelyi, 1981). Without recourse to semantics on the taxonomy of the dorsal horn cells, we prefer to denote these neurons as convergent, as their major characteristic seems to be a marked convergence of various excitatory and inhibitory influences.

Studies in the cat (Wall, 1967) have emphasized the concentration of this type of cell in a zone centered on lamina V (nomenclature of Rexed, 1954), although cells were also located in lamina IV or VI. Similarly, in nucleus caudalis of the trigeminal complex, these cells have been frequently encountered in the deep layers of the magnocellular region (see Dubner *et al.*, Chapter 13). However, it is now apparent that these neurons also exist in the most superficial layers of the dorsal horn (Handwerker *et al.*, 1975; Cervero *et al.*, 1976; Giesler *et al.*, 1976; Menétrey *et al.*, 1977; Price *et al.*, 1978, 1979; Bennett *et al.*, 1979, 1980).

Convergent neurons usually have excitatory peripheral fields larger than those of the nociceptive-specific neurons, although they are still compatible with a reasonable degree of stimulus location (Willis, 1981). As noted by many authors, the capability of encoding the intensity of noxious stimuli (criterion 2) is most often verified when studied with a single modality of stimulus and under standardized temporal conditions: examples are the graded responses to temperature (Handwerker *et al.*, 1975; Price and Browe, 1975; Kenshalo *et al.*, 1979; Menétrey *et al.*, 1979) or the increasing discharges to mechanical stimuli applied to the receptive fields (Mendell and Wall, 1965; Mendell, 1966; Wall, 1967; Hillman and Wall, 1969; Wagman and Price, 1969). Studies in the awake monkey again illustrate the ability of these neurons to code noxious stimuli (Hoffman *et al.*, 1981). Furthermore, these neurons are strongly activated by the administration of algogenic compounds into the arterial supply of the body area containing the receptive field (Besson *et al.*, 1972, 1975; Levante *et al.*, 1975).

By using direct nerve stimulation, it is possible to ascertain the afferent fiber groups activating the neuron. Convergent cells receive Aα-, Aδ-, and C-fiber inputs (Wagman and Price, 1969; Price and Wagman, 1970; Price *et al.*, 1971; Gregor and Zimmermann, 1972). The application of repetitive electrical stimuli at C-fiber strength frequently produces the phenomenon of "wind up" (Mendell, 1966; Price and Wagman, 1970), which consists of a progressive increase in discharge with each stimulus. This effect is reminiscent of certain observations in humans, where repetitive stimuli produce an increasing sensation of pain (see Price, Chapter 18).

Sidestepping the issue of the ascending tracts involved in nociceptive processing, we should note that numerous convergent neurons have been identified by antidromic activation techniques as giving rise to ascending axons (criterion 3). These cells are involved in the spinothalamic, spinoreticular, and spinocervical tracts (see Willis, Chapter 11). In a recent review, Willis (1982) has considered the percentages of different neurons projecting in the spinothalamic tract of the monkey from three separate studies: 55% of the total were convergent cells, 32% were nociceptive specific, and the rest were either cells activated by innocuous mechanical stimuli (2%) or cells with deep receptive fields (11%).

Most of the procedures that result in hypoalgesia or analgesia in humans also result in a reduction in the responses of convergent cells to noxious stimulus (criterion 4): these include systemic (Kitahata *et al.*, 1974; Le Bars *et al.*, 1975, 1976, 1979c; Calvillo *et al.*, 1979; Johnson and Duggan, 1981; Woolf and Fitzgerald, 1981) or intrathecal (Homma *et al.*, 1983) morphine, dorsal column stimulation (Hillman and Wall, 1969; Handwerker *et al.*, 1975; Foreman *et al.*, 1976; Lindblom *et al.*, 1977), transcutaneous electrical stimulation (Mendell, 1966; Wagman and Price, 1969; Price and Wagman, 1970; Gregor and Zimmermann, 1972; Brown *et al.*, 1973; Handwerker *et al.*, 1975; Cervero *et al.*, 1976), and stimulation of periaqueductal and periventricular structures (Guilbaud *et al.*, 1972; Liebeskind *et al.*, 1973; Oliveras *et al.*, 1974; Carstens *et al.*, 1979, 1980, 1981; Duggan and Griersmith, 1979; Hayes *et al.*, 1979b; Yezierski *et al.*, 1982).

In addition, an important property of these convergent cells, in the light of the frequent incidence in clinical practice of pain originating from muscle and visceral structures, is their activation by stimuli to these structures. Viscero-somatic convergence has been demonstrated by visceral afferent nerve stimulation, injection of algogenic compounds into the mesenteric circulation, and nociceptive stimuli applied to the heart, bladder, and testicle (see Foreman, Chapter 10). This property of the convergent cells may represent the functional basis for referred pain (Ruch, 1949, 1979). Convergent cells are, furthermore, equally well activated by nociceptive muscle afferents (Pomeranz *et al.*, 1968; Foreman *et al.*, 1977, 1979; Kniffki *et al.*, 1977; Hong *et al.*, 1979).

The first criterion (criterion 1: discrimination of nociceptive from non-nociceptive information) has not yet been discussed for these convergent cells, as we believe an important problem exists, as illustrated by the example in Figure 1. This convergent neuron increased its discharge rate in relation to the heating steps applied to the center of its receptive field and gave maximal discharges when the stimulus intensities reached the noxious range. The observation illustrates the capability of this neuron to code noxious thermal information (see above). However, as illustrated on the right of Figure 1, extremely high levels of firing could also be produced by repetitive innocuous stimulation of the same area. This finding was systematically confirmed in a recent study performed on 30 convergent neurons in the rat (Le Bars and Chitour, 1983). Along the same lines, it has been reported (Price *et al.*, 1976) that in trigeminal nucleus caudalis of the monkey, the firing frequencies of convergent neurons evoked by 44–48°C radiant heat application could often also be attained by innocuous mechanical stimuli, but such an observation was attributed to the effects of anesthetics. However, our observations in the rat (Le Bars and Chitour, 1983) were identical in the anesthetized "intact" animal

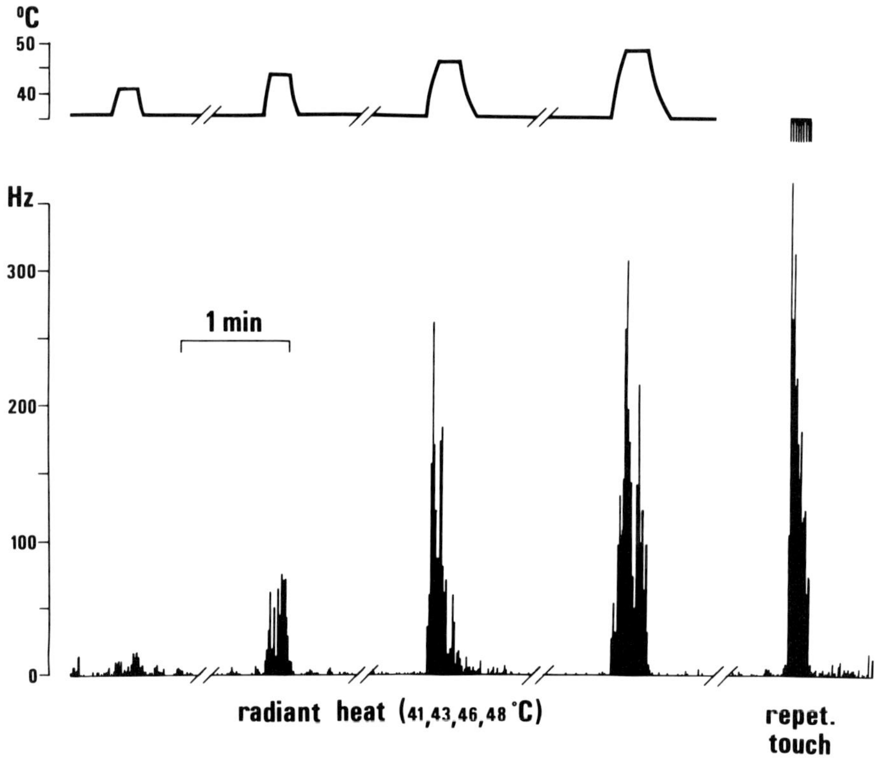

FIGURE 1. Rate meter record of a lumbar convergent neuron studied in the rat. The four sequences to the left show the responses of the neuron to radiant heat application (heating steps depicted above) to its peripheral excitatory field; note that the neuron responded in the noxious range with an increasing firing rate as the applied temperature was increased. A response of the neuron evoked by a repetitive innocuous stimulus (light pressure applied by means of a blunt probe) is shown on the extreme right; note the high level of firing achieved with this stimulus. (From Le Bars and Chitour, 1983.)

and in the unanesthetized "spinal" animal, suggesting that the level of anesthesia is not an explanation.

Thus, convergent neurons largely fulfill the last three principal criteria (Table I), which seem to be requirements for a role of a neuron in nociception. Adding the further complementary criteria in Table I, the conclusions seem to strongly support the proposition that convergent neurons are of great importance in the transmission of nociceptive information towards the higher centers.

With regard to the first criterion, it has been long known that convergent cells respond to stimuli ranging from weak to intense. Although the increasing neuronal responses with increasing stimuli applied in standardized conditions indicate a role in nociception (criterion 2), we consider this criterion insufficient, since it is hard to ignore the relationships between the temporal occurrence of somatic stimuli and the resultant organization of the neuronal responses and, furthermore, the differences between the discharges evoked by different sensory modalities. Hence, since noxious stimuli do not obviously occur in a standardized fashion in normal (nonexperimental) environmental conditions, a rather more precise definition of the first criterion would also include that all nociceptive stimuli produce a neuronal discharge greater than any form of nonnoxious stimulus whatever the nature and duration of both types of stimulus (criterion 1). As shown in Figure 1, this is clearly not the case for convergent cells.

If, however, one accepts that convergent neurons participate in the transfer of information from nociceptors to the higher centers, these studies indicate that the intensity of discharge cannot alone provide information on the nociceptive character of the stimulus. In other words, the proposition that "the signal which triggers the action system responsible for pain experience and response occurs when the output of the trigger cells reaches or exceeds a critical level" (Melzack and Wall, 1965) is unlikely, at least in terms of frequency of discharge of the cells. It must be stressed that the responses to innocuous stimuli consist of high-frequency bursts of activity; this point has been raised by Melzack and Wall (1965), who stated:

> We presume that the action system requires a definite time period for integrating the total input from the trigger cells. Small, fast variations of the temporal pattern produced by the trigger cells might be ineffective, and the smoothed envelope of the frequency of impulses—which contains information on the rate of rise and fall, the duration, and the amplitude of firing—would be the effective stimulus that initiates the appropriate sequence of activities in the cells that comprise the action system (see also Wall, 1973, 1978).

Equally, one cannot reject other theories of varying complexities proposing patterns of discharge in the processing of painful information.

C. Complex Mechanisms for Information Coding

It is possible that the significant messages from the dorsal horn result from simultaneous activity in several neuronal classes. The activity transmitted by the convergent cells might then serve a role as a comparison signal, aiding the extraction of certain qualities of sensation from messages emanating from cells activated by innocuous mechanical stimuli or nociceptive-specific neurons. Several systems exist that might subserve the modulatory processes mediating the extraction of the sensory message. They can be considered as (1) those that involve segmental interactions, (2) propriospinal, and (3) a more generalized system involving supraspinal centers, which is essentially based on the concept of diffuse noxious inhibitory controls (DNIC).

These hypotheses are not mutually exclusive.

1. Role of Segmental Convergence

As pointed out by many authors, the excitatory receptive fields of convergent neurons often show a gradient of responsiveness, with the center responding to both noxious and innocuous stimuli and the remaining area responding only to strong stimuli (Wall, 1967; Wall *et al.*, 1967; Hillman and Wall, 1969; Applebaum *et al.*, 1975; Menétrey *et al.*, 1977; Price *et al.*, 1977, 1978; See Willis, Chapter 11, and Cervero, Chapter 9). It is commonly observed that the "center" is restricted in comparison with the remaining area (Figure 2A). In view of this, as already proposed (Hillman and Wall, 1969; Price *et al.*, 1978), an innocuous stimulus would excite a few neurons, whereas a noxious one applied on the same somatic area would excite all the neurons showing an overlapping of receptive fields (Figure 2B); one could therefore easily imagine that pain processes are triggered when a liminal number of neurons reach a liminal firing rate. At that stage, one could argue on the basis of such a hypothesis that the multiplication of innocuous stimuli applied over a large area, including a sufficient number of "centers" of receptive fields, would induce pain. No such observation has been made, at least in nonpathological conditions.

Nevertheless, this hypothesis cannot be rejected, since many convergent neurons also have an adjacent inhibitory receptive field distinct from the excitatory one. The majority of mechanical stimuli applied to this inhibitory field, particularly weak repetitive stimuli, are able to inhibit convergent neuronal activity (Wall, 1967; Hillman and Wall, 1969; Wagman and Price, 1969; Besson *et al.*, 1974).

This is illustrated in Figure 3A, where the firing of a convergent neuron induced by a sustained pinch applied in the center of its excitatory field was strongly depressed by light repetitive touch applied in its inhibitory receptive field. The natural stimulation within the cutaneous inhibitory receptive field was found equally potent in blocking neuronal phasic discharges induced by microelectrophoretic injection of glutamate (Figure 3B). Since it is generally well accepted that the major part of intense neuronal firing seen during glutamate application results from a direct drug action on cell bodies (Curtis

FIGURE 2. Theoretical spatial organization of the excitatory receptive fields of convergent neurons. A: Noxious stimuli applied to any part of the excitatory receptive field excite convergent neurons, whereas the "center" (black area) is sensitive to both noxious and innocuous stimuli (experimental conditions in which a single neuron is recorded). B: In fact, because of the overlapping of fields, a noxious stimulus is applied not only to the centers of a certain number of receptive fields (e.g., area 1) but also to the edges of other receptive fields (e.g., those receptive fields centered on areas 2, 3, and 4), with the resulting activation of a large number of convergent neurons. The application of an innocuous stimulus to the same area (1) would only affect those receptive fields centered on that area and would result in the firing of fewer neurons. (From Le Bars and Chitour, 1983.)

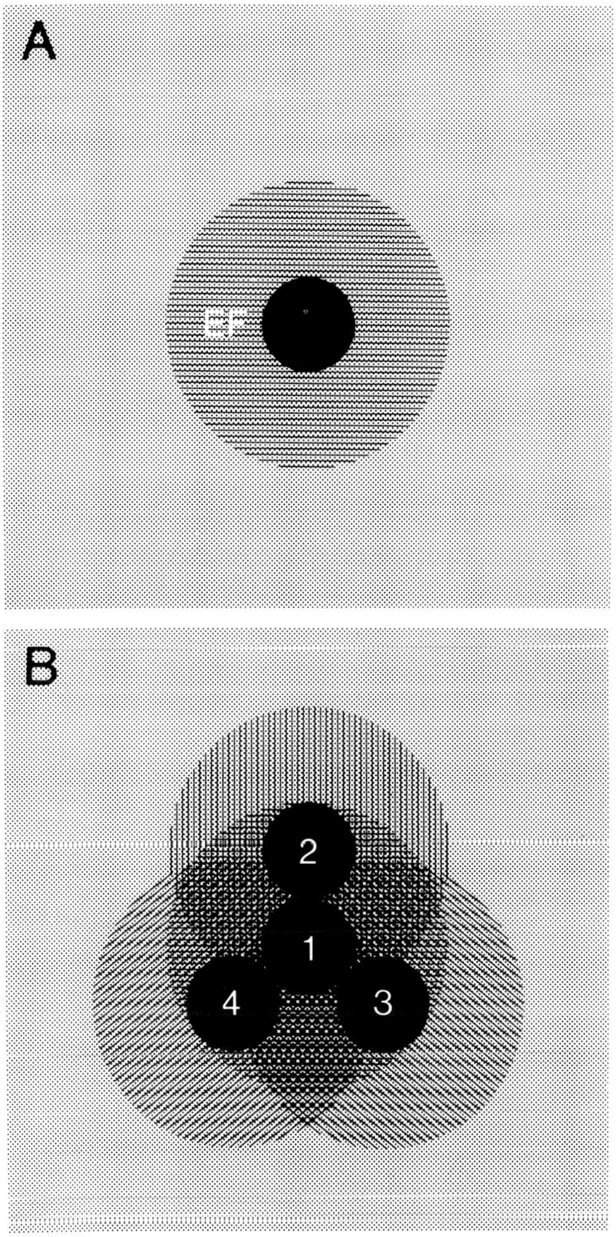
A
EF
B
2
1
4
3

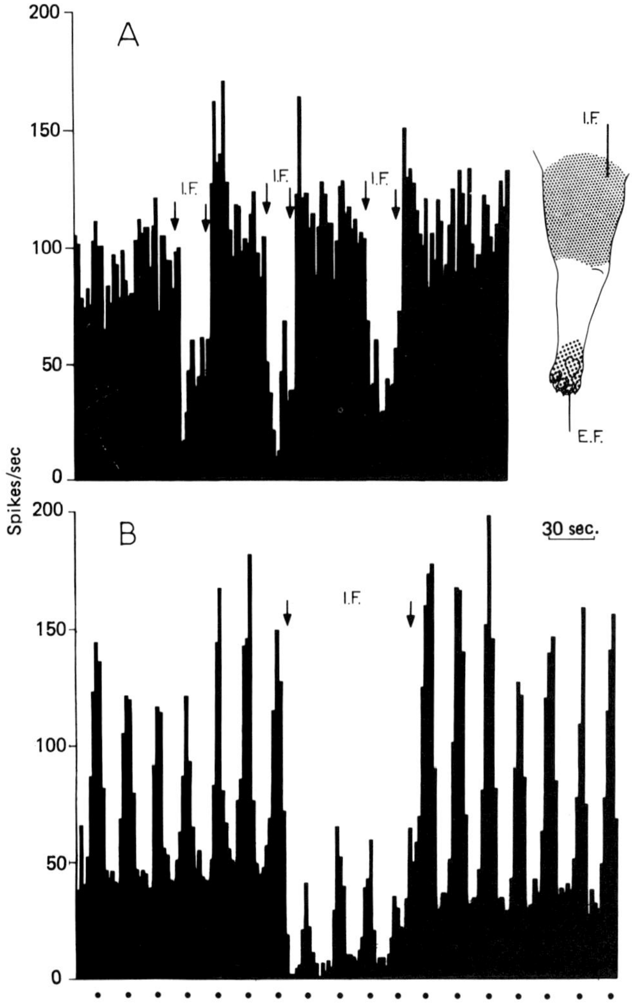

FIGURE 3. Rate meter record of a lumbar convergent neuron studied in the cat: synaptically mediated and chemically induced firing, which is influenced by natural stimulation within an inhibitory receptive field. The positions of excitatory (EF) and inhibitory (IF) receptive fields on the hindlimb are shown. A: Firing frequency chart recording showing tonic discharge in response to sustained pinch in the excitatory field and interruption of discharge while the inhibitory field is stimulated (between arrows). B: Firing depression by inhibitory field stimulation (IF) of glutamate-evoked phasic discharges (peaks) on top of tonic discharge (about 50 spikes/s) induced synaptically during maintained pinch in the excitatory field. Circles indicate the sequence of periodic injections of glutamate by 10-s and 25-nA current pulses. (From Besson *et al.*, 1974.)

and Watkins, 1960; Krnjević and Phillis, 1963; Galindo *et al.*, 1967, 1968; see Puil, 1981), such an observation suggests the existence of inhibitory postsynaptic potentials in response to natural stimulation within the cutaneous inhibitory receptive field. This assertion is strongly supported by the type of observation illustrated in Figure 4.

These experiments, although they do not exclude the existence of presynaptic inhibitions produced by stimulation of the inhibitory receptive fields, demonstrate the strength of these postsynaptic inhibitions. If one refers to the theoretical model in Figure 5A, one could see that the inhibitory fields could restrict the efficacy of such stimuli by reducing the firing of a large number of convergent neurons (Figure 5B). The fact that inhibitory receptive fields are generally larger than the excitatory ones supports this functional potency. It is worth emphasizing the fact that such a view is fully compatible with the proposal (Noordenbos, 1959; Melzack and Wall, 1965) of an interaction between nociceptive and nonnociceptive messages at the spinal level and is therefore supported by the relevant clinical data.

In addition to the hypothesis of local controls acting to alter or restrict the modalities of information emanating from convergent neurons, a second scheme can be put forward whereby a clear nociceptive message is somehow extracted from the output of the whole population of convergent neurons. This is discussed in the following sections.

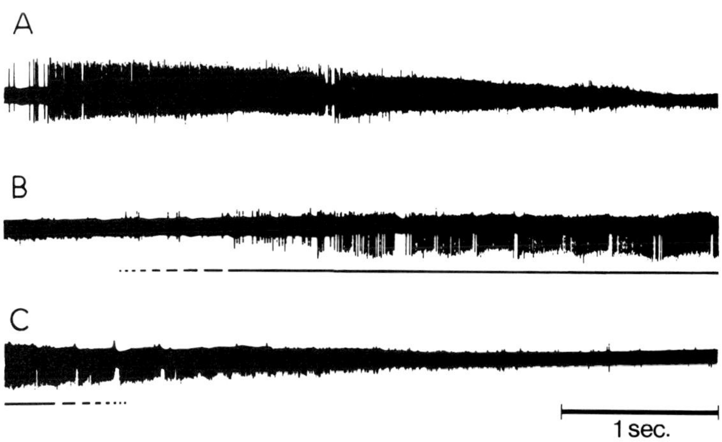

FIGURE 4. Hyperpolarizing effect of natural stimulation within the inhibitory receptive field. A: Neuronal firing induced by a continuous injection of 110 nA of glutamate with final firing blockade by excessive depolarization (Curtis *et al.*, 1960). B, C: Glutamate injection was maintained and the firing restored (B) by stimulation of the inhibitory receptive field (horizontal lines); renewal of firing blockade (C) when stimulation of inhibitory receptive field is withdrawn. (From Besson *et al.*, 1974.)

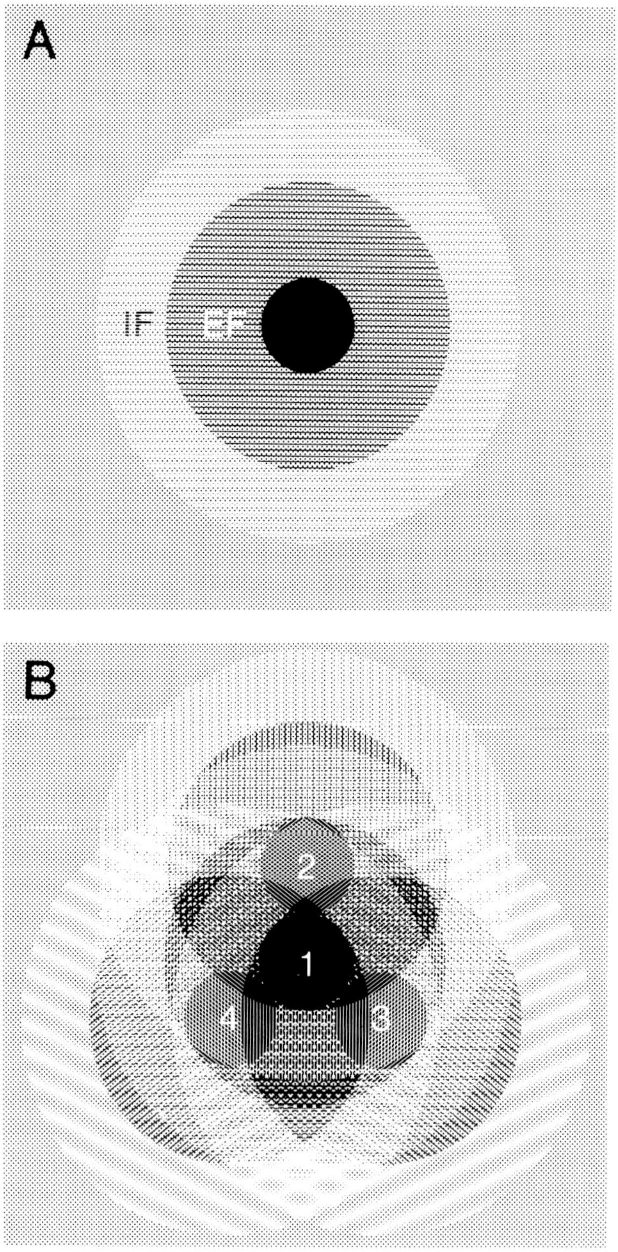

FIGURE 5. Theoretical spatial organization of the excitatory and inhibitory receptive fields of convergent neurons. A: In addition to an excitatory receptive field (EF), convergent neurons often show a surrounding inhibitory field (IF, white area) mainly activated by nonnoxious stimuli. B: The application of innocuous stimuli on a wide surface of the body would not only affect the centers of excitatory fields (e.g., areas 1, 2, 3, and 4) but also several inhibitory fields, thus resulting in an attenuation of the global response. (From Le Bars and Chitour, 1983.)

2. *Propriospinal Inhibitory Mechanisms Triggered by Noxious Stimuli*

In addition to the excitatory and inhibitory influences of segmental origin that we have reported above, there is evidence that convergent neurons can be inhibited by nociceptive stimuli applied to areas of the body remote from the excitatory and inhibitory fields. These effects are mediated by various mechanisms, one of which involves supraspinal structures and is described in the following section devoted to diffuse noxious inhibitory controls (DNIC); the second involves propriospinal mechanisms (Cadden *et al.*, 1983), since such inhibitions could be observed in the dorsal horn of spinal animals. In both cases, inhibitions are only triggered by noxious stimuli.

Examples of results obtained from four neurons in spinal rats are shown in Figure 6. It can be seen from these examples that the inhibitions, when present, were relatively weak and generally of shorter duration than the conditioning period. The inhibitions in spinal unanesthetized rats were observed on fewer than half of the convergent neurons studied and were more often produced by stimulation of parts of the body proximal to the excitatory receptive field than by stimulation of more distal structures. These effects were less powerful than those in the intact animal (see below), generally adapted rapidly, and were never followed by posteffects. In addition, it was found that although inhibitions could repeatedly be produced for a given cell, the strength of these inhibitions exhibited a noticeable variability.

These findings in the spinal preparation are in keeping with the earlier reports of Gerhart *et al.* (1981b) in the monkey and of Fitzgerald (1982) in the rat. In view of the marked differences between the inhibitions observed in intact animals (see below) and those observed in spinal animals, it is most likely that the mechanisms involved are different.

3. *Diffuse Noxious Inhibitory Controls*

Convergent neurons in the dorsal horn or the spinal trigeminal nucleus are practically all influenced by powerful inhibitory controls, which have been termed diffuse noxious inhibitory controls (DNIC). Convergent neurons recorded in the lumbar dorsal horn of the intact anesthetized rat are strongly inhibited by intense stimuli applied to various areas of the body (Le Bars *et al.*, 1979a). Examples of these areas include the tail, nose, ears, forepaws, the hindpaw contralateral to the receptive field, and viscera. The stimuli that produce these inhibition are equally varied, the only condition being that they are frankly noxious. With regard to the convergent neurons located in the trigeminal nucleus caudalis, a clear confirmation of the existence of these inhibitions has been published together with evidence for very similar characteristics of the inhibitions at both levels (Dickenson *et al.*, 1980).

The strength of the observed inhibitions is directly related to the strength of the conditioning stimuli (see below), and frequently long-lasting inhibitory

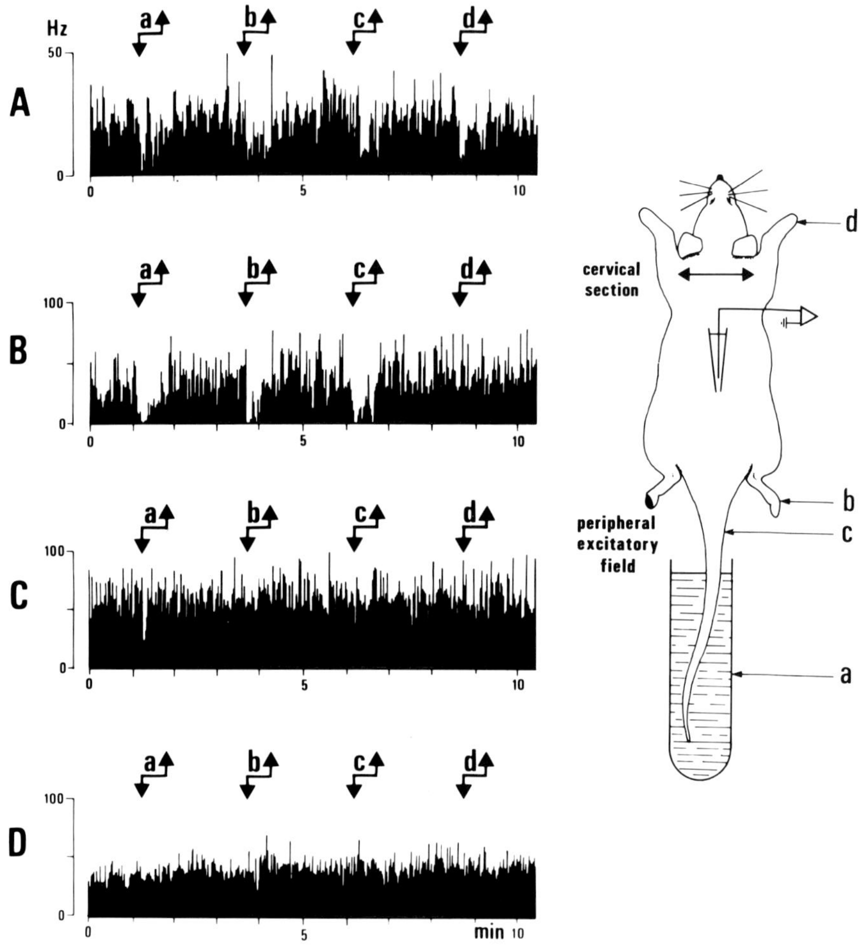

FIGURE 6. Examples of tonic discharges from four different convergent neurons (A, B, C, D) recorded in spinal unanesthetized rats, against which various conditioning stimuli were tested. The discharges were induced by the application of a sustained pinch on their hindpaw peripheral excitatory field. As depicted on the insert on the right, four noxious conditioning stimuli were applied: (a) immersion of the tail in a 52°C water bath; (b) pinch of the contralateral hindpaw; (c) pinch of the tail; (d) pinch of a forepaw. Depression of activity was obtained with all four conditioning stimuli for neuron A, with three for neuron B, and with only one for neuron C. Note in every case the rapid recovery of the neuronal activity. Neuron D was not affected by any of those conditioning stimuli. (From Cadden *et al.*, 1983.)

effects are observed. Evoked activity produced by natural stimuli, noxious or not, is equally influenced by these conditioning stimuli; an example is given in Figure 7 by a recording of a convergent neuron with activity evoked by moderate pinch applied to the receptive field. The effect of DNIC on the responses produced by transcutaneous electrical stimuli applied to the receptive field has been similarly studied. Such stimuli produce an activation of

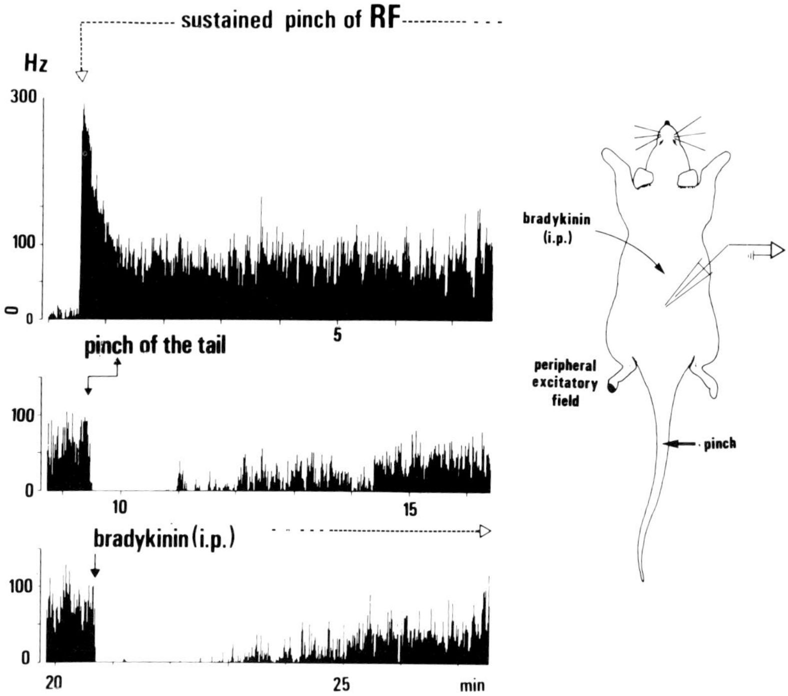

FIGURE 7. Example of inhibitory effects induced by two heterotopic noxious stimuli in the intact anesthetized rat (continuous record). The application of sustained pinch (open arrowhead, broken line) to the peripheral excitatory field of the convergent neuron resulted in a phasic response followed by a tonic discharge (upper histogram). A pinch applied to the tail (middle histogram) or an intraperitoneal injection of bradykinin (8 μg in 1 ml saline, lower trace) both resulted in a blockade of firing. Note the long-lasting post-effects (full recovery about 5 min).

large (A) and fine (C) fibers, and systematic studies have been done using suprathreshold currents because of the ease of producing a reproducible C-fiber response to this stimulation. All noxious conditioning stimuli tested induced marked inhibitions of these responses. Figure 8 summarizes these findings using a single modality of conditioning stimulation, namely, hindpaw pinch. This figure is based on four experiments in which four convergent cells were recorded in four different loci: nucleus caudalis ipsilateral and contralateral to the site of pinch application, the lumbar cord contralateral to the site of pinch application, and the sacral spinal cord. Note how the conditioning stimuli block the evoked responses irrespective of the recording site. Figure 9 illustrates the converse, a convergent neuron recorded in nucleus caudalis, the responses of which were conditioned by a thermal stimulus (52°C) applied to three different body areas.

On the basis of the influence of DNIC on practically all convergent neurons, both spinal and trigeminal, and the number of these cells with thalamic projections (see Willis, Chapter 11), it seems likely that these controls can

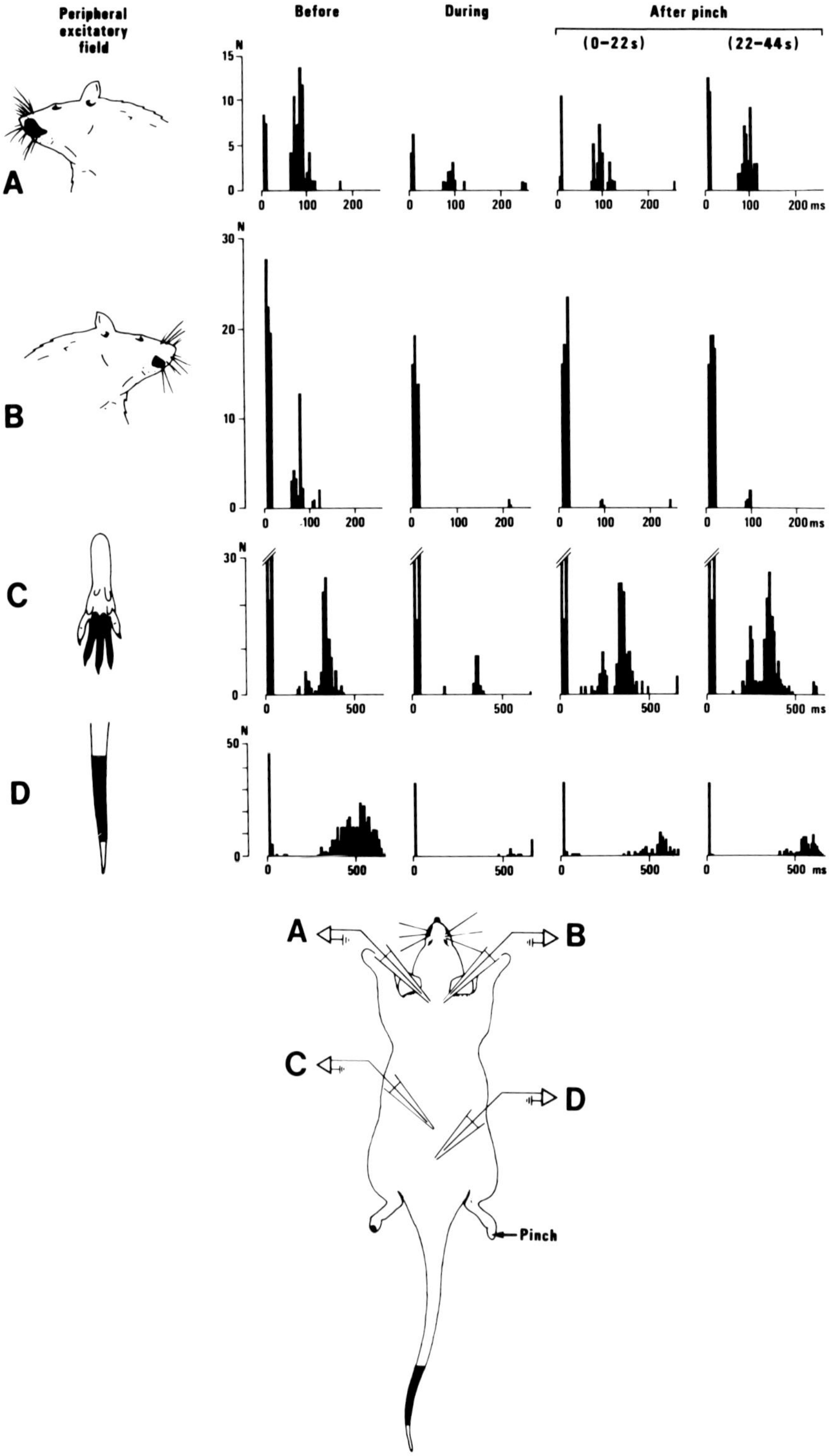

Peripheral excitatory field
Before
During
After pinch
(0-22s)
(22-44s)
N
A
B
C
D
ms
Pinch

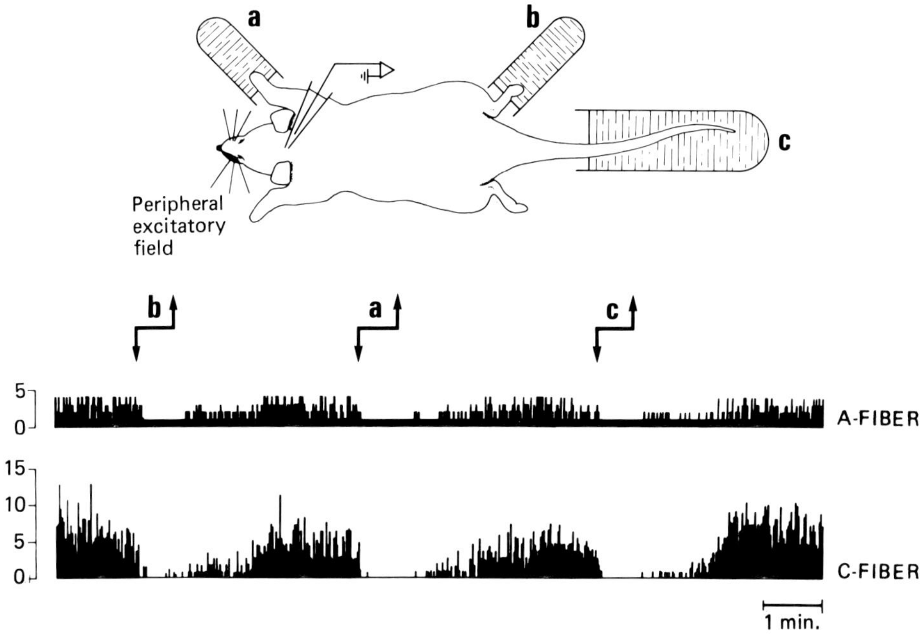

FIGURE 9. Examples of inhibitory effects induced by a noxious thermal stimulus (52°C) applied on various parts of the body (a, forepaw; b, hindpaw; c, tail) on the Aα- and C-fiber responses of a trigeminal convergent neuron to electrical stimulation of its peripheral excitatory receptive field. Electrical shocks were applied every 1500 ms, and individual responses to Aα- and C-fiber activation (see Figure 8) were monitored continuously (abscissa, time; ordinate, number of spikes per stimulus). Note the profound inhibitions followed by long-lasting post-effects triggered by each of the conditioning stimuli.

influence the ascending information from these neurons that can reach supraspinal structures. This has been directly demonstrated by the effect of DNIC on all spino- and trigeminothalamic convergent cells recorded in a recent study (Dickenson and Le Bars, 1983a).

The influence of DNIC on these convergent cells is a specific effect, as other classes of neurons (noxious only, nonnoxious, proprioceptive, and cold-

FIGURE 8. Examples of inhibitory effects induced by a pinch applied on the right hindpaw on the responses of four convergent neurons (A, B, C, D) to suprathreshold transcutaneous electrical stimulation of their excitatory fields (depicted on the left). Poststimulus histograms (PSH; 15 trials; bin width 2 ms for neurons A and B and 5 ms for neurons C and D) built just before (left PSH), during (middle PSH), and after (two right PSHs) the application of a strong pinch on the right hindpaw. Each neuron responded by a short-latency Aα-fiber response (truncated for neuron C) followed by a long-latency C-fiber response. Note that this latter response disappeared almost completely during pinch application; because of the suprathreshold nature of the electrical shocks, Aα responses were affected to a lesser extent.

responsive cells) are not modulated by these controls (Le Bars *et al.*, 1979b; Dickenson *et al.*, 1980; and see Figure 11).

The studies presented so far in this chapter illustrate the profound inhibitions of convergent neurons by the application of noxious stimuli to diverse areas of the body. Although our observations did not seem to have been previously reported, there are hints in the literature of electrophysiological findings that may well be related. For example, certain responses of convergent neurons in the monkey can be reduced by pinch of the contralateral paw (Wagman and Price, 1969); similarly, stimulation of the infraorbital nerve can inhibit some mechanical responses of spinothalamic neurons in the cat (McCreery and Bloedel, 1976).

Diffuse noxious inhibitory controls cannot be demonstrated in the anesthetized animal in which the spinal cord has been sectioned (Le Bars *et al.*, 1979b). The mechanisms underlying DNIC are therefore obviously not confined to the spinal cord, and supraspinal structures are implicated in the circuits. They are therefore very different from the propriospinal-mediated inhibitions described above. In this respect, the following differences between the propriospinal effects and the effect of DNIC are important to note: (1) practically all convergent neurons are under the influence of DNIC, whereas inhibitions in spinal animals were observed on fewer than half of them; (2) both the maximal and mean inhibitory effects are much greater in intact than in spinal animals; (3) the inhibitory effects in the intact animals are sustained throughout the conditioning period, whereas in the spinal animals the effects begin to adapt, normally within the first 10 s, and with few exceptions disappear before the end of the conditioning period; and (4) the inhibitions in the intact animals always outlast the period of conditioning, whereas such posteffects are never observed in the spinal animals. Figure 10 clearly illustrates these marked differences (compare also Figures 6 and 7). However, we have to mention the observations of Gerhart *et al.* (1981b), who reported similar patterns of inhibition triggered by heterotopic noxious stimuli in both spinal and intact monkeys in that these inhibitions were always of relatively short duration, adapted, and generally had no posteffects (resembling those that we observed in the spinal rat). The contrast between our results in the intact rat and those of Gerhart *et al.* in the monkey may be related to species and/or methodological (e.g., anesthetic regimen) differences.

Because of the involvement of supraspinal areas in DNIC, obvious candidate structures are regions in which electrical stimulation produces particularly strong inhibitions of dorsal horn convergent neurons (see Gebhart, Chapter 16). Serotonergic bulbospinal pathways would therefore seem likely to be involved in DNIC. This idea has been tested by several complementary experiments, which have been reviewed recently (Le Bars *et al.*, 1982). In summary, anatomic, biochemical, and electrophysiological substrates do exist for the possibility that peripheral noxious stimuli trigger complex loops ascending from and, via 5-HT NRM neurons, descending to the dorsal horn for inhibiting convergent neurons (see Hammond, Chapter 15).

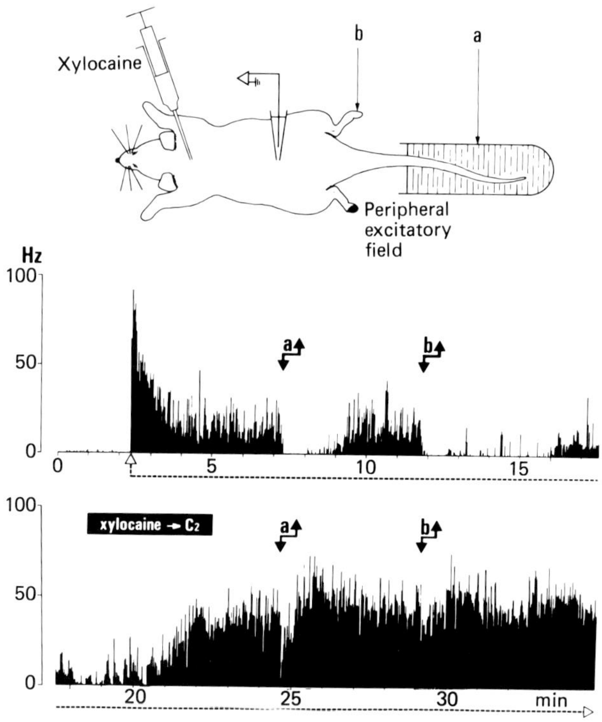

FIGURE 10. Example of a functional block [lidocaine (xylocaine) infusion] of the cervical spinal cord on the tonic discharge of a lumbar dorsal horn convergent neuron and on the depression of such activity by noxious conditioning stimuli. The discharge was induced by the sustained application (dotted line, open arrows) of a pinch on the receptive field of the neuron located on the extremity of one hindpaw. Before the infusion of lidocaine, the noxious conditioning stimuli (a, immersion of the tail in a 52°C water bath; b, pinch of the contralateral hindpaw) produced strong, long-lasting depressions of the neuronal activity. The infusion of 25 μl of 5% lidocaine (solid bar) resulted both in a large increase in the activity of the neuron and in marked decreases in the magnitude and duration of the effects of the noxious conditioning stimuli (virtually abolishing those produced by noxious pinch of the contralateral hindpaw). (From Cadden *et al.*, 1983.)

The previous sections demonstrate the action of DNIC on all responses of convergent neurons, equally effective against the activity produced by Aα-fiber stimulation as on C-fiber responses. These properties of DNIC suggest a postsynaptic inhibitory influence.

As an alternative to the technically difficult procedure of recording intracellularly from dorsal horn neurons, we used the microelectrophoretic application of glutamate ions (see Puil, 1981) to excite identified neurons and then investigated the effects of noxious conditioning stimuli applied to various parts of the body on the glutamate-induced activity (Villanueva *et al.*, 1984a). As illustrated in upper parts of Figure 11, DNIC very markedly reduced the neuronal excitations produced by glutamate. Similar observations were made

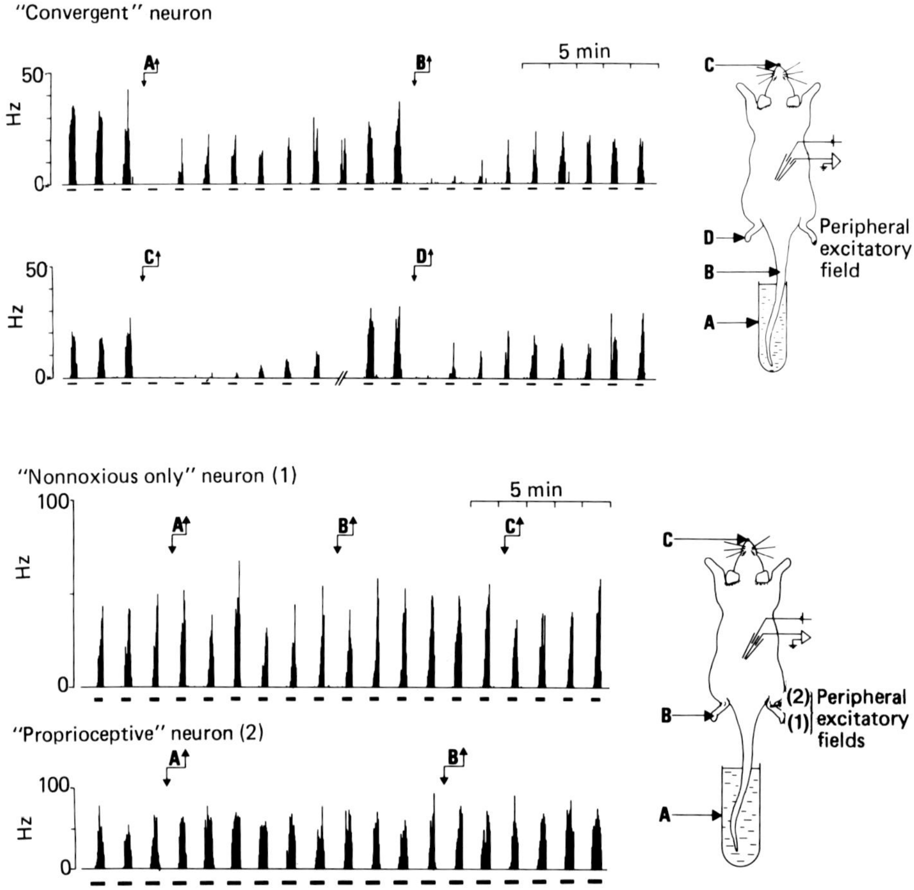

FIGURE 11. Example of the effect of various nociceptive conditioning stimuli on glutamate-induced activities of lumbar neurons: upper parts, convergent neuron; middle part, "nonnoxious-only" neuron; lower part, "proprioceptive" neuron. The electrophoretic current (convergent neuron, 20 nA; "nonnoxious-only" neuron, 30 nA; proprioceptive neuron, 45 nA) was regularly applied (horizontal bars) every 1 min. Conditioning stimuli (arrows), as depicted on the insert drawing, were immersion of the tail in a 52°C water bath or pinch of the tail, the contralateral hindpaw, or the muzzle. Note that in the case of the convergent neuron, all these conditioning stimuli virtually blocked the glutamate-induced firing, with these inhibitions remaining for several minutes in most cases. (From Villanueva *et al.*, 1984a.) No such effects were observed for the two other types of neuron.

for all convergent neurons whether recorded in the dorsal cord or the nucleus caudalis of the trigeminal system. In contrast, as shown in the middle part of Figure 11 for a "nonnoxious only" cell and in the lower part for a "proprioceptive" cell, no clear effects of the conditioning stimuli were obtained for the glutamate-evoked activity of the other types of neuron.

It seems likely that the neuronal processes responsible for the effects observed on convergent neurons involve postsynaptic inhibitory mechanisms (Curtis *et al.*, 1959; see Besson *et al.*, 1974; Belcher *et al.*, 1978; Jordan *et al.*, 1978), but in order to obtain further support for such a proposition, we tested the effects of noxious conditioning stimuli during periods of excessive depolarization induced by the continuous electrophoretic application of glutamate using large currents. A typical example is illustrated in Figure 12. During the recording of this lumbar convergent neuron, the progressive administration of glutamate, using a current much greater than the threshold for evoking a response, induced intense firing followed by a progressive decrease in spike amplitude and finally a blocking of the spike discharge (upper traces), which, in the absence of any other manipulation, would last as long as the current ejection was sustained; such an effect is a typical example of excessive depolarization (Curtis *et al.*, 1960). Noxious pinch of the muzzle resulted in a progressive recovery of firing (middle trace), which lasted throughout and outlasted the period of conditioning stimulation by several seconds (lower trace). Similar findings were made at the trigeminal level. The fact that heterotopic noxious stimuli were able to restore extracellularly recorded spike discharges, most probably reflecting a repolarization of the neuronal membrane, strongly suggests that inhibitory postsynaptic potentials were being triggered by such stimuli. Furthermore, the fact that on several occasions this repolarization clearly outlasted the period of noxious conditioning stimulation is reminiscent of the characteristic posteffects that are a major feature of DNIC.

These results, although not excluding the possibility of presynaptic inhibitions triggered by heterotopic noxious stimuli, further illustrate the strength

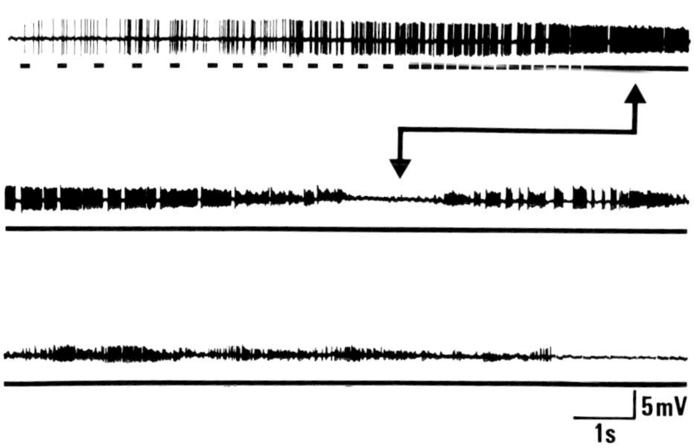

FIGURE 12. Hyperpolarization of a convergent neuron produced by noxious pinch of the muzzle (continuous record; see text). Upper trace: Progressive application (dotted line) of a large dose of glutamate induced an increased firing of the neuron. Middle trace: The sustained application of a 100-nA current (solid line) resulted in a progressive blocking of activity; the application (arrow) of a noxious pinch to the muzzle induced recovery of the extracellular recorded activity. Lower trace: Burst of activity outlasted the period of conditioning stimulation by several seconds; such an effect is reminiscent of the posteffects illustrated in Figure 11.

of DNIC. It is obviously difficult to deny some functional role for such a powerful modulation.

D. *Diffuse Noxious Inhibitory Controls and the Coding of Nociceptive Information*

The fact that a noxious stimulus seems able to activate certain brainstem structures to hyperpolarize spinal and trigeminal convergent neurons but only when the stimulus is such as to be perceived as noxious by the experimenter suggests that DNIC could play a role in nociception.

A clear correlation between the intensity of a noxious stimulus and the resultant strength of DNIC would seem an important piece of evidence in this respect, allowing the possibility of a coding of the nociceptive information by inhibitory phenomena such as DNIC. For simplicity and technical ease, we have considered the effect of various temperatures applied to the tail on the responses of trigeminal and lumbar convergent neurons activated by transcutaneous electrical stimulation of their facial and hindpaw receptive fields (Le Bars *et al.*, 1981a; Villanueva and Le Bars, 1985). These studies are summarized in Figure 13. It should be noted that the threshold for producing DNIC is between 40 and 44°C, and above this temperature in the range 44–52°C, a highly significant correlation exists between the conditioning temperature and the degre of inhibition. In addition, analogous results were obtained when identical thermal stimuli were tested against activities evoked by microelectrophoresis of an excitatory amino acid (Villanueva and Le Bars, 1985).

As stated previously, the inhibitory effects of DNIC obviously impinge on supraspinal structures. What then could be the mechanism(s) by which DNIC could code nociceptive information? In other words, how can descending inhibitory controls, the functinal role of which would intuitively seem to be in analgesic phenomena, play a role in nociception?

This proposition, which at first sight might seem illogical, becomes realistic when one considers the paradoxical property of convergent neurons that we have discussed previously, i.e., the ease with which the convergent neurons can be activated by innocuous stimuli (e.g., see Figure 1). Since such stimuli are a common and frequent occurrence in everyday life, it is possible to safely predict that the total population of spinal and trigeminal convergent neurons will be active to a marked degree as a result of activity in cutaneous mechanoreceptors. This activity can be considered as a "somesthetic background noise" from within which the higher centers must attempt to recognize a significant nociceptive message. The term "noise" refers only to nociception in that somesthetic activity will mask information emanating from nociceptors; this does not preclude a functional role of this "noise" (see below).

Diffuse noxious inhibitory controls may provide a means by which an unequivocal nociceptive signal can be recognized from the nonspecific so-

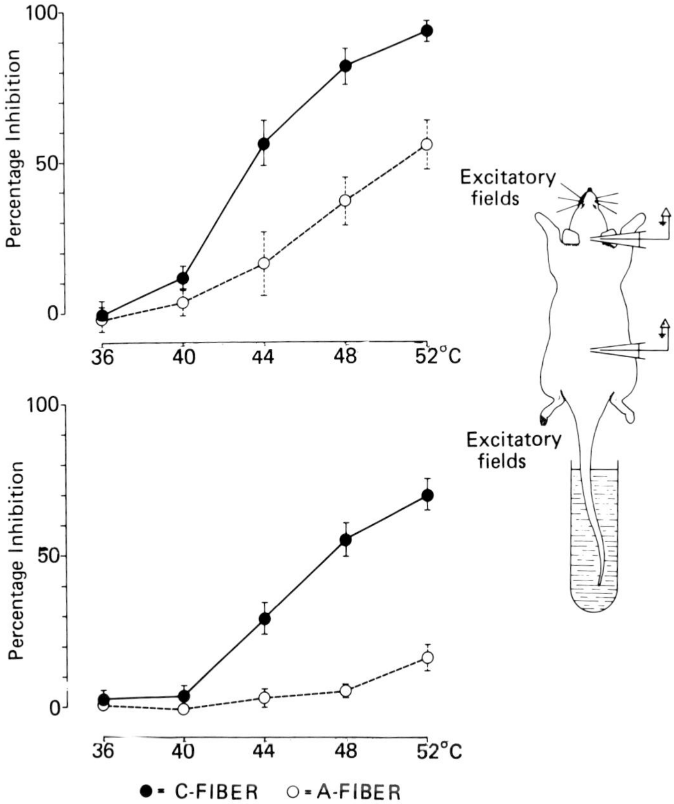

FIGURE 13. Mean percentages of inhibition (ordinate) of A- (dotted line) and C (solid line)-fiber-evoked responses of trigeminal (upper curves) and lumbar (lower curves) convergent neurons induced by the immersion of the tail in water baths at various temperatures (abscissa). Note that no significant effects were observed when 36° or 40°C was applied on the tail; then there was a highly significant correlation between noxious temperatures (44–52°C) and the degree of inhibition, especially in the case of C-fiber responses. A-fiber responses were affected to a lesser extent because of the suprathreshold nature of the conditioned stimulus.

mesthetic activity arising from convergent neurons (Le Bars *et al.*, 1979b). As detailed earlier, DNIC inhibits all activities of these convergent cells, notably in this context the spontaneous and innocuous activities. If one accepts the existence of a relatively high order of somesthetic noise in the absence of a noxious stimulus (Figure 14A), the experimental situations illustrated can be interpreted in the following way: as an intense noxious stimulus is applied to an area of the body, the convergent and nociceptive-specific neurons in the corresponding segmental zone will be activated (Figure 14B) and then give rise to excitatory messages transmitted to higher centers (Figure 14C). This signal will then, in turn, induce DNIC (Figure 14D), which will inhibit those convergent spinal and trigeminal neurons not directly influenced by the initial

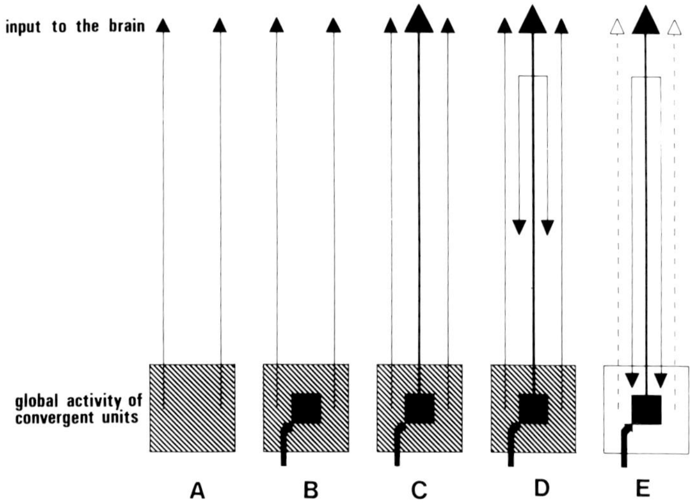

FIGURE 14. Hypothetical interpretation of the global activity of spinal and trigeminal neurons involved in nociception at spinal and trigeminal levels. Taken as a whole, this activity would be of a reasonably high order in freely moving animals because of the properties of convergent neurons, sending a kind of "noise" toward the brain (A). A noxious stimulus activates both noxious-only and convergent neurons (B), which send an excitatory input to the brain (C). These inputs trigger the DNIC system (D), with a consequent reduction of the activity of the remaining nonsegmental convergent units not directly affected by the initial stimulus (E). Hence, a contrast signal is set up. (From Le Bars *et al.*, 1983a.)

stimulus (Figure 14E). By these means, a high level of contrast will be attained between the activities of the excited segmental neurons and the depressed activity of the rest of the pool of convergent cells.

The existence of this contrast message is not in doubt. What remains unknown is the mechanisms of recognition and eventual processing of this signal by the higher centers. We have proposed that the brain is able to recognize this contrast message and that DNIC can consequently be interpreted as a filter, allowing the extraction of a nociceptive message from the overall activity of convergent neurons. Figure 15 illustrates this idea of a double process of coding of the nociceptive information, an excitatory and an inhibitory facet, the latter produced by DNIC. If the brain is able to recognize such a contrasted picture as a pain-signaling message, then DNIC could be interpreted not only as a filter that allows the extraction of a meaningful nociceptive message from the nonspecific activities of convergent neurons but also, and perhaps more importantly, as an additional amplifier favoring the basic gain system (Figure 15B) and, therefore, the "alarm" function of nociceptive messages. On the basis of this hypothesis, the complexity of certain forms of clinical pains and the variety and range of syndromes observed could be as a result of this dual signal transmission of nociceptive information.

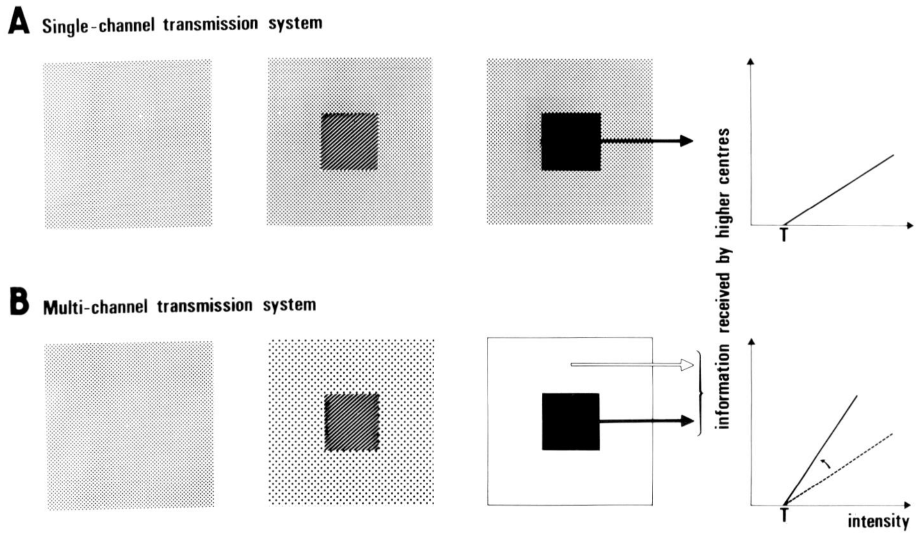

FIGURE 15. Hypothetical coding of the intensity of nociceptive stimuli by both excitatory responses and silencing of the remaining population of neurons. A: The application of an increasing noxious stimulus on a somatic area would result in an increase of the activity of the corresponding segmental pool of convergent and noxious-specific neurons (from left to right). B: Such a stimulus would also trigger the DNIC system (see Figure 14), inducing a progressive decrease of the random activity of the convergent neuronal population (from left to right). In this hypothesis of a multichannel transmission system, the complementary action of excitatory and inhibitory events would produce a contrasted picture, which would be sent to the brain, and which could be the source of an amplification of the gain of the transmission system (right; T, threshold). (From Le Bars and Chitour, 1983.)

It should be clearly stated that this hypothesis does not resolve the problem of the initial transmission of noxious messages at the spinal level, which is necessary for activation of DNIC, and does not deny a role for nociceptive-specific cells.

It is obviously extremely difficult to directly verify this model of pain transmission. One can, however, derive certain theoretical implications of the model that can then be tested experimentally. The following section considers first clinical and behavioral and then pharemacological evidence for this proposition.

E. *Diffuse Noxious Inhibitory Controls and the Phenomenon of Counterirritation*

We have already stressed the effect of DNIC on all activities of convergent neurons including that produced by noxious stimuli. An example in the lower part of Figure 9 illustrates a convergent neuron activated by C-fiber stimulation, a stimulus presumably able to produce a sensation of pain in man, inhibited by an intense noxious stimulus applied to areas of the body far from the peripheral receptive field of the neuron. Quite simply, when two noxious stimuli are applied to two distant areas of the body, the pool of neurons activated by the weaker stimulus is inhibited. If, and it seems likely (see Table I), these convergent neurons are involved in the transmission of a nociceptive message towards supraspinal structures, the result of simultaneous application of two noxious stimuli will, in terms of pain sensation, depend on a balance between the activities of the two pools of active neurons (Figure 16), the net result being an attenuation of the pain produced by the weaker stimulus.

This prediction of our model has its roots in historical observations and can be expressed as "one pain can mask another." A good number of practices in popular medicine are founded on this principle (counterirritation), which most probably dates from ancient times (see Le Bars *et al.*, 1984). Despite the advent of modern medicine, these practices still continue in certain countries, presumably as a result of their beneficial therapeutic effects. Although the techniques differ from one society to another (discharge of electric fish, cupping, scarring, moxibustion, hot plasters, hot irons), the principle remains to produce a marked pain in an attempt to reduce a preexisting pain. For example, the therapy of hot irons is the chosen treatment for some forms of pain in Algeria (D. Chitour, personal communication). The best indications

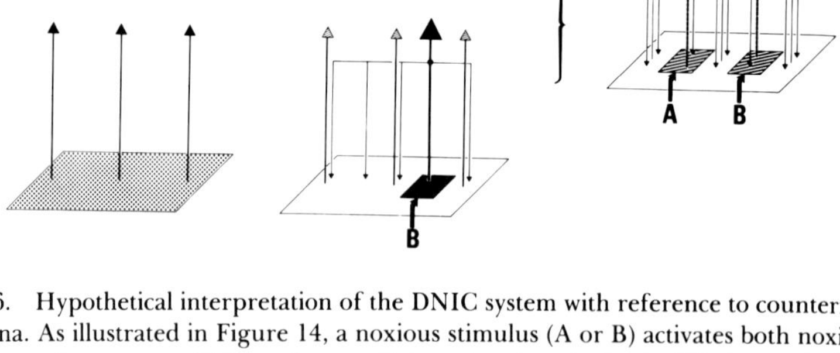

FIGURE 16. Hypothetical interpretation of the DNIC system with reference to counterirritation phenomena. As illustrated in Figure 14, a noxious stimulus (A or B) activates both noxious-only and convergent neurons, which send an excitatory signal to the brain (filled arrow); this input triggers the DNIC system (downwards arrows) with a consequent reduction of the activity of the remaining population of convergent units not directly affected by the stimulus. In this model, the concomitant application of two noxious stimuli, i.e, A and B (right), would mutually influence the neuronal responses, with the final output depending on the relative strength of the stimuli. (From Le Bars *et al.*, 1984.)

are rheumatic or visceral pain, often diffuse, deep, chronic, and highly disagreeable. The technique consists of the application of a red hot rod to the abdomen, usually at about 3 Hz, which produces an acute pain, progressively, at the limit of the patient's tolerance. The frequency of treatment depends on the duration and degree of the beneficial effects.

Although this description of counterirritation is purely qualitative, it agrees well with the results of many quantitative studies, demonstrating that it is possible to attenuate preexisting pain by applying a more intense noxious stimulus (Duncker, 1937; Hardy *et al.*, 1940; Gamon and Starr, 1941; Parsons and Goetzl, 1945; Pertovaara *et al.*, 1982; Le Bars *et al.*, 1983b; Willer *et al.*, 1984).

More recently, these traditional practices have been reintroduced under the term "hyperstimulation analgesia," covering certain therapeutic methods (Melzack, 1975; Jeans, 1979). It is of great interest to note the parallels between the phenomenon of counterirritation and the hypoalgesic effects obtained using both traditional forms of acupuncture and the contemporary electroacupuncture, as noted by certain authors (Wand-Tetley, 1956; Fox and Melzack, 1976a,b; Levine *et al.*, 1976; Melzack *et al.*, 1977; Han and Terenius, 1982). The conclusions reached by Mann (1974) on the basis of a large number of clinical observations were that acupunctural stimuli must be painful and even only just tolerable by the subject to be efficacious. Furthermore, it has been reported that organic pain is accompanied by an elevation of the threshold for experimental pain applied elsewhere on the body (Hazouri and Mueller, 1950; Merskey and Evans, 1975).

These clinical observations are corroborated by behavioral studies in animals. In the rat, for example, it has been shown that various nociceptive stimuli (intraperitoneal injection of algogenic compounds, pinch applied to the tail or paws, intense electrical stimulation of the same areas) produce a reduction in the responses of the animals to noxious stimuli applied to other body areas (see Curzon and Tricklebank, 1984). Similarly, in the cat, electrical stimulation of the tooth pulp produces a considerable increase in the threshold for escape behavior induced by electrical stimulation of the paws (Anderson *et al.*, 1976).

We believe that DNIC could be the neuronal substrate for these hypoalgesic effects (Le Bars *et al.*, 1979b). This proposition is borne out not only by the preceding analysis but also by the fact that, in man, the pain-relieving effects of heterotopic nociceptive stimuli are extremely well correlated with a concomitant depression of a spinal nociceptive reflex (Le Bars *et al.*, 1983b; Willer *et al.*, 1984). In an electrophysiological and psychophysiological study of these phenomena in man, the sural nerve was stimulated, and the variations in the pain sensation and a nociceptive reflex (flexion reflex R III) produced by various noxious conditioning stimuli applied elsewhere on the body were studied. For example, the thresholds for sensation and the reflex are highly significantly increased in a correlated way by hot water ($\geq$45°C) applied to the hand contralateral to the foot stimulated. These data suggest that the modulation of pain by heterotopic nociceptive stimuli can be explained, at least in part, by a depression in the transmission of nociceptive messages at the spinal level. Related results have been obtained in the rat, where concurrent with the depression by tail or nose pinch of convergent neuronal activity produced by C-fiber-strength stimulation of the sural nerve, the flexion reflex activity is similarly reduced by the conditioning stimulus (Schouenborg and Dickenson, 1985).

It is apparent, then, that as two noxious stimuli are applied to distinct areas of the body, a competitive effect is induced, with the stronger stimulus able to limit the perceptual and motor responses induced by the second stimulus.

In this context, it is important to note that the nociceptive-specific neurons are not influenced by DNIC, at least neurons of this class in the marginal layer of the rat. If these findings are confirmed in other species, it is suggestive that the activation alone of a pool of nociceptive-specific neurons does not produce a nociceptive process sufficient to counter the inhibition of the pool of convergent cells that, initially, were concurrently activated. It also follows that the activation of both types of neurons is more effective in triggering integrative processes leading to the sensation of pain than is the unique activation of the marginal zone nociceptive-specific cells.

F. Diffuse Noxious Inhibitory Controls and Morphine

We have explained at length the reasons for believing that DNIC may be involved in the coding of nociceptive information. On the basis of the hypothesis that certain neural events leading to recognition of a painful sensation could be induced by a gradient of activity between a pool of activated neurons and the relative silence of the rest of the population of cells, one could envisage that any enhancement of this contrast would result in hyperalgesia, whereas interfering with the contrast would lead to hypoalgesia or even analgesia if the contrast were abolished. A direct consequence of this model is that pharmacological manipulations of this gradient of activity should lead to corresponding changes in pain sensation. These manipulations could equally involve the active pool and the concomitantly inhibited pool of neurons. Thus, a depression of the messages emanating from the activate cells could lead to hypoalgesia, and a facilitation could correspondingly result in hyperalgesia; an increase in the "background noise" (by a reduction in DNIC) could produce hypoalgesia, and a decrease in this activity (by a facilitation of DNIC) should result in hyperalgesia.

On this theoretical basis, we investigated the effect of morphine on DNIC (Le Bars *et al.,* 1981b). This subject has been reviewed recently (Le Bars *et al.,* 1983a), and only a brief account is presented below.

The essential finding was the pronounced sensitivity of DNIC to morphine: very low doses (0.1–1 mg/kg i.v.) that were ineffective in producing a significant direct depressive effect at the spinal level very significantly decreased the effects of DNIC. This effect was observed irrespective of the nature of the convergent neuronal activity against which DNIC was tested. Several findings affirm the receptor specificity of the observed effects: the increase in DNIC by morphine was dose dependent, naloxone reversible, and stereospecific.

The site of this action of morphine most probably resides within supraspinal structures; supporting this is the demonstration that 5 μg of morphine in 0.2 μl saline can very significantly reduce DNIC when microinjected into certain ventral parts of the periaqueductal gray matter of the rat (Dickenson and Le Bars, 1983b).

These results agree with the predictions of our model (Figure 17): if the gradient of activity between two pools of neurons, one inhibited, one excited, gives rise to a final sensation of pain (Figure 17B), then morphine analgesia could result from a restoration of the background noise (Figure 17C) or by a depression of the excited neurons (Figure 17D). We have proposed that the low doses of morphine, via a reduction in DNIC, restore the background noise towards its original level; with higher doses, an inhibition of the segmental pool of active neurons (direct spinal action, see Yaksh, Chapter 20) is superimposed on this primary mechanism. The summation of these two effects (Figure 17C,D) reduces considerably the contrast between the levels of activity of the two groups of neurons, resulting in a profound analgesia.

This view is in accord with clinical and behavioral studies of the characteristic of morphine analgesia. In man, morphine is analgesic at low doses (0.15 mg/kg), similar to those that lift DNIC (ED_{50} about 0.6 mg/kg) or almost identical to the doses that block the inhibitory posteffects (ED_{50} 0.13 mg/kg).

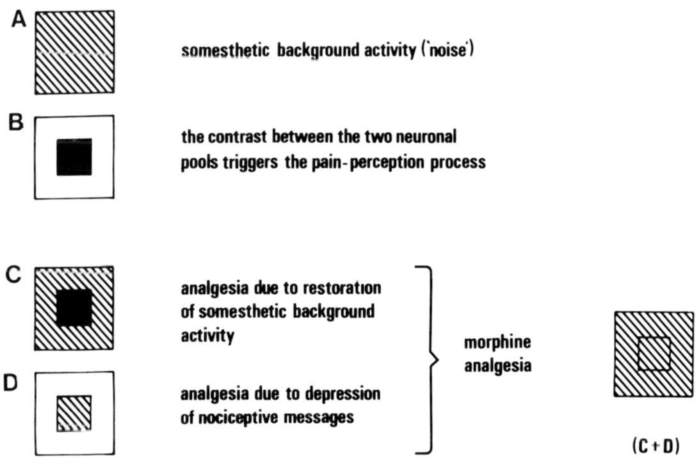

FIGURE 17. Hypothetical interpretation of the direct and indirect effects of morphine at the spinal level (see text). (From Le Bars *et al.*, 1983a.)

It is interesting to note that these low doses are without effect on the behavioral tests in animals in which threshold measurements are made using epicritic nociceptive stimuli but are clearly effective against nociceptive reactions induced by stimuli such as experimental arthritis (Pircio *et al.*, 1975) or intraperitoneal injection of algogenic agents (Niemegeers *et al.*, 1975).

In fact, morphine analgesia in man is frequently characterized by a perceptual alteration of the nociceptive message, which maintains its sensory qualities but does not induce the usual affective and emotional reactions associated with pain. This dissociation leads to an indifference of the subject to the stimulus, which, however, he still feels. A straightforward block of the excitatory message cannot underlie these characteristics of the analgesia, which are more probably caused by complex integrative mechanisms; the lifting of DNIC may be one of these. When morphine and other opiates are given at higher doses, in anesthesiology for example, all pain, especially sharp pain, which can be considered as epicritic, disappears. In this case, a block of nociceptive information seems likely to account for this form of analgesia. Recall that the well-demonstrated direct spinal action of morphine (see Yaksh, Chapter 20) in inhibiting this nociceptive information occurs at systemic doses of an order ten times those capable of reducing DNIC.

Additionally, the direct spinal action of morphine, far from counteracting the supraspinal action, tends to amplify it for two major reasons. It is generally agreed that morphine acts on the noxious-related activities of convergent cells without altering their responses to innocuous stimuli. This property would not have a functional significance if the convergent neurons were able to discriminate the two types of information (criterion 1). By contrast, this observation is particularly significant in the light of our hypothesis, as the spinal action will not hinder or counteract the supraspinal effect of morphine in restoring the "background noise" from the sensory milieu. Furthermore, it is clear that the direct depression of activity in the spinal cord by morphine will lead to a reduced activation of the loop subserving DNIC and so result in a recovery of the level of somesthesic noise. This will facilitate the supraspinal effect of lifting DNIC and signifies that the spinal and supraspinal actions will not be simply additive but synergistic. Behavioral studies (Yeung and Rudy, 1980) have clearly demonstrated that the analgesia produced by the intracerebroventricular administration of morphine is potentiated by the intrathecal injection of morphine, confirming this hypothesis.

G. *Summary and Conclusions*

The studies presented in this chapter illustrate the complexity of the mechanisms regulating the activity of convergent neurons of the spinal cord and trigeminal nucleus caudalis. Their properties are such as to suggest a strategic position in the reception and transmission towards higher centers of certain somesthetic information from the environment.

It should be recalled that this system is entirely separate from the lemniscal system, which, according to the evidence, is perfectly adapted to receive discrete point-to-point information. The dorsal horn of the spinal cord is, however, not merely the parallel of such specific systems. The existence of multiple mechanisms of modulation indicates a site of elaboration of more integrative processes.

For example, the convergence of very varied information of cutaneous, visceral, and muscular origins onto the population of convergent neurons predisposes these to a global reception of sensory information that could be interpreted by the higher centers as basic somesthetic activity (BSA), indicating that no one perturbation is produced by the internal or external environment. It is not impossible that this BSA has a functional role, for example, in assisting the specific somatosensory system in elaboration of a "body representation" in terms of a continual and global reception of information relevant to the integrity of the body. In this regard, the functional significance of the mixing of cutaneous, muscular, and visceral information should be considered. Along the same lines, it is interesting to note that a certain number of convergent neurons are able to code innocuous temperatures ("warming/noxious heat convergent neurons," Burton, 1975; Price and Browe, 1975; Menétrey *et al.*, 1979), and that some respond to cooling (Burton, 1975; Menétrey *et al.*, 1979), such that the ambient temperature also can contribute to the BSA. It is worth noting that the contribution of cutaneous low-threshold mechanoreceptors to the BSA is generally problematical, and there is probably a local autolimitation from the powerful segmental control mechanisms (see Figure 5).

The arrival of a nociceptive occurrence completely perturbs this BSA in two ways, which we consider complementary. The first is the activation of a pool of specific nociceptive and convergent neurons. The second event is more complex, since propriospinal mechanisms and, above all, mechanisms of integration from supraspinal sites are brought into play. The result is that the activity of the pool of neurons affected by the nociceptive event emerges clearly as a result of a nullifying of the noise constituting the BSA (see Figure 14). Whatever the cause or the interpretation of the BSA, it is clear from the electrophysiology that all the convergent neurons, spinal and trigeminal, are implicated when a noxious stimulus is applied, no matter the body area stimulated, the segmental pool is depolarized and the rest of the neuronal population is hyperpolarized.

Furthermore, we have seen the strong correlation between the strength of DNIC and the intensity of stimulation, such that one could envisage that the transmission of nociceptive messages at the spinal level depends not only on a system the gain of which is regulated by the excitation of a pool of neurons but is equally a function of dynamic events resulting in an amplification of the initial gain by a secondary system represented by DNIC (see Figure 15). Such a mechanism of autoamplification of the nociceptive message accords well with the idea of nociception subserving an alarm function.

The paradoxical phenomenon of counterirritation fits perfectly with this model since it is a result (see Figure 16) of the mechanisms described above. It is as if the CNS, because of difficulties in discriminating or integrating several nociceptive stimuli emanating simultaneously from different areas, temporarily eliminates, in the same manner as the BSA, the transmission of the less urgent weaker stimulus.

The effects of morphine on DNIC (see Figure 17) are educative, since low but analgesic doses of the drug are able to restore the BSA without inhibiting the spinal transmission of excitatory nociceptive messages to the higher centers; morphine hence blocks the autoamplification processes we have postulated. As previously stressed, this effect fits very well with the particular characteristics of morphine analgesia producing an indifference of the recipient to the stimulus, which he is still able to recognize. From a theoretical viewpoint, we find ourselves in a situation in which a stimulus, although recognized as nociceptive, is not painful; one could speculate whether a nociceptive state becomes a painful one when the classic excitatory mechanisms of nociception are augmented by the disappearance of the BSA caused by DNIC. Added to this, the spinal action of morphine, produced by higher doses that block all nociceptive sensations, not only does not hinder the restoring of the BSA but acts synergistically with it.

In conclusion, it could be rather disconcerting that two opposite manipulations, the activation of DNIC counterirritation and its blocking by morphine, lead in therapeutic terms to the same end point, i.e., hypoalgesia. We feel, however, that this seeming anomaly reflects the complexity of the spinal systems and provides insight into the likely role of the convergent neuron in the encoding of nociceptive and nonnociceptive sensory information.

ACKNOWLEDGMENT. This work was supported by l'Institut National de la Santé et de la Recherche Médicale (INSERM), CRL 82 60 29. The authors are very grateful to Drs. Cadden, Calvino, Catchlove, Chitour, Feltz, and Kraus for their contributions to some aspects of this work, to Mrs. M. Hoch for the dactylography, and to E. Dehausse for the photography.

References

ANDERSON, K. V., PEARL, G. S., AND HONEYCUTT, C. Behavioural evidence showing the predominance of diffuse pain stimuli over discrete stimuli in influencing perception. *J. Neurosci. Res.* 2:283–289, 1976.

APPLEBAUM, A. E., BEALL, J. E., FOREMAN, R. D., AND WILLIS, W. D. Organization and receptive fields of primate spinothalamic tract neurons. *J. Neurophysiol.* 38:572–586, 1975.

BELCHER, G., RYALL, R. W. AND SCHAFFNER, R. The differential effects of 5-hydroxytryptamine, noradrenaline and raphé stimulation on nociceptive and non nociceptive dorsal horn interneurons in the cat. *Brain Res.* 151:307–321, 1978.

BENNETT, G. J., HAYASHI, H., ABDELMOUMENE, M., AND DUBNER, R. Physiological properties of stalked cells of the substantia gelatinosa intracellularly stained with horseradish peroxidase. *Brain Res.* 164:285–289, 1979.

BENNETT, G. J., ABDELMOUMENE, M., HAYASHI, H., AND DUBNER, R. Physiology and morphology of substantia gelatinosa neurons intracellularly stained with horseradish peroxidase. *J. Comp. Neurol.* 194:809–827, 1980.

BESSON, J. M., CONSEILLER, C., HAMMANN, K. F., AND MAILLARD, M. C. Modifications of dorsal horn cell activities in the spinal cord, after intra-arterial injection of bradykinin. *J. Physiol. (Lond.)* 221:189–205, 1972.

BESSON, J. M., CATCHLOVE, R. F. H., FELTZ, P., AND LE BARS, D. Further evidence for postsynaptic inhibitions on lamina V dorsal horn interneurons. *Brain Res.* 66:531–536, 1974.

BESSON, J. M., GUILBAUD, G., AND LE BARS, D. Descending inhibitory influences exerted by the brain stem upon the activities of dorsal horn lamina V cells induced by intra-arterial injection of bradykinin into the limbs. *J. Physiol. (Lond.)* 248:725–739, 1975.

BROWN, A. G., AND RÉTHELYI, M. (eds.) *Sensory Cord Sensation,* Scottish Academy Press, Edinburgh, 1981, pp. 331–336.

BROWN, A. G., HAMMANN, W. C., AND MARTIN, H. F. Interactions of cutaneous myelinated (A) and non myelinated (C) fibres on transmission through the spinocervical tract. *Brain Res.* 53:222–226, 1973.

BURTON , H. Responses of spinal cord neurons to systematic changes in hindlimb skin temperatures in cats and primates. *J. Neurophysiol.* 38:1060–1079, 1975.

CADDEN, S. W., VILLANUEVA, L., CHITOUR, D., AND LE BARS, D. Depression of activities of dorsal horn convergent neurones by propriospinal mechanisms triggered by noxious input; comparison with diffuse noxious inhibitory controls (DNIC). *Brain Res.* 275:1–11, 1983.

CALVILLO, O., HENRY, J. L., AND NEUMAN, R. S. Actions of narcotic analgesics and antagonists on spinal units responding to natural stimulation in the cat. *Can. J. Physiol. Pharmacol.* 57:652–663, 1979.

CARSTENS, E., YOKOTA, T., AND ZIMMERMANN, M. Inhibition of spinal neuronal responses to noxious skin testing by stimulation of mesencephalic periaqueductal gray in the cat. *J. Neurophysiol.* 42:558–568, 1979.

CARSTENS, E., KLUMPP, D., AND ZIMMERMANN, M. Differential inhibitory effects of medial and lateral midbrain stimulation on spinal neuronal discharges to noxious skin heating in the cat. *J. Neurophysiol.* 43:332–342, 1980.

CARSTENS, E., BIHL, H., IRVINE, D. R. F., AND ZIMMERMANN, M. Descending inhibitions from medial and lateral midbrain of spinal dorsal horn neuronal responses to noxious and nonnoxious cutaneous stimuli in the cat. *J. Neurophysiol.* 45:1029–1042, 1981.

CERVERO, F., IGGO, A., AND OGAWA, H. Nociceptor-driven dorsal horn neurons in the lumbar spinal cord of the cat. *Pain* 2:5–24, 1976.

CHRISTENSEN, B. N., AND PERL, E. R. Spinal neurons specifically excited by noxious or thermal stimuli: Marginal zone of the dorsal horn. *J. Neurophysiol.* 33:293–307, 1970.

CURTIS, D. R., AND WATKINS, J. C. The excitation and depression of spinal neurones by structurally related amino acids. *J. Neurochem.* 6:117–141, 1960.

CURTIS, D. R., PHILLIS, J. W., AND WATKINS, J. C. Chemical excitation of spinal neurones. *Nature* 183:611–612, 1959.

CURTIS, D. R., PHILLIS, J. W., AND WATKINS, J. C. The chemical excitation of spinal neurones by certain acidic amino-acids. *J. Physiol. (Lond.),* 150:656–682, 1960.

CURZON, G., AND TRICKLEBANK, M. D. (eds.) *Stress-Induced Analgesia,* John Wiley & Sons, London, 1984.

DICKENSON, A. H., AND LE BARS, D. Diffuse noxious inhibitory controls (DNIC) involve trigemino- and spinothalamic neurones in the rat. *Exp. Brain Res.* 49:174–180, 1983a.

DICKENSON, A. H., AND LE BARS, D. Morphine microinjections into periaqueductal grey matter of the rat: Effects on dorsal horn neuronal responses to C-fibre activity and diffuse noxious inhibitory controls. *Life Sci.* 33(S1):549–554, 1983b.

DICKENSON, A. H., LE BARS, D., AND BESSON, J. M. Diffuse noxious inhibitory controls (DNIC). Effects on trigeminal nucleus caudalis neurones in the rat. *Brain Res.* 200:293–305, 1980.

DUGGAN, A. W., AND GRIERSMITH, B. T. Inhibition of the spinal transmission of nociceptive information by supraspinal stimulation in the cat. *Pain* 6:149–161, 1979.

DUNKER, K. Some preliminary experiments on the mutual influence of pains. *Psychol. Forsch.* 21:311–326, 1937.

FITZGERALD, M. The contralateral input to the dorsal horn of the spinal cord in the decerebrate spinal rat. *Brain Res.* 236:275–287, 1982.

FOREMAN, R. D., BEALL, J. E., APPLEBAUM, A. E., COULTER, J. D., AND WILLIS, W. D. Effects of dorsal column stimulation on primate spinothalamic tract neurons. *J. Neurophysiol.* 39:534–546, 1976.

FOREMAN, R. D., SCHMIDT, R. F., AND WILLIS, W. D. Convergence of muscle and cutaneous input onto spinothalamic tract neurons. *Brain Res.* 124:555–560, 1977.

FOREMAN, R. D., SCHMIDT, R. F., AND WILLIS, W. D. Effects of mechanical and chemical stimulation of fine muscle afferents upon primate spinothalamic tract cells. *J. Physiol. (Lond.)* 286:215–231, 1979.

FOREMAN, R. D., HANCOCK, M. B., AND WILLIS, W. D. Responses of spinothalamic tract cells in the thoracic spinal cord of the monkey to cutaneous and visceral inputs. *Pain* 11:149–162, 1981.

FOX, E. J., AND MELZACK, R. Comparison of transcutaneous electrical stimulation and acupuncture in the treatment of chronic pain. *Adv. Pain Res. Ther.* 1:797–801, 1976a.

FOX, E. J., AND MELZACK, R. Transcutaneous electrical stimulation and acupuncture: Comparison of treatment for low-back pain. *Pain* 2:141–148, 1976b.

GALINDO, A., KRNJEVIĆ, K., AND SCHWARTZ, S. Microiontophoretic studies on neurones in the cuneate nucleus. *J. Physiol. (Lond.)* 192:359–377, 1967.

GALINDO, A., KRNJEVIĆ, K., AND SCHWARTZ, S. Patterns of firing in cuneate neurons and some effects of Flaxedil. *Exp. Brain Res.* 5:87–101, 1968.

GAMMON, G. D., AND STARR, I. Studies on the relief of pain by counterirritation. *J. Clin. Invest.* 20:13–20, 1941.

GERHART, K. D., WILCOX, T. K., CHUNG, J. M., AND WILLIS, W. D. Inhibition of nociceptive and non-nociceptive responses of primate spinothalamic cells by stimulation in medial brainstem. *J. Neurophysiol.* 45:121–136, 1981a.

GERHART, K. D., YEZIERSKI, R. P., GIESLER, G. J., JR., AND WILLIS, W. D. Inhibitory receptive fields of primate spinothalamic tract cells. *J. Neurophysiol.* 46:1309–1325, 1981b.

GIESLER, G. J., JR., MENÉTREY, D., GUILBAUD, G., AND BESSON, J. M. Lumbar cord neurons at the origin of the spinothalamic tract in the rat. *Brain Res.* 118:320–324, 1976.

GREGOR, M., AND ZIMMERMANN, M. Characteristics of spinal neurones responding to cutaneous myelinated and unmyelinated fibres. *J. Physiol. (Lond.)* 221:555–576, 1972.

GUILBAUD, G., BESSON, J. M., LIEBESKIND, J. C., AND OLIVERAS, J. L. Analgésie induite par stimulation de la substance grise périaqueducale chez le chat: Données comportementales et modifications de l'activité des interneurones de la corne dorsale de la moelle. *C. R. Acad. Sci. [D] (Paris)* 275:1055–1057, 1972.

HAN, L. S. AND TERENIUS, L. Neurochemical basis of acupuncture analgesia. *Annu. Rev. Pharmacol. Toxicol.* 22:193–220, 1982.

HANDWERKER, H. O., IGGO, A., AND ZIMMERMANN, M. Segmental and supraspinal actions on dorsal horn neurons responding to noxious and non-noxious skin stimuli. *Pain* 1:147–165, 1975.

HARDY, J. D., WOLFF, H. G., AND GOODELL, H. Studies on pain. A new method for measuring pain threshold: Observations on spatial summation of pain. J. Clin. Invest. 19:649–657, 1940.

HAYES, R. L., PRICE, D. D., AND DUBNER, R. Behavioural and physiological studies of sensory coding and modulation of trigeminal nociceptive input. *Adv. Pain Res. Ther.* 3:219–243, 1979a.

HAYES, R. L., PRICE, D. D., RUDA, M., AND DUBNER, R. Suppression of nociceptive responses in the primate by electrical stimulation of the brain or morphine administration: Behavioral and electrophysiological comparisons. *Brain Res.* 167:417–421, 1979b.

HAZOURI, L. A., AND MUELLER, A. D. Pain threshold studies on paraplegic patients. *Arch. Neurol. Psychiatry* 64:607–613, 1950.

HILLMAN, P., AND WALL, P. D. Inhibitory and excitatory factors influencing the receptive fields of lamina 5 spinal cord cells. *Exp. Brain Res.* 9:284–306, 1969.

HOFFMAN, D. S., DUBNER, R., HAYES, R. L., AND MEDLIN, T. P. Neuronal activity in medullary dorsal horn of awake monkeys trained in a thermal discrimination task. I. Response to innocuous and noxious thermal stimuli. *J. Neurophysiol.* 46:409–427, 1981.

HOMMA, E., COLLINS, J. G., AND KITAHATA, L. M. Effects of intrathecal morphine on activity of dorsal horn neurons activated by noxious heat. *Adv. Pain Res. Ther.* 5:481–486, 1983.

HONG, S. K., KNIFFKI, K. D., MENSE, S., SCHMIDT, R. F., AND WENDISH, M. Descending influences on the responses of spinocervical tract neurons to chemical stimulation of fine muscle afferents. *J. Physiol. (Lond.)* 290:129–140, 1979.

IGGO, A. Activation of cutaneous nociceptors and their action on dorsal horn neurons. *Adv. Neurol.* 4:1–9, 1974.

JEANS, M. E. Relief of chronic pain by brief, intense transcutaneous electrical stimulation: A double blind study. *Adv. Pain Res. Ther.* 3:601–606, 1979.

JOHNSON, S. M., AND DUGGAN, A. W. Evidence that the opiate receptors of the substantia gelatinosa contribute to the depression by intravenous morphine of the spinal transmission of impulses in unmyelinated primary afferents. *Brain Res.* 207:223–228, 1981.

JORDAN, L. M., KENSHALO, D. R., MARTIN, R. F., HABER, L. H., AND WILLIS, W. D. Depression of primate spinothalamic tract neurons by iontophoretic application of 5-hydroxytryptamine. *Pain* 5:135–142, 1978.

KENSHALO, D. R., LEONARD, R. B., CHUNG, J. M. AND WILLIS, W. D. Responses of primate spinothalamic neurons to graded and to repeated noxious heat stimuli. *J. Neurophysiol.* 42:1370–1389, 1979.

KITAHATA, L. M. KOSAKA, Y., TAUB, A., BONIKOS, K., AND HOFFERT, M. Lamina specific suppression of dorsal-horn unit activity by morphine sulfate. *Anesthesiology* 41:39–48, 1974.

KNIFFKI, K. D., MENSE, S., AND SCHMIDT, R. F. The spinocervical tract as a possible pathway for muscular nociception. *J. Physiol. (Paris)* 73:359–366, 1977.

KRNJEVIĆ, K., AND PHILLIS, J. W. Iontophoretic studies of neurones in the mammalian cerebral cortex. *J. Physiol. (Lond.) 165:274–304, 1963.*

LE BARS, D., AND CHITOUR, D. Do convergent neurones in the spinal dorsal horn discriminate nociceptive from non-nociceptive information? *Pain* 17:1–19, 1983.

LE BARS, D., MENÉTREY, D., CONSEILLER, C., AND BESSON, J. M. Depressive effects of morphine upon lamina V cells activities in the dorsal horn of the spinal cat. *Brain Res.* 98:261–277, 1975.

LE BARS, D., GUILBAUD, G., JURNA, I., AND BESSON, J. M. Differential effects of morphine on response of dorsal horn lamina V type cells elicited by A and C fibre stimulation in the spinal cat. *Brain Res.* 115:518–524, 1976.

LE BARS, D., DICKENSON, A. H., AND BESSON, J. M. Diffuse noxious inhibitory controls (DNIC). I—Effects on dorsal horn convergent neurones in the rat. *Pain* 6:283–304, 1979a.

LE BARS, D., DICKENSON, A. H., AND BESSON, J. M. Diffuse noxious inhibitory controls (DNIC). II—Lack of effect on non convergent neurones, supraspinal involvement and theoretical implications. *Pain* 6:305–327, 1979b.

LE BARS, D., RIVOT, J. P., GUILBAUD, G., MENÉTREY, D., AND BESSON, J. M. The depressive effect of morphine on the C fibre response of dorsal horn neurones in the spinal rat pretreated or not by pCPA. *Brain Res.* 176:337–353, 1979c.

LE BARS, D., GUILBAUD, G., CHITOUR, D., AND BESSON, J. M. Does systemic morphine increase descending inhibitory controls of dorsal horn neurones involved in nociception? *Brain Res.* 202:223–228 1980.

LE BARS, D., CHITOUR, D., AND CLOT, A. M. The encoding of thermal stimuli by diffuse noxious inhibitory controls (DNIC). *Brain Res.* 230:394–399, 1981a.

LE BARS, D., CHITOUR, D., KRAUS, E., CLOT, A. M., DICKENSON, A. H., AND BESSON, J. M. The effect of systemic morphine upon diffuse noxious inhibitory controls (DNIC) in the rat: Evidence for a lifting of certain descending inhibitory controls of dorsal horn convergent neurones. *Brain Res.* 215:257–274, 1981b.

LE BARS, D., DICKENSON, A. H., AND BESSON, J. M. The triggering of bulbo-spinal serotonergic inhibitory controls by noxious peripheral inputs, in: *Brainstem Control of Spinal Mechanisms*, Fernström Foundation Series 1 (B. SJÖØLUND AND A. BJÖRKLUND, eds.), Elsevier, Amsterdam 1982, pp. 381–410.

LE BARS, D. DICKENSON, A. H., AND BESSON, J. M. Opiate analgesia and descending control systems. *Adv. Pain Res. Ther.* 5:341–372, 1983a.

LE BARS, D., ROBY, A., AND WILLER, J. C. Effects of heterotopic thermal stimuli on a nociceptive flexion reflex and the related pain sensation in man. *J. Physiol. (Lond.)* 336:31–32P, 1983b.

LE BARS, D., CALVINO, B., VILLANUEVA, L., AND CADDEN, S. Physiological approaches to counter-irritation phenomena, in: *Stress-Induced Analgesia* (G. CURZON AND M. D. TRICKLEBANK, eds.), John Wiley & Sons, London, 1984, pp. 67–101.

LEVANTE, A., LAMOUR, Y., GUILBAUD, G., AND BESSON, J. M. Spinothalamic cell activity in the monkey during intense nociceptive stimulation; intra-arterial injection of bradykinin into the limbs. *Brain Res.* 88:550–554, 1975.

LEVINE, J. D., GORMLEY, J., AND FIELDS, H. L. Observations on the analgesic effects of needle puncture (acupuncture). *Pain* 2:149–159, 1976.

LIEBESKIND, J. C., GUILBAUD, G., BESSON, J. M., AND OLIVERAS, J. L. Analgesia from electrical stimulation of the periaqueductal gray matter in the cat: Behavioral observations and inhibitory effects on spinal cord interneurons. *Brain Res.* 50:441–446, 1973.

LINDBLOM, U., TAPPER, D. N., AND WIESENFIELD, Z. The effect of dorsal horn column stimulation on the nociceptive response of dorsal horn cells and its relevance to pain suppression. *Pain* 4:133–144, 1977.

MANN, F. Acupuncture analgesia, report of 100 experiments. *Br. J. Anaesth.* 46:361–364, 1974.

MC CREERY, D., AND BLOEDEL, J. R. Effect of trigeminal stimulation on the excitability of cat spinothalamic neurons. *Brain Res.* 117:136–140, 1976.

MELZACK, R. Prolonged relief of pain by brief, intense transcutaneous somatic stimulation. *Pain* 1:357–373, 1975.

MELZACK, R., AND WALL, P. D. Pain mechanisms: A new theory. *Science* 150:971–979, 1965.

MELZACK, R., STILLWELL, D. M., AND FOX, E. J. Trigger points and acupuncture points for pain: Correlations and implications. *Pain* 3:3–24, 1977.

MENDELL, L. M. Physiological properties of unmyelinated fiber projections to the spinal cord. *Exp. Neurol.* 16:316–332, 1966.

MENDELL, L. M., AND WALL, P. D. Responses of single dorsal cord cells to peripheral cutaneous unmyelinated fibers. *Nature* 206:97–99, 1965.

MENÉTREY, D., GIESLER, G. J., JR., AND BESSON, J. M. An analysis of responses properties of spinal cord dorsal horn neurones to non-noxious and noxious stimuli in the spinal rat. *Exp. Brain Res.* 27:15–33, 1977.

MENÉTREY, D., CHAOUCH, A., AND BESSON, J. M. Responses of spinal cord dorsal horn neurons to non noxious and noxious cutaneous temperature changes in the spinal rat. *Pain* 6:265–282, 1979.

MERSKEY, H., AND EVANS, P. R. Variation in pain complaint threshold in psychiatric and neurological patients with pain. *Pain* 1:73–79, 1975.

MILNE, R. J., FOREMAN, R. D., GIESLER, G. J., JR., AND WILLIS, W. D. Convergence of cutaneous and pelvic visceral nociceptive inputs onto primate spinothalamic neurons. *Pain* 11:163–183, 1981.

NIEMEGEERS, C. J. E., VAN BRUGGEN, J. A. A., AND JANSSEN, P. A. J. Suprofen, a potent antagonist of acetic-induced writhing in rat. *Arzneim. Forsch.* 25:1505–1509, 1975.

NOORDENBOS, W. *Pain*, Elsevier, Amsterdam, 1959.

OLIVERAS, J. L., BESSON, J. M., GUILBAUD, G., AND LIEBESKIND, J. C. Behavioral and electrophysiological evidence of pain inhibition from midbrain stimulation in the cat. *Exp. Brain Res.* 20:32–44, 1974.

PARSONS, C. M., AND GOETZL, F. R. Effect of induced pain on pain threshold. *Proc. Soc. Exp. Biol.* 60:327–329, 1945.

PEERTOOVARA, A., KEMPPAINEN, P., JOHANSSON, G., AND KARONEN, S. L. Ischemic pain non segmentally produces a predominant reduction of pain and thermal sensitivity in man: A selective role for endogenous opioids. *Brain Res.* 251:83–92, 1982.

PIRCIO, A. W., FEDELE, C. I., AND BIERWAGEN, M. E. A new method for the evaluation of analgesic activity using adjuvant-induced arthritis in the rat. *Eur. J. Pharmacol.* 31:207–215, 1975.

POMERANZ, B., WALL, P. D., AND WEBER, W. V. Cord cells reponding to fine myelinated afferents from viscera, muscle and skin. *J. Physiol. (Lond.)* 199:511–532, 1968.

PRICE D. D., AND BROWE, A. C. Responses of spinal cord neurons to graded noxious and non noxious stimuli. *Exp. Neurol.* 48:201–221, 1975.

PRICE, D. D., AND MAYER, D. J. Physiological laminar organization of the dorsal horn of *M. mulatta. Brain Res.* 79:321–325, 1974.

PRICE, D. D., AND WAGMAN, I. H. The physiological roles of A and C fiber inputs to the dorsal horn of *M. mulatta. Exp. Neurol.* 29:373–390, 1970.

PRICE, D. D., HULL, C. D., AND BUCHWALD, N. A. Intracellular responses of dorsal horn cells to cutaneous and sural nerve A and C fiber stimuli. *Exp. Neurol.* 33:291–309, 1971.

PRICE, D. D., DUBNER,R., AND HU, J. W. Trigeminothalamic neurons in nucleus caudalis responsive to tactile, thermal and nociceptive stimulation of monkey's face. *J Neurophysiol.* 39:936–953, 1976.

PRICE, D. D., HU, J. W., DUBNER, R., AND GRACELY, R. Pain suppression of first pain and central summation of second pain evoked by noxious heat pulses. *Pain* 3:57–68, 1977.

PRICE, D. D., HAYES, R. L., RUDA, M. A., AND DUBNER, R. Spatial and temporal transformation of input to spinothalamic tract neurons and their relation to somatic sensations. *J. Neurophysiol.* 41:933–947, 1978.

PRICE, D. D., HAYASHI, H., DUBNER, R., AND RUDA, M. A. Functional relationships between neurons of the marginal and substantia gelatinosa layers of the primate dorsal horn. *J. Neurophysiol.* 42:1590–1608, 1979.

PUIL, E. *S*-Glutamate: Its interactions with spinal neurons. *Brain Res. Rev.* 3:229–322, 1981.

REXED, B. A cytoarchitectonic atlas of the spinal cord in the cat. *J. Comp. Neurol.* 100:297–380, 1954.

RUCH, T. C. Visceral sensation and referred pain, in: *Howell's Textbook of Physiology* (J. F. BULTON, ed.), W. B. Saunders, Philadelphia, 1949, pp. 360–374.

RUCH, T. C. Pathophysiology of pain, in: *Physiology and Biophysics,* Vol. 1 (T. C. RUCH AND H. D. PATTON, eds.), W. B. Saunders, Philadelphia, 1979, pp. 309–316.

SCHOUENBORG, J., AND DICKENSON, A. H. The effects of a distant noxious stimulation on A and C fibre evoked flexion reflexes and neuronal activity in dorsal horn of the rat. *Brain Res.* 328:23–32, 1985.

VILLANUEVA, L., AND LE BARS, D. The encoding of thermal stimuli applied to the tail of the rat by lowering the excitability of trigeminal convergent neurones. *Brain Res.* 330:245– 251, 1985.

VILLANUEVA, L., CADDEN, S. W., AND LE BARS, D. Evidence that diffuse noxious inhibitory controls (DNIC) are mediated by a final post-synaptic inhibitory mechanism. *Brain Res.* 298:67– 74, 1984a.

VILLANUEVA, L., CADDEN, S. W., AND LE BARS, D. Diffuse noxious inhibitory controls (DNIC): Evidence for post-synaptic inhibition of trigeminal nucleus caudalis convergent neurones. *Brain Res.* 321:165–168, 1984b.

WAGMAN, I. H., AND PRICE, D. D. Responses of dorsal horn cells of *M. mulatta* to cutaneous and sural nerve A and C-fiber stimulation. *J. Neurophysiol.* 32:803–817, 1969.

WALL, P. D. Cord cells responding to touch, damage and temperature of skin. *J. Neurophysiol.* 23:197–210, 1960.

WALL, P. D. The laminar organizaton of dorsal horn and effects of descending impulses. *J. Physiol. (Lond.)* 188:403–423, 1967.

WALL, P. D. Dorsal horn electrophysiology, in: *Handbook of Sensory Physiology,* Vol. II, *Somatosensory System* (A. IGGO, ed.), Springer Verlag, New York, 1973, pp. 253–270.

WALL, P. D. The gate control theory of pain mechanisms. *Brain* 101:1–18, 1978.

WALL, P. D., FREEMAN, J., AND MAJOR, D. Dorsal horn cells in spinal and in freely moving rats. *Exp. Neurol.* 19:519–529, 1967.

WAND-TETLEY, J. I. Historical methods of counter-irritation. *Ann. Phys. Med.* 3:90–98, 1956.

WILLER, J. C., ROBY, A., AND LE BARS, D. Psychophysical and electrophysiological approaches to the pain-relieving effects of heterotopic nociceptive stimuli. *Brain* 107:1095–1112, 1984.

WILLIS, W. D. Ascending pathways from the dorsal horn, in: *Spinal Cord Sensation* (A. G. BROWN AND M. RETHELYI, eds.) Scottish Academy Press, Edinburgh, 1981, pp. 169–178.

WILLIS, W. D. Control of nociceptive transmission in the spinal cord, in: *Progress in Sensory Physiology,* vol. 3 (D. OTTOSON, ed.), Springer-Verlag, New York, 1982, pp. 1–155.

WILLIS, W. D., TREVINO, D. L., COULTER, J. D., AND MAUNZ, R. A. Responses of primate spinothalamic tract neurons to natural stimulation of hindlimb. *J. Neurophysiol.* 37:358–372, 1974.

WOOLF, C. J., AND FITZGERALD, M. Lamina-specific alteration of C-fibre evoked activity by morphine in the dorsal horn of the rat spinal cord. *Neurosci. Lett.* 25:37–41, 1981.

YEUNG, J. C., AND RUDY, T. A. Multiplicative interaction between narcotic agonisms expressed at spinal and supraspinal sites of antinociceptive action as revealed by concurrent intrathecal and intracerebroventricular injections of morphine. *J. Pharmacol. Exp. Ther.* 215:633–642, 1980.

YEZIERSKI, R. P., WILCOX, T. K., AND WILLIS, W. D. The effects of serotonin antagonists on the inhibition of primate spinothalamic tract cells produced by stimulation in nucleus raphé magnus or the periaqueductal gray. *J. Pharmacol. Exp. Ther.* 220:266–277, 1982.

ZIMMERMANN, M. Encoding in dorsal horn interneurons receiving noxious and nonnoxious afferents. *J. Physiol. (Paris)* 73:221–232, 1977.

20
The Effects of Intrathecally Administered Opioid and Adrenergic Agents on Spinal Function

TONY L. YAKSH

A. Introduction

From the preceding chapters of this book, it is clear that the basic experimental work carried out during the past 10–15 years has led to a remarkable growth in our appreciation of the anatomic and biochemical complexity of the afferent systems through which sensory information in general and that associated with pain in particular is processed.

Conceptually, a major insight has been the growing application of the idea that processing at the spinal cord level is subject to a powerful modulation by a variety of anatomically and pharmacologically distinct systems (see Hammond, Chapter 15; Ruda, Chapter 7). The conceptualization of the "gate-control theory" by Melzack and Wall (1965), the "postsynaptic inhibitory balance theory" of Kerr (1975; 1976), and more recently the "diffuse noxious inhibitory control (DNIC)" of Le Bars and Besson and colleagues (see Chapter 19) all suggest the presence of intrinsic systems that modulate spinal function. As reviewed in previous chapters, several lines of physiological and biochemical evidence have accumulated pointing to the identity of several such neurotransmitter systems that may indeed alter the characteristics of the sensory

TONY L. YAKSH • Departments of Neurosurgery and Pharmacology, Mayo Clinic, Rochester, Minnesota 55905.

message related to pain transmission. Two such systems are those that release endorphins, for which opioid receptors serve to mediate the effect, and the spinopetal adrenergic systems (see LaMotte, Chapter 5; Ruda, Chapter 7; Seybold, Chapter 6). The ability of such systems to modulate physiological indices of spinal activity evoked by small-fiber input leads naturally to the question of whether such spinal receptor systems may alter the behavior consequences of high-intensity somatic/visceral stimuli. In the following sections I wish to review (1) the characteristics of the action of opioid and adrenergic agonists on spinal function, particularly as it pertains to pain transmission, and (2) the pharmacological characteristics of the receptor acted on by the agents to alter nociceptive transmission.

B. *Spinal Opioid Receptor Systems*

1. *Effects of Opioid Agonists on Spinal Neuronal Function*

Systemic administration of opiates in spinally transected animals attenuates the polysynaptic ventral root reflex (Wikler, 1950) and selectively suppresses activity in dorsal horn neurons evoked by the stimulation of Aδ/C-fiber afferents or the activity induced by a variety of somatic and visceral stimuli that evoke pain behavior (Le Bars *et al.*, 1975; Yaksh, 1978a, b; Einspahr and Piercey, 1980). In paraplegic man, morphine has been reported to block the polysynaptic reflex evoked by sural nerve stimulation of the tibialis anterior muscle with no effect on the monosynaptic H reflex (Willer and Bussel, 1980). Three questions are raised. Are these effects selective for noxious stimuli? Are the neurons whose activity is affected by spinal opiates actually projection neurons, or is the opioid effect limited to an effect on segmentally processed information. Is the effect of spinal opiates mediated by an "opioid receptor"?

With regard to the question of selectivity, although the effects noted above were observed to be preferential for nociceptive input, measurable effects on receptor field size and on the response to nonnoxious stimuli have also been described, though at generally higher doses (Yaksh, 1978b; Einspahr and Piercey, 1980). Secondly, neurons that were demonstrated to project into the ventrolateral tract and whose activity was evoked by noxious stimuli were indeed suppressed by systemically administered opiates (Jurna and Grossman, 1976). Thus, some neurons whose activity was affected by opiates indeed projected suprasegmentally. Finally, the effects of systemically administered opiates in spinal-transected animals on nociceptive evoked discharge are mediated by an opioid receptor as defined by the following criteria: (1) the rank order of activity (i.e., the structure–activity relationship) was in accord with the expected efficacy of these agents in receptor bioassay systems, etorphine > fentanyl > levorphanol ⩾ morphine ⩾ *d,l* methadone ⩾ U50488H ⩾ meperidine ⩾ dextrorphan = naloxone = 0) (Iwata and Sakai,

1971; Jurna and Heinz, 1979; Piercey *et al.*, 1982a; T. L. Yaksh, unpublished observations); and (2) the effects were readily antagonized by systemically administered naloxone in a dose-dependent fashion (Yaksh, 1978).

2. *Substrates on Which Spinal Opioids May Act*

Iontophoretic application of opiates into the dorsal horn will suppress the activity evoked by a variety of noxious thermal or mechanical stimuli applied to the cutaneous receptive field of the cells being examined (Calvillo *et al.*,1979; Zieglgansberger and Bayerl, 1976). Although application near the cell body in the nucleus proprius would inhibit evoked activity, significant suppressant effects were more readily demonstrated when the opiate was given into the substantia gelatinosa, where the dendritic arbors of the primary afferents and the more deeply lying neurons were spatially congruent (Duggan *et al.*, 1981. Naloxone given either systemically or iontophoretically could frequently antagonize the suppression (but see Davies and Dray, 1978).

Such observations indicated that opiates acting within the dorsal gray matter of the spinal cord suppressed activity evoked by stimuli that would support escape behavior in the unanesthetized animal. Moreover, by virtue of the pharmacological characteristics relating the action of drugs to the observed physiological endpoint, it appeared likely that the local drug effect is mediated by an action on opioid receptors.

An important question is by what mechanisms opiates act to alter nociceptive processing in the spinal cord.

Binding studies reviewed by Seybold (see Chapter 6) demonstrated that (1) rhizotomies would produce a significant but subtotal reduction in opioid binding in the dorsal horn (LaMotte *et al.*, 1976), (2) opioid binding sites could be found in dorsal roots and on dorsal root ganglion cells (Fields *et al.*, 1980; Ninkovic *et al.*, 1982), and (3) capsaicin, a neurotoxin that primarily destroys small or unmyelinated primary afferents (see Yaksh, Chapter 8), produced a reduction in opioid ligand binding in rat spinal cord that is comparable to that seen with rhizotomy (Gamse *et al.*, 1979). These results suggest that a proportion of the opioid binding sites in the dorsal horn is associated with small afferents that may serve in part to transmit nociceptive information.

The likelihood of a presynaptic action of opiates mediated by primary afferent binding sites is indeed supported by several physiological observations: (1) opiates have a powerful receptor-mediated effect on electrical activity in dorsal root ganglion cultures (Mudge *et al.*, 1979; MacDonald and Nelson, 1978; Werz and MacDonald, 1983); (2) opiates decrease the excitability of primary afferent terminals (Carstens *et al.*, 1979; Sastry, 1980); and (3) release of substance P from small primary afferents is inhibited *in vivo* and *in vitro* by morphine and DAla^2-DLeu^5-enkephalin in a naloxone-reversible fashion (see Yaksh, Chapter 8).

Alternatively, a postsynaptic action of opiates also appears likely. First, rhizotomy produces only a partial loss of dorsal horn opiate binding (see above). Secondly, opiates can suppress the postsynaptic EPSP evoked by iontophoretically administered excitatory amino acids, which are thought to exert a direct effect in the membrane postsynaptic to the primary afferent (Zieglgansberger and Bayerl, 1976).

3. Analgesic Effects Mediated by Spinal Opioid Receptors

The potent action of opioid ligands on nociceptive reflexes and the activity in spinal cord neurons provoked by nociceptive stimulation along with the clear pharmacology characterizing these effects suggest that opioids in the cord may significantly alter the processing of nociceptive information. Such observations provide, however, no insight as to the relevance of these opiate-receptor-linked systems to pain-evoked behavior. At one time, we considered it possible that these effects on spinal systems were related to substrates that regulated autonomic or somatomotor processing but not necessarily to spinal systems that were relevant to pain-processing behavior. For that reason, early studies were carried out to determine whether an action of opiates limited to the spinal cord in the unanesthetized and intact animal would produce a change in the nociceptive threshold. The advances in these studies were facilitated by the demonstration that a small polyethylene catheter could be passed atraumatically to various levels of the intrathecal space in the spinal cords of a variety of species ranging from the rat to the primate (Yaksh and Rudy, 1976; Yaksh and Reddy, 1981).

The phenomenon of analgesia may be described as the absence of an organized pain response in the presence of otherwise adequate stimuli in an organism otherwise capable of responding to all stimuli. The principal consideration is that peripheral information must reach supraspinal levels to evoke the pain state. In animal studies, the endpoint that signifies analgesia is the failure by the organism to respond in an organized behavioral response such as a bar press or jump escape response to remove itself from the presence of an unconditioned stimulus that would otherwise evoke that behavior. Spinally mediated responses such as the tail flick and the skin twitch, though convenient, can never alone be taken to indicate "analgesia," as many factors may alter motor tone either physiologically (as by an alteration in extensor–flexor tone, e.g. Straub tail in the rat after morphine) or by altering motor neuron excitability or synergy between extensor/flexor pools of motor horn cells. Thus, although inhibition of a spinal flexor reflex may covary with inhibition of an interneuron relevant to the transmission of an ascending sensory message, it is clear that the loss of the reflex can occur in the absence of an effect on the ascending sensory system (see Gebhart, Chapter 16, for further comments).

Table I presents the effect of spinally administered morphine on a wide variety of spinal or supraspinally organized pain models in man and animal.

TABLE I
Summary of Experimental Models of Pain Behavior

Pain model	Species	Spinal morphine[a] dose (nmol)	References[e]
Experimental			
Temperature			
Thermal spinal reflex			
Tail flick	Mouse	0.9– 2.4[b]	1
	Rat	1.3–11.9	2
Skin twitch	Cat	120[b]	3
Thermal supraspinal			
Hot plate	Mouse	1.5– 5.7[b]	1
	Rat	0.9–12.7[b]	1
Cold supraspinal			
Limb immersion	Human	30,000[c]	
Electrical			
Shock vocalization	Rat	90[c]	5
Shock titration	Rat	135[c]	6
	Primate	3,000[d]	7
Pressure			
Pinch	Rat	0.8– 3.5[b]	8
Tourniquet pressure	Human	10,500[c]	9
Inflammatory			
Writhing	Mice	0.08–0.21[b]	1
	Rat	0.3–12.1[b]	2
Clinical			
Postoperative, thoracic/upper abdominal		2–8 mg	
Visual analogue scale			10,11,12
Modified McGill pain questionnaire			10
Mobilization scale			13
Duration or time to first analgesia[c] (>10 h)			14,15,16
Cumulative consumption of additional analgesics			14,16
Respiratory function			
Peak expiratory flow rate			12,13
Vital capacity			12,17
Forced expiratory volume at 1 s			13,16,17
CO_2 response curves			18
Pulmonary X-ray changes			13,17
Terminal cancer			
Visual analogue scale			18
McGill pain questionnaire			18
Consumption of additional analgesics			18,19,20
Time between doses			18,19,21

[a] Intrathecal in animals; epidural in man.
[b] 95% CI of ED_{50}.
[c] Dose that produces a significant increase over base line.
[d] Dose that just produces the maximum increase in the shock titration response.
[e] 1, Piercey *et al.*, 1982a,b; 2, Schmauss and Yaksh, 1984; 3, Yaksh, 1978a,b,c; 4, Bromage *et al.*, 1980; 5, Tang and Schoenfeld, 1978; 6, Yaksh and Rudy, 1977; 7, Yaksh, 1983; 8, Kuraishi *et al.*, 1980; 9, Thompson *et al.*, 1981; 10, Anderson *et al.*, 1981; 11, Cahill *et al.*, 1983; 12, Torda and Pybus, 1984; 13, Rawal *et al.*, 1984; 14, Nordberg, 1984; 15, Torda and Pybus, 1982; 16, Bromage *et al.*, 1980; 17, Rybro *et al.*, 1982; 18, Coombs *et al.*, 1984; 19, Müller *et al.*, 1982; 20, Onofrio *et al.*, 1981, 21, Zenz, 1985.

Though not an exhaustive summary, it emphasizes that morphine with an action limited to the spinal cord will produce a powerful alteration in responses otherwise evoked by high-intensity stimuli. As indicated, spinal morphine will produce a significant increase in the latency of spinally and supraspinally mediated responses (tail flick/skin twitch or hot plate, respectively), attenuate the magnitude of the response to mechanical stimuli (pressure) applied to the paws and limbs, increase the intensity of shock required to evoke an operant response such as the bar press or an evoked response such as a squeak, and reduce the response evoked by visceral irritants.

Though experimental pain models in man have not proven as useful as in animals, spinal opiates have been shown to increase the ability to tolerate cold-water immersion and a pressure torniquet applied to the limbs. In man, spinal morphine in postoperative patients or in patients suffering from cancer will produce a powerful analgesia as measured by a wide variety of behavioral endpoints including the visual analogue scale, the McGill pain questionnaire, and scales indicating postoperative mobility. Physiological indices such as respiratory function also indicate significant improvement in performance secondary to a reduction in the pain stimulus. In groups receiving spinal opioid administration, there is (1) an increase in the time to the administration of the first alternative analgesic, and (2) the cumulative consumption of the parenternal analgesic otherwise expected in the postoperative course is remarkably reduced. Comparable results have been reported with patients suffering from metastatic disease although the interpretation of such data over long periods of time is rendered difficult by both the possible day-to-day variation in the pain and the problems of tolerance that are associated with long-term use of opiates whether by a systemic or spinal route.

4. *Effect of Spinal Opiates on Non-Pain-Related Behaviors*

In view of the effect of spinal opiates on pain behavior, it is important to consider whether these suppressed effects are limited to a certain class of stimulus–response relationships. Doses of spinally administered opiates that produce a significant inhibition of reflex and nonreflexively mediated nociceptive responses have been reported to have no effect on placing, stepping, or tendon reflexes (Yaksh and Rudy, 1977; Yaksh and Reddy, 1981). In operant studies, spinal morphine given at analgesic doses will have no detectable effect on nonnociceptive modalities. Thus, monkeys with intrathecal catheters trained to respond to avoid shock delivered to the ear cued by a tactile stimulus applied to the foot showed no loss of the ability to detect the tactile cue in the presence of maximally analgesic doses of spinal morphine (Yaksh and Reddy, 1981). In man, no significant effect of morphine on two-point thresholds has been observed.

5. *Pharmacology of Opioid Agonists in the Spinal Cord*

As reviewed elsewhere (W. R. Martin, 1983; Yaksh, 1984a,b; see Seybold, Chapter 6), there appear to be several populations of opioid receptors. Following the description by Martin and colleagues (see Martin, 1983) of three classes of receptors (μ, κ and σ), the discovery of the opioid peptides led to the subsequent derivation of two other populations: δ (Lord *et al.*, 1977) and ε (Schulz *et al.*, 1979). More recently, multiple subpopulations of μ sites and κ sites have also been postulated (Pasternak *et al.*, 1980; Attali *et al.*, 1982). As discussed by Seybold (Chapter 6), significant levels of μ, δ and κ selective ligand binding sites have been demonstrated in the spinal cord, with the highest levels commonly being observed in the dorsal gray matter.

Although these binding studies suggest the presence of recognition sites, an important question is which (if any) of these defined sites are relevant to the processing of pain-related behavior? The characteristics of the opiate receptors that may modulate the processing of nociceptive transmission may be defined in terms of three properties: (1) the structure–activity relationship, (2) the characteristics of the antagonism by an appropriate receptor antagonist such as naloxone, and (3) the characteristics of the cross tolerance between families of the spinally administered opiates.

a. *Structure–Activity Relationship of Spinally Administered Opioid Agonists*

Table II presents the structure–activity series for a variety of opioids, alkaloids, and peptides given intrathecally in three species including the mouse (tail flick and hot plate), the rat (hot plate, tail flick, and writhing), and the primate (shock titration). Several points may be emphasized regarding the data presented in Table II. Intrathecal injection of a series of opioid alkaloids in these different species will result in a suppression of the behavioral responses evoked by high-intensity thermal, mechanical, and chemical stimuli. The maximum inhibition of the response on each of the measures is achieved in a monotonic dose-dependent fashion by opioid alkaloids and peptides whose relative spinal analgetic potency (as indicated by their respective ED_{50} values) on the several tests may differ by as much as 3–4 orders of magnitude (e.g., lofentanil versus codeine or metkephamid versus met-enkephalin). Moreover, the rank ordering of potency in the primate and the rat on the several tests is comparable and suggests that the relative activity on cutaneous thermal and foot-shock titration stimulus-related tests could not be distinguished, although such results do not imply that the relevant receptor populations acted on by these spinally administered agents are homogeneous. The rank ordering of activity on the several cutaneous thermal tests suggests that agents classified by *in vitro* bioassay and binding systems as having high affinity or efficacy at both μ and δ receptors (for example metkephamid and β-endorphin) as opposed to μ (morphine, sufentanil) or δ (DADL/DPE_2) receptors alone are

TABLE II
Potencies Relative to Morphine of Intrathecally Administered μ, δ, κ, and σ Agonists in the Rat and Primate

Ligand and putative receptor selectivity	Rat[a]			Primate[b]: shock titration
	Tail flick	Hot plate	Writhing	
μ				
Morphine	1.0	1.0	1.0	1.0
Lofentanil	98.6	118.2	—[c]	2100.0
Sufentanil	15.0	27.7	—	—
Levorphanol	8.1	10.2	7.8	—
Fentanyl	2.0	1.7	—	—
Alfentanil	0.9	0.76	—	—
D/L-Methadone	0.1	0.6	—	1.0
Meperidine	0.07	0.05	—	0.2
Codeine	<0.01	<0.01	—	—
δ				
DADL	1.5	1.0	<0.1	—
DPE_2	1.3	1.0	<0.06	—
Met-enkephalin	0.03	0.02	<0.01	—
Leu-enkephalin	<0.01	<0.01	<0.01	—
DSTLE	—	—	<0.1	—
μ/δ				
D-Ala^2-MEA	42.0	33.0	0.04	2.3
β-Endorphin	33.0	25.0	2.6	27.0
Metkephamid	21.0	21.0	1.4	35.0
Etorphine	18.1	22.3	—	—
D-Ala^2-Met-enkephalin	0.7	0.9	—	—
κ				
U-50488H	<0.01	<0.01	0.03	—
Bremazocine	<0.01	0.05	0.09	—
EKC	<0.01	0.03	0.18	—
Dynorphin$_{1-10}$	<0.1	<0.1	1.1	—
σ				
SKF10047	<0.01	<0.01	<0.01	—
Partial agonists				
Nalbuphine	<0.01	<0.01	0.03	—
Buprenorphine	0.2	—	0.2	—
Nallorphine	<0.01	<0.01	—	—
Pentazocine	<0.01	<0.01	0.1	—
D-isomers				
D-Methadone	<0.01	<0.01	<0.01	<0.01
Dextrorphan	<0.01	<0.01	<0.01	—

[a] Yaksh and Rudy, 1977; Yaksh *et al.*, 1977a, 1978; Yaksh and Henry, 1978; Tung and Yaksh, 1982; Schmauss *et al.*, 1983, 1984; Schmauss and Yaksh, 1984; Schmauss *et al.*, 1985; T. L. Yaksh and colleagues, unpublished observations; Russell and Yaksh, 1981.
[b] Yaksh and Reddy, 1981; Yaksh, 1983; T. L. Yaksh, G. Harty and K. Gross, unpublished observersations.
[c] Not tested.

among the most active. These observations are consistent with the hypothesis that coactivation of μ and δ spinal receptor sites will result in a synergistic interaction (Larson *et al.*, 1980).

κ Ligands such as U50488H or partial agonists such as buprenorphine and partial agonists/antagonists such as nalbuphine in general show limited activity in the cutaneous thermal test when administered spinally. Ethylketocyclazocine, which has been reported to be weakly active on hot plate and tail flick (but see Wood *et al.*, 1981), has been shown by *in vitro* binding and studies in bioassay analysis to possess significant μ receptor activity (see Yaksh, 1984a,b, for review). Agents having purportedly significant degrees of κ selectivity such as U50488H appeared devoid of any effect on hot plate and tail flick in the rat when given spinally (Schmauss and Yaksh, 1984). More recently, dynorphinlike peptides have been shown to have κ receptor selectivity and have been shown after spinal administration to produce significant effects on several nociceptive reflexes (Piercey *et al.*, 1982a,b, Przewlocki *et al.*, 1983; Herman and Goldstein, 1985). It should be noted, however, that such effects often were obtained only at doses at which significant signs of hindlimb dysfunction were present (Kaneko *et al.*, 1983).

With regard to visceral chemical stimuli, Table II indicates that the relative potencies of intrathecal morphine on hot plate, tail flick, and writhing are very similar. It should be stressed that such similarity is fortuitous, as the exact ED_{50} on a given measure will vary with the endpoint selected. Nevertheless, in comparison, agents that by virtue of bioassay and binding studies, are designated as δ receptor ligands, such as the dimer peptides (DPE_n; Krumins *et al.*, 1982) or DAla^2-D-Leu^5-enkephalin, given intrathecally in the rat were considerably less active than morphine on the writhing test. Indeed, effects on this response were not obtained at doses that did not produce effects on hindlimb function. In contrast, κ ligands that were inactive on the hot-plate and tail-flick response became measurably more active on the visceral chemical writhing response. Consistent with the apparent lack of δ receptor-mediated activity in the visceral chemical writhing test in the rat, agents such as metkephamid and β endorphin with high levels of both μ and δ activity show a marked attenuation in their measured potency after intrathecal administration on the writhing test as compared to the relatively pure μ agonists such as sufentanil and morphine, which show essentially no change in relative activity between visceral chemical and cutaneous thermal tests. Thus, the loss of activity relative to morphine shown by agents with mixed μ/δ activity on visceral chemical versus the cutaneous thermal tests is consistent with the apparent lack of effect of δ ligands such as DADL or the dimer peptides, DPE_2.

b. *Antagonism by Naloxone of the Effects Produced by Intrathecal Opioids*

Changes in the nociceptive threshold evoked by intrathecal administration of opioid alkaloids and peptides can be antagonized in a dose-dependent fashion by systemic or intrathecally administered naloxone. Naloxone produces parallel shifts in the dose–response curve of the agonists, with the magnitude of the shift in the agonist dose–response curve being proportional to the logarithm of the antagonist dose (Yaksh and Rudy, 1977). The results of systematic examination of the ability of systemically administered antagonists to antagonize the effect curves of intrathecal opioid agonists have been employed to derive Schild plots (Tallarida *et al.*, 1979). This analysis permits the estimation of the apparent affinity of the antagonist for the receptor acted on by the agonist to produce the measured effect. Table III lists a summary of the results of current studies in which a systematic pA_2 analysis has been carried out in the rat with intrathecal opioids on the hot plate and tail flick and in the primate on the shock titration. As indicated, the estimated pA_2 value for the antagonism by naloxone and the antinociceptive effects of intrathecal morphine, sufentanil, alfentanil, fentanyl, β-endorphin, and EKC are similar, suggesting that on hot plate and tail flick, these agents given intrathecally act on a local population of spinal receptors that cannot be distinguished.

TABLE III
Apparent pA_2 Values for Systemic Naloxone in Antagonizing the Effect of Intrathecal Opioid Alkaloids and Peptides in the Rat and Primate

	Naloxone pA_2[a]			
	Rat			Primate: shock titration[f]
	Writhing[c,d]	Hot plate[d,e]	Tail flick[d,e]	
μ				
Morphine	7.2	7.0	7.0	6.7
Sufentanil	7.0	7.0	6.8	—
δ				
DADL	NA[c]	6.2	6.2	(—)
μ/δ				
β-Endorphin	7.4	7.3	7.1	6.8
DAME	—	7.0	7.2	(—)
κ				
U50488H	6.4	(—)[b]	(—)	—
EKC	5.9	(—)	(—)	—
Bremazocine	6.1	(—)	(—)	(—)
Partial agonists				
Nalbuphine	8.02	NA[b]	NA	(—)

[a] pA_2 values are derived from experiments in which the effect of the agonists administered intrathecally on the hot plate and tail flick (rat) and shock titration (primate) are examined in the presence of systemically administered antagonist. Injections were ordered such that responses were assessed at the time of peak effect of either agent.
[b] NA, not active as an agonist; (—), not tested.
[c] Schmauss and Yaksh, 1984.
[d] Noueihed *et al.*, 1984.
[e] Yaksh and Rudy, 1977; Tung and Yaksh, 1982; Yaksh and Henry, 1978; Schmauss and Yaksh, 1984.
[f] Yaksh and Reddy, 1981; Yaksh *et al.*, 1982a; Yaksh, 1983.

Relatively few studies have been carried out to assess the characteristics of the antagonism by naloxone of the spinal inhibition of the writhing response. Nevertheless, morphine, sufentanil and β-endorphin show a relative sensitivity to naloxone antagonism that is comparable to the effects observed on the hot plate and tail flick, suggesting that the receptor site acted on spinally by these two agents in altering the writhing response is not distinguishable from the receptor site acted on by these agents in blocking the hot plate and tail flick. In contrast, the antagonism by naloxone of DADL and metkephamid yields pA_2 values that are approximately 0.5 to 1 log unit less than those observed with spinally administered morphinelike agents. These results suggest, therefore, that the spinal receptor acted on by DADL resembles the system found in mouse vas deferens, where the enkephalinoid peptides are resistant to naloxone antagonism. With regard to the kappa agonist, the agents that are active on the writhing test are also antagonized by naloxone, but they show a similar resistance to naloxone antagonism. It should be pointed out that whereas EKC shows a pA_2 of around 7 in its effects on hot plate and tail flick, its effects on writhing are relatively resistant to naloxone antagonism, which supports the speculation that EKC may work on both μ and κ receptors with the effects of the μ receptor predominating on those cutaneous thermal measures, whereas the κ sites mediate those systems that are involved in the processing of visceral chemical information.

c. *Tolerance and Cross Tolerance among Spinally Administered Opioid Ligands and between Spinally Administered and Systemically Administered Agents*

Systemically administered morphine possesses a pharmacology that indicates that it produces analgesia by an action on an opioid receptor. Early studies indicated that animals rendered tolerant to systemic morphine showed a diminished response to intrathecal morphine (Yaksh *et al.*, 1977b; DeLander and Takemori, 1983), suggesting that the effects of intrathecal morphine are mediated by a receptor that is comparable to that acted on by systemic morphine. If prolonged exposure of the spinal cord is made with repeated intrathecal administrations of opiates, comparable tolerance also develops. This phenomenon is clearly evident in the rat and primate following intrathecal administration of a variety of opioid alkaloids and peptides, including morphine (Yaksh *et al.*, 1977,a,b; Yaksh and Reddy, 1981) or peptides such as β-endorphin (Yaksh *et al.*, 1982b; Tung and Yaksh, 1982), metkephamid, and DADL (Yaksh, 1983). A loss of the effects produced by otherwise equiactive doses of other agents has been observed in rats and primates rendered tolerant to intrathecal morphine. Thus, if the ED_{50} values are examined after an animal is rendered tolerant to intrathecal morphine, either by daily intrathecal injections or the implantation of pellets or the daily systemic administration of morphine, a relative loss of activity is observed such that morphine ≥ β-endorphine ≥ meperidine ≫ metkephamid ≥ DADL = 0 (Tung and Yaksh, 1982; Schmauss and Yaksh, 1984; Yaksh, 1983; Schmauss *et al.*, 1985; Yaksh *et al.*,

1984. T. L. Yaksh, unpublished observations). Agents that have a relative selectivity for the δ receptor as evidenced by *in vitro* binding studies and as evidenced by the pA_2 data obtained with systemic naloxone against intrathecal ligands showed little or no loss of effect in animals rendered tolerant to morphine. Asymmetry in cross tolerance has been reported in animals rendered tolerant to δ ligands such as DADL (Tseng, 1982) or metkephamid (Yaksh, 1983) such that these animals showed a significant loss in the response evoked by otherwise active doses of morphine and β-endorphin.

I stress that the cross-tolerance experiments are not without controversy. Thus, β-endorphin is thought to have mixed μ/δ receptor activity (see Yaksh, 1984a,b). Yet there is a significant loss of activity in morphine-tolerant animals. In contrast, metkephamid, which also is thought to have mixed μ/δ activity, was relatively resistant to the loss of activity in morphine-tolerant animals. Similarly, according to the loss of activity in the writhing test, a significant proportion of metkephamid activity may originate from a synergistic interaction between μ and δ receptors. It is likely that cross-tolerance studies do provide valuable information but are subject to a significant number of variables that are not currently understood, such as dose and time of exposure to the tolerance-producing agent. High doses of a given agonist will give rise to actions that are not specific to the receptor thought to be under investigation. No systematic studies have yet been reported addressing these considerations. The asymmetric cross-tolerance data thus may reflect this particular difficulty.

In summary, in the spinal cord, the different structure–activity relationships on different types of nociceptive measures (e.g., cutaneous thermal versus visceral chemical), the distinguishability of pA_2 values for naloxone in antagonizing the effects of the intrathecally administered agent, and the different degrees of cross tolerance all provide lines of evidence that argue persuasively for distinguishable populations of opioid receptors that modulate spinal nociceptive processing. Interpretation of these data vis-á-vis conventionally accepted receptor profiles strongly suggests that μ and δ type systems may mediate effects observed on the primate shock titration and in the rat hot plate and tail flick. In contrast, κ-receptor profiles appear to be largely directed toward those systems that are activated by visceral chemical stimulation. Other stimulus modalities such as pressure and so forth have not been systematically examined in these models, but κ agonists have classically been known to affect pressure evoked paw withdrawal (see Section B.3).

d. Characteristics of the Spinal Opioid Receptors in Man

Although the pharmacological investigations carried out in animal models cannot be repeated with the same degree of preciseness in man, considerable information may be derived from the characteristics of the spinal receptors that modulate pain transmission in man. Virtually all of the criteria that were addressed in the previous section on animal models, have partial data support in humans as well.

Structure–Activity Relationship. Spinally administered opioids produce a powerful analgesia, which demonstrates a monotonic dose dependency, although no systematic comparison is possible because of varying paradigms. The approximate rank order of potency seen in man, however, resembles that observed after spinal injection in rat and primate animal models. As summarized in Table IV, on a molar basis, β-endorphin ⩾ DADL ⩾ fentanyl > morphine > pentazocine > meperidine. The observation that D-Ala^2-D-leu^5-enkephalin given spinally in terminal cancer patients produces a powerful analgesia supports the concept that δ receptors are potentially active in the human spinal cord (Onofrio and Yaksh, 1983; Moulin *et al.*, 1985). The reported activity of buprenorphine and pentazocine also appears to suggest a receptor-type interaction that resembles that displayed by these agents in visceral chemical tests. It is important to consider the fact that κ binding sites

TABLE IV
Summary of Clinical Studies Showing the Range of Doses of Epidurally Administered Opioids Required to Produce "Acceptable" Analgesia in Man

Drug	Clinical situation	Dose range (mg)	Reference[c]
Morphine	Upper abdominal/thoracic	4–10	1[a],2,3,4[a]
	C-section/gynecologic	4–8	5[a],6,7[a]
	Lower abdominal/orthopedic	2–4	8,9[a]
	Terminal cancer[b]		10,11,12
Methadone	Upper abdominal/thoracic	9	3
Diamorphine	Lumbar laminectomy, major abdominal vascular surgery	5	13,14
β-Endorphin	Terminal cancer pain	3	15
Meperidine	Upper abdominal/thoracic	50–60	16,17
Alfentanil	Orthopedic/abdominal	0.015–0.3	18
Pentazocine	Gynecologic/abdominal	10–15	19,20
Fentanyl	Upper abdominal/thoracic	0.06	21
Bupenorphine	Major abdominal, orthopedic	0.06–0.3	22

[a] Dose–response curves were generated.
[b] Doses required are variable, depending on state of tolerance. Doses as high as 175 mg have been reported (Coombs, 1983).
[c] References: 1, Pybus and Torda, 1982; 2, Torda and Pybus, 1984; 3, Bromage *et al.*, 1980; 4, Nordberg, 1984; 5, Cahill *et al.*, 1983; 6, Kotelko *et al.*, 1984; 7, Rosen *et al.*, 1983; 8, Gustafsson *et al.*, 1982; 9, R. Martin *et al.*, 1982; 10, Coombs *et al.*, 1983; 11, Müller *et al.*, 1982; 12, Zenz, 1985; 13, Cowen *et al.*, 1982; 14, Malins *et al.*, 1984; 15, Oyama *et al.*, 1982; 16, Torda and Pybus, 1982; 17, Rutter *et al.*, 1981; 18, Chauvin *et al.*, 1983; 19, Mori, 1982; 20, Kalsa *et al.*, 1983; 21, Welchew, 1983; 22, Rondomanska *et al.*, 1982.

have been reported to be predominant in human spinal cord (Czlonkowski *et al.*, 1983), and it is argued by some investigators that κ binding sites predominate in other species as well (see Gouarderes *et al.*, 1982).

Naloxone Antagonism. Though systematic studies have not been carried out for ethical reasons, the effects of spinally administered opiates are antagonized by naloxone (Bromage *et al.*, 1980; Struppler *et al.*, 1983).

Cross Tolerance. Patients exposed to continued administration of morphine as in chronic infusion or by daily spinal administration by percutaneous catheters display a significant increase over time in the dose of drug required to produce a given effect (i.e., the effects of spinal opiates are subject to the development of tolerance). Patients exposed to high doses of systemically administered opiates, as in terminal cancer, invariably show a diminished response to the effects of a given dose of intrathecal morphine (Müller *et al.*, 1982). These observations suggest that patients rendered tolerant to systemic morphine show a loss of response at the receptors acted on by the spinally administered morphine. It should be noted that although the phenomenon of tolerance is real, the rate at which it occurs is subject to a number of variables. It is certain that tolerance develops more rapidly in animal models than in clinical pain situations. Thus, chronic spinal administration of opiates has been shown to produce adequate analgesia for extended periods of time (Onofrio *et al.*, 1981; Müller *et al.*, 1982; Zenz, 1985; Coombs *et al.*, 1983). In recent systematic studies, we have studied 14 patients suffering from metastatic carcinoma (chordoma). The chronic infusion of morphine (by an implanted pump system) resulted in adequate relief. Statistical analysis reveals no significant escalation in dose requirements up to 3 months. Longer periods of analysis suggest incrementation, but the diminishing population precludes a statistical analysis (B. M. Onofrio and T. L. Yaksh, unpublished observations).

This consideration of the structure–activity relationship of spinal opiates in man is not trivial. The likelihood of a nonspecific action is one of considerable importance in view of the high local concentration of drugs that are administered into the spinal space. Given the fact that all agents have local anesthetic properties at high concentrations, it is important to consider the fact that the ordering of the structure–activity of these three agents as local anesthetics is: naloxone = meperidine > morphine (Staiman and Seemans, 1974). Yet the pharmacological profile of an opiate receptor is exactly the reverse. Thus, though it may seem trivial, this exercise indicates that opiates administered spinally indeed are acting on a specific receptor site and in general are not acting as local anesthetics. It should be stressed that although this holds for these agents, novel compounds such as peptides and other agents must always be considered in light of the receptors on which they are thought to act.

6. *Effects of Intrathecal Opiates on Other Measures Mediated by Spinal Cord Processing*

a. Motor

Early studies demonstrated that opiates do have an effect on somatomotor outflow. In spinal-transected animals, morphine will depress monosynaptic flexion reflexes (Jurna and Schafer, 1965; Jurna, 1966) and attenuate the firing of α-motor neurons evoked by muscle stretch (Krivoy *et al.*, 1973). Morphine has been observed to enhance the firing of populations of extensor motor neurons (Kuschinsky *et al.*, 1978; Jurna *et al.*, 1978). Single-unit studies have indicated that opiates have a direct effect on the glutamate-evoked excitation of motor neurons (Zieglgansberger and Bayerl, 1976). Also, Renshaw inhibition and to a lesser extent inhibitions mediated by interneurons acted on by large primary afferents are also suppressed by systemically administered opiates (Kruglov, 1964). At spinal doses that produce analgesia, such phenomena do not appear relevant for μ and δ ligands. Nevertheless, at doses that are 10–15 times that required to produce significant analgesia on thermal nociceptive measures, intrathecally administered morphine in rats will produce several syndromes including convulsive seizure of the hindquarters coupled with hyperreflexia secondary to cutaneous stimuli and intense motor rigidity. Neither phenomenon appears antagonized by naloxone (Tang and Schoenfeld, 1978).

The mechanism of such effects are not clear but may occur secondary to the ability of morphine to block the action of glycine (Curtis and Duggan, 1969). Intrathecal delta ligands such as DADL at doses significantly higher than those required to produce analgesia result in a loss of hindlimb placing and stepping reflexes, with the limbs showing motor tone but no voluntary movement. This phenomenon is not antagonized by naloxone. Intrathecal dynorphin has been shown to produce a comparable syndrome in doses that are slightly higher than that required to produce some degree of analgesia, and this phenomenon is not antagonized by naloxone (Herman and Goldstein, 1985; Kaneiko *et al.*, 1983; C. W. Stevens, G. J. Harty, and T. L. Yaksh, unpublished observations). Motor dysfunction such as is observed with high doses in animal models after intrathecal administration has not as yet been reported in man after either intrathecal μ or δ agonists.

It should be stressed that the pharmacology of the motor effects is distinguishable from that associated with analgesia. The failure of naloxone to antagonize is the principal example. Finaly, because the motor phenomenon occurs after intrathecal administration only at higher doses, the possibility that a portion of the motor effect may be mediated by a supraspinal redistribution represents a very real concern. The syndrome observed after high doses of intrathecal morphine in which the rat shows truncal rigidity can be induced by injections into supraspinal structures.

b. Cardiovascular

Intrathecally administered opioids given into unanesthetized rat, cat, dog, and man (Bromage *et al.*, 1980; Yasuoka and Yaksh, 1983; Atchison *et al.*, 1984), have no effect on resting heart rate or blood pressure. In dogs either anesthetized with halothane or unanesthetized, intrathecal morphine or DADL has no effect on cardiac output or peripheral resistance (Atchison *et al.*, 1984; R. Noueihed and T. L. Yaksh, unpublished observations). Spinal opiates in man have no effect on skin temperature or sudomotor activity and, unlike spinal anesthetic, do not diminish the magnitude of the valsalva maneuver (Bromage *et al.*, 1980). Spinal morphine in man or intrathecal DADL in dogs (R. Noueihed and T. L. Yaksh, unpublished observations) will often produce a significant but variable reduction in autonomic outflow as measured by markers of pituitary, adrenal medullary, and sympathetic activity evoked by high-intensity somatic/visceral stimulation (Bormann *et al.*, 1983; El-Baz and Goldin, 1983; Rutberg *et al.*, 1984, R. Noueihed and T. L. Yaksh, unpublished observations).

c. Gastrointestinal Function

Intrathecally administered μ and δ ligands in mice will produce a dose-dependent slowing of the transitive radioactive stomach load, which is naloxone reversible, and this suppressive effect remains in the presence of spinal transection. κ ligands such as EKC or dynorphin were inactive (Porrecca *et al.*, 1982, 1983; Porrecca and Burks, 1983). Recently, we have observed that intrathecal morphine does not suppress the migrating motor complex in unanesthetized dogs (G. Telford, J. H. Szurszewski, and T. L. Yaksh, unpublished observations) but did evoke an unfed pattern that was otherwise suppressed after a meal (J. R. Malagelada, M. Camilleri, and T. L. Yaksh, unpublished observations). In man, no systematic studies have been carried out with spinal opiates on gastric motility, but ileus, a finding associated with the action of local anesthetics, or constipation has not been reported as a principal side effect.

d. Bladder Function

Intrathecally administered opiate alkaloids will produce an inhibition of the volume evoked micturition reflex in man (Rawal *et al.*, 1983; Aoki *et al.*, 1982) and animals (Brent *et al.*, 1983; De Groat *et al.*, 1983). This has been shown to be reversed by systemically administered naloxone. Cystometrograms in man display an increase in bladder capacity with unchanged urethral pressures and an increase in external sphincter tone. In unanesthetized dogs, intrathecal morphine was observed to result in an increased threshold pressure required to evoke a micturition reflex (Bolam *et al.*, 1984). Cystometrograms carried out in unanesthetized rats with chronic bladder catheters revealed that intrathecal opiates produced a significant dose-dependent inhibition of the volume-evoked micturition reflex in this model. Dose–response curves carried out in unanesthetized rats with these indwelling bladder catheters revealed a clear structure–activity relationship with β-endorphin $\geqslant$ DADL $\geqslant$ morphine > EKC $\gg$ U50488H > SKF10047 = 0. Animals rendered tolerant to the micturition-suppressing effects of spinal morphine showed no change in the ED_{50} of intrathecal DADL (Brent *ewt al.*, 1983). In anesthetized models with urethral catheterization, intrathecal met-enkephalin, leu-enkephalin, and D-Ala^2-met-enkephalinamide were observed to reduce spontaneous bladder contraction (De Groat *et al.*, 1983). Although the mechanisms of these effects on bladder function are not clear, the observations made in man and animals suggest a vesicle sphincter dysynergia and are consistent with the inhibition by opiates of firing in vesicular postganglionic nerves.

C. *Spinal α-Adrenoceptor Systems*

1. *Effects of Adrenergic Agonists on Spinal Neuronal Function*

Weber (1904) demonstrated that the application of epinephrine to the spinal cord would produce an attenuation of the thermally evoked withdrawal response in the cat.

Microinjection of norepinephrine into the dorsal gray matter of the cat spinal cord produces a significant depression of C-fiber reflexes evoked by either electrical stimulation of cutaneous nerve or noxious radiant heat applied to the foot pad (Bell and Matsumiya, 1981). Such microinjections carried out in the ventral horn result in a significant facilitation of these C-fiber-evoked ventral root reflexes. Iontophoretically administered norepinephrine will suppress in a relatively selective fashion activity in dorsal horn neurons evoked by noxious (heat) but not nonnoxious (hair deflection) stimuli (Belcher *et al.*, 1978; Headley *et al.*, 1978; Fleetwood-Walker *et al.*, 1985). The most profound inhibition is observed in the deeply lying wide-dynamic-range neurons when norepinephrine is iontophoresed into the vicinity of the terminals of the primary afferents that excite the dendritic tree of the underlying neuron. By virtue of its selective inhibition, the inhibitory effects appear largely mediated by an α_2 type receptor (Fleetwood-Walker *et al.*, 1984).

Localization of the site of this inhibition has been a point of considerable interest. Unilateral sensory ganglionectomy resulted in a 20–30% decrease in dorsal horn α_2 binding at 7–21 days. This observation, in conjunction with the finding that significant levels of α_2 binding can be found in dorsal root ganglion cells, suggests the likelihood that a proportion of the α_2 binding in spinal cord may in fact be found on primary afferent terminals (J. R. Howe and T. L. Yaksh, unpublished data).

These observations suggesting α binding sites on primary afferents indicate the possibility of an action of α-adrenergic compounds on the primary afferent terminal. On the basis of excitability-testing procedures, it has been reported (Jeftinija *et al.*, 1981) that the norepinephrine applied into the dorsal gray resulted in increases in the threshold current required for the antidromic activation of C fibers. This effect was antagonized by phentolamine but not naloxone. Comparable results have been reported by Zimmermann and colleagues (1983). Similarly, in hemisected frog spinal cord, the application of norepinephrine resulted in a significant hyperpolarization of primary afferent terminals. These effects were reduced by the application of manganese, tetrodotoxin, or mephenesin, suggesting that the effect was mediated by an interneuron. The hyperpolarization produced by the adrenergic agent was antagonized by yohimbine and piperoxin but not by prazosin or the β antagonists sotalol and propranolol. This effect was potentiated by catecholamine uptake blockers (Wohlberg *et al.*, 1983). The possibility of a presynaptic action is further suggested by the work of Dunlap and Fischbach (1979) in dorsal root ganglion cell culture, in which it was observed that norepinephrine resulted in a decrease in the inward calcium current of the soma membrane.

As with opiates, a postsynaptic action cannot be excluded. The fact that norepinephrine served to inhibit the effects of excitatory amino acids suggests that it likely possesses a postsynaptic site of action.

In *in vitro* studies, Yoshimura and North (1983) observed that norepinephrine evoked hyperpolarization of gelatinosa neurons in rat spinal cord slices. The effect appeared mediated by the opening of potassium channels and was the result of a direct membrane action, as the hyperpolarization remained after the introduction of cobalt, magnesium, or low-calcium solutions. Importantly, these effects were antagonized by yohimbine and phentolamine but not by either prazosin or propranolol.

The iontophoretic effects of norepinephrine are not antagonized by naloxone (Headley *et al.*, 1978), bicuculline, or strychnine (Fleetwood-Walker *et al.*, 1983) and are not mimicked by iontophoretically applied GABA (Headley *et al.*, 1978). This suggests that the local effects of adrenergic agents are not mediated by these known inhibitory systems.

It should be stressed that although spinal noradrenergic receptors can influence sensory processing, these systems also exert a powerful effect on motor horn function. Thus, the iontophoretic administration of norepinephrine onto spinal motor neurons results in a significant depression of their activity associated with the hyperpolarization (Engberg and Ryall, 1966; Weight and Salmoiraghi, 1966). Jordan *et al.*, (1977) observed significant inhibition of interneurons in the vicinity of motor nuclei and suggested that this might explain a hyperpolarizing effect on motor horn cells. Alternatively, it has been demonstrated that although norepinephrine may not uniformly excite motor neurons (McCall and Aghajanian, 1979; White and Neuman, 1980), its local application can facilitate the depolarizing effects of excitatory drive or the effects of excitatory neurotransmitters. This effect appears to be mediated by a subthreshold depolarization and an increase in input resistance (Vandermaelen and Aghajanian, 1980). These observations are consistent with the complex effects on motor reflex tone observed after systemic administration of L-DOPA or α agonists (Anden *et al.*, 1964, 1966, 1972; Kawasaki *et al.*, 1978).

2. *Analgesic Effects Mediated by Spinal Adrenergic Receptors*

Although it is clear that α-adrenergic receptors in spinal cord produce an alteration in the processing of nociceptive information, an important question is whether these spinal effects are relevant to the pain behavior of the intact and unanesthetized animal. With the intrathecal injection model, it has been shown that spinal administration of adrenergic agonists will produce a powerful inhibition of the animal's response in a variety of nociceptive measures. These antinociceptive effects have been observed following spinal administration in mouse, rat, cat, and primate.

Table V lists the tests in which the spinal effects of adrenergic agonists have been so examined. The suppressive effects of intrathecally administered norepinephrine on all of these measures demonstrate monotonic dose–response curves (see below) in which the maximum inhibition can be achieved in the absence of significant signs of motor dysfunction. As indicated in Table V, the effects of spinally administered α agonists have been demonstrated to alter the nociceptive response not only on spinal nociceptive reflexes but also on tests in which the response substrate involves complex coordinated behaviors having supraspinal components. Thus, the primate shock titration, the rat hot plate, the tail shock vocalization, and the coordinated paw withdrawal to pinch are examples of tests that are altered by intrathecally administered α agonists. In man, intrathecally administered clonidine will produce a powerful analgesia as defined by verbal report in terminal cancer patients who have been rendered refractory to spinal morphine by the prior chronic infusion of the opioid (D. Coombs, personal communication, 1984). These data together offer clear support for the concept that in all species tested, including man, the spinal action of α agonists produces a powerful analgesia.

With regard to other sensory functions, adequate data do not exist, but these suppressive effects appear selective. At analgetically effective doses, there are no changes in nonnociceptive reflexes such as placing or stepping (Reddy and Yaksh, 1980; Reddy *et al.*, 1980), and the orientation response to light brushing of the flank is unaltered. In studies carried out in primates, doses of intrathecal clonidine that maximally elevated the shock-titration threshold had no effect on the avoidance of ear shock cued by light pressure applied to the analgesic hindpaw (Yaksh and Reddy, 1981).

TABLE V
Experimental Pain Models in Which Intrathecally Administered α-Adrenergic Agonists Have Been Examined

Species	References[a]
Mouse	1
Tail flick	
Paw lick, response to hypertonic saline	
Intrathecal substance-P-evoked scratching response	
Rat	2,3,4,5
Hot plate	
Tail Flick	
Writhing	
Hind-paw pinch	
Tail withdrawal	
Cat	4
Skin twitch	
Monkey	6
Shock titration	
Man	7
Terminal cancer	

[a] 1, Hylden and Wilcox, 1983; 2, Kuraishi *et al.*, 1979; 3, Reddy *et al.*, 1980; 4, Reddy and Yaksh, 1980; 5, Yaksh, 1985; 6, Yaksh and Reddy, 1981; 7, D. Coombs, personal communication, 1984.

3. *Pharmacology of α-Adrenergic Agonists in Spinal Cord*

Characterization of the receptors in the spinal cord that mediate the antinociceptive effects of intrathecally administered adrenergic agonists have been carried out by examining (1) the agonist structure–activity relationship; (2) the antagonist structure–activity relationship; (3) the effect of altering spinal norepinephrine disposition (metabolism, uptake, and release); and (4) tachyphylaxis.

a. Structure–Activity Relationship of Spinally Administered α Agonists

In rodents, intrathecal administration of adrenergic agonists yields a dose-dependent increase in the response latency on the hot plate and tail flick with the duration of the drug effect proportional to the intrathecal dose (Reddy *et al.*, 1980). These antinociceptive effects are produced by a variety of adrenoceptor agents, including L-norepinephrine, DL-epinephrine, DL-α-methylnorepinephrine, ST-91, clonidine, L-phenylephrine, 3,4-dihydroxytolazoline, oxymetazoline, methoxamine, and cirazoline (Kuraishi *et al.*, 1979; Reddy and Yaksh, 1980; Reddy *et al.*, 1980; Howe *et al.*, 1983). β-agonists such as isoproterenol are without effect. With few exceptions, all agents with the exception of the α_1 agonists were observed to produce monotonic increases in the dose–response curves, with each agent able to produce maximum response suppression (Reddy *et al.*, 1980; Howe *et al.*, 1983). α_1 agonists (methoxamine, cirazoline) failed to produce a maximum effect on the tail flick. These agents also evoke a dose-dependent cutaneous hyperreflexia and a tendency to spontaneous movements of the tail (see below). Based on these systematic studies, the structure–activity series for adrenoceptor agonists in the cutaneous thermal measures of the hot plate and tail flick is: ST-91 = norepinephrine > methoxamine ≫ isoproterenol = 0 (*vide supra*). In the acetic acid writhing test, monotonic dose–response curves have also been obtained, with the relative ordering of activity being ST-91 ≥ norepinephrine > methoxamine ≫ isoproterenol = 0 (Yaksh, 1985).

On the shock titration task in the primate, the rank order of drug potency in producing a just-maximum increase in the tolerated titration level after intrathecal injection is clonidine = ST-91 > methoxamine > isoproterenol = 0 (Yaksh and Reddy, 1981; T. L. Yaksh and G. Harty, unpublished obserations). As in the rat, a maximum inhibition could not be achieved with methoxamine because of a dose-dependent motor dysfunction that consisted of hyperreflexia and hindlimb stiffness.

b. Structure–Activity Relationship of Spinally Administered Antagonists

The effects of intrathecal norepinephrine on the nociceptive threshold appear to be mediated by an α-adrenergic receptor. Thus, a dose-dependent inhibition of the effect can be achieved by phentolamine but not propranolol administered intrathecally (Kuraishi *et al.*, 1979; Reddy *et al.*, 1980; Reddy and Yaksh, 1980). The interaction of phentolamine with intrathecal norepinephrine, consistent with classical pharmacology, displays a competitive antagonism of the antinociceptive effects of intrathecal norepinephrine and produces a parallel shift in the norepinephrine dose–response curve (Reddy *et al.*, 1980).

The question of whether the spinal α-receptor effect is α_1 or α_2 in nature has been assessed in studies examining the ability of α_1 and α_2 selective antagonists to alter the effects of intrathecally administered α agonists. Howe and colleagues (1983) observed that the α_2 antagonist yohimbine will attenuate in a dose-dependent fashion the antinociceptive effects produced on hot plate and tail flick of intrathecal ST-91. The ID_{50} for yohimbine was observed to be approximately one-tenth that of prazosin, an α_1 antagonist. This is consistent with the known α_2 selectivity of ST-91. In the antagonism of the antinociceptive effects of intrathecal norepinephrine and methoxamine, the ordering of activity is reversed, such that prazosin is approximately ten times more effective in antagonizing the effects of intrathecal norepinephrine and methoxamine than yohimbine. More recently, we have extended these studies to examine the relative potency of the stereoisomers of yohimbine (α_2), rauwolscine (α_2), and corynanthine (α_1) in antagonizing the intrathecal effects of

ST-91 and norepinephrine. Table VI presents the relative ordering of activity of intrathecal α_1 and α_2-preferring antagonists in reversing the tail-flick inhibition produced by intrathecal norepinephrine; this sequence is prazosin, phentolamine, rauwolscine, yohimbine, corynanthine, propranolol (= 0). The ordering of activity for antagonizing intrathecal ST-91 is yohimbine, rauwolscine, prazosin, phentolamine, corynanthine, propranolol (= 0). Comparable results were observed with the hot-plate test.

It thus appears likely that a spinal receptor population with a pharmacological profile comparable to that of an α_2 site mediates analgesia as measured by a wide variety of tests in a variety of species. To summarize, the support for this derives from (1) the rank ordering of agonist activity on several nociceptive measures in several species and (2) the preferential antagonism of the spinal effects of α_2 agonists on pain-evoked behavior by agents with a relative selectivity for the α_2 receptor. The fact that this ordering of antagonist potency was observed with yohimbine, rauwolscine, and corynanthine, three agents that are stereoisomers with identical physicochemical properties, indeed suggests that the selective inhibition reflects their relative affinity for the spinal α_2 receptor.

Agonists such as methoxamine and cirazoline with α_1 receptor selectivity were also observed to produce a suppression of the nociceptive response, but in all measures these agents were characterized by less activity. In view of the relatively lower activity of these agonists, it is possible that at higher doses the effects may be mediated by an action on α_2 receptors. This, however, appears

TABLE VI
ID_{50} Values (nM)[a] for Intrathecal Adrenergic Antagonists on Tail-Flick Responses Elevated by Prior Treatment with Periaqueductal Gray Morphine or Intrathecal Injection of Norepinephrine

	IT NE[c]			IT ST-91[c]		
Drug	*N*	ID_{50} (nM)	(95% CI)	*N*	ID_{50} (nM)	(95% CI)
Phentolamine	19	26	(18–43)	26	18	(12–31)
Yohimbine	35	43	(18–100)	35	1.1	(0.8–1.5)
Rauwolscine	14	39	(23–58)	30	2.3	(1.0–3.8)
Corynanthine	22	98	(65–154)	18	249	(205–378)
Prazosin	24	2.4	(0.4–15)	27	10	(3.6–30)
Propranolol	8	>386		8	>386	
Vehicle[b,c]	6	—		—	—	

[a] ID_{50} values represent the dose of intrathecally administered antagonists that produced a 50% reduction in the antinociceptive effects of intrathecally administered ST-91 or norepinephrine (10 μg/10 μl). In all work, the intrathecal agent was administered 5 min after the intrathecal α agonist. Each entry presents the mean ID_{50} calculated from the regression equation and the 95% dose confidence interval.
[b] No reversal of the response inhibition was observed; 10 μl of 50% DMSO–saline.
[c] Howe *et al.*, 1983; Yaksh, 1984a,b.

unlikely, as the effects of methoxamine were more potently antagonized by the α_1 selective (e.g., prazosin) than α_2 selective antagonists. That α_1 receptors are "analgetically coupled" is also suggested by the observation that norepinephrine can produce a very significant elevation in the nociceptive threshold and that this effect is potently antagonized by prazosin. It should be noted that if populations of α_1 and α_2 receptors both contribute to the antinociceptive effect of spinal norepinephrine, then both receptor populations would have to be affected to alter the norepinephrine effect. As intrathecal prazosin is equipotent in antagonizing agonists that are thought to act at one or the other population of receptors, i.e. α_1 and α_2 (see Table VI), it would likely display a similar potency against norepinephrine, as it does. Alternatively, the α_2 antagonist yohimbine against norepinephrine appears to have an apparent potency at the receptors acted on by norepinephrine, for which it is least potent. Thus, against norepinephrine, yohimbine appears to have the same potency it would have against α_1 receptors.

The effects of norepinephrine on hot plate and tail flick in the rat were not antagonized by methysergide, phentolamine, picrotoxin, or strychnine (Reddy *et al.*, 1980). These data suggest that spinal norepinephrine does not exert its effect through an opioid intermediary or by the release of a potential inhibitory neurotransmitter in the spinal cord (GABA or glycine) or indirectly through a local action on serotonergic terminals. These observations are consistent with the results produced on single spinal neurons by iontophoretically applied norepinephrine.

c. Alterations of the Disposition of Intrathecally Administered Norepinephrine

The duration of action of intrathecal norepinephrine is relatively short, with the interval of activity being on the order of between 30 and 60 min. Administration of a monoamine oxidase inhibitor or monoamine uptake blocker results in a significant facilitation of the intrathecal effect at doses of the drugs that by themselves have no effect (Reddy *et al.*, 1980).

d. Tachyphylaxis Secondary to Repeated Spinal Administration

Repeated intrathecal administration at 30-min intervals of norepinephrine in doses that initially blocked the hot-plate and tail-flick response showed a significant reduction after seven or eight injections, a period of approximately 4 h (Reddy and Yaksh, 1980). Comparable results were also seen with repeated injections of intrathecal ST-91 in which the drug was given on a daily basis for a period of 7 days (T. L. Yaksh, J. Wang, and G. Harty, unpublished observations). At this time, the injection of morphine was observed to produce an effect that was indistinguishable from that produced in animals that had received intrathecal injections of saline.

4. Effects of Intrathecal Adrenergic Agonists on Motor Function

A powerful suppression of the response of the animal otherwise evoked by a high-intensity stimulus is produced by intrathecal adrenoceptor agonists in the absence of any detectable effect on motor function. In rats receiving antinociceptive doses of intrathecal norepinephrine or α_2 agonists, no effect on placing, stepping or pinna twitch reflexes are observed (Reddy *et al.*, 1980; Reddy and Yaksh, 1980). No effect on hindlimb withdrawl strength is observed in primates (Yaksh and Reddy, 1981). Nevertheless, α-adrenoceptor agonists can markedly influence motor tone. In doses considerably in excess of those required to block the hot-plate and tail-flick response, intrathecal norepinephrine or α_2 agonists will produce flaccidity of the tail and hindlimb (Howe *et al.*, 1983; Yaksh and Reddy, 1981). In primates, α_1 agonists at doses required to increase the nociceptive threshold result in hindlimb tremor and an exaggerated reflex withdrawal response to brisk but noninjurious scratching of the foot pad (T. L. Yaksh, unpublished observations). In rat, α_1 agonists in doses that inhibit the hot-plate and tail-flick responses will result in a dose-dependent cutaneous hyperreflexia, clonic flexion of the hindlimbs, rigidity, and serpentine movements of the tail.

These different motor syndromes produced by α_1 and α_2-selective agents offer further support for distinguishable spinal adrenergic receptor systems. As noted above, norepinephrine injected into the ventral horn principally facilitated ventral root reflexes (Bell and Matsumiya, 1981). These effects on motor function observed with intrathecally administered α_1 agonists are consistent with the effects of high doses of clonidine on tail-flexion reflex evoked by pinch (Kawasaki *et al.*, 1978) and the facilitating effects noted above at intravenous L-DOPA. Davis and colleagues (Davis and Astrachan, 1981; Astrachan *et al.*, 1983) have provided convincing evidence that spinal α_1 and not α_2 receptors will produce a powerful dosedependent facilitation of the auditory evoked startle reflex. Thus, the effects are selectively antagonized by α_1 receptor antagonists such as WB40101.

D. Characteristics of the Interaction of Spinal α-Adrenergic and Opioid Receptor Systems

Early data suggested that α agonists potentiated the effects of systemically administered morphine (Sigg *et al.*, 1958; Spaulding *et al.*, 1979). Recent studies with intrathecally administered agents have indicated that there is a very signficant shift in the opioid dose response for coadministered morphine and α_2 agonists such as ST-91, clonidine, or norepinephrine (Wang *et al.*, 1980, Yaksh and Reddy, 1981; Hylden and Wilcox, 1983) in mouse, rat, and primate. It is unlikely that the α_2 agonists produced a significant alteration in the clearance of the opiate drug, as the clearance of morphine from the intrathecal space is relatively slow, and the effects of the α agonist are manifested immediately and do not reflect a simple increase in the duration of action. This may reflect a synergistic interaction between α_2 receptors and opiates in the spinal cord (Yaksh, 1981).

It is interesting that where examined, opiates and α-adrenergic agonists tend to have comparable effects on neural sysems, e.g., dorsal root ganglion cells, dorsal horn neurons, and primary afferent excitability (see preceding discussion in this chapter). Opiates and clonidine both prolong the afferent hyperpolarization observed in guinea pig mesenteric plexuses at doses considerably lower than those required to hyperpolarize the resting membrane (Tokimasa *et al.*, 1981). This would effectively limit the frequency of activity of discharge in these neurons in the absence of any effect on resting potential. Nevertheless, it is clear that α_2 agonists do not act by an opiate receptor, and morphine does not act by a clonidine receptor. Such observations are not supported by efforts to antagonize intrathecal morphine with phentolamine or intrathecal α agonists with naloxone (Reddy *et al.*, 1980; Reddy and Yaksh, 1980). In primates rendered tolerant to intrathecal morphine, there was no loss of response to the intrathecally administered ST-91 (Yaksh and Reddy, 1981; but see Paalzow *et al.*, 1978). We have thus speculated that this interaction between α_2 receptors and opiates reflects a synergistic interaction.

It is significant that earlier studies directed at investigating the spinal and supraspinal actions of opiates reported that supraspinal opiates would synergize with the effects of spinal opiates in altering the nociceptive threshold. This speculative hypothesis put forth first by Yaksh and Rudy (1978) was based on the observation that the effects of systemically administered morphine on hot-plate and tail-flick tests could be shifted to the right by intrathecally or intracerebrally administered naloxone. At the higher opioid doses, the dose–response curves could not be further shifted, suggesting that an action on opiate receptors in either the brain or the spinal cord was sufficient at high systemic doses to produce analgesia. It was later shown that the dose response isobols for intraventricular and intrathecal morphine were hyperbolic, suggesting that there was a nonlinear interaction between the effects of morphine at supraspinal (after intraventricular injection) and spinal (intrathecal) actions of morphine (Yeung and Rudy, 1980). Given the literature that some of the effects of brainstem morphine may act on spinal function by the activation of descending noradrenergic pathways (see Hammond, Chapter 18), it was reasonable to consider the likelihood that intrathecal α-adrenergic agents, which mimic the activation of these descending pathways, should synergize in a comparable fashion with intrathecally administered morphine. As described above, such synergy has indeed been noted. The important consideration arising from the apparent synergy is that significant physiological effects (analgesia) can be achieved with doses of either agent that alone produce minimal receptor activation.

A second important consideration that arises from the synergy relates to the development of tolerance. In contrast to the rapid (3–5 days) loss of analgesia potency observed with intrathecal morphine in primates (Yaksh,

1983), equiactive dose combinations of morphine and ST-91 showed no apparent loss of activity over a 21-day period (Yaksh and Reddy, 1981). Yaksh and Reddy (1981) speculated that if the rate of tolerance development were proportional to the degree of receptor activation, and if the adrenergic and opiate receptors were independent, then the ability to produce a long-term analgesia was consistent with the minimum degree of activation of either receptor required concurrently to produce the maximum physiological effect. In other words, as the level of drug at the receptor is minimized, the rate of tolerance development at the receptor will be less for a given endpoint when the endpoint is achieved by two independent receptor systems being activated concurrently. It is significant that the ability to reverse the effects of combined α-adrenergic and opioid activity can be achieved with either naloxone or phentolamine alone (Yaksh and Reddy, 1981; T. L. Yaksh and G. Harty, unpublished observations). This suggests that the effect is indeed dependent on the coactivation of the two sets of receptors and is not caused by an alteration in clearance of one of the other drug *per se*. This interesting interaction between these different classes of agents in the spinal cord is a subject of considerable interest, and more work is clearly required.

E. *Future Directions in the Use of Receptor-Selective Agents in the Spinal Cord*

The discussion in this chapter has been directed at the concept that opiates and α-adrenoceptor agonists with an action limited to the spinal cord produce a powerful elevation in the nociceptive threshold. It is of primary significance (1) that these effects are mediated by selective classes of receptors and (2) that these receptors are apparently associated with anatomic systems that process different types of sensory information. Although the emphasis in this chapter was on opioid and α-adrenoceptor systems that modulate pain processing in the spinal cord, a comparable analysis could have been similarly carried out with other systems that we now know also modulate spinal sensory processing, including neurotensin (G. E. Martin and Naruse, 1982; Yaksh *et al.*, 1982b; Hylden and Wilcox, 1983), acetylcholine (Yaksh *et al.*, 1985), serotonin (Yaksh and Wilson, 1979), and GABA (Wilson and Yaksh, 1978).

It should be stressed in light of this knowledge, that in our desire to advance the cause of the patient, we do not lose sight of the fact that the administration of drugs into the spinal space is potentially a risky business. The placement of high concentrations of receptor-active drugs and agents with significant degrees of membrane activity (i.e., with high lipid partition coefficients) offers the possibility of significant and untoward effects being exerted. The ability to do systematic toxicological investigations in well-defined animal models precludes the excuse that it is not easily possible to study the action of new agents in the spinal space of animals. Clinically, the relevance of such observations is evident. The ability to provide alternative pharmacological modalities that produce such a selective modulation of nociceptive transmission offers hope for the possibility that long-term analgetic therapy may be achieved by pharmacological intervention and not neurolysis.

In addition to sensory modulation, however, these studies also indicate that certain spinal receptor systems are likely associated with spinal substrates including the motor horn and the sacral/thoracic intermediolateral cell column, which mediate other physiological functions. Indeed, the association of these receptors with other neuronal substrates accounts for some of the "side effects" produced when these drugs are given spinally. Nevertheless, these very same phenomena, which are currently regarded as side effects, indeed may reflect drug–system interactions that signal potential advances in aspects of therapeutic modalities other than those related to pain transmission.

The effects of α-adrenoceptor agents on motor horn function indicate the possible relevance of these receptor systems in motor outflow. The distinctive effects of α_1 versus α_2 agonists on motor tone suggest a possible role of such receptor systems in motor dysfunctions such as spasticity. The likelihood is that partial cord lesions give rise to changes in segmental and bulbospinal activity that result in changes in motor neuron tone whereas long-term lesions give rise to increases in spinal α_2 binding (J. R. Howe and T. L. Yaksh, unpublished observations). These changes may be relevant to the time course of motor changes observed after such lesions. Similarly, inhibition of the volume-evoked micturition reflex by spinal opiates is an untoward phenomenon when the therapeutic use of these agents is considered. However, such observations clearly indicate that there is a selective pharmacology associated with the central link in the bladder–spinal–bladder reflex arc that is opioid in character. It is significant that the depressant effect of spinal morphine on spontaneous bladder tone has been used successfully to manage bladder spasm (Baxter and Kiruluta, 1984) and that naloxone has been observed to augment the micturition reflex in spinally transected animals (Thor *et al.*, 1983). The possibility of regulating bladder function pharmacologically in manners other than the gross manipulation of sympathetic and parasympathetic systems is therefore an exceedingly important consideration, particularly in view of the relevance of bladder dysfunction in various disorders such as cord injury, parkinsonism, or aging. As discussed elsewhere (see Hammond, Chapter 15; Seybold, Chapter 6), bulbospinal amine receptor systems play an interactive role in the thoracic and sacral autonomic plexi. The likelihood that these receptors also interact with bladder tone is a subject we are currently examining.

Finally, in a philosophical sense, one may ask what role these intrinsic receptor systems normally perform. The comments in this chapter should not be construed to imply that the spinal terminal receptors, even those associated with small primary aferents, constitute a natural "antinociceptive system." As argued elsewhere (Yaksh and Hammond, 1982; see Yaksh, Chapter 8) several more subtle functions are likely involved. Thus, the selective inhibition of A-δ/C-fiber stimulation in fact converts a polymodal wide-dynamic-range neuron (responding to Aβ/Aδ and C fibers) into a modality-selective neuron responding only to Aβ input. Thus, these modulatory systems may be considered modality selector mechanisms. Similarly, many of these systems act to reduce the "gain" of the stimulus–response relationship. This in itself would permit these systems to transmit the maximum amount of information while maintaining the maximum range of dynamic response. Thus, in the aferent side of the spinal processing, these systems likely play a natural role in the coding of dorsal horn sensory processing, allowing for the large number of polymodal neurons to be specifically coded for different modalities depending on circumstances in a way similar to a "user-defined" computer keyboard.

In summary, a basic understanding of the spinal cord has led, I think, to very significant advances in the therapeutic management of pain. In a more general sense, however, such investigations have led us to broaden our views to appreciate that this analysis of pain processing is a template for the study of many physiological systems that share the circuitry of the spinal gray. As documented by the contributions of the several neurobiologists in this volume, advances in our understanding of pain processing are providing insights into the mechanisms of sensory coding, processing of autonomic reflexes, and the organization of motor function. The understanding of the pharmacology and physiology of these systems under normal circumstances is necessary for the evaluation of the mechanisms underlying pathological circumstances. Such understanding must precede rational advances in therapy. Our growing appreciation of the complex pharmacology of these systems promises that many functions may be selectively altered by the local action of appropriate agents.

As Fred Kerr often said, it is an exciting time to be studying brain function. As is usual in these matters, I have never found him to be in error. God bless you Fred Kerr.

ACKNOWLEDGMENTS. Work cited herein was supported by grants DA02110, NS16541, and NS19650. I would like to thank Ms. Ann Rockafellow for her patience and skilled assistance. I would like to particularly note the extensive and valuable contributions during the past several years of Drs. Donna Hammond, Jim Howe, Frederick W. L. Kerr, Paul Micevych, S. V. Ramana Reddy, Gertrude Tyce, and Mr. Paul Camarata to the work, thinking, and ideas discussed herein.

References

ANDEN, N.-E., ENGEL, J., AND RUBENSON, A. Mode of action of L-DOPA on central noradrenaline mechanisms. Naunyn Schmiedebergs Arch. Pharmakol. 273:1–10, 1972.

ANDEN, N.-E., JUKES, M. G. M., AND LUNDBERG, A. Spinal reflexes and monoamine liberation. *Nature* 202:1222–1223, 1964.

ANDEN, N.-E., JUKES, M. G. M., AND LUNDBERG, A. The effect of DOPA on the spinal cord. 2. A pharmacological analysis. *Acta Physiol. Scand.* 67:387–397, 1966.

ANDERSON, I., THOMPSON, W. R., VARKEY, G. P. AND KNILL, R. L. Lumbar epidural morphine as an effective analgesic following cholecystectomy. *Can. Anesth. Soc. J.* 28:523–529, 1981.

AOKI, M., WATANABE, H., NAMIKI, A., TAKAHASI, T., YOKOYAMA, E., AND HURUYA, S. Mechanism of urinary retention following intrathecal administration of morphine. *Masui* 31:939–943, 1982.

ASTRACHAN, D. I., DAVIS, M., AND GALLAGER, D. W. Behavior and binding: Correlations between α_1-adrenergic stimulation of acoustic startle and α_1-adrenoceptor occupancy and number in rat lumbar spinal cord. *Brain Res.* 260:81–90, 1983.

ATCHISON, S. R., YAKSH, T. L. AND DURANT, P. Cardiovascular and respiratory effects of intrathecal DADL in awake dogs. *Anesthesiology* 61:A219, 1984.

ATTALI, B., GOUARDERES, C., MAZARGUIL, H., AUDIGIER, Y., AND CROS, J. Differential interaction of opiates to multiple "kappa" binding sites in the guinea-pig lumbosacral spinal cord. *Life Sci.* 31:1371–1375, 1982.

BAXTER, A. D., AND KIRULUTA, G. Detrusor tone after epidural morphine. *Anesth. Analg.* 63:464, 1984.

BELCHER, G., RYALL, R. W., AND SCHAFFNER, R. The differential effects of 5-hydroxytryptamine, noradrenaline and raphe stimulation on nociceptive and non-nociceptive dorsal horn interneurones in the cat. *Brain Res.* 151:307–321, 1978.

BELL, J. A., AND MATSUMIYA, T. Inhibitory effects of dorsal horn and excitant effects of ventral horn intraspinal microinjections of norepinephrine and serotonin in the cat. *Life Sci.* 29:1507–1514, 1981.

BOLAM, J. M., ROBINSON, C. J., AND WURSTER, R. D. Micturition in conscious dogs following spinal opiate administration. *Soc. Neurosci. Abstr.* 10:1108, 1984.

BORMANN, B., WEIDLER, B., DERNHARDT, R. STRUM, G. SCHELD, H. H. AND HEMPELMANN, G. Influence of epidural fentanyl on stress-induced elevation of plasma vasopressin (ADH) after surgery. *Anesth. Analg.* 62:727–732, 1983.

BRENT, C. R., HARTY, G., AND YAKSH, T. L. The effects of spinal opiates on micturition in unanesthetized animals. *Soc. Neurosci. Abstr.* 9:743, 1983.

BROMAGE, P. R., CAMPORESI, E., AND LESLIE, J. Epidural narcotics in volunteers: Sensitivity to pain and carbon dioxide. *Pain* 9:145–160, 1980.

CAHILL, J., MURPHY, D., O'BRIEN, D., MULHRALL, J., AND FITZPATRICK, G. Epidural buprenorphine for pain relief after major abdominal surgery: A controlled comparison with epidural morphine. *Anaesthesia* 38:760–764, 1983.

CALVILLO, O., HENRY, J. L., AND NEUMAN, R. S. Actions of narcotic analgesics and antagonists on spinal units responding to natural stimulation in the cat. *Can. J. Physiol. Pharmacol.* 51:652–663, 1979.

CARSTENS, E., TULLOCH, I., ZIEGLGANSBERGER, W., AND ZIMMERMAN, M. Presynaptic excitability changes induced by morphine in single cutaneous afferent C- and A-fibers. *Pflugers Arch.* 379:143–147, 1979.

CHAUVIN, M., SALBAING, J., PERRIN, D., LEVON, J. C., AND VIARS, P. Comparison between intramuscular and epidural administration of alfentanil for pain relief and plasma kinetics. *Anesthesiology* 59:A197, 1983.

COOMBS, D. Mechanism of epidural lidocaine reversal of tachyphylaxis to epidural morphine analgesia. *Anesthesiology* 59:486–487, 1983.

COOMBS, D. W., SAUNDERS, R. L., GAYLOR, M. S., BLOCK, A. R., COLTON, T., HARBAUGH, R., PAGEAU, M. G., AND MROZ, W. Relief of continuous chronic pain by intraspinal narcotics infusion via an implanted reservoir. *JAMA* 250:2336–2339, 1983.

COWEN, M. J. BULLINGHAM, R. E. S., PATERSON, G. M. C. MC QUAY, H. J., AND TURNER, M. *Anesth. Analg.* 61:15–18, 1982.

CURTIS, D. R., AND DUGGAN, A. W. The depression of spinal inhibition by morphine. *Agents Actions* 1:14–19, 1969.

CZLONKOWSKI, A., COSTA, T., PRZEWLOCKI, R., PASI, A., AND HERZ, A. Opiate receptor binding sites in human spinal cord. *Brain Res.* 267:392–396, 1983.

DAVIES, J., AND DRAY, A. Pharmacological and electrophysiological studies of morphine and enkephalin on rat supraspinal neurones and cat spinal neurones. *Br. J. Pharmacol.* 63:87–96, 1978.

DAVIS, M., AND ASTRACHAN, D. I. Spinal modulation of acoustic startle: Opposite effects of clonidine and D-amphetamine. *Psychopharmacology* 75:219–225, 1981.

DE GROAT, W. C., KAWATANI, M. HISAMITSU, T., LOWE, I., MORGAN, C. ROPPOLO, J., BOOTH, A. M., NADELHAFT, I., KUD, D. AND THOR, K. The role of neuropeptides in the sacral autonomic reflex pathways of the cat. *J. Autonom. Nerv. Syst.* 7:339–350, 1983.

DELANDER, G.E., AND TAKEMORI, A.E. Spinal antagonism of tolerance and dependence induced by systemically administered morphine. *Eur. J. Pharmocol.* 94:35–42, 1983.

DUGGAN, A. W., JOHNSON, S. M., AND MORTON, C. R. Differing distributions of receptors for morphine and Met^5-enkephalinamide in the dorsal horn of the cat. *Brain Res.* 229:379–387, 1981.

DUNLAP, K., AND FISCHBACH, G. D. Neurotransmitter modulation of voltage-sensitive calcium currents in sensory neurons. *Neurosci. Abstr.* 5:291, 1979.

EINSPAHR, F. J., AND PIERCEY, M. F. Morphine depresses dorsal horn neuron responses to controlled noxious and non-noxious cutaneous stimulation. *J. Pharmacol. Exp. Ther.* 213:456–461, 1980.

ELBAZ, N., AND GOLDIN, M. D. Continuous epidural morphine infusion for pain relief after open heart surgery. *Anesthesiology* 59:A193, 1983.

ENGBERG, I., AND RYALL, R. W. The inhibitory action of noradrenaline and other monoamines of spinal neurones. *J. Physiol. Lond.* 185:298–322, 1966.

FIELDS, H. L., EMSON, P. C., LEIGH, B. K., GILBERT, R. F. T., AND IVERSEN, L. L. Multiple opiate receptor sites on primary afferent fibres. *Nature* 284:351–353, 1980.

FLEETWOOD-WALKER, S. M., HOPE, P. J., MITCHELL, R., AND MOLONY, V. Investigation of interactions between descending and noradrenaline-mediated and local GABA- and glycine-mediated influences on spinocervical tract neurons of the cat. *J. Physiol. Lond.* 346:498, 1983.

FLEETWOOD-WALKER, S. M., MITCHELL, R., HOPE, P. J. MOLONY, V., AND IGGO, A. An α_2 receptor mediates the selective inhibition by noradrenaline of nociceptive responses of identified dorsal horn neurons. *Brain Res.* 334:243–254, 1985.

GAMSE, R., HOLZER, P., AND LEMBECK, F. Indirect evidence for presynaptic location of opiate receptors in chemosensitive primary sensory neurones. *Naunyn Schmiedbergs Arch. Pharmacol.* 308:281–285, 1979.

GOUARDERES, C., AUDIGIER, Y., AND CROS, J. Benzomorphan binding sites in rat lumbo-sacral spinal cord. *Eur. J. Pharmacol.* 78:483–486, 1982.

GUSTAFSSON, L. L., FRIBERG-NIELSEN, S., GARLE, M., MOHALL, A., RANE, A. SCHILDT, B., AND SYMRENG, T. Extradural and parenteral morphine kinetics and effects in postoperative pain. A controlled clinical study. *Br. J. Anesth.* 54:1167–1174, 1982.

HEADLEY, P. M., DUGGAN, A. W., AND GRIERSMITH, B. T. Selective reduction by noradrenaline and 5-hydroxytryptamine of nociceptive responses of cat dorsal horn neurones. *Brain Res.* 145:185–189, 1978.

HERMAN, B., AND GOLDSTEIN, A. Antinociception and paralysis induced by intrathecal dynorphin A. *J. Pharmacol. Exp. Ther.* 232:27–32, 1985.

HOWE, J. R., WANG, J.-Y., AND YAKSH, T. L. Selective antagonism of the antinociceptive effect of intrathecally applied alpha adrenergic agonists by intrathecal prazosin and intrathecal yohimbine. *J. Pharmacol. Exp. Ther.* 224:552–558, 1983.

HYLDEN, J. L. K., AND WILCOX, G. L. Antinociceptive action of intrathecal neurotensin in mice. *Peptides* 4:517–520, 1983.

HYLDEN, J. L. K., AND WILCOX, G. L. Pharmacological characterization of substance P-induced nociception in mice: Modulation by opioid and noradrenergic agonists at the spinal level. *J. Pharmacol. Exp. Ther.* 226:398-404, 1983.

IWATA, N., AND SAKAI, Y. Effects of fentanyl upon the spinal interneurons activated by Ad afferent fibers of the cutaneous nerve of the cat. *Jpn. J. Pharmacol.* 21:413–426, 1971.

JEFTINIJA, S., SEMBA, K., AND RANDIC, M. Norepinephrine reduces excitability of single cutaneous primary afferent C-fibers in the cat spinal cord. *Brain Res.* 219:456–463, 1981.

JORDAN, L. M., MMCREA, D. A., STEEVES, J. D., AND MENZIES, J. E. Noradrenergic synapses and effects of noradrenaline on interneurons in the ventral horn of the cat spinal cord. *Can. J. Physiol. Pharmacol.* 55:399–412, 1977.

JURNA, I. Inhibition of the effect of repetitive stimulation on spinal motoneurones of the cat by morphine and pethidine. *Int. J. Neuropharmacol.* 5:117–123, 1966.

JURNA, I., AND GROSSMANN, W. The effect of the activity evoked in ventrolateral tract axons of the cat spinal cord. *Exp. Brain Res.* 24:473–484, 1976.

JURNA, I., AND HEINZ, G. Differential effects of morphine and opioid analgesics on A and C fiber-evoked activity in ascending axons of the rat spinal cord. *Brain Res.* 171:573–576, 1979.

JURNA, I., AND SCHAFER, H. Depression of post tetanic potentiation in the spinal cord by morphine and pethidine. *Experientia* 21:226-227, 1965.

JURNA, I., HEINZ, G. BLINN, G., AND NELL, T. The effect of substantia nigra stimulation and morphine on α-motoneurones and the tail flick response. *Eur. J. Pharmacol.* 51:239–250, 1978.

KALSA, P., MADAN, R., SABSENA, R., BATRA, R., AND GODE, G. Epidural pentazocine for post-operative pain relief. *Anesth. Analg.* 52:949–950, 1983.

KANEIKO, T., NAKAZAWA, T., IKEDA, M., YAMATSU, K., IWAMA, T. WADA, T., SATOH, M., AND TAKAGI, H. Sites of analgesic action of dynorphin. *Life Sci.* 33:661–664, 1983.

KAWASAKI, K., TAKESUE, H., AND MATSUSHITA, A. Modulation of spinal reflex activities in acute spinal rats with α-adrenergic agonists and antagonists. *Jpn. J. Pharmacol.* 28:165–168, 1978.

KERR, F. W. L. Pain: A central inhibitory balance theory. *Mayo Clin. Proc.* 50:685–690, 1975.

KERR, F. W. L. Segmental circuitry and spinal cord nociceptive mechanisms. *Adv. Pain Res. Ther.* 1:75–89, 1976.

KOTELKO, D. M., DAILEY, P. A., SHNIDER, S. M., ROSEN, M. A., HUGHES, S. C., AND BRIZGYS, R. V. Epidural morphine analgesia after caesarean delivery. *Obstet. Gynecol.* 63:409–413, 1984.

KRIVOY, W., KROEGER J., D., AND ZIMMERMANN, E. Actions of morphine on the segmental reflex of the decerebrate spinal cat. *Br. J. Pharmacol.* 47:457–464, 1973.

KRUGLOV, N. A. Effect of morphine group analgesics on the central inhibitory mechanisms. *Int. J. Neuropharmacol.* 3:197–203, 1964.

KRUMINS, S. A., COSTA, T., SHIMOHIGASHI, Y., MUNSON, P. J., AND RODBARD, D. Differential effects of GTP and cations on binding of labeled dimeric and monomeric enkephalins to neuroblastoma–glioma cell delta opiate receptors. *Biochem. Biophys. Res. Commun.* 108:406–413, 1982.

KURAISHI, Y., HARADA, Y., AND TAKAGI, H. Noradrenaline regulation of pain-transmission in the spinal cord mediated by :ga-adrenoceptors. *Brain Res.* 174:333–336, 1979.

KURAISHI, Y., SATON, M., HARADA, Y., AKAIKE, A., AND SHIBATA, T. Analgesic action of intraspinal and intracerebral β-endorphin in rats: Comparison with morphine. Eur. J. Pharmacol. 67:143–146, 1980.

KUSCHINSKY, K., SEEBER, U., LANGER, J., AND SONTAG, K. H. Effects of opiates and of neuroleptics on alpha-motoneurones in rat spinal cord: Possible correlations with muscular rigidity and akinesia, in: *Characteristics and Function of Opioids* (J. M. VAN REE AND L. TERENIUS, eds.), Elsevier-North Holland, Amsterdam, 1978, pp. 431–435.

LAMOTTE, C., PERT, C. B., AND SNYDER, S. H. Opiate receptor binding in primate spinal cord: Distribution and changes after dorsal root section. *Brain Res.* 112:407–412, 1976.

LARSON, A. A., VAUGHT, J. L., AND TAKEMORI, A. E. The potentiation of spinal analgesia by leucine enkephalin. *Eur. J. Pharmacol.* 61:381–383. 1980.

LE BARS, D., MENETREY, D., CONSEILLER, C., AND BESSON, J. M. Depressive effects of morphine upon lamina V cell activities in the dorsal horn of the spinal cat. *Brain Res.* 93:261–277, 1975.

LORD, J. A. H., WATERFIELD, A. A., HUGHES, J., AND KOSTERLITZ, H. W. Endogenous opioid peptides: Multiple agonists and receptors. *Nature* 267:495–499, 1977.

MACDONALD, R. L., AND NELSON, P. G. Specific opiate-induced depression of transmitter release from dorsal root ganglion cells in culture. *Sciences* 199:1449–1451, 1978

MALINS, A. F., GOODMAN, N. W., COOPER, G. M., PRYS-ROBERTS, C., AND BAIRD, R. N. Ventilatory effects of pre and postoperative diamorphine. A comparison of extradural with intramuscular administration. *Anaesthesia* 39:118–125, 1984.

MARTIN, G. E., AND NARUSE, T. Differences in the pharmacological actions of intrathecally administered neurotensin and morphine. *Regul. Peptides* 3:97–103, 1982.

MARTIN, R., SALBAING, J., BLAISE, G., TETRAULTj, J. P., AND TETREAULT, L. Epidural morphine for postoperative pain relief: A dose response curve. *Anesthesiology* 56:423–426, 1982.

MARTIN, W. R. Pharmacology of opioids. *Pharmacol. Rev.* 35:283–323, 1983.

MCCALL, R. B., AND AGHAJANIAN, G. K. Serotonergic facilitation of facial motoneuron excitation. *Brain Res.* 169:11–27, 1979.

MELZACK, R., AND WALL, P. D. Pain mechanisms: A new theory. *Science* 150:971–979, 1965.

MORI, T. Studies on comparison of the postoperative analgesic method between epidural morphine HCl and pentazocine. *Acta. Obstet. Gynaecol. Jpn.* 34:1819–1826, 1982.

MOULIN, D., MAX, M., KAIKO, R., INTURRISI, C., MAGGARD, J., YAKSH, T. L. AND FOLEY, K. Analgesic efficacy of IT *d*-Ala^2*d*-Leu^5-enkephalin (DADL) in cancer patients with chronic pain. *Pain* (in press), 1985.

MUDGE, A. W., LEEMAN, S. E., AND FISCHBACH, G. D. Enkephalin inhibits release of substance P from sensory neurons in culture and decreases action potential duration. *Proc. Natl. Acad. Sci. U.S.A.* 76:526–530, 1979.

MÜLLER, H., STOYANOV, M., BÖRNER, U., AND HEMPELMAN, G. Epidural opiates for relief of cancer pain, in *Spinal Opiate Analgesia* (T. L. YAKSH AND H. MÜLLER, eds.) Springer-Verlag, Berlin-Heidelberg, New York, 1982. pp, 125–137.

NINKOVIC, M., HUNT, S. P., AND GLEAVE, J. R. W. Localization of opiate and histamine H_1-receptors in the primate sensory ganglia and spinal cord. *Brain Res.* 241:197–206, 1982.

NORDBERG, G. Pharmacokinetic aspects of spinal morphine analgesia. *Acta Anesthesiol. Scand.* 79(Suppl):7–37, 1984.

NOUEIHED, R., DURANT, P., AND YAKSH, T. L. Studies on the effects of intrathecal sufentanil, fentanil and alfentanil in rats and cats. *Anesthesiology* 61:A218, 1984.

ONOFRIO, B. M., AND YAKSH, T. L. Intrathecal delta-receptor ligand produces analgesia in man. *Lancet* 1:1386–1387, 1983.

ONOFRIO, B. M., YAKSH, T. L., AND ARNOLD, L. E. Continuous low dose intrathecal morphine administration in the treatment of chronic pain of malignant origin. *Mayo Clin. Proc.* 56:516–520, 1981.

OYAMA, T., FUKUSHI, S., AND JIN, T. Epidural β-endorphin in treatment of pain. *Can. Anaesth. Soc. J.* 29:24–26, 1982.

PAALZOW, G. Development of tolerance to the analgesic effect of clonidine in rats cross-tolerance to morphine. *Naunyn Schmiedebergs Arch. Pharmacol.* 304:1–4, 1978.

PASTERNAK, G. W., CHILDERS, S. R., AND SNYDER, S. H. Opiate analgesia: Evidence for mediation by a subpopulation of opiate receptors. *Science* 208:514–516, 1980.

PIERCEY, M. F., LAHTI, R. A. SCHROEDER, L. A., EINSPAHR, F. J., AND BARSAHN, C. U-50488H, a pure kappa receptor agonist with spinal analgesic loci in the mouse. *Life Sci.* 31:1197–1200, 1982a.

PIERCEY, M. F., VARNER, K., AND SCHROEDER, L. A. Analgesic activity of intraspinally administered dynorphin and ethylketocyclazocine. *Eur. J. Pharmacol.* 80:283–384, 1982b.

PORRECA, F., AND BURKS, T. F. The spinal cord as a site of opioid effects on gastrointestinal transit in the mouse. *J. Pharmacol. Exp. Ther.* 227:22–27, 1983.

PORRECA, F., FILLA, A., AND BURKS, T. F. Spinal cord-mediated opiate effects on gastrointestinal transit in mice. *Eur. J. Pharmacol.* 86:135–136, 1982.

PORRECA, F., FILLA, A., AND BURKS, T. F. Studies *in vivo* with dynorphin(1–9): Analgesia but not gastrointestinal effects following intrathecal administration to mice. *Eur. J. Pharmacol.* 91:291–294, 1983.

PRZEWLOCKI, B., SHEARMAN, G. T., AND HERZ, A. Mixed opioid/non opioid effects of dynorphin related peptides after intrathecal injection in the rat. *Neuropeptides* 3:233–240, 1983.

PYBUS, D. A., AND TORDA, T. A. Dose–effect relationships of extradural morphine. *Br. J. Anaesth.* 54:1259–1262, 1982.

RAWAL, N., MÖLLEFORS, K., AXELSSON, K., LINGARDH, G., AND WIDMAN, B. An experimental study of urodynamic effects of epidural morphine and of naloxone reversal. *Anesth. Analg.* 62:641–647, 1983.

RAWAL, N., SJÖSTRAND, U., CHRISTOFFERSSON, E., DAHLSTRÖM, B., ARVILL, A., AND RYDMAN, H. Comparison of intramuscular and epidural morphine for postoperative analgesia in the grossly obese: Influence on postoperative ambulation and pulmonary function. *Anesth. Analg.* 63:583–592, 1984.

REDDY, S. V. R., AND YAKSH, T. L. Spinal noradrenergic terminal system mediates antinociception. *Brain Res.* 189:391–401, 1980.

REDDY, S. V. R., MADERDRUT, J. L., AND YAKSH, T. L. Spinal cord pharmacology of adrenergic agonist-mediated antinociception. *J. Pharmacol. Exp. Ther. 213:525–533, 1980.*

RONDOMANSKA, M., DECASTRO, J., AND LECRON, L. The use of epidural buprenorphine for the treatment of postoperative pain, in: *Spinal Opiate Analgesia* (T. L. YAKSH AND H. MÜLLER, eds.), Springer-Verlag, Berlin, Heidelberg, New York, 1982, pp. 91–94.

ROSEN, M. A., HUGHES, S. C., SHNIDER, S. M., ABBOUD, T. K., NORTON, M. DAILEY, P. A. AND CURTIS, J. D. Epidural morphine for the relief of postoperative pain after caesarean delivery. *Anesth. Analg.* 62:666–672, 1983.

RUSSELL, B., AND YAKSH, T. L. Antagonism by phenoxybenzamine and pentazocine of the antinociceptive effects of morphine in the spinal cord. *Neuropharmacology* 20:575–579, 1981.

RUTBERG, H., HAKANSON, E., ANDERBERG, B., JORFELDT, L., MARTENSSON, J. AND SCHILDT, B. Effects of the extradural administration of morphine, or bupivacaine, on the endocrine response to upper abdominal surgery. *Br. J. Anesth.* 56:233–238, 1984.

RUTTER, D. V., SKEWES, D. G., AND MORGAN, M. Extradural opioids for postoperative analgesia. *Br. J. Anesth.* 53:915–920, 1981.

RYBRO, L., SCHURIZEK, A., PETERSEN, T. K., AND WERNBERGER, M. Postoperative analgesia and lung function: A comparison of intramuscular with epidural morphine. *Acta Anaesth. Scand.* 26:514–518, 1982.

SASTRY, B. R. Potentiation of presynaptic inhibition of nociceptive pathways as a mechanism for analgesia. *Can. J. Physiol. Pharmacol.* 58:97–100, 1980.

SCHMAUSS, C., AND YAKSH, T. L. *In vivo* studies on spinal opiate receptor systems mediating antinociception. II. Pharmacological profiles suggesting a differential association of mu, delta and kappa receptors with visceral chemical and cutaneous thermal stimuli in the rat. *J. Pharmacol. Exp. Ther.* 228:1–12, 1984.

SCHMAUSS, C., DOHERTY, C., AND YAKSH, T. L. The analgetic effects of an intrathecally administered partial opiate agonist, nalbuphine hydrochloride. *Eur. J. Pharmacol.* 86:1–7, 1983.

SCHMAUSS, C., SHIMOHIGASHI, Y., JENSEN, T. S., RODBARD, D., AND YAKSH, T. L. Studies on spinal opiate receptor pharmacology. III. Analgetic effects of enkephalin dimers as measured by cutaneous thermal and visceral chemical evoked responses. *Brain Res* 337:209–215, 1985.

SCHULZ, R. E., WÜSTER, M., AND HERZ, A. Pharmacological characterization of the ε-opiate receptor. *J. Pharmacol. Exp. Ther.* 215:604–606, 1981.

SIGG, E. B., CAPRIO, G., AND SCHNEIDER, J. A. Synergism of amines and antagonism of reserpine to morphine analgesia. *Proc. Soc. Exp. Biol. Med.* 97:97–100, 1958.

SPAULDING, T. C., FIELDING, S., VENAFRO, J. J., AND LAL, H. Antinociceptive activity of clonidine and its potentiation of morphine analgesia. *Eur. J. Pharmacol.* 58:19–25, 1979.

STAIMAN, A., AND SEEMAN, P. The impulse blocking concentrations of anesthetics, alcohols, anticonvulsants, barbiturates and narcotics on phrenic and sciatic nerves. *Can. J. Physiol. Pharmacol.* 52:535–550, 1974.

STRUPPLER, A., BURGMAYER, B., OCHS, G. B., AND PFEIFFER, H. G. The effect of epidural application of opioids on spasticity of spinal origin. *Life Sci.* 33:607–610, 1983.

TALLARIDA, R. J., COWAN, A., AND ADLER, M. W. pA_2 and receptor differentiation: A statistical analysis of competitive antagonism. *Life Sci.* 25.637–654, 1979.

TANG, A. H., AND SCHOENFELD, M. J. Comparison of subcutaneous and spinal subarachnoid injections of morphine and naloxone in analgesic tests in the rat. *Eur. J. Pharmacol.* 52:215–223, 1978.

THOMPSON, W. R., SMITH, P. T., HIRST, M., VARKEY, G. P., AND KNILL, R. L. Regional analgesic effects of epidural morphine in volunteers. *Can. Anaesth. Soc. J.* 28:530–536, 1981.

THOR, K. B., ROPPOLO, J. R., AND DEGROAT, W. C. Naloxone-induced micturition in unanesthesized paraplegic cats. *J. Urol.* 129:202–205, 1983.

TOKIMASA, T., MORITA, K., AND NORTH, A. Opiates and clonidine prolong calcium-dependent after-hyperpolarizations. *Nature* 294:162–163, 1981.

TORDA, T. A., AND PYBUS, D. A. Comparison of four narcotic analgesics for extradural analgesia. *Br. J. Anesth.* 54:291–295, 1982.

TORDA, T. A., AND PYBUS, D. A. Extradural administration of morphine and bupivacaine: A controlled comparison. *Br. J. Anesth.* 56:141–146, 1984.

TSENG, L.-F. Tolerance and cross tolerance to morphine after chronic spinal D-Ala^{2}D-Leu^5-enkephalin infusion. *Life Sci.* 31:987–992, 1982.

TUNG, A. S., AND YAKSH, T. L. *In vivo* evidence for multiple opiate receptors mediating analgesia in the rat spinal cord. *Brain Res.* 247:75–83, 1982.

VANDERMAELEN, C. P., AND AGHAJANIAN, G. K. Intracellular studies showing modulation of motoneurone excitability by serotonin. *Nature* 287:346–347, 1980.

WANG, J.-Y., YASUOKA, S., AND YAKSH, T. L. Studies on the analgetic effect of intrathecal ST-91 (2-[2,6-diethyl-phenylamino]-2-imidazoline): Antagonism, tolerance and interaction with morphine. *Pharmacologist* 22:302, 1980.

WEBER, H. Uber Anästhesie durch Adrenalin. *Verh. Deut. Ges. Inn. Med.* 21:616–619, 1904.

WEIGHT, F. F., AND SALMOIRAGHI, G. C. Responses of spinal cord interneurons to acetylcholine, norepinephrine and serotonin administered by microelectrophoresis. *J. Pharmacol. Exp. Ther.* 153:420–427, 1966.

WELCHEW, E. A. The optimum concentration for epidural fentanyl. A randomized double-blind comparison with and without 1 : 200000 adrenalin. *Anaesthesia* 38:1037–1041, 1983.

WERZ, M. A., AND MACDONALD, R. L. Opioid peptides with differential affinity for mu and delta receptors decrease sensory neuron calcium-dependent action potentials. *J. Pharmacol. Exp. Ther.* 227:394–402, 1983.

WHITE, S. R., AND NEUMAN, R. S. Facilitation of spinal motorneurone excitability by 5-hydroxytryptamine and noradrenaline. *Brain Res.* 188:119–127, 1980.

WIKLER, A. Sites and mechanisms of action of morphine and related drugs in the central nervous system. *Pharmacol. Rev.* 2:435–506, 1950.

WILLER, J. C., AND BUSSEL, B. Evidence for a direct spinal mechanism in morphine-induced inhibition of nociceptive reflexes in humans. *Brain Res.* 287:212–215, 1980.

WILSON, P. R., AND YAKSH, T. L. Baclofen is antinociceptive in the spinal intrathecal space of animals. *Eur. J. Pharmacol.* 51:323–330, 1978.

WOHLBERG, C. J., HACKMAN, J. C., RYAN, G. P., AND DAVIDOFF, R. A. Hyperpolarization of primary afferent terminals mediated by α_2-adrenoceptors. *Soc. Neurosci. Abstr.* 9:1001, 1983.

WOOD, P. L., RACKHAM, A., AND RICHARD, J. Spinal analgesia: Comparison of the mu agonist morphine and the kappa agonist ethylketocyclazocine. *Life Sci.* 28:2119–2125, 1981.

YAKSH, T. L. Opiate receptors for behavioral analgesia resemble those related to the depression of spinal nociceptive neurons. *Science* 199:1231–1233, 1978a.

YAKSH, T. L. Inhibition by etorphine of the discharge of dorsal horn neurons: Effects upon the neuronal response to both high- and low-threshold sensory input in the decerebrate spinal cat. *Exp. Neurol.* 60:23–40, 1978b.

YAKSH, T. L. Analgetic actions of intrathecal opiates in cat and primate. *Brain Res.* 153:205–210, 1978c.

YAKSH, T. L. Spinal opiate analgesia: Characteristics and principles of action. *Pain* 11:293–346, 1981.

YAKSH, T. L. *In vivo* studies on spinal opiate receptor systems mediating antinociception. I. Mu and delta receptor profiles in the primate. *J. Pharmacol. Exp. Ther.* 226:303–316, 1983.

YAKSH, T. L. Multiple opiate receptor systems in brain and spinal cord: Part I. *Eur. J. Anaesthesiol.* 1:171–199, 1984a.

YAKSH, T. L. Multiple opiate receptor systems in brain and spinal cord: Part II. *Eur. J. Anaesthesiol.* I:201–243, 1984b.

YAKSH, T. L. Pharmacology of spinal adrenergic systems which modulate spinal nociceptive processing. *Pharmacol. Biochem. Behav.* 22:845–858, 1985.

YAKSH, T. L., AND HAMMOND, D. L. Peripheral and central substrates involved in the rostrad transmission of nociceptive information. *Pain* 13:1–85, 1982.

YAKSH, T. L., AND HENRY, J. L. Antinociceptive effects of intrathecally administered human β-endorphin in the rat and cat. *Can. J. Physiol. Pharmacol.* 56:754–760, 1978.

YAKSH, T. L., AND REDDY, S. V. R. Studies in the primate on the analgetic effects associated with intrathecal actions of opiate, α-adrenergic agonists and baclofen. *Anesthesiology* 54:451–467, 1981.

YAKSH, T. L., AND RUDY, T. A. Chronic catheterization of the spinal subarachnoid space. *Physiol. Behav.* 17:1031–1036, 1976.

YAKSH, T. L., AND RUDY, T. A. Studies on the direct spinal action of narcotics in the production of analgesia in the rat. *J. Pharmacol. Exp. Ther.* 202:411–428, 1977.

YAKSH, T. L., AND RUDY, T. A. Narcotic analgesics: CNS sites and mechanisms of action as revealed by intracerebral injection techniques. *Pain* 4:299–359, 1978.

YAKSH, T. L., AND WILSON, P. R. Spinal serotonin terminal system mediates antinociception. *J. Pharmacol. Exp. Ther.* 208:446–453, 1979.

YAKSH, T. L., HUANG, S. P., RUDY, T. A., AND FREDERICKSON, R. C. A. The direct and specific opiate-like effect of Met^5-enkephalin and analogues on the spinal cord. *Neuroscience* 2:593–596, 1977a.

YAKSH, T. L., KOHL, R. L., AND RUDY, T. A. Induction of tolerance and withdrawl in rats receiving morphine in the spinal subarachnoid space. *Eur. J. Pharmacol.* 42:275–284, 1977b.

YAKSH, T. L., FREDERICKSON, R. C. A., HUANG, S. P., AND RUDY, T. A. *In vivo* comparison of the receptor populations acted upon in the spinal cord by morphine and pentapeptides in the production of analgesia. *Brain Res.* 148:516–520, 1978.

YAKSH, T. L., GROSS, K. E., AND LI, C. H. Studies on the intrathecal effect of β-endorphin in primate. *Brain Res.* 241:261–269, 1982a.

YAKSH, T. L., SCHMAUSS, C., MICEVYCH, P. E., ABAY, E. O., AND GO, V. L. W. Pharmacological studies on the application, disposition and release of neurotensin in the spinal cord. *Ann. N.Y. Acad. Sci.* 400:228–242, 1982b.

YAKSH, T. L., HOWE, J. R., AND HARTY, G. J. Pharmacology of spinal pain modulatory systems. *Ad. Pain Res. Ther.* 7:57–70, 1984.

YAKSH, T. L., DIRKSEN, R., AND HARTY, G. J. Antinociceptive action of intrathecally administered cholinomimetics in rat and cat. *Eur. J. Pharmacol.*, (in press), 1985.

YASUOKA, S., AND YAKSH, T. L. Effects on nociceptive threshold and blood pressure of intrathecally administered morphine and α-adrenergic agonists. *Neuropharmacology* 22:309–315, 1983.

YEUNG, J. C., AND RUDY, T. A. Multiplicative interaction between narcotic agonisms expressed at spinal and supraspinal sites of antinociceptive action as revealed by concurrent intrathecal and intracerebroventricular injections of morphine. *J. Pharmacol. Exp. Ther.* 215:663–642, 1980.

YOSHIMURA, M., AND NORTH, A. R. Hyperpolarization of substantia gelatinosa neurons *in vitro* by enkephalin and noradrenaline. *Soc. Neurosci. Abstr.* 9:1129, 1983.

ZENZ, M. Epidural opiates for the treatment of cancer pain in: *Recent Advances in Pain Therapy* (M. Zimmerman, ed.), Springer-Verlag, Berlin Heidelberg New York, (in press), 1985.

ZIEGLGANSBERGER, W., AND BAYERL, H. The mechanisms of inhibition of neuronal activity by opiates in the spinal cord of the cat. *Brain Res. 115:111–128, 1976.*

ZIMMERMANN, M., CARSTENS, E., SCHREIBER, H., AND GILLY, H. Excitability changes at intraspinal terminals of afferent C- and A-fibers produced by midbrain stimulation and iontophoretic application of transmitters in cat. *Soc. Neurosci. Abstr.* 9:254, 1983.

Index